Ethics in Palliative Care

Ethics in Palliative Care

A Complete Guide

Robert C. Macauley

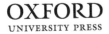
OXFORD
UNIVERSITY PRESS

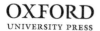

OXFORD
UNIVERSITY PRESS

Oxford University Press is a department of the University of Oxford. It furthers
the University's objective of excellence in research, scholarship, and education
by publishing worldwide. Oxford is a registered trade mark of Oxford University
Press in the UK and certain other countries.

Published in the United States of America by Oxford University Press
198 Madison Avenue, New York, NY 10016, United States of America.

Library of Congress Cataloging-in-Publication Data
Names: Macauley, Robert C., author.
Title: Ethics in palliative care / Robert C. Macauley.
Description: New York, NY : Oxford University Press, [2018] |
Includes bibliographical references and index.
Identifiers: LCCN 2017047687 (print) | LCCN 2017048448 (ebook) | ISBN 9780190652340 (epub) |
ISBN 9780190652357 (online content) | ISBN 9780190652364 (online content) |
ISBN 9780190652333 (updf) | ISBN 9780199313945 (pbk. : alk. paper)
Subjects: | MESH: Palliative Care—ethics
Classification: LCC R726 (ebook) | LCC R726 (print) | NLM WB 310 | DDC 616.02/9—dc23
LC record available at https://lccn.loc.gov/2017047687

9 8 7 6 5 4 3 2

Printed by Webcom, Inc., Canada

For Canoluchapa, the sweetest sound in the world

Contents

Preface

No specialty faces more complex and diverse ethical dilemmas than palliative medicine. From acute issues ranging from fractured communication to limitation of life-sustaining treatment to ongoing discussions regarding goals of care for seriously ill patients—as well as hot-button social issues such as physician-assisted dying and so-called "death panels"—palliative care clinicians frequently face dilemmas that call for ethical analysis, clinical expertise, and historical and legal perspective. It is no surprise, then, that ethical and legal aspects of care were identified as one of the eight core domains of palliative medicine by the National Consensus Project, which established the expectation that a "palliative care program [be] aware of and [address] the complex ethical issues arising in the care of people with life-threatening debilitating illness" (Colby, Dahlin, Lantos, Carney, & Christopher, 2010).

Textbooks have attempted to address these complex issues but often fail to do so in a comprehensive manner. Clinical texts, for instance, provide realistic portrayals of practical dilemmas yet frequently suffer from a lack of philosophical nuance. Conversely, philosophical explorations offer rigorous analysis but often fail to appreciate the clinical context or implication of specific decisions.

Beyond philosophical rigor and clinical realism, a thorough discussion of ethical issues in palliative care requires two additional elements. The first is context, for ethical issues do not exist in historical isolation. Many have been around for thousands of years—such as the question of what constitutes a "good death"—while others have arisen more recently (such as whether medically administered nutrition and hydration constitutes a medical treatment or ordinary care). Even supposedly novel questions are often specific applications of more universal principles—such as what physicians are obligated to provide a patient and what he or she[1] has the right to refuse—and as such benefit from historical perspective.

The second additional element is an assessment of the medicolegal landscape. While often related, ethics and the law are not synonymous. An action may be legal but not ethical—lying, for instance—while another may be ethical but not legal, as in the case of nonviolent civil disobedience. Certain ethically charged practices (such as physician-assisted dying) are legal in some jurisdictions but not in others, but it would be hard to argue that ethics change at a national or state/provincial boundary. Ultimately, the fact that an action is illegal in a specific jurisdiction is relevant to determining whether one should commit it—given the stakes involved in committing an illegal action—but not necessarily determinative (Macauley, 2005).

This textbook examines fundamental ethical issues in palliative care from each of these four critically important vantage points. Chapters generally include at least one paradigmatic case and proceed to explore the historicolegal evolution of the primary issue raised by the case.[2] Next, the clinical context is explored, using technical terms insofar as they are necessary and beneficial. Ethical arguments for and against a certain practice are then examined in detail. While one could read the book from cover to cover, each chapter provides a stand-alone comprehensive analysis of a specific dilemma, so as to provide the reader with a thorough and multifaceted appreciation of its complexity and potential resolutions.

It should be noted that this is a single-author textbook. This was a conscious choice, borne of my experience studying ethics in college and graduate school, which I confess to finding rather frustrating, primarily because there appeared to be no conclusion. It seemed that the purpose of ethical deliberation was to take a complex issue, explore it for an extended period of time, and ultimately concede that the issue was much more complex than one had originally given it credit for.

Clinical ethics, by contrast, is a branch of applied ethics whereby a decision—with its inherent strengths and weaknesses—must be reached. When someone (whether a physician, nurse, other staff person, patient, or family member) requests ethical assistance, they are looking for both analysis and recommendation. The ethics consultant whose only conclusion is that the precipitating question was, indeed, very complex will likely not receive many repeat requests for consultation.

---

1. On a stylistic note, in order to avoid the cumbersome repetition of "he or she," chapters will alternate between using a male or female pronoun to refer to the patient. For the sake of clarity, the other pronoun will generally be used to refer to the physician.

2. Admittedly, this exploration largely reflects American law and culture, as that is the context in which I work and write, and taking into consideration every cultural or legal setting would be impractical. Distinctions are therefore drawn between the concepts of hospice and palliative care, which are often synonymous in other parts of the world. The ethical perspective may feel to some readers from other countries as heavily weighted toward patient autonomy, but within the landscape of American bioethics—which often prioritizes autonomy to an extreme—it actually is rather moderate.

A single-author textbook can present a clear and consistent narrative voice throughout. Unlike books that strive for neutrality—and often leave readers with more questions than answers—this book puts forth a position on each issue, inviting readers to form their own opinions in response to it. The position taken is admittedly biased, simply because we all have our own biases (which necessarily contribute to our views and opinions). Rather than attempting the impossible task of eradicating those biases, the most we can hope for is to be aware of them and take steps to compensate for the ways they might lead us to jump to conclusions. By the end of the textbook, readers will likely be able to predict the conclusions of each chapter (based on the common narrative thread) and also weigh the cumulative argument against their own opinions (and personal biases).

I certainly do not expect every reader to agree with my conclusions, and I do not claim divine wisdom or authority. The most I aspire to is presenting an informed, consistent, and cogent approach to important issues, with clear conclusions that readers can evaluate and critique as they see fit. I also recognize that the disadvantage to this approach is that, unlike an edited collection, such a textbook cannot avail itself of the wisdom of respected authorities on every issue. (Although the reviewers noted in the acknowledgment section are surely an impressive lot.)

In terms of audience, this volume is directed at professionals already in the field who seek deeper grounding in the ethical dilemmas specific to palliative care, as well as those new to the field. Given the transdisciplinary nature of palliative care, by *professional* I do not just mean physicians but also nurses, social workers, chaplains, psychotherapists, physical therapists, occupational therapists, expressive therapists, and child life workers (as well as any other disciplines I may have overlooked, with apologies). Given the wide range of disciplines involved, I have attempted to tone down the technical language—both medicalese as well as philosophical jargon—that pervades many books related to bioethics. I have also provided a glossary and list of abbreviations at the end of the book, to provide further explanation of terms that are frequently used in the clinical practice of palliative care. This makes the text more accessible to the lay public, many of whom have an interest in palliative care, often for very personal reasons.

The great philosopher Ludwig Wittgenstein once wrote that "what can be said at all can be said clearly; and what we cannot talk about we must pass over in silence" (Wittgenstein, 1922). Many of the topics in this book inspire silence, for most of us would prefer to discuss almost anything more than death and dying. But that does not mean they *cannot* be spoken of, only that it is hard to do so. And to speak of them fully means going beyond philosophical argument or clinical assessment to the profoundly human stories and relationships that undergird every decision related to serious illness. The ethics of palliative care are not only complex but also frequently gut-wrenching, describing impossible choices that patients, their families, and the medical professionals caring for them face. The personal anecdotes and patient stories that permeate this volume are, therefore, not merely practical illustrations; they are the reason this textbook was written. Without them, it would be impossible to appreciate the depth of the questions, and there would also be insufficient reason to spend so much time and energy in search of the answers.

References

Colby, W. H., Dahlin, C., Lantos, J., Carney, J., & Christopher, M. (2010). The National Consensus Project for Quality Palliative Care Clinical Practice Guidelines Domain 8: Ethical and legal aspects of care. *HEC Forum, 22*(2), 117–131. doi:10.1007/s10730-010-9128-3

Macauley, R. (2005). The Hippocratic underground: Civil disobedience and health care reform. *Hastings Cent Rep, 35*(1), 38–45.

Wittgenstein, L. (1922). *Tractatus logico-philosophicus.* New York: Harcourt, Brace & Company.

Acknowledgments

This book would not have happened without the contributions of a great many people. I wouldn't be where—or who—I am today without the support, guidance, and friendship of an amazing team at the University of Vermont, including Bob Orr, Sally Bliss, Gail Cashman, Shaden Eldakar-Hein, and Gordon Meyer. Special thanks to Sally, who was my partner-in-crime for nearly a decade and made coming to work a joy. After years of "Hey, Sal" prefacing a request for her to do something, now I can simply say, "Hey, Sal, thank you for everything."

My deepest thanks goes to my mentor, Bob Orr, who has made so many things possible for me—both personally and professionally—and many others through his wisdom, generosity, and professionalism. No aspiring ethicist could ask for a better role model.

I'm so very fortunate to now be part of a wonderful team at Oregon Health and Science University and Doernbecher Children's Hospital, including Dana Braner, Kathy Perko, Hannah Holiman, Monica Holland, Anat LeBlanc, Sara Taub, Greg Thomas, and Lindsay Wooster-Halberg. And we wouldn't be able to do what we do without the remarkable generosity of the Cambia Health Foundation—led by Mark Ganz and Peggy Maguire—which has been instrumental in promoting palliative care in Oregon and beyond.

A cadre of wonderful palliative care clinicians and ethicists generously gave of their time and expertise to offer thoughtful criticism of individual chapters: Armand Antommaria, Bob Arnold, Jim Bernat, Jeff Berger, Brian Carter, Jacob Dahlke, Doug Diekema, Chris Feudtner, Lauris Kaldjian, Marcia Levetown, Mark Mercurio, Sean Morrison, Bob Orr, Tim Quill, Francine Rainone, Bob Truog, and Gregg VandeKieft. Richard Hain "took it all in," reading the entire manuscript and offering truly insightful feedback not only on structure and theme but also on individual arguments. I am honored to have all these good folks as colleagues and blessed to call them friends.

The staff at Oxford University Press have been so supportive (not to mention patient!) throughout the conceiving of this textbook book and the writing process. Special thanks to Abby Gross for inviting me to write the book and to Andrea Knobloch, Rebecca Suzan, Hannah Doyle, and Lucy Randall for shepherding it through to completion.

A big thanks to the wonderful folks at Clare Hall, Cambridge, who provided a home for me and my family while a large part of this book was composed.

And most of all I thank my family. My mother showed me the importance of hard work and helped me believe in myself. And my amazing wife and kids support me every step of the way, especially in the writing of this book, even when I felt like giving up. Most of what I know I learned from them, and this book—not to mention the very best parts of my life—never would have happened without them.

Overview and Introduction

Ethics and Palliative Care

Ethics and palliative care have always been a part of medicine. Twenty-five hundred years ago, the Hippocratic Oath laid out specific expectations for what physicians must do (such as maintaining patient confidentiality) and what they must avoid (such as intentionally causing harm), which are still relevant today (Hippocrates, 1923). For all the wonders of modern medicine—especially the relatively recent discoveries of anesthesia, antibiotics, and other technological interventions—for most of medicine's history palliative care was the only thing physicians had to offer, in the form of compassionate presence. Indeed, Robert Buckman once referred to palliative care as "what, 150 years ago, was simply known as *good doctoring*" (personal communication, 2008).

As formal medical specialties, however, ethics and palliative care are relatively new, and both evolved over a similar period of time. The first textbook on medical ethics was published in 1803 (Percival, 1803), and the first American Medical Association Code of Ethics was published in 1847 (American Medical Association, 1847). The broader term "bioethics"—which takes into account additional issues in the life sciences, incorporating considerations of philosophy, law, and politics—did not appear in the literature until 1970 (Potter, 1970). Codification of the field (in the form of peer-reviewed journals and a national society) soon followed.

Hospice and palliative medicine also established its own identity over the second half of the twentieth century. The pioneering work of Dame Cicely Saunders (1960, 1963) ushered in "the modern hospice movement." And only four years after the term "bioethics" was coined, so too was "palliative care," by Balfour Mount, to counteract the negative connotations of the term "hospice"—a much older term initially used more broadly than it is today—in French-speaking society (Mount, 1997). A similar process of recognition and codification ensued, with the first American Board of Medical Specialties–certified palliative care board exam taking place in 2008. (By contrast, the debate about how—or even whether—to certify clinical ethicists rages on [Kodish et al., 2013].)

So why, over approximately the same period of time, did these two fields finally come to be recognized as distinct specialties? The reason has much to do with the things that medicine should have been doing but was not (i.e., honoring patient autonomy and attending to suffering at the end of life) and was doing that it should not have been (i.e., unethical practices, in both clinical treatment and research). Through scientific discoveries—such as the benefits of opioids at the end of life—and recognition of evolving clinical complexities, palliative care came to be recognized as more than hand-holding and ethics as something more than upright character. Each established an evidence base and demanded specific training and skills to address the needs of patients and their families. From a largely common foundation, two distinct specialties sprang forth, often with overlapping purposes involving a similar—though not identical—cadre of patients. This offered both the potential for collaboration and the possibility of conflict, as the two specialties sought to understand their proper scope.

Evolution of the Fields

Ethics

With regard to an individual patient, there are two basic ethical obligations in the practice of medicine: to do what the patient wants—or, more narrowly, to *not* do anything the patient has not consented to—and to do what is good for the patient. In philosophical terms, the former is called autonomy and the latter beneficence (or, in the case of refraining from doing something that would be harmful to the patient, nonmaleficence).

For most of the history of Western medicine, there was not much of a balance between these two principles. The physician's focus was almost exclusively on beneficence, which—when taken to an extreme—is known as paternalism (or, more inclusively, parentalism). Physicians were tasked with doing what was right for the patient and also trusted to determine what exactly that was.

In one respect, this does not seem problematic. It is a virtue to act beneficently toward others, and the word "paternal" generally carries positive connotations of caring and protection. Certainly when a patient is unable—or unwilling—to offer an opinion about various medical treatments, acting in the patient's best interests can be appropriate. But parentalism generally refers to the more extreme practice of not respecting—or even soliciting—the patient's goals or decisions related to medical treatment.

This was very much the norm in the age of Hippocrates, who urged his followers to "[conceal] most things from the patient, while you are attending to him. Turn his attention away from what is being done to him . . . revealing nothing of the patient's future or present condition" (Hippocrates, 1923). Lest this be viewed as a vestige of antiquity, it is important to recognize that the American Medical Association's Code of Ethics for many years endorsed "beneficent deception for gloomy prognostications" in order to "avoid all things which have a tendency to discourage the patient and to depress his spirits" (American Medical Association, 1847). When placed in this historical context, it is not surprising that 90% of oncologists in an oft-cited midcentury study would not tell a patient that she had cancer, so as "to sustain and bolster the patient's hope" (Oken, 1961).

One of the reasons that a beneficence-based model functioned so well for so long was that patients were willing to entrust physicians with decisions about their care. (The absence of the Internet probably helped, too, making physicians' medical knowledge proprietary.) But in the twentieth century, the legal and ethical landscape began to change. In an increasingly multicultural society, it was becoming clear that there was not always "one right answer" to a treatment question and that, even if there was, the physician was not the appropriate person to identify it. So instead of physicians unilaterally making decisions, patients themselves began to demand the right to be informed of their options and choose among them.

This transition from parentalism to patient autonomy in the United States can be charted through seminal court cases. The earliest landmark decision was *Schloendorff v. Society of New York Hospital* (1914), which dealt with the case of a patient who agreed to an "ether examination" but not to surgery. Surgery was nevertheless performed, however, prompting the patient to sue. Justice Benjamin Cardozo's oft-cited opinion is the first—and perhaps still the best—legal encapsulation of the concept of informed consent: "Every human being of adult years and sound mind has a right to determine what shall be done with his own body; and a surgeon who performs an operation without his patient's consent commits an assault, for which he is liable in damages."

While *Schloendorff* applies to cases where a physician does something which the patient had not been informed would be done, other cases arose over the course of the century which specified the requirements of disclosure of risks and benefits to ensure the patient truly understands what is being proposed. In *Salgo v. Leland Stanford, Jr. University Board of Trustees* (1957) the Court heard a case of a patient who was paralyzed as a result of a procedure, although this risk had never been discussed. The court held that physicians have a duty to disclose "any facts which are necessary to form the basis of an intelligent consent by the patient to proposed treatment."

This decision was based in battery law, but a subsequent decision shifted the focus to negligence law. *Natanson v. John R. Kline and St. Francis Hospital and School of Nursing* (1960) reviewed the case of a woman who experienced burns as a result of cancer treatment, after having been told there were no risks associated with the treatment. The court held that a patient must be informed of collateral hazards that any "reasonable medical practitioner" would disclose.

These seminal cases focused on the need for disclosure, leaving later decisions to determine what extent of disclosure was required. In *Canterbury v. Spence* (1972) the Court—responding to a patient partially paralyzed from a procedure without foreknowledge of the risk—articulated an obligation on physicians to help patients make decisions based on the patient's interests. The Court deemed this a basic obligation of the medical professional and thus not dependent on the patient's explicit request for information. *Canterbury*—along with *Cobbs v. Grant* (1972)—also went beyond the *Natanson* assertion of a "reasonable physician" standard of disclosure to establish a "reasonable patient" standard (i.e., the physician is obligated to disclose information that a reasonable patient would want to know). Currently twenty-five states (plus the District of Columbia) use the reasonable patient standard, with twenty-three using the reasonable physician standard and the final two (Colorado and Georgia) not easily classifiable (Studdert et al., 2007).

The final landmark case of the twentieth century regarding informed consent was *Lane v. Candura* (1978), which evaluated an elderly patient's refusal of amputation of a gangrenous leg. The Court found that the patient appreciated the consequences of her action, establishing the right of competent adult patients to make health care decisions even when these decisions do not seem to be in their own best interests.

Over the course of a century, therefore, the pendulum swung all the way from physicians being advised to engage in "beneficent deception" to being required to disclose risks that a reasonable patient would want to know (and to respect a patient's refusal after being so informed). This right to make potentially "bad decisions" coincided with rights movements of various kinds—such as those related to race and gender—which emphasized minimizing hierarchies and maximizing self-determination (Fins, 2006). Internal factors within the practice of medicine also led to a diminution in the physician's role in decision-making. For instance, evolving residency work hour limits and the rise of hospitalist medicine led to frequent hand-offs from one clinician to another, rendering individual parentalism less practical. Less than twenty years after 90% of physicians had said they would not inform a patient that she had cancer, the same proportion proclaimed that they *would* (Novack et al., 1979).

In addition to the patient's right to make her own treatment decisions, a second reason for the birth of bioethics was the advent of new and complex questions in the field of medicine. With advancing technology came new applications of established questions such as the distribution of scarce resources, which now included modalities such as dialysis machines (Alexander, 1962) as well as solid organs for transplantation.

These discoveries also prompted novel questions. Prior to the discovery of mechanical ventilation, the question of how to define and determine death was rather straightforward. But once it was possible to physiologically maintain a patient who lacked brain function, this question became much more complex (Ad Hoc Committee of the Harvard Medical School to Examine the Definition of Brain Death, 1968).

The same decade saw the first report of closed-chest cardiac resuscitation, now known as cardiopulmonary resuscitation (Kouwenhoven, Jude, & Knickerbocker, 1960). What has since become a cultural rite of passage started off as a novel intervention that showed high levels of success in the operating room. That success prompted expansion to the rest of the hospital and beyond—even though its probability of success plummeted in those contexts (Mozaffarian, 2015)—and its emergent nature led to its adoption as the only treatment that a patient has to refuse in order *not* to receive it.

Such expansion without full consideration of the relative burdens and benefits illustrates what Victor Fuchs has called the "technological imperative": the impulse to do everything one is trained to do, regardless of the cost/benefit or the burden/benefit ratio (Fuchs, 1975). Clinical medicine understandably tends to focus on what can be done to help patients, but just because something is possible does not mean it is advisable. Clinical ethics provides a crucial counterbalance to the technological imperative by focusing on what *should* be done for a patient. As Jonsen (2003) writes, "In large part, the appearance of a new medicine that offered promise of great benefit initiated the examination of medicine's conscience."

The third reason for the rise of bioethics was the recognition that physicians—even if they were granted the right to make treatment decisions and even if the questions were not novel—sometimes did not make the right choice. Prior to the twentieth century, it was not uncommon for physicians to be viewed not only as content experts but moral experts as well. (Historically, the role of priest and physician were closely intertwined.) The twentieth century, however, brought many examples of clearly unethical behavior on the part of physicians, beginning in the 1940s with the Nuremberg trials. The world was confronted with evidence of atrocities perpetrated by Nazi physicians on prisoners of war, prompting the development of the Nuremberg Code, the first official statement on research ethics (Beals, Sebring, and Crawford, 1946–1949).

Unethical behavior by physicians was not limited to wartime. In 1966, for instance, Henry Beecher (1966) published his famous "twenty-two examples" of unethical research that had been published over the past two decades in seminal medical journals, including the *New England Journal of Medicine*. Examples included developmentally disabled patients being inoculated with active hepatitis virus and elderly patients injected with live cancer cells.

While Beecher's report may not have been widely recognized outside the medical community, the revelation in 1972 of the Tuskegee syphilis study was. For over forty years investigators monitored African Americans infected with syphilis and did not treat them with antibiotics, which had been discovered after the beginning of the study in the late 1930s. This revelation prompted intense examination of research ethics in particular, leading to the publication of the Belmont Report (National Commission for the Protection of Human Subjects of Biomedical and Behavioral Research, 1978).

For all these reasons, the field of bioethics came to be recognized in the 1970s, with the term coined in the first year of that decade. The following year both the *Hastings Center Report* and the Kennedy Institute of Ethics were founded, providing a forum and venue for discourse. Given the impetus of empowering patients and concern for unethical behavior on the part of physicians, one of the field's initial focuses was on protecting patients from physicians.

It therefore should not come as a surprise that the earliest bioethicists tended to be non-physicians. Theologians (such as Joseph Fletcher, Paul Ramsay, and Richard McCormick), philosophers (such as Tristram Engelhardt, K. Danner Clouser, and Daniel Callahan), and attorneys (such as Luis Kutner) came together to support the rights of patients to make their own decisions, and explore new issues that had never been faced before (Caplan & Callahan, 1981; Clouser, 1980; Engelhardt, 1986; Fletcher, 1954; Kutner, 1969; McCormick, 1981; Ramsey, 1970). As Rothman (2008) writes, "The changes that came to medicine generally came over the strenuous objections of doctors, giving the entire process an adversarial quality . . . Outsiders crossed over into medicine to correct what they perceived as wrongs."

Part of the early bioethicists' task was to determine how—beyond thinktanks, books, and journal articles—to actually "do" ethics. The establishment of institutional review boards was a logical response to violations of research ethics, but clinical ethics required a different model. Hospital ethics committees therefore began to proliferate (Teel, 1975), although at first their prognosis was guarded (Purtilo, 1984). Most of the dilemmas they addressed had to do with end-of-life decision-making, especially regarding requests to forgo[1] treatment (an area that palliative care—then barely a term and certainly not a field—now specializes in).

At first, these dilemmas were often misdiagnosed as psychiatric in nature, rather than ethical. It was assumed that a patient refusing life-sustaining medical treatment (LSMT) must have a mental illness, thus prompting psychiatric consultation. Eventually it came to be recognized that this assumption was "masking moral dilemmas" (Perl & Shelp, 1982), and formal ethics consultations were (reluctantly) requested (Siegler, 1978).

Both legal and regulatory steps spurred patient empowerment during this period. In 1976, the California Natural Death Act codified the right of patients to refuse un-wanted treatment, and the first article appeared describing a "do not resuscitate," or DNR, order (Rabkin, Gillerman, & Rice, 1976).[2] That same year saw the case of Karen Ann Quinlan, the first to declare that patients had the right to refuse LSMT and also that their surrogates could make that decision on their behalf if they lacked decision-making ca-pacity. (Other cases over the prior two decades had explored similar issues, but due to their idiosyncrasies none had codified the evolving societal consensus [Meisel, 2016].)

Karen Ann was a young woman who was ventilator-dependent and in a persistent vegetative state. Her parents requested that the doctors discontinue mechanical ventila-tion, but the trial court in New Jersey refused their request, deeming it a violation of state homicide statutes. On appeal, though, the New Jersey Supreme Court overturned the lower court decision, deeming the request an appropriate extension of Karen Ann's right of privacy (In re Quinlan, 1976).

Her physicians resisted, however, asserting that "in this hospital we don't kill people" (Quinlan, Quinlan, & Battelle, 1977). Forced to comply with the order, the physicians did

---

1. "Forgo" will be used to describe either withholding a treatment, or withdrawing a treatment already in use. The ethical equivalence of the latter two concepts is explored in chapter 5.

2. While DNR is the more common abbreviation, this textbook generally uses the abbreviation DNAR—for Do Not Attempt Resuscitation—to refer to the order instructing medical personnel to forgo further medical treatment for a patient who is pulseless and is not breathing. The term "DNR" is still used on occasion when it is temporally accurate or to emphasize misunderstandings specifically related to it.

not immediately extubate her but rather weaned her gradually from the ventilator on which she was thought to be dependent. To everyone's surprise, she was able to breathe on her own and went on to survive for nearly a decade in a nursing home, before eventually dying of pneumonia. (Her parents never requested discontinuation of medically administered nutrition and hydration [MANH], believing that unlike mechanical ventilation this was "ordinary" treatment.) As her mother later said, "We never asked to have her die. We just asked to have her put back in a natural state so she could die in God's time" (Nessman, 2006).

The right to refuse LSMT was soon reflected in position statements of governmental commissions (President's Commission for the Study of Ethical Problems in Medicine and Biomedical and Behavioral Research, 1983) and academic task forces (The Hastings Center, 1987). The *Quinlan* case also shifted the locus of decision-making regarding forgoing LSMT from the courts to ethics committees: "Physicians should consult with [the] hospital ethics committee and if [the] committee should agree with physicians' prognosis, the life-support systems may be withdrawn" (*In re Quinlan*, 1976).

Such reliance on hospital ethics committees was not universally embraced, however. The following year another state supreme court—this time in Massachusetts in the case of *Superintendent of Belchertown State School v. Saikewicz* (p. 68)—identified the judicial system as the locus of decision-making in end-of-life cases. Confronted with this disagreement, other states hurried to pass their own laws on the matter, and the President's Commission was established in 1978 to help settle the issue. The Commission's findings (President's Commission for the Study of Ethical Problems in Medicine and Biomedical and Behavioral Research, 1983)—in concert with the majority of state court decisions—ultimately established a consensus that physicians and patients (with the assistance of ethics committees where available) were equipped to handle most situations, although the courts were the last recourse in cases of intractable disagreement.

There was only one problem: at that time, a mere 1% of hospitals actually had an ethics committee (McGee, Caplan, Spanogle, & Asch, 2001). Once these were identified as appropriate forums for resolution, however, that number dramatically increased. Only four years later, the majority of hospitals had their own ethics committees (Fleetwood, Arnold, & Baron, 1989).

Physicians also became more involved in ethics consultation and education. This stemmed both from a recognition that clinical ethics required clinical expertise, as well as a less insular environment whereby physicians dared to be critical of the establishment of which they were a part. Medical students and residents were exposed to ethical decision-making, and advanced certification in ethics came to be available to clinicians and not only academics (Siegler, 1982). In addition to philosophically rigorous bioethics textbooks—such as *Principles of Biomedical Ethics* (Beauchamp & Childress, 2009), which is considered by many to be the "gold standard"—practical clinical guides were formulated, such as *Clinical Ethics*, which is now in its eighth edition (Jonsen, Siegler, & Winslade, 2015).

During this period advance directives (ADs)—initially proposed in 1969 (Kutner, 1969) and first established in state law in California in 1976 (Natural Death Act, 1976)—were gaining greater recognition. At first these were of questionable legality, though, and in order to honor a patient's right of refusal of LSMT families often had to bring lawsuits or rely on the press to appeal their case. To remedy this, the Patient Self-Determination Act (Omnibus Budget Reconciliation Act of 1990) was passed. It required that patients, upon hospital admission, be given a written summary of their health care decision-making rights and asked if they have an AD (without concern for discrimination if they do). It also required health care facilities to educate staff and community about ADs. Within the next two years every state as well as the District of Columbia had passed legislation recognizing the right of patients to express in advance their wishes regarding medical treatment in writing.

That same year, the case of Nancy Cruzan was decided by the US Supreme Court (*Cruzan v. Director, Missouri Department of Health*, 1990). She, like Karen Ann Quinlan, was a young woman in a persistent vegetative state, but unlike Karen Ann she was not ventilator-dependent, and her family did request discontinuation of MANH. As noted in more detail later (p. 185), the US Supreme Court concluded that MANH was a medical intervention that (like any other medical intervention) could be limited, but individual states could apply higher evidentiary standards to this determination. In addition, the *Cruzan* decision also addressed the Rule of Double Effect (p. 209) and, in Justice O'Connor's concurring opinion, embraced the use of ADs.

Recognizing the expanding ethical complexity that pervades all aspects of medicine, the following year the Joint Commission on Accreditation of Healthcare Organizations (now known simply as the Joint Commission) mandated that certified hospitals have a "mechanism" for "the consideration of ethical issues arising in the care of patients and ... provide education to caregivers and patients on ethical issues in health care" (Joint Commission, 2011). Generally this is accomplished by a hospital ethics committee, which is traditionally tasked with responsibility for clinical consultation, education, and policy development. Despite the Joint Commission's mandate, however, ethics committees are often underutilized, with half of hospitals performing three or fewer consultations annually (Fox, Myers, & Pearlman, 2007).

One would think that with all the emphasis on patient autonomy and advance care planning (ACP) that patients' wishes would be respected. The Study to Understand Prognoses and Preferences for Outcomes and Risks of Treatments (SUPPORT)—which involved over 9,000 patients—sadly dispelled this optimistic belief. The first phase of the study was observational and took place over two years in five major teaching hospitals. It found that nearly half of physicians did not know that their patient did not want CPR, and a similar percentage of DNR orders were written within two days of death. Over a third of study subjects who died spent ten or more days in the intensive care unit, and half of conscious patients reported moderate or severe pain more than half the time in the days leading up to their deaths (SUPPORT Principal Investigators, 1995).

Having identified significant problems, the second phase of the study attempted to remedy these. In a randomized trial, the experimental group received specific interventions to identify patient goals, improve patient understanding and pain control, and facilitate ACP. Despite these very thoughtful interventions, however, the concerning findings noted in the observational phase did not improve, suggesting that medical professionals were content with the status quo.

The SUPPORT study highlighted deficiencies in the ACP process, prompting more innovative approaches that have shown remarkable success in some areas (Hammes & Kane, 1998). It also documented grossly inadequate symptom management—especially at the end of life—which prompted remedial steps such as the Joint Commission's publication of Pain Management Standards (Berry & Dahl, 2000). This established pain as "the fifth vital sign," hoping to improve pain management but unintentionally perhaps contributing to overuse (and ultimately abuse) of opioid medications (Fiore, 2016).

As bioethics became more established as a field, diverse professional advocacy groups consolidated. In 1998 the Society for Health and Human Values, the Society for Bioethics Consultation, and the American Association of Bioethics merged to form a unified voice. The American Society for Bioethics and Humanities now represents mainstream practice in the field.

With the dawn of the Internet and the increased use of social media, bioethics also made the headlines, notably in the case of Terri Schiavo, which may be the most litigated medical ethics case in US history. Like Karen Ann Quinlan and Nancy Cruzan, Terri was a young woman in a persistent vegetative state and like Nancy was not ventilator-dependent. Unlike the Cruzans, however, Terri's family was not unified in their view of MANH. Her husband (and guardian) favored discontinuation, while her parents adamantly opposed this plan.

From a legal (and ethical) point of view, the appropriate response seemed clear: her appropriate surrogate, using substituted judgment (p. 61), had the right to refuse LSMT including MANH. In reality, though, the case was drawn out through legal and legislative battles, extending beyond state lines to include Congress and even the president. What distinguished this case—along with more recent high-profile cases such as Jahi McMath (Gostin, 2014)—was the 24/7 news coverage and impassioned social media advocacy of her parents, as well as the political maneuvering of various parties.

As the role of the bioethicist became more accepted, the need for bioethicists has become increasingly recognized (Toulmin, 1982). In the field's nascent days bioethicists had largely been philosophers or theologians who had garnered some clinical experience, later adding clinicians with specialized training in bioethics such as at the University of Chicago fellowship program (Siegler, 1982). Responding to increased need, there are now over thirty-five online graduate degree programs in ethics, open to professionals (and non-professionals) of every stripe. Barely half a century ago there was no such thing as a "bioethicist," but now a debate rages on about whether all who claim this mantle truly merit it (Kodish et al., 2013).

Palliative Care

The word "hospice" is derived from two Latin words: *hospis* (referring to both host and guest) and *hospitium* (referring to the location where hospitality was offered). As such, it did not initially refer to caring for people at the end of life. At first it was much broader, dating back as far as the fourth century to Fabiola, a matron and follower of Saint Jerome, who provided strangers in need with food, drink, clothing, and shelter. The tradition continued in the form of monastic hospices in the Middle Ages, catering to pilgrims and other travelers. It was only in the nineteenth century that the term was increasingly used for the care of dying patients, with facilities focusing on this group opening in France and in Ireland (Hallenbeck, 2003).

This coincided with a change in the societal view of death. Phillippe Ariès, in his classic study *Western Attitudes toward Death: From the Middle Ages to the Present* (Ariès, 1974), traces this evolution. Initially death was "tamed," meaning that it was accepted, communal and prepared for. This gradually yielded to an increased focus on "one's own death" (emphasizing personal responsibility and questions of salvation). The eighteenth and early nineteenth centuries brought the concept of the "beautiful death," a joyous transition to the afterlife extolled in famous works such as *Jane Eyre* and *War and Peace*.

Over the course of the nineteenth century, however, this gave way to the modern conception of "forbidden death," characterized by the concealment and medicalization of death. Whereas people previously had usually died suddenly, at home, and at a younger age, people were now surviving longer, and dying later and in institutions (i.e., out of public view). Antibiotics made it increasingly possible to delay death, essentially eradicating what had been the three most common causes of death (Figure 1.1). In a matter of decades, pneumonia went from being "the old man's best friend" (Osler, 1901) to a treatable infection.

Improved treatment modalities did not just cure disease; they also paved the way for chronic illness, prolonged hospitalizations, and the assumption that all available resources would be brought to bear to prevent death from occurring (i.e., the "technological imperative"). The focus of medicine began to shift from healing to curing, with relatively little attention focused on the quality of life of dying patients.

As noted previously, the first half of the twentieth century heralded the shift from parentalism to patient autonomy, as evidenced in the United States by court cases beginning with *Schloendoerff*. A focus on the rights of patients near the end of life marked the beginning of the modern hospice movement, beginning with the work of Dame Cicely Saunders in the United Kingdom in the 1950s. She was one of the first modern clinicians to not only recognize the suffering of dying patients but also to explore specific ways to ameliorate it (Saunders, 1960, 1963). In 1967 the first modern hospice (St. Christopher's) opened in London. Two years later Elizabeth Kübler-Ross (1969) published her influential work *On Death and Dying*, bringing an analytic approach to the process of dying and paving the way for further studies in this area. Remarkably, she said that the greatest barrier to her initial request to speak with dying hospital patients was a denial they even existed!

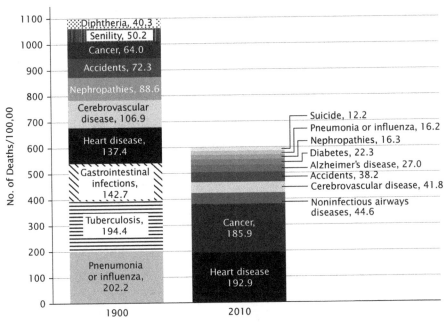

FIGURE 1.1 Epidemiology of death over the course of the twentieth century (Jones, Podolsky, & Greene, 2012)

The hospice movement crossed the Atlantic in the early 1970s, with the first hospice in North America opening in 1974 in Branford, Connecticut, followed a year later by one in Montreal (Stoddard, 1978). It shared the same mission as St. Christopher's and other hospices in Britain, but unlike the European hospice model—which evolved within the health care system—"the American hospice . . . was outside the medical mainstream and a reaction to its excesses, notably the overuse of medical technology" (Fins, 2006). In addition, whereas in many parts of the Western world a hospice is a structure which cares for patients with serious—although not always terminal—illness, in the United States "hospice" is more accurately considered a philosophy, or an approach to care. Barely one in four hospice patients in America die in a residential hospice, with approximately two-thirds dying in what they consider "home" (i.e., private residence, nursing home, or residential facility) (National Hospice and Palliative Care Organization, 2014).

It was around this time that Balfour Mount coined the term "palliative care," primarily as a cultural and linguistic necessity in Quebec (where he practiced). The word "hospice" in French referred to nursing homes—often repositories of neglect—and *soins palliatifs* constituted a fitting translation of the English term, both literally and in spirit (Hallenbeck, 2003). While not initially intended as being distinctive from hospice, over time (and especially with the establishment of the Medicare Hospice Benefit in 1982 [Davis, 1988]) the term "palliative care" has taken on a broader meaning than hospice, including patients not within the last six months of life.

The word "palliate" is derived from the Latin *pallium,* an ancient scarf or cloak. It literally means to cover or clothe and in common usage refers to the prevention and relief of suffering. The World Health Organization (2002) has defined palliative care as

> [A]n approach that improves the quality of life of patients and their families facing the problems associated with life-threatening illness, through the prevention and relief of suffering by means of early identification and impeccable assessment and treatment of pain and other problems, physical, psychosocial and spiritual.

Some have gone further and distinguished palliative care from palliative *medicine,* which has been defined as the "study and management of patients with active, progressive, far-advanced disease for whom the prognosis is limited and the focus of care is the quality of life" (Doyle, Hanks, Cherny & Calman, 2004). Palliative medicine therefore exists more within the explicitly medical model.

It is important to note that palliative care is appropriate for anyone with "life-threatening" illness, not only those patients at the end of their lives. To restrict palliative care to patients who are imminently dying would deprive patients of the benefit of palliative care in goal-setting, psychosocial support, and symptom management in the earlier stages of their illness. Sadly, though, palliative care is often misunderstood (Meier, 2011). Many patients, upon being offered palliative care consultation, immediately assume that they are dying. This is a major reason that patients suffering from serious illness though still hoping for a cure may be reluctant to engage in discussions related to palliative care.

During this period there were further advances in pain management. These included the invention of patient-controlled analgesia in the 1970s (Forrest, Smethurst, & Kienitz, 1970) and the publication of the World Health Organization (1986) analgesic ladder. An expert committee was formed, tasked with disseminating knowledge of pain management and palliative care throughout the world (World Health Organization, 1990). The Centers for Medicare & Medicaid Services sponsored hospice demonstration projects to assess the efficacy and cost of enhanced care at the end of life. Positive results led to the Medicare Hospice Benefit in 1982, which provided Medicare funding for hospice care that previously was provided by non-profit groups through philanthropic support. The only requirements were that a patient be a Medicare beneficiary, have a prognosis of six months or less if the disease ran its natural course, and decline disease-modifying treatment for the terminal diagnosis. Private insurers soon followed suit in providing a hospice benefit, and currently nearly all state Medicaid programs offer some form of hospice benefit for the nonelderly as well.

Ongoing societal and personal struggles with death and dying became better known during this period. The *Quinlan* and *Cruzan* decisions codified the rights of patients and surrogates to refuse unwanted treatment, including MANH. The first American academic hospital palliative care program was established in 1987 at the Cleveland Clinic, and the first major textbook was published in 1993 (Doyle, Hanks, & MacDonald, 1993).

The Project on Death in America (1994–2003) provided research funding to investigators focused on end-of-life care and in the process created a nexus of leaders in the field. The Institute of Medicine published its seminal report *Approaching Death: Improving Care at the End of Life* (Field, Cassel, & Institute of Medicine Committee on Care at the End of Life, 1997), reflecting the growing importance of end-of-life care within the US health care system. Public awareness was heightened by media attention, such as Bill Moyers' "On Our Own Terms," which premiered in 2000. Many cross-over books during this period helped increase public awareness about palliative and end-of-life care, including *How We Die* (Nuland, 1994) and *Dying Well* (Byock, 1997).

During this period, the field of palliative care continued to expand. The American Board of Hospice and Palliative Medicine was formed in 1995 to implement standards of certification. In light of the evolving evidence base and relevant scholarship, the American Board of Medical Specialties recognized hospice and palliative medicine as a subspecialty in 2006, nineteen years after such recognition in the United Kingdom.

The year 2010 brought with it huge advances in both the professional and lay arenas. The first randomized controlled trial of palliative care was published in the *New England Journal of Medicine* (Temel et al., 2010). The fact that patients with advanced non-small cell lung cancer who were randomized to receive a mandatory palliative care consultation had better symptom control was not surprising. What was surprising, however, is that they lived longer than patients receiving usual care, thus debunking (at least in this population) the conventional belief that patients who opt for a more palliative course of treatment die sooner, though more comfortably. Subsequent studies have yielded similar results with other terminal diagnoses (Bakitas et al., 2015; Rugno, Paiva, & Paiva, 2014), prompting major organizations to proclaim early palliative care as standard cancer care (Ferrell et al., 2017).

The other major development of that year was the publication of "Letting Go," an article by Atul Gawande in *The New Yorker* (Gawande, 2010). Subsequently incorporated into the best-selling book *Being Mortal* (Gawande, 2014), this article highlighted the benefits of palliative care and confronted common myths (including that palliative care and hospice represented "giving up"). It also revealed how much a professor at Harvard Medical School still had to learn about palliative care.

With the growth of professional groups—such as the National Hospice and Palliative Care Organization (formed in 1978) and the American Academy of Hospice and Palliative Medicine (founded in 1988)—as well as advocacy groups (such as the Center to Advance Palliative Care, founded in 1998), the field of palliative care has increasingly solidified itself within the US health care system. This includes specific palliative care certification by the Joint Commission (Buck, 2013) and report cards offered by the Center to Advance Palliative Care (2015).

With greater visibility has also come the potential for criticism of the field of hospice and palliative medicine. The concept of reimbursing physicians for having goals-of-care conversations with patients has been labeled "death panels" (Kenny, 2012). The evolution of for-profit hospices has led to increased regulatory scrutiny regarding extended lengths of stay (Whoriskey & Keating, 2014).

To be sure, the field still has a long way to go. Hospice utilization—both whether and how early a patient enrolls in hospice—varies widely (Dartmouth Institute for Health Policy and Clinical Practice, 2016). The requirement to decline disease-modifying therapy limits access to hospice while not necessarily decreasing costs (Spettell et al., 2009). And there exists a severe palliative care workforce shortage, highlighting the need for broader education and the provision of "generalist palliative care" (Quill & Abernethy, 2013).

Relationship of Ethics and Palliative Care

As should be evident, ethics and palliative care share a common history. Both evolved out of a recognition that patients have the right to make informed decisions about their care and ultimately have a dignified death on their own terms where suffering is controlled. Both address difficult situations involving serious illness, complex social situations, organizational implications, and cultural issues. The names Schloendoerff and Quinlan—and the terms "advance directive" and the "Rule of Double Effect"—are common parlance in both fields.

Since bioethics emerged as a field slightly earlier than palliative care, some of the work of palliative care originally was done by ethicists. Prior to the early 2000s, ethicists often facilitated goals of care conversations (and continue to do so in contexts without palliative care support). The converse is also true, for at institutions without a dedicated department of ethics, palliative care clinicians are often viewed as the local ethics experts, frequently serving on or chairing the institution's ethics committee. It is understandable, then, that the departments of ethics and palliative care are combined at some major medical centers (University of Pittsburgh, 2016).

Reflecting the overlap between the two, each one talks about the other. The American Academy of Hospice and Palliative Medicine has an Ethics Special Interest Group, and the American Society for Bioethics and Humanities hosts a Hospice and Palliative Medicine affinity group. Both could also be said to have unfortunate or misunderstood names: ethics conjuring judgment and moral "holy rollers," and palliative care either not being understood—as the word "palliative" is infrequently used in its nontechnical sense—or inaccurately conjuring images of imminent death (Reich, 1994).

Despite the areas of commonality, the two fields are distinct. Not every ethical dilemma involves the end of life, nor does every palliative care situation involve an ethical dilemma. The two fields could, therefore, be said to have "parallel and intersecting domains" (Carter & Wocial, 2012).

Background, training, and practice also differ. Bioethicists represent many different disciplines, ranging from law to philosophy to theology to medicine. Generally patients are not billed for an ethics consult, and the approval of the attending physician is not required. Ethics consultations may or may not be documented in the patient's chart and may not even involve direct patient contact (Rhodes & Alfandre, 2007).

Palliative care teams, on the other hand, are made up of several distinct disciplines, each with clearly defined training and skill sets. Existing squarely within the medical model, palliative care clinicians usually require the attending physician's approval before consulting on a patient. The end result is that a proportion of ethics consultations may be more appropriate for palliative care consultation, save for the fact that the attending will not approve the latter. Often the work of ethics consultation in these cases is persuading the attending to consent to the palliative care consultation, or at least recommending this in the consultation note. In one study of oncology patients who had both ethics and palliative consultations, for instance, half of the palliative care consultations came about as a result of a preceding ethics consultation (Shuman et al., 2013).

This necessarily raises the question of how to tell whether a dilemma is primarily ethical or palliative. While it true that ethicists generally focus on resolving conflict whereas palliative care clinicians provide psychosocial support and symptom management (Reich, 1994), many complex cases involve all these components, raising the question of which consultant is best equipped to assist the patient, family, and clinical team. Regrettably, interprofessional tensions may come into play, given palliative care's assuming what once was considered ethics' "market share" (i.e., guidance and clarification in end-of-life decision-making) (Aulisio, Chaitin, & Arnold, 2004). The fact that palliative care—unlike ethics—can bill for its consultations creates expectations but also opportunities, making the former more attractive to hospital administrations.

When deciding whether to seek bioethics or palliative care consultation for a patient with life-threatening illness, three aspects are relevant: knowledge, perspective, and role (Figure 1.2). With regard to knowledge, palliative care is the only field of medicine that explicitly includes ethics knowledge and skills as one of its core domains. That this knowledge is focused on palliative care issues is not a disadvantage given the area of concern, but one should not conclude that a palliative care clinician's ethics knowledge

	Ethics	Palliative care
Require attending approval?	No	Yes
Bill for servicess	No	Yes
Patient population	All	Patients with life-limiting illness
Goal with patients/families	Impartiality	Building alliances
Involvement	Moment in time	Longitudinal
Focus	Conflict resolution	Symptom management; psychosocial support
Role	Outsiders	Members of care team
Primary concern	Precedent	Individual case

FIGURE 1.2 Differences between ethics and palliative care

and skill is equivalent to that of a well-trained, experienced ethicist (whose sole focus is ethics). There could be times when the complexity of an ethical dilemma might exceed the abilities of a skilled palliative care practitioner, requiring external consultation. For this reason the National Consensus Project recommends that "appropriate referrals are made to ethics consultants or a committee for case consultation and assistance in conflict resolution" (Colby, Dahlin, Lantos, Carney, & Christopher, 2010).

With regard to perspective, ethicists and palliative care clinicians often approach clinical situations from different vantage points. Depending on their background, ethicists tend to focus more on philosophical principles (such as autonomy and beneficence) and specific duties (such as that of relieving suffering). Palliative care clinicians, on the other hand, often focus more on the concrete details of a specific case. From personal experience, ethicists often seem more concerned about precedent (i.e., if they do something for one patient, they would have to do it for *all* patients), while palliative care clinicians tend to reason one case at a time, more focused on the well-being of an individual patient or family than the broader ramifications of an action.

Finally, there is the question of role. Ethicists often encounter patients and families at one moment in time, often after many discussions (and treatments) have already occurred. In that context, ethicists generally strive for impartiality, bringing a fresh eye to a complex situation As such, they are often something of "outsiders" in the midst of the care team.

Palliative care clinicians, on the other hand, tend to have a longitudinal relationship with patients and families, focusing more on empathetic engagement than impartiality. While some situations require an answer to a moment-in-time question, many others require ongoing relationship, support, and clarification.

In determining which service to consult, the context is as important as the question. Questions about whether there is an ethical obligation to provide treatment considered inappropriate is an ethical question. Questions about whether treatment is inappropriate in relation to the overall goals of care is more of a palliative care question. Ultimately, both clinical ethics and palliative care deal with several key domains—such as communication, suffering, distress, end-of-life decisions, and appropriateness of treatment—but each has a unique and valuable perspective on those domains (Figure 1.3).

Often what may appear to be an ethical dilemma is really a failure of communication. This is not hard to understand, for in modern health care the stakes are high and emotions run strong. Unless conflict is addressed and the lines of communication are open, it will be impossible to provide optimal care to a patient and family. Since both ethicists and palliative care clinicians are acknowledged experts in communication, each be helpful in such stressful situations. The primary consideration here is what the *goal* of enhanced communication is. Clarifying goals of care? Identifying professional obligation? Providing psychosocial support? Resolving interpersonal conflict?

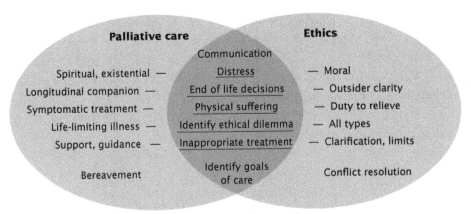

FIGURE 1.3 Overlapping domains of ethics and palliative care

When deciding which service to consult, the decision may largely be a practical one. If the attending physician will not approve a palliative care consultation, an ethics consultation—with subsequent palliative care involvement—remains an option. Ethics involvement also avoids any confusion about the authority for clinical care, while palliative care consultation allows for the possibility of the consultant assuming that very authority, if desired. Ultimately, when the most appropriate resource is unclear, it may simply come down to a question of which service a patient or family is most likely to accept and work with (Aulisio et al., 2004; Carter & Wocial, 2012).

The choice of ethics or palliative is not mutually exclusive. In some situations, it is appropriate to consult both services. Ideally they will work in concert, utilizing their specific gifts while deferring to the specific skills of the other. Such collaboration may be required because of distinct tasks which lend themselves specifically to each skill set. Alternatively the two services might sequentially address the same task, perhaps because the first attempt was unsuccessful, a new aspect of the task arose, or additional conflict resolution is necessary (Childers, Demme, Greenlaw, King, & Quill, 2008). This is especially true when a surrogate decision-maker demands continued aggressive treatment when the clinical team feels the goal should be comfort, and when intensive symptom management is necessary to continue burdensome treatments (Lantos, 2011).

Summary Points

- Ethics and palliative care have both long been a part of clinical medicine but have only recently come to be formally recognized.
- Increased interest in clinical ethics was prompted by technological advances, a shift from parentalism to autonomy, and decreasing confidence that physicians knew what the "right" thing to do was (and would do it).

- Increased interest in palliative care was prompted by evidence of significant suffering at the end of life, which could be ameliorated with targeted interventions.
- There is some degree of overlap between clinical ethics and palliative care. In some situations one consultation service is required and in others both are (either simultaneously or sequentially).
- Generally it is better to identify the pressing question and target the consultation to the service best equipped to address it.

References

Ad Hoc Committee of the Harvard Medical School to Examine the Definition of Brain Death. (1968). A definition of irreversible coma. Report of the Ad Hoc Committee of the Harvard Medical School to Examine the Definition of Brain Death. *JAMA, 205*(6), 337–340.

Alexander, S. (1962). They decide who lives, who dies. *Life, 53*(19), 102–124.

American Medical Association. (1847). *Code of medical ethics of the American Medical Association.* Chicago: American Medical Association Press.

Ariès, P. (1974). *Western attitudes toward death: From the Middle Ages to the present.* Baltimore: Johns Hopkins University Press.

Aulisio, M. P., Chaitin, E., & Arnold, R. M. (2004). Ethics and palliative care consultation in the intensive care unit. *Crit Care Clin, 20*(3), 505–523, x–xi. doi:10.1016/j.ccc.2004.03.006

Bakitas, M. A., Tosteson, T. D., Li, Z., Lyons, K. D., Hull, J. G., Li, Z., . . . Ahles, T. A. (2015). Early versus delayed initiation of concurrent palliative oncology care: Patient outcomes in the ENABLE III randomized controlled trial. *J Clin Oncol, 33*(13), 1438–1445. doi: 10.1200/JCO.2014.58.6362

Beauchamp, T. L., & Childress, J. F. (2009). *Principles of biomedical ethics* (6th ed.). New York: Oxford University Press.

Beals W.B., Sebring H.L., and Crawford J.T. (1946–1949). Permissible medical experiments. In: *Trials of War Criminals Before the Nuremberg Military Tribunals.* Vol 2. Washington, DC: US Government Printing Office.

Beecher, H. K. (1966). Ethics and clinical research. *N Engl J Med, 274*(24), 1354–1360. doi:10.1056/NEJM196606162742405

Berry, P. H., & Dahl, J. L. (2000). The new JCAHO pain standards: Implications for pain management nurses. *Pain Manag Nurs, 1*(1), 3–12. doi:10.1053/jpmn.2000.5833

Buck, H. G. (2013). The Joint Commission "speaks up" for palliative care. *Nursing, 43*(5), 14. doi:10.1097/01.NURSE.0000428707.96625.67

Byock, I. (1997). *Dying well: The prospect for growth at the end of life.* New York: Riverhead Books.

Canterbury v. Spence. (1972). 464 F.2d 772 (D.C. Cir.).

Caplan, A. L., & Callahan, D. (1981). *Ethics in hard times.* New York: Plenum Press.

Carter, B. S., & Wocial, L. D. (2012). Ethics and palliative care: Which consultant and when? *Am J Hosp Palliat Care, 29*(2), 146–150. doi:10.1177/1049909111410560

Center to Advance Palliative Care. (2015). America's care of serious illness. Retrieved from https://reportcard.capc.org/

Childers, J. W., Demme, R., Greenlaw, J., King, D. A., & Quill, T. (2008). A qualitative report of dual palliative care/ethics consultations: Intersecting dilemmas and paradigmatic cases. *J Clin Ethics, 19*(3), 204–213.

Clouser, K. D. (1980). *Teaching bioethics: Strategies, problems, and resources.* New York: Hastings Center, Institute for Society, Ethics, and the Life Sciences.

Cobbs v. Grant. (1972). 8 Cal. 3d 229, 502 P.2d 1, 104 Cal. Rptr. 505.

Colby, W. H., Dahlin, C., Lantos, J., Carney, J., & Christopher, M. (2010). The National Consensus Project for Quality Palliative Care Clinical Practice Guidelines Domain 8: Ethical and legal aspects of care. *HEC Forum, 22*(2), 117–131. doi:10.1007/s10730-010-9128-3

Cruzan v. Director, Missouri Department of Health, 497 261 (S.Ct. 1990).

Dartmouth Institute for Health Policy and Clinical Practice. (2016). The Dartmouth atlas of health care. Retrieved from http://www.dartmouthatlas.org/

Davis, F. A. (1988). Medicare hospice benefit: Early program experiences. *Health Care Financ Rev, 9*(4), 99–111.

Doyle, D., Hanks, G. W. C., Cherny, N.I. & Calman, K. (2004). Introduction. In D. Doyle, G. W. C. Hanks, Cherny, N.I. & Calman, K (Eds.), *Oxford textbook of palliative medicine* (pp. 1–4). Oxford: Oxford University Press.

Doyle, D., Hanks, G. W. C., & MacDonald, N. (1993). *Oxford textbook of palliative medicine*. Oxford: Oxford University Press.

Engelhardt, H. T. (1986). *The foundations of bioethics*. New York: Oxford University Press.

Ferrell, B. R., Temel, J. S., Temin, S., Alesi, E. R., Balboni, T. A., Basch, E. M., . . . Smith, T. S. (2017). Integration of palliative care into standard oncology care: American Society of Clinical Oncology clinical practice guideline update. *J Clin Oncol, 35*, 96–112.

Field, M. J., Cassel, C. K., & Institute of Medicine Committee on Care at the End of Life. (1997). *Approaching death: Improving care at the end of life*. Washington, DC: National Academy Press.

Fins, J. (2006). *A palliative ethic of care: clinical wisdom at life's end*. Sudbury, MA: Jones and Bartlett.

Fiore, K. (2016). Opioid crisis: Scrap pain as 5th vital sign? Retrieved from http://www.medpagetoday.com/publichealthpolicy/publichealth/57336

Fleetwood, J. E., Arnold, R. M., & Baron, R. J. (1989). Giving answers or raising questions? The problematic role of institutional ethics committees. *J Med Ethics, 15*(3), 137–142.

Fletcher, J. F. (1954). *Morals and medicine: The moral problems of the patient's right to know the truth, contraception, artificial insemination, sterilization, euthanasia*. Princeton, NJ: Princeton University Press.

Forrest, W. H. Jr., Smethurst, P. W., & Kienitz, M. E. (1970). Self-administration of intravenous analgesics. *Anesthesiology, 33*(3), 363–365.

Fox, E., Myers, S., & Pearlman, R. A. (2007). Ethics consultation in United States hospitals: A national survey. *Am J Bioeth, 7*(2), 13–25. doi:10.1080/15265160601109085

Fuchs, V. R. (1975). *Who shall live? Health, economics, and social choice*. New York: Basic Books.

Gawande, A. (2010, August 2). Letting go. *The New Yorker*.

Gawande, A. (2014). *Being mortal: Medicine and what matters in the end* (1st ed.). Toronto: Doubleday.

Gostin, L. O. (2014). Legal and ethical responsibilities following brain death: The McMath and Munoz cases. *JAMA, 311*(9), 903–904. doi:10.1001/jama.2014.660

Hallenbeck, J. (2003). *Palliative care perspectives*. Oxford; New York: Oxford University Press.

Hammes, B. J., & Kane, R. S. (1998). CPR practices in Wisconsin long-term care facilities. *WMJ, 97*(1), 55–57.

Hippocrates. (1923). *Hippocrates*. London, New York: W. Heinemann; G. P. Putnam's Sons.

In re Quinlan, 70 10 (N.J. 1976).

Joint Commission. (2011). *Comprehensive accreditation manual for hospitals (CAMH): The official handbook*. Oakbrook Terrace, IL: Joint Commission Resources.

Jones, D. S., Podolsky, S. H., & Greene, J. A. (2012). The burden of disease and the changing task of medicine. *N Engl J Med, 366*(25), 2333–2338. doi:10.1056/NEJMp1113569

Jonsen, A. R. (2003). *The birth of bioethics*. New York: Oxford University Press.

Jonsen, A. R., Siegler, M., & Winslade, W. J. (2015). *Clinical ethics: A practical approach to ethical decisions in clinical medicine* (8th ed.). New York: McGraw-Hill Medical.

Kenny, N. P. (2012). Debunking "death panels": Unfounded assumptions undercut planning for a "good death." *Health Prog, 93*(1), 48–56.

Kodish, E., Fins, J. J., Braddock, C., 3rd, Cohn, F., Dubler, N. N., Danis, M., . . . Kuczewski, M. G. (2013). Quality attestation for clinical ethics consultants: A two-step model from the American Society for Bioethics and Humanities. *Hastings Cent Rep, 43*(5), 26–36. doi:10.1002/hast.198

Kouwenhoven, W. B., Jude, J. R., & Knickerbocker, G. G. (1960). Closed-chest cardiac massage. *JAMA, 173*, 1064–1067.

Kübler-Ross, E. (1969). *On death and dying*. New York: Macmillan.

Kutner, L. (1969). Due process of euthanasia: The living will a proposal. *Indiana Law J, 44*.

Lane v. Candura. (1978). 6 Mass. App. Ct. 377, 383.

Lantos, J. (2011). The interface of ethics and palliative care. In J. Wolfe, P. S. Hinds, & B. M. Sourkes (Eds.), *Textbook of interdisciplinary pediatric palliative care* (pp. 119–124). Philadelphia: Elsevier/Saunders.

McCormick, R. A. (1981). *How brave a new world? Dilemmas in bioethics* (1st ed.). Garden City, NY: Doubleday.

McGee, G., Caplan, A. L., Spanogle, J. P., & Asch, D. A. (2001). A national study of ethics committees. *Am J Bioeth, 1*(4), 60–64. doi:10.1162/152651601317139531

Meier, D.E. (2011). Training doctors, combating myths. *Health Prog, 92*(1), 54–57.

Meisel, A. (2016). Legal issues in death and dying. In S. J. Youngner & R. M. Arnold (Eds.), *The Oxford handbook of ethics at the end of life* (pp. 7–26). Oxford: Oxford University Press.

Mount, B. M. (1997). The Royal Victoria Hospital palliative care service: A Canadian experience. In C. M. Saunders & R. Kastenbaum (Eds.), *Hospice care on the international scene* (pp. 73–85). New York: Springer Pub. Co.

Mozaffarian, D., Benjamin, E. J., Go, A. S., Arnett, D. K., Blaha, M. J., Cushman, M., . . . Stroke Statistics, S. (2015). Heart disease and stroke statistics—2015 update: a report from the American Heart Association. *Circulation, 131*(4), e29–322. doi: 10.1161/CIR.0000000000000152

Natanson v. John R. Kline and St. Francis Hospital and School of Nursing. (1960). 187 Kan. 186; 354 P.2d 670.

National Commission for the Protection of Human Subjects of Biomedical and Behavioral Research. (1978). *The Belmont report: Ethical principles and guidelines for the protection of human subjects of research.* Washington, DC: US Government Printing Office.

National Hospice and Palliative Care Organization. (2014). Facts and figures: Hospice care in America. Retrieved from https://www.nhpco.org/sites/default/files/public/Statistics_Research/2014_Facts_Figures.pdf

Natural Death Act, 7, California Health and Safety Code § 7185-95, 1 Stat. (1976).

Nessman, R. (2006). Karen Ann Quinlan's parents reflect on painful decision 20 years later. Associated Press. Retrieved from http://articles.latimes.com/1996-04-07/news/mn-55744_1_karen-ann-quinlan

Novack, D. H., Plumer, R., Smith, R. L., Ochitill, H., Morrow, G. R., & Bennett, J. M. (1979). Changes in physicians' attitudes toward telling the cancer patient. *JAMA, 241*(9), 897–900.

Nuland, S. B. (1994). *How we die: Reflections on life's final chapter* (1st large print ed.). New York: Random House Large Print.

Nuremberg Code. (1996). *JAMA, 276*(20), 1691.

Oken, D. (1961). What to tell cancer patients. A study of medical attitudes. *JAMA, 175,* 1120–1128.

Omnibus Budget Reconciliation Act of 1990, Pub. L. No. 101-508 § 4206 & 4751 (1990).

Osler W. (ed.) (1901). *The principles and practice of medicine,* 4th edn. New York: Appleton.

Percival, T. (1803). *Medical ethics, or, A code of institutes and precepts adapted to the professional conduct of physicians and surgeons.* London: W. Jackson.

Perl, M., & Shelp, E. E. (1982). Sounding board. Psychiatric consultation masking moral dilemmas in medicine. *N Engl J Med, 307*(10), 618–621. doi:10.1056/NEJM198209023071011

Potter, V. R. (1970). Bioethics, the science of survival. *Perspect Biol Med, 14,* 127–153.

President's Commission for the Study of Ethical Problems in Medicine and Biomedical and Behavioral Research. (1983). *Deciding to forego life-sustaining treatment: A report on the ethical, medical, and legal issues in treatment decisions.* Washington, DC: U.S. Government Printing Office.

Purtilo, R. B. (1984). Ethics consultations in the hospital. *N Engl J Med, 311*(15), 983–986. doi:10.1056/NEJM198410113111511

Quill, T. E., & Abernethy, A. P. (2013). Generalist plus specialist palliative care—creating a more sustainable model. *N Engl J Med, 368*(13), 1173–1175. doi:10.1056/NEJMp1215620

Quinlan, J., Quinlan, J., & Battelle, P. (1977). *Karen Ann: The Quinlans tell their story* (1st ed.). Garden City, NY: Doubleday.

Rabkin, M. T., Gillerman, G., & Rice, N. R. (1976). Orders not to resuscitate. *N Engl J Med, 295*(7), 364–366. doi:10.1056/NEJM197608122950705

Ramsey, P. (1970). *The patient as person: Explorations in medical ethics.* New Haven, CT: Yale University Press.

Reich, W. T. (1994). The word "bioethics": Its birth and the legacies of those who shaped it. *Kennedy Inst Ethics J, 4*(4), 319–335.

Rhodes, R., & Alfandre, D. (2007). A systematic approach to clinical moral reasoning. *J Clin Ethics, 18*(2), 66–70.

Rothman, D. J. (2008). *Strangers at the bedside: A history of how law and bioethics transformed medical decision making.* New Brunswick, NJ: AldineTransaction.

Rugno, F. C., Paiva, B. S., & Paiva, C. E. (2014). Early integration of palliative care facilitates the discontinuation of anticancer treatment in women with advanced breast or gynecologic cancers. *Gynecol Oncol, 135*(2), 249–254. doi:10.1016/j.ygyno.2014.08.030

Salgo v. Leland Stanford, Jr. University Board of Trustees. (1957). 152 Cal.App.2d 560, 317 P.2d 170.

Saunders, C. (1960). Drug treatment of patients in the terminal stages of cancer. *Curr Med Drugs, 1,* 16–28.

Saunders, C. (1963). The treatment of intractable pain in terminal cancer. *Proc R Soc Med, 56,* 195–197.

Schloendorff v. Society of New York Hospital. (1914). 211 NY 125, 105 NE 92.

Shuman, A. G., Montas, S. M., Barnosky, A. R., Smith, L. B., Fins, J. J., & McCabe, M. S. (2013). Clinical ethics consultation in oncology. *J Oncol Pract, 9*(5), 240–245. doi:10.1200/JOP.2013.000901

Siegler, M. (1978). A legacy of Osler. Teaching clinical ethics at the bedside. *JAMA, 239*(10), 951–956.

Siegler, M. (1982). Decision-making strategy for clinical-ethical problems in medicine. *Arch Intern Med, 142*(12), 2178–2179.

Spettell, C. M., Rawlins, W. S., Krakauer, R., Fernandes, J., Breton, M. E., Gowdy, W., . . . Brennan, T. A. (2009). A comprehensive case management program to improve palliative care. *J Palliat Med, 12*(9), 827–832. doi:10.1089/jpm.2009.0089

Stoddard, S. (1978). *The hospice movement: A better way of caring for the dying.* New York: Stein and Day.

Studdert, D. M., Mello, M. M., Levy, M. K., Gruen, R. L., Dunn, E. J., Orav, E. J., & Brennan, T. A. (2007). Geographic variation in informed consent law: Two standards for disclosure of treatment risks. *J Empir Leg Stud. 4*(1), 103–124.

SUPPORT Principal Investigators. (1995). The study to understand prognoses and preferences for outcomes and risks of treatments (SUPPORT). *JAMA, 274*(20), 1591–1598.

Teel, K. (1975). The physician's dilemma: A doctor's view—what the law should be. *Bayl Law Rev, 27*(1), 6–9.

Temel, J. S., Greer, J. A., Muzikansky, A., Gallagher, E. R., Admane, S., Jackson, V. A., . . . Lynch, T. J. (2010). Early palliative care for patients with metastatic non-small-cell lung cancer. *N Engl J Med, 363*(8), 733–742. doi:10.1056/NEJMoa1000678

The Hastings Center. (1987). *Guidelines on the termination of life sustaining treatment and the care of the dying.* Bloomington: Indiana University Press.

Toulmin, S. (1982). How medicine saved the life of ethics. *Perspect Biol Med, 25*(4), 736–750.

University of Pittsburgh. (2016). Section of palliative care and medical ethics. Retrieved from https://www.dom.pitt.edu/dgim/spc/index.html

Whoriskey, P., & Keating, D. (2014, December 26). Dying and profits: The evolution of hospice. *Washington Post.*

World Health Organization. (1986). *Cancer pain relief.* Retrieved from http://apps.who.int/iris/bitstream/10665/43944/1/9241561009_eng.pdf

World Health Organization. (1990). *Cancer pain relief and palliative care.* Retrieved from http://apps.who.int/iris/bitstream/10665/39524/1/WHO_TRS_804.pdf

World Health Organization. (2002). WHO definition of palliative care. Retrieved from www.who.int/cancer/palliative/definition/en/

2

Overview of Ethical Approaches

For most of the history of Western medicine, ethics received relatively little attention because the right course of action seemed obvious. A short list of basic rules (e.g., do no harm, put the patient's welfare before one's own) sufficed to guide medical professionals. Parentalism reigned supreme, placing responsibility for medical decision-making entirely in the hands of physicians.

Over time, however, the situation has become substantially more complicated. There are several reasons for this. First, some historic assumptions have not translated well into the modern world. For instance, the overriding emphasis on beneficence—taken to its extreme in the form of parentalism—has gradually given way over the last century to a respect for patient rights and personal choice (i.e., autonomy). Second, in the aftermath of events such as the Nazi prisoner experiments and the Tuskegee syphilis study, physicians can no longer be assumed to do the right thing, even when it is obvious. And, finally, technological developments in the practice of medicine have created an unprecedented level of complexity, such that well-intentioned, principled clinicians can reasonably disagree as to the best course of actions in ethically fraught situations (Thomasma, 1983).

In the midst of technological progress and increasing reliance on evidence-based medicine—where decisions are reached and treatment plans implemented based on empirical data—ethical dilemmas stand out because they deal with conflicts of values, which are neither measurable nor externally verifiable (Jonsen, Siegler, & Winslade, 2015). Unlike other decision-making fields which emphasize quantitative, structured analysis (Hunink, 2001), ethical decision-making is qualitative and narrative (Stiggelbout, Elstein, Molewijk, Otten, & Kievit, 2006). This opens ethical deliberation to criticisms of lack of intellectual rigor, whether by virtue of the absence of established algorithms to follow or quantitative values to analyze (Engelhardt, 2012), or accusations of personal bias (Scofield, 1993). Indeed, surveys of ethicists reveal wide diversity of opinion as to the optimal course of action (Fox & Stocking, 1993). As one critic has stated, "One man's categorical imperative is another man's heresy" (Shalit, 1997).

Even though ethics is taught at all US medical schools (Eckles, Meslin, Gaffney, & Helft, 2005) and most residency programs (Forrow, Arnold, & Frader, 1991), many physicians possess only a rudimentary appreciation of the subject. The four principles of bioethics (Beauchamp & Childress, 2009) and the four-quadrant approach to ethical dilemmas (Jonsen et al., 2015) may be easy to remember, but applying these constructs to real-life situations requires nuance, expertise, and wisdom. Sometimes the constructs are so theoretical as to defy application to particular situations, and at other times the obligations that flow from them are clear but conflict with other obligations (Callahan, 1996). An effective method of resolving ethical dilemmas must take theories into account but more importantly provide practical guidance to patients, families, and medical professionals (LaPuma, 1990).

This chapter attempts to dispel the common misperception that ethical analysis is idiosyncratic or overly theoretical by providing a structured approach for analyzing moral problems in the practice of medicine. The approach presented bears striking (and intentional) resemblance to the systematic evaluation of patients used by clinicians. In addition, this approach provides a method for resolving ethical disagreements, which often persist following a thoughtful and comprehensive analysis of a clinical situation. For unlike academic discussions of hypothetical ethical dilemmas, clinical ethics involves the very real problems facing patients, families, and clinicians. As such, it is not sufficient to recognize the complexity of a given situation by highlighting the respective arguments for and against a proposed course of action. A decision must be made, often choosing between alternatives of varying degrees of undesirability. As such, clinical ethics has been described as the search for the "least bad option" (Powderly, 2003), since if a good option were available, someone would have already identified it.

Over the past three decades, many approaches to analyzing clinical ethical dilemmas have been proposed (Arnlov, Ingelsson, Sundstrom, & Lind, 2010; Doukas, 1992; Doukas & McCullough, 1991; Finnerty, Pinkerton, Moreno, & Ferguson, 2000; Fletcher & Boyle, 1997; Gillon, 1994; Jonsen, Siegler, & Winslade, 2006; Kaldjian, Weir, & Duffy, 2005; Siegler, Pellegrino, & Singer, 1990; Thomasma, 1978). As will be evident from the ensuing discussion, there are profound similarities between these methods, especially in the preliminary steps they advocate. Thus, while some might reasonably question the applicability and generalizability of the conclusions reached by these methods, the *method* of reaching these conclusions is remarkably standardized and thus not open to accusations of idiosyncrasy.

In order to maximize applicability in the day-to-day practice of medicine, the method proposed tends to bear significant resemblance—often with explicit recognition of this fact (Kaldjian, Weir, & Duffy 2005; Thomasma 1978)—to the time-proven clinical assessment of a patient: subjective report (medical history), acquisition of clinical data (through physical exam and laboratory and radiological evaluation), assessment, and plan. As such, this method should appear familiar and reasonable to clinicians, as it brings to bear well-honed skills traditionally used for diagnosis and treatment, now applied to the task of identifying and resolving ethical dilemmas.

Published approaches to potential ethical dilemmas generally involve the following components (Figure 2.1).

1. Clarify and classify of the dilemma
2. Review existing information
3. Acquire additional, relevant information
4. Analyze the ethical issue, with reference to relevant legal and professional considerations
5. Formulate response, consider criticisms, and identify lessons learned

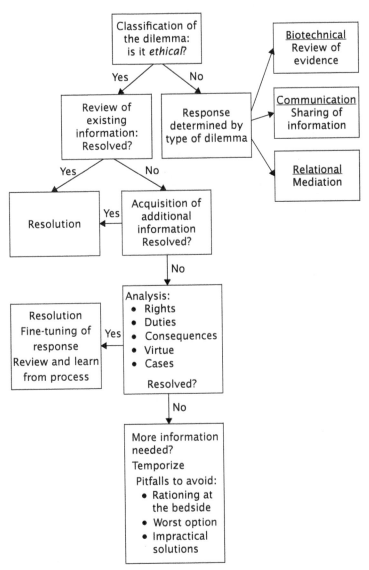

FIGURE 2.1 Algorithm for analysis and resolution of potential ethical dilemmas

Clarify and Classify the Dilemma

An ethical dilemma involves a conflict of *values*, where there is more than one acceptable course of action or, more often, there are mutually exclusive goods, thus forcing the clinician to choose among them (Thomasma, 1978). Situations where clinicians are unsure what to do—or where they are sure what to do but something is preventing them from doing it—often appear, at first glance, to be ethical in nature. The first step in addressing a perceived dilemma is to clarify the question to be answered and then to determine if it is, indeed, *ethical* in nature.

In some cases, this can be quite a challenge. A patient, family, or staff person may raise a profound concern, but they may not be able to articulate the precise nature of their discomfort. "This just feels wrong," they might say. In the language of the classic medical model, this is akin to a patient presenting with a chief complaint, not yet knowing its cause (Kaldjian et al., 2005). The person's feelings are valid and certainly merit further analysis as well as clarification of the medical facts. But this may not represent an ethical dilemma (Ahronheim, Moreno, & Zuckerman, 2005).

Consider, for example, a family member who is incensed that the patient's antibiotics have been discontinued, claiming that the physicians are discriminating against the patient by virtue of his race, ethnicity, or disability. At first glance this may seem clearly a matter of ethics or professionalism, but there are several other possible interpretations. The antibiotics may not have been indicated for the patient's condition or had proven to be ineffective. The reason they were withdrawn is therefore *biotechnical*, rather than ethical (Lo, 2009).

The conflict may also stem from a failure of *communication* (DuVal, Sartorius, Clarridge, Gensler, & Danis, 2001; Fetters & Brody, 1999; Kelly, Marshall, Sanders, Raffin, & Koenig, 1997). The family member clearly believes—perhaps as a result of independent research or media reports—that the antibiotics were beneficial. Perhaps the team did not adequately explain why they were discontinued or what better alternatives would be. In such situations, additional conversation or review of all available information can resolve the perceived dilemma.

Alternatively, the family member may feel ignored or not taken seriously, and the treatment in question may be the occasion for expressing their underlying feelings. The issue, therefore, is more *relational* than informational, based on interpersonal conflict between the patient, family, and health care team. In situations such as this, mediation of the conflict can be helpful (Orr & deLeon, 2000), through acknowledgment of the autonomy of all parties, informed decision-making, and assurance of confidentiality (Dubler & Liebman, 2004).

Situations such as this are so common that some have even claimed that most conflicts encountered in the practice of medicine are apparent or false dilemmas (Fins, 1996). Conversely, some dilemmas which are, indeed, ethical in nature may not initially be acknowledged as such. Parties involved may fail to recognize either the overriding importance of one value or that the fact that two or more values are in conflict (Forrow et al., 1991). For instance, a clinician's reluctance to continue a specific treatment for a patient certainly could initially be framed in terms of probability of success (a biotechnical question), but it could also be due to that clinician's belief that the patient's potential quality of life is not sufficient to justify the treatment (a profoundly ethical question). Only in situations where the question is crisply framed and determined to be ethical in nature is further ethical analysis indicated.

Proposed structures of ethical analysis differ as to the degree to which the question needs to be "classified" at this stage. Some advocate "[identifying] the basic principles involved and [explaining] how they relate to the case" (Rhodes & Alfandre, 2007), thus making it possible to distinguish between conflicting principles and uncertainty as to what a specific principle requires. Other experts consider identifying the conflicting principles to be premature at this stage, potentially leading to an exaggerated use of principles in problem-solving (Fletcher & Boyle, 1997).

While the first approach may be appropriate for trained ethics consultants, it is not reasonable to expect clinicians to classify ethical dilemmas at this early stage. Instead, it is enough to simply identify the competing goods—such as increased likelihood of survival, optimal comfort, respect for patient wishes, and proper use of scarce resources— that appear to be in conflict and which render the dilemma ethical in nature. While the professional ethicist might tend to apply technical terms such as "autonomy" and "beneficence" to these goods, it is sufficient at this point to admit that all goods cannot be simultaneously achieved, forcing the patient and the medical team to make a difficult choice about which informed, well-intentioned people could reasonably disagree (Doukas, 1992; Forrow et al., 1991; Siegler et al., 1990; Thomasma, 1978).

Review Existing Information

As the old saying goes, "Good ethics begin with good facts" (Sujdak Mackiewicz, 2016). A review of existing information relating to the perceived dilemma will not only help clarify whether the dilemma is ethical in nature; it is also integral to resolving the dilemma. Throughout this review, it is crucial to keep an open mind regarding the competing issues at play, in order not to leap prematurely to a conclusion. As John Dewey writes, "The essence of critical thinking is suspended judgment; and the essence of this suspense is inquiry to determine the nature of the problem before proceeding to attempts at its solution" (Dewey, 1991).

A thorough understanding of the clinical situation is the universal starting point for all proposed systems of ethical analysis, although the terminology varies slightly with references to "medical factors" (Thomasma, 1978), "medical indications" (Jonsen et al., 2015), "medical facts and goals" (Kaldjian et al., 2005), and the like. This necessarily involves a detailed review of the patient's medical record and discussion with the professionals involved in the patient's care. The end result is a comprehensive understanding of the patient's current condition, prognosis, and treatment options, with attendant risks and benefits.

The next step should be to identify the patient's goals (Kaldjian et al., 2005), what others have called "patient preferences" (Jonsen et al., 2015) or "human factors" (Thomasma, 1978). Patients who possess sufficient decision-making capacity (DMC) may be able to directly express their goals and values. In situations where DMC is impaired or absent, the patient may have expressed his wishes at an earlier point in time, perhaps in the form of an advance directive. Additionally, loved ones (whether family or friends) may have a sense of the patient's goals and values, gleaned from prior conversations or interactions, and thus are able to offer "substituted judgment" as to what the patient would want (Beauchamp & Childress, 2009).

Here it is critical to distinguish—in the terminology of mediation—between positions and interests (Fisher, Ury, & Patton, 1997). Some patients say they want to be "full code" or have "everything done." Strictly speaking, though, no one *wants* to receive CPR or be intubated, as both are highly burdensome. In addition, it is logistically impossible to do every possible medical procedure to a single patient. A request to have "everything done" is therefore a position that may—or may not—reflect the patient's true goals.

"Patient preferences," on the other hand, are interests, which refer to human hopes and longings. As such, they are not inherently linked to specific medical procedures. Viewed in these terms, "full code" may represent a fervent wish to survive despite significant burden and low probability of success. It is crucial at this stage of analysis to identify the patient's interests in nonmedical terminology, which allows them to be analyzed in light of the specific medical situation.

In the well-known "four quadrant approach" (Jonsen et al., 2015) (Figure 2.2), medical indications and patient preferences represent the upper two quadrants which, when not in conflict, are often sufficient to resolve perceived dilemmas. However, when the patient (or the surrogate decision-maker) disagrees with the medical team as to what should be done—in ethical terminology, when autonomy and beneficence are in conflict—then further information is necessary. The third "quadrant" deals with the patient's quality of life, both prior to the current situation and in the future (to the degree that that can be predicted). Specific attention must be paid to the patient's goals and values and how they relate to projected quality of life. It is imperative here to use the patient's own measure of an acceptable quality of life, given that physicians tend to underestimate patients' quality of life, especially in subjective domains such as emotion and pain (Janse et al., 2004; Saigal et al., 1999).

The fourth quadrant is "contextual features," which takes into account familial, social, religious, cultural, and financial factors. Attention to these factors recognizes that a variety of considerations play into a patient or surrogate's decision. In addition, it acknowledges that most patients have substantive personal relationships, such that what happens to the patient influences others as well. And while some might argue that the medical team's concern should be solely focused on the patient, even a modest recognition of

4 Box Method

Medical Indications	Patient Preferences
Principles of Beneficence and Nonmaleficence	*Principle of Respect for Autonomy*
What are the goals of treatment? What are the probabilities of success? Is the problem acute? chronic? reversible, emergent?	Is patient mentally capable and legally competent? Evidence of incapacity? Has patient been informed and understands? Is patient unwilling or unable to cooperate? Why?
Quality of Life	Contextual or External
Principles of Beneficence and Nonmaleficence and Respect for Autonomy	*Principles of Loyalty and Fairness*
What are prospects for return to normal life? Are there biases which might prejudice provider's evaluation of patient's quality of life? Are there plans for comfort and palliative care?	Are there family issues that might influence treatment decisions? Are there financial and economic factures? Are there limits on confidentiality? Are there religious or cultural factors? Problems with allocation of resources?

Jonsen, A.R., Siegler, M. & Winslade, W.J. (2010) *Clinical Ethics: A Practical Approach to Ethical Decisions in Clinical Medicine.* 7th Ed. New York: McGraw-Hill

FIGURE 2.2 Four-quadrant approach to ethical decision-making

interrelationship necessitates consideration of other people's feelings, beliefs, and values as well (McCullough, 1984).

Acquire Additional Relevant Information

In many situations, a review of available data reveals that some pertinent information has not yet been obtained. There are several reasons for this. First, the situation may be sufficiently critical that the medical team has been so caught up in stabilizing the patient that they have not had the time or resources to acquire supporting information. Alternatively, the additional information may lie outside the traditional realm of data acquired in the care of a patient, especially one who is critically ill. For instance, it is not uncommon for the clinical team to focus on the patient's chief complaint and history of present illness, delving into the patient's goals and values only insofar as necessary to establish a "code status" (p. 101). In such situations, it can be invaluable to obtain further information as to the patient's beliefs and goals—such as by taking a "values history" (Doukas & McCullough, 1991)—which can then inform decision-making in ethically complex situations.

In situations where the patient is not able to provide such a history—or where the patient is espousing goals or values which seem in conflict with his long-standing beliefs, leading to concern regarding his DMC—it is critically important to engage the patient's family and friends in the discussion. Just as prior discussions with the patient concerning values may have been rather cursory, the same may have been the case with friends and family. If they were previously asked simply whether the patient wanted "everything done," in the face of ethical complexity more details must be acquired. In addition, some individuals who know the patient well may not have previously been involved in the discussions. Steps should be taken to ensure that all relevant members of the patient's family and other loved ones have the opportunity to share their perspectives (Levine & Zuckerman, 1999), with primary focus on the patient's goals and values.

Preliminary explorations of ethical dilemmas also frequently overlook nonphysician medical staff who may be able to provide significant input regarding the patient's frame of mind and prognosis. For instance, nurses (especially the primary nurse) generally spend significantly more time with a patient and family than do physicians. Therapists (whether psychological, physical, or occupational) have valued windows into the patient's mental and functional state. Chaplains may have had the opportunity to spend significant time with the patient exploring nontechnical issues, including hopes, goals, and beliefs. In the case of hospitalized patients, outpatient clinicians (such as the patient's primary care provider or staff from a nursing home or visiting nurse association, if applicable) can offer a perspective not otherwise available to hospital staff (Orr & Shelton, 2009).

In addition to information regarding the patient in question, it may also be necessary to acquire additional information about the dilemma which the patient is facing. For instance, professional oaths or codes of ethics may refer to the clinical situation (American Medical Association, 2016; Turton & Snyder, 2008), although frequently such comments are too vague to be of assistance with specific decisions (Veatch, 2006). Specific hospital or institutional policies may address the particular situation. While these policies may not be determinative, at least they will provide a context for the decision to be made and additional perspective as to how similar situations have been resolved in the past. Finally, there may be legal ramifications to various courses of action, which would require a review of relevant statutes and case law, on both federal and state levels.

Analyze the Ethical Issue

Essentially every published approach to resolving clinical ethical dilemmas advocates delineation of the question and acquisition of all relevant information, both already existing and such that additional exploration is required. In the process, many dilemmas are shown not to be ethical in nature, and the appropriate method of resolution becomes clear. In situations where the dilemma *is* an ethical one, these steps ensure that any proposed resolution will be, at the very least, fully informed. In addition, they achieve the basic task of ensuring that moral perceptions—which may have previously been unspoken or even unrecognized, yet nevertheless prompted ethical examination of the case—are made explicit and transparent (Brody, 1989).

At this point, however, the various approaches diverge as to how to resolve an ethical dilemma once all relevant information is in hand. Some advocate a particular paradigm by which ethical decisions can be made, such as principlism (Beauchamp & Childress, 2009). The four core principles of biomedical ethics are autonomy, beneficence, nonmaleficence (i.e., do no harm), and justice. Some argue that after identifying what each of these principles would obligate a person to do in a given situation, a solution to the dilemma will emerge.

There are two major drawbacks to relying on a particular paradigm, however. In the first place, it is no guarantee of resolution. In the case of principlism, for instance, if autonomy and beneficence are in conflict, it is not entirely clear how to decide which principle takes precedence (Thomasma, 1978).

Second, even if the paradigm generates a conclusion, exclusive reliance on one theory will limit the applicability and generalizability of that conclusion. As a result, the most one can hope for is a measured conclusion that "the principlist would do this, and the consequentialist would do that" (Finnerty et al., 2000). A solution might therefore be identified, but it would not necessarily be embraced by all involved parties.

Indeed, the very act of applying a theory—*any* theory—is open to criticism because it assumes a deductive approach to the problem, through reliance on universal rules that may not pay sufficient attention to the details of a particular case (Jecker, 1997). Recognizing this potential drawback, some experts limit the use of principles to hypothetical—rather than determinative—guides (Fins, Bacchetta, & Miller, 1997).

Others go further in recommending an explicitly inductive approach to ethical decision-making, whereby the case in question is compared with similar cases in order to determine where the limits of acceptability reside (Jonsen & Toulmin, 1988). On such an approach, the rules are generated by a thoughtful analysis of cases, instead of the analysis of the case following logically from predetermined rules. This represents a practical recognition that specific facts about the world and people in it affect—perhaps even determine—the principles we choose to apply to a particular situation (Hare, 1981).

Rather than appealing to one specific ethical theory—or to any theory at all—it is more practical as well as more generalizable to draw from a variety of approaches in addressing ethical dilemmas. In so doing, a wide swath of relevant concerns can be taken into consideration in the formulation of what has been called—in keeping with the parallel structure of the clinical work-up—an "ethical differential diagnosis" (Fins et al., 1997). Examples of such an eclectic, broad-based approach include Rhodes and Alfandre's consideration of "principles/duties/concepts of medical ethics" (Rhodes & Alfandre, 2007) (Figure 2.3), as well as Doukas' consideration of "ethical norms," such as autonomy, beneficence, contract keeping, honesty, and justice (Doukas, 1992).

The strength of this approach is its comprehensiveness. By balancing not only deductive approaches (such as principlism and consequentialism) but also inductive ones (such as casuistry), this approach strives for coherence between theories that describe how one should act and practical examples of ethically appropriate actions (Beauchamp & Childress, 2009).

However, such comprehensiveness is also potentially its greatest drawback. For if principlism, for example, can be criticized for not providing a method of adjudicating between four competing principles, how much more could an eclectic approach be criticized

- duty to provide care
- assess decisional capacity
- confidentiality
- assess surrogate appropriateness
- truth telling
- respect for autonomy (patient goals)
- minimize harms
- beneficence/caring (team goals)
- duty to warn
- nonjudgmental regard
- professionalism
- trust/fiduciary responsibility
- informed consent
- justice (fair allocation of scarce resources)
- justify parentalism
- futility (furthers no goals)
- no conflict of interest
- professional competence
- evidence-based practice
- responsibilities to peers and institutions

FIGURE 2.3 Principles/duties/concepts of medical ethics (adapted from Rhodes & Alfandre, 2007)

for not providing a clear-cut mechanism for balancing competing considerations drawn from numerous rights, duties, consequences, virtues, and cases?

This criticism can be answered in two ways. First, it is important to recognize that such complexity is intrinsic to the endeavor of ethical deliberation, lacking as it is in quantitative or objective measures. Any approach that is not complex is overly simplistic and likely to ignore salient considerations.

Further, the approaches included in this method are more complementary than competitive and thus provide a well-rounded and comprehensive assessment of complex issues. To enhance applicability, specific concerns within each "consideration" that typically take precedence are highlighted, in order to streamline the process of ethical decision-making.

Relevant Legal and Professional Considerations
Rights

While there has long been a recognized need for clinicians and patients to engage in shared decision-making (National Commission for the Protection of Human Subjects of Biomedical and Behavioral Research, 1978), nevertheless situations occur where patients and clinicians disagree as to the appropriate course of action. In such situations, the rights of the patient and family may conflict with the rights of the professionals involved. While one could generate a long list of relevant human and professional rights (Freeden, 1991), this discussion focuses on patient autonomy and physician conscience.

Patient Autonomy

In modern American culture, autonomy is now preeminent, often to the same extreme that parentalism formerly ruled medical decision-making (Veatch, 2009). The right of competent patients to refuse essentially any treatment is clearly codified in the law (*Cruzan v. Director, Missouri Department of Health*, 1990) and in standard bioethics treatises (Beauchamp & Childress, 2009). The application of this right is not as clear-cut as it first appears, however (Schneider, 2002).

One reason for this is that "autonomy" can be understood in two different senses. Classically, an autonomous choice was not only a freely made choice but also a *rational* one. As such, it would not be impacted by personal desires or self-interest but rather based on the "categorical imperative," meaning that it is worthy of becoming a universal role that every person in a similar situation should follow (Kant, 1998). On this understanding, an ill-considered, impetuous decision would not be considered truly autonomous. As such, seemingly irrational decisions—which could merely reflect not accepting medical recommendations—could be overridden without concern for violating any sacred ethical principle. Clearly, this would make a sham of the right of patients to disagree with their physicians, essentially compelling patients to accept the recommended treatment plan.

The other sense of autonomy—which is predominant in the medical literature—refers to a choice made without coercion and without significant cognitive impairment, regardless of the negative consequences for the patient. On this understanding, no ethical dilemma can exist when the patient's wishes are clearly known. Indeed, some clinical ethicists seem to be no more than protectors of the patient's right to choose, rather than experts in negotiating moral ambiguity (Gorovitz, 1986).

This notion of autonomy is overly simplistic. It often can overlook the crucial distinction between positive and negative rights (as noted later) in its emphasis on giving the patient "what he wants." It also pays insufficient attention to the goals and values that undergird treatment decisions. Recalling the distinction between positions and interests (p. 30), it is not enough to know what treatments the patient wants or does not want. The reasons for those decisions—and the extent to which they will help the patient achieve his deeper goals—must also be explored.

There are specific situations where the patient's DMC warrants more in-depth evaluation, in order to be sure that the decision truly reflects the patient's goals and values (however rational or irrational those may appear to be). Situations where the decision is extremely complex, the consequences of the decision are especially grave, or the decision is contrary to what a "reasonable" person would typically want require the physician to be certain that the patient has sufficient DMC to make that decision (Buchanan, 2004). Such a sliding-scale approach either to the patient's capacity (Buchanan & Brock, 1989; Grisso & Appelbaum, 1998) or *evidence* of that capacity (Beauchamp & Childress, 2009) recognizes both the importance of respecting autonomy, as well as the consequences of decisions made in the context of uncertain decisional capacity (Pellegrino & Thomasma, 1988).

The right of autonomy is also relevant to patients who can no longer exercise that right (*In re Quinlan*, 1976). For a patient who lacks DMC, those who know the patient well—whether named by the patient in a Durable Power of Attorney for Health Care, appointed guardian by a court, or else identified as an appropriate surrogate according to relevant state law (Pope, 2011)—provide "substituted judgment" based on what the patient would have wanted. This necessarily injects an additional layer of complexity, given the inherent uncertainty as to what another person might choose (Shalowitz, Garrett-Mayer, & Wendler, 2006), not to mention the potential for the surrogate's own feelings or beliefs to influence her decision (Fagerlin, Ditto, Danks, Houts, & Smucker, 2001). So just as the capacity of a patient must be taken into account in respecting the patient's autonomy, so must the reliability of a surrogate in estimating what that patient would want.

The concept of autonomy also needs to be applied differently in situations where a patient is requesting a treatment, compared with one where the patient is refusing a treatment. Here the distinction between positive and negative rights is critical (Feinberg, 1973). A negative right is one of noninterference, according to which others cannot stand in the way of a person's obtaining something. This right is expressed in the Fourteenth Amendment to the Constitution, which bars the government from depriving a person of "life, liberty, or property" without due process of law. A positive right, on the other hand, is a right of entitlement, which necessarily incurs an obligation on the part of another (often the government) to help people obtain that to which they have a right, if they are unable to do so on their own. Because positive rights are so broad, there are relatively few in American society: education through grade twelve, police protection, fire protection, and military protection are among them. Notably absent on this list is the universal right to health care, which every other member nation of the Organisation for Economic Co-operation and Development—with the exception of Mexico—provides (Organisation for Economic Co-operation and Development, 2014).

In a medical context, the "right" of autonomy is predominantly a negative right. That is to say, patients with sufficient DMC have the right to refuse unwanted treatment, even one that is life-sustaining. However, patients do not have the right to receive any treatment they request. Plentiful reasons exist—such as lack of benefit, disproportionate burden, and scarcity of resources—for not providing a requested treatment. Indeed, the American Medical Association clearly states that "respecting patient autonomy does not mean that patients should receive specific interventions simply because they (or their surrogates) request them" (American Medical Association, 2016). Thus a patient's "right" to a requested treatment is less compelling than his "right" to refuse unwanted treatment, causing the clinician to take multiple other factors into account.

Professional Autonomy

The right to decide for oneself is a basic human right (Freeden, 1991), and thus the negative right of autonomy (i.e., to refuse treatment) is essential. The positive right is narrower, as it incurs an obligation on the part of physicians to provide the care that is requested. This raises the question of *professional* rights, which are based on the social contract under which that profession functions. If patients do not have an absolute right to any treatment they request, to what degree should the physician's own moral beliefs be taken into consideration when determining whether to provide a specific treatment (Wardle, 1993)?

Often a physician's refusal to provide a specific treatment is a biotechnical decision that is defensible based on the best available evidence (Cassel & Guest, 2012). In other cases, however, the physician's refusal is based on ethical rather than empirical grounds. The classic example of this is termination of pregnancy, leading many health care facilities to develop "conscience clauses" which allow staff who have moral objections to abortion to not participate in the procedure. In palliative care practice, some clinicians have moral objections to physician-assisted dying (chapter 8) and, to a lesser degree, palliative sedation (chapter 9).

While some defend the physician's right to refuse (Berlinger, Jennings, & Wolf, 2013; Wicclair, 2008), others assert that someone who is unwilling to provide requested procedures (which are neither illegal nor proscribed) should essentially choose another profession (Savulescu, 2006). A more thoughtful position would be to identify those practices which are generally accepted and integral to palliative care practice (such as intensive symptom management at the end of life), requiring all clinicians to take part in these.

In situations where true moral ambiguity exists about a specific practice, a physician is often able to transfer care of the patient to a colleague who does not hold the same moral reservations about the requested procedure (Curlin, Lawrence, Chin, & Lantos, 2007). Where that is not possible—such as emergent situations or where no other physician is available—the physician may be obligated to provide the treatment, as long as it is legal and consistent with the standard of care.

Duties

In addition to the rights of patients as human beings and of physicians as conscientious moral individuals, there are also specific duties which the physician owes to the patient by virtue of the professional relationship (Gert, Culver, & Clouser, 2006). The physician-patient relationship is a fiduciary one, meaning that it is based on trust and focused on the interests of the more vulnerable party (i.e., the patient) (Dorr Goold & Lipkin, 1999). Several of these duties are directly relevant to the resolution of ethical dilemmas.

Nonmaleficence

Perhaps the most compelling duty of a physician to a patient is to "first do no harm" (Beauchamp & Childress, 2009). There may exist debate as to a patient's right to a certain intervention and whether that intervention holds out the prospect of benefit, but before proceeding with any intervention the physician must be confident that it will not cause undue harm to the patient. This duty applies to nearly all medical procedures, since it is difficult to imagine a procedure that does not hold out some risk of injury or suffering, however minor.

The duty of nonmaleficence is an important counterbalance to physicians' recognized tendency toward action, which some have termed "commission bias" (Groopman, 2007). This tendency—especially when coupled with the patient's autonomous request for a specific treatment—can make it very difficult for the physician to decline. Yet when there exists a significant risk of harm—especially without prospect of proportionate benefit—physicians are permitted (even obligated) to decline from acting, or at least defer action until the risk/benefit ratio improves.

Truth-Telling

Another duty the physician has toward patients and family is that of veracity, or truth-telling. This duty relates to the patient's right of autonomy, since it is not possible to exercise that right if the patient does not have an accurate sense of the present situation, future prognosis, and options available. One can imagine situations, however, when this duty seems to conflict with other duties or responsibilities. For instance, in situations where certain information is deemed potentially detrimental to a patient, some physicians have invoked "therapeutic privilege" in withholding that information. This principle was established in *Canterbury v. Spence*, which held that "patients occasionally become so ill or emotionally distraught on disclosure as to foreclose a rational decision" (*Canterbury v. Spence*, 1972). Subsequently, however, courts began to look with disfavor upon this practice (*Rogers v. Whitaker*, 1992; *Thornburgh v. American College of Obstetricians*, 1986), and recent revisions of the AMA Code of Ethics have deemed the practice "ethically unacceptable" (American Medical Association, 2010–2011).

Other challenging situations include potential pressures to withhold or alter information provided to a third party, such as an insurance company, in order to procure needed services for a patient (Morreim, 1991). While the pressures are real and the motivations for considering such a course of action may be noble, there is no ethical justification for lying.

However, there may be situations where complete disclosure is not required and may even be contraindicated. For instance, patients may waive their right to informed consent, if they freely choose not to know the risks, benefits, and alternatives of a given procedure (Faden, Beauchamp, & King, 1986). In certain cultures, the locus of decision-making is not so much the patient (as it is under the autonomy-dominated American model) but rather the family (p. 484). In such cases, it is appropriate to ask the patient how much information he would like to receive and whom he would want to make medical decisions. In so doing, patients' autonomy as well as their cultural background are respected (Searight & Gafford, 2005).

Confidentiality

Treating patient information as confidential has been an integral part of medicine since the age of Hippocrates (Moskop, Marco, Larkin, Geiderman, & Derse, 2005) and is also explicit in the law (Health Insurance Portability and Accountability Act, 1996). There are, however, specific legal obligations which supersede the patient's right of confidentiality. One is the duty to warn or protect others at risk of harm, which is an important consideration in psychiatric practice (Soulier, Maislen, & Beck, 2010). Another exception to the rule of confidentiality is the duty to report certain situations or results, such as specific communicable diseases or the abuse or neglect of a child or vulnerable adult (Mathews & Kenny, 2008). Generally speaking, the duty of confidentiality is compelling unless there is a specific legal requirement to breach that duty.

Consequences
Beneficence

In addition to the rights of patients and physicians, and the professional duties of physicians toward their patients, another major consideration in examining an ethical decision is the expected outcome of that decision (Smart & Williams, 1973). Physicians are tasked with determining a course of treatment that not only reflects the patient's goals but also represents the optimal balance of benefits and burdens. While the future cannot be known with certainty, recommendations should be based on the best available evidence.

Arguably most ethical dilemmas stem from a conflict between what the patient wants—and may or may not have a right to—and what the physician believes is best for the patient (i.e., the principle of beneficence). When parentalism reigned supreme, this conflict did not represent a problem, for patients' wishes were not solicited nor their consent for treatment sought. In the era of patient autonomy, however, physicians are often faced with situations where the patient is refusing something potentially beneficial or requesting something that is potentially harmful.

In autonomy-dominated American society, the refusal of a fully informed patient with sufficient DMC must be respected, even if this trumps the duty of beneficence (McCullough, 1984). To be sure, this can cause significant distress among the medical staff, as they watch the patient suffer needlessly. But the alternative (i.e., to override a capacitated refusal "for the patient's own good") runs the risk of sliding down the slippery slope back to parentalism, as physicians' judgments about suffering and quality of life take precedence over the patient's own goals and values.

When patients request a treatment of uncertain benefit, the proper response is less obvious. If the harms are well-known and disproportionate, the physician's obligation of nonmaleficence takes precedence. But what of situations where the patient is requesting something that *might* work but is suboptimal, or for which the balance of benefits and burdens is generally unfavorable? Here one might imagine an experimental treatment, or one which merely sustains the patient in a compromised condition with slim hope of subsequent improvement. The issue here is not the physician's personal moral objections (discussed previously) but rather professional disagreement as to the most beneficial course of action.

Clearly, a wide variety of other concerns are relevant to the provision of treatment of questionable benefit, such as resource allocation, creation of false hope, and potential harm to the patient. In general, though, where the burden/benefit balance is not overwhelmingly negative and the related costs (both monetary and material) are not exorbitant, and where there exists the potential for improvement, the physician should initiate the treatment. This can be done on a time-limited basis (p. 118), in order to gauge the efficacy of the intervention. Especially in terms of life-sustaining medical treatment, this also preserves options, since it is possible to subsequently scale back treatment, but it is not always possible to escalate it. In addition, it provides the patient and family reassurance that all potentially beneficial measures have been used (Kasman, 2004) and also hopefully brings them to a point where they clearly recognize that the treatment in question is not providing benefit.

Virtues

Up to this point, the analysis has focused on rights, obligations, and outcomes, without taking into account the motivation behind a specific action. Some commentators, however, place virtue in a preeminent position in evaluating the propriety of a certain decision, citing specific qualities of exemplary physicians. These include compassion, fidelity to trust, and practical wisdom (Pellegrino & Thomasma, 1993). Others situate virtue in a confirmatory position, asking whether a presumptive decision is what "a consensus of exemplary doctors would agree to" (Rhodes & Alfandre, 2007). Even those who are associated with supposedly "rival" methodologies, such as principlism, recognize the importance of virtue in determining an appropriate course of action (Beauchamp & Childress, 2009).

At the very least, an analysis of motivation can serve to either clarify, confirm, or nullify a proposed response to an ethical dilemma. In certain situations, the complexity of the ethical analysis may be overwhelming, thus making it impossible to settle on any specific conclusion. Interpreting the situation in light of the motivations that would drive a person to pursue competing options may reframe the discussion in a way that permits additional progress and, eventually, resolution. In other contexts, an analysis of virtue can confirm the appropriateness of a certain course of action, based on its alignment with what a virtuous physician would do. Finally, there may be instances where a virtue-based analysis nullifies a proposed resolution dilemma, if one is unable to conceive of an exemplary physician acting in such a fashion.

As with all the other methodologies noted so far, a virtue-based approach is susceptible to internal tension or disagreement. Two or more virtues may appear to be in conflict with each other, such as compassion and fidelity to trust in the case of patient with a newly diagnosed terminal illness whom the physician is reluctant to inform of his diagnosis. Even when a specific virtue is acknowledged as most compelling, there may be disagreement as to what actions that virtue should lead to. By referencing virtues along with the other considerations noted previously, however, a balanced and comprehensive response can be reached.

Cases

Some approaches to ethical dilemmas do not emphasize principles at all (DuBose, Hamel, & O'Connell, 1994). Casuistry, for instance, reasons inductively from "paradigmatic cases," using analogy to determine whether a proposed course of action is ethically acceptable (Jonsen & Toulmin, 1988). While some criticize such an approach because it appears to be devoid of any ethical theory, others appropriately claim that casuistry is "theory-modest" (Arras, 1991), in that it takes a structured approach based on the belief that ethics is "a series of practices that arise from human moral experience" (Ahronheim et al., 2005). As Jonsen and Toulmin describe it:

> The heart of moral experience does not lie in a mastery of general rules and theoretical principles, however sound and well reasoned those principles may appear. It is located, rather, in the wisdom that comes from seeing how the ideas behind those rules work out in the course of people's lives: in particular, seeing more exactly what is involved in insisting on (or waiving) this or that rule in one or another set of circumstances. (Jonsen & Toulmin, 1988)

Casuistry offers many potential benefits. First, like virtue ethics, casuistry offers valuable confirmation and/or clarification of a presumptive decision, by placing that decision on a spectrum of similar dilemmas. Casuistry can also provide guidance in situations where the competing ethical theories, duties, and obligations are so complex that it is difficult to even generate a presumptive resolution. Finally—and here casuistry distinguishes itself from virtue ethics—case-based reasoning recognizes that sometimes it is easier to agree on a practical resolution than on the ethical underpinnings of that solution.

There are plentiful examples of groups reaching consensus as to the appropriate course action, only to devolve into fervent dissent when attempting to identify the appropriate *rationale* for the consensus (National Commission for the Protection of Human Subjects of Biomedical and Behavioral Research, 1978). Irrespective of the route that brought involved parties to a given decision, if that decision represents consensus—and meets the requirements of the respective ethical models used to reach it—then that decision should be accepted.

Narrative

Principlism grew out of a period of conflict between physicians and patients and thus understandably focuses on judicial standards such as disclosure and informed consent. Some have argued that it is therefore poorly equipped to deal with collaborative, trusting relationships in an era of shared decision-making (Charon, 2006). A more productive and positive approach may focus less on general rules and more on the particularity of individual human relationships. Decisions may be guided by principles, but ultimately they are determined by specific circumstances.

One such approach is "narrative ethics." Mirroring the emphasis on narrative in other fields—ranging from theology (Frei, 1974) to cultural studies (Schiffrin, De Fina, & Nylund, 2010) to psychology (Sarbin, 1986)—narrative ethics holds that "meaning in human life emerges not from rules given but from lived, thick experience and that determinations of right and good by necessity arise from context, perspective, culture, and time" (Charon, 2006).

The approach set forth in this chapter pays specific attention to narrative and context. Each person and situation demands analysis and reflection, as the physician-writer Oliver Sacks famously did in his "clinical tales" (Sacks, 2006). For while it is important to appreciate basic principles and the rationale that undergirds them, particular situations demand analysis and resolution that take the details into account. Especially in clinical ethics—where the stakes are high and complexity significant—rote application of general rules will not sufficiently take into account the nuances of an individual case. Thus Charon writes,

> If another kind of ethicist could fulfill his or her duty by hearing, in the safety of a conference room, the report of the patient's predicament and somehow making judgments from afar about the proper action to pursue, the narrative bioethicist must sit by the patient, lean forward toward the person who suffers, and offer the self as an occasion for the other to tell and therefore comprehend the events of illness. This ethicist does his or her work by absorbing and containing the singular patient's plight, soliciting others' perspectives on the situation, being the flask in which these differing points of view can mingle toward equilibrium. (Charon, 2006)

Formulate Response, Consider Criticisms, and Identify Lessons Learned

The more comprehensive an approach one takes to an ethical dilemma, the more cumbersome and potentially conflicting the results will be. As Beauchamp and Childress note, "No theory approximates [the ideal of putting] enough content in its norms to escape conflicts and dilemmas in all contexts" (Beauchamp & Childress, 2009). The approach outlined here attempts to divide considerations into manageable and applicable divisions—rights, duties, consequences, virtues, and cases—while prioritizing arguably the most important elements within each category (such as the right of patient autonomy, the duty of nonmaleficence, and the goal of maximizing beneficial outcomes). Such a structure is helpful in identifying the nature of an ethical dilemma by delineating relevant considerations and generating potential responses.

Because this approach does not rely exclusively on one methodology, it is valuable in forging consensus. It also resembles the "clinical pragmatism" approach of John Dewey, which "treats moral rules and principles as hypothetical guides that identify a range of reasonable moral choices for the deliberations of patients, families, and clinicians"

(McGee, 2003). Drawn from the tradition of Oliver Wendell Holmes Jr., Charles Sanders Peirce, and William James, this is an applied approach which focuses on inductive reasoning. Rather than viewing ethical principles as immutable and eternal, pragmatism recognizes the evolutionary state of our knowledge. Ethical deliberation takes place regarding particular cases, which may then require some reassessment of guiding principles (Fins et al., 1997).

Even when a decision is reached in response to a dilemma, the process of ethical deliberation is not finished. At this point, it is crucial to explore the potential criticisms of the proposed course of action, which can serve to identify previously unrecognized concerns and potential drawbacks to the proposed solution (McCullough, 1984). In addition, once the solution has been enacted, it is important to observe the results and continue to modify future responses in light of them. Proposed ethical resolutions, therefore, represent "hypotheses to be worked out in practice, and to be rechecked, corrected and expanded as they fail or succeed in giving our present experience the guidance it requires" (Dewey, 2004). This process also builds greater expertise in addressing future ethical dilemmas, based on the skills and experience acquired.

Next Steps in the Absence of Resolution

Despite its comprehensiveness, this approach is no guarantee of reaching consensus regarding an ethical dilemma. In such cases, it is important to review the steps noted previously to determine if any relevant considerations have been overlooked. Can more information as to the patient's preferences or the medical context be acquired? Have all persons with relevant knowledge (whether personal or professional) been consulted? Have any relevant considerations been overlooked or misprioritized? If resolution is still not possible, certain intermediate steps can be taken while the process of ethical deliberation continues.

Temporize

The first step is to buy time, if possible. Some situations are not critical and thus deferring a decision may be the wisest course of action. While this runs counter to the "commission bias" noted earlier, it is often the most prudent response which may spare the patient from potentially unnecessary harm.

In situations that do appear critical, erring on the side of overtreatment—assuming that the burdens of that treatment are not overwhelming—keeps multiple avenues of response open. For instance, if there exists debate as to whether to intubate a patient with impending respiratory failure, proceeding with mechanical ventilation preserves future options. As the US Supreme Court observed, "An erroneous decision not to terminate results in maintenance of the status quo. . . . An erroneous decision to withdraw . . . is not susceptible of correction" (*Cruzan v. Director, Missouri Department of Health*, 1990). It is well-accepted in both ethics and the law that there is no distinction between withdrawing and withholding (American Medical Association, 2010–2011), and thus if it is determined at a later time that the patient would not want mechanical ventilation, then this can be discontinued (p. 156).

Options to Avoid

Clinical ethics tends to focus on identifying a range of ethically permissible options, rather than one clearly superior option (Orr & Shelton, 2009). Even if it is not clear what the optimal course of action is, it may nevertheless be clear what some clearly *unacceptable* responses are. Identifying these responses prevents obvious errors and at the same time narrows the remaining list of possibilities.

Worst Option

While most potential responses to an ethical dilemma can be ranked on a spectrum of varying propriety or acceptability, there may be some options that definitely violate sacred oaths or considerations and thus can be excluded from consideration. Among these are overriding the informed, voluntary refusal of a patient with clearly intact DMC (a violation of autonomy), putting a patient at disproportionate risk of harm (a violation of nonmaleficence), and explicitly lying to a patient (a failure of veracity). While it is true that duties are generally *prima facie* in nature—in other words, they are compelling unless another more pressing duty supersedes them (Beauchamp & Childress, 2009)—one could reasonably argue that some obligations are so sacred that it is difficult (or perhaps impossible) to imagine a realistic situation when that duty would not take precedence.

Impractical Solutions

An appropriate solution to an ethical dilemma must not only be ethically acceptable; it must also be practical. It is all well and good, for instance, to conclude that a reluctant adolescent patient should be compelled to undergo chemotherapy for a treatable malignancy, but that does not answer the question of *how* to achieve this goal over the patient's objections (p. 346). Overreliance on theory to the exclusion of logistical considerations is not helpful.

Limiting Options

In addition to avoiding impractical solutions, it is also important not to overlook any potential alternatives (Kaldjian et al., 2005). This may involve "thinking outside the box" to identify previously unconsidered options and at other times carving out a middle ground. For instance, a family may be requesting maximal treatment for a patient whose quality of life is severely diminished and whose prognosis is guarded. The treating team, on the other hand, may feel that a change of goals to comfort measures only is indicated. In addition to likely attendant communication—perhaps stemming from a common misperception that DNR means "do not respond" (p. 383)—and interpersonal challenges, the primary issue here is the unwillingness to consider a compromise option. Some limitation of treatment—such as DNR status, or a "Do Not Escalate" order if the patient's condition were to worsen (p. 119)—might be acceptable to both the team and the family. In such cases, the dilemma is not so much choosing between Option A and B but rather identifying Option C, which (at least temporarily) avoids the pitfalls of the other two.

Rationing at the Bedside

The last pitfall to avoid is allocation at the bedside. The rising cost of medical care in the United States is well known (Swensen et al., 2011), with over one-quarter of Medicare expenditures devoted to care in the last six months of life (Hogan, Lunney, Gabel, & Lynn, 2001). It is tempting, therefore, to ration expensive but potentially beneficial health care on a case-by-case basis. In situations where ethical consensus is not currently achievable, the drive to rein in costs or shift resources to patients with a better prognosis may seem compelling.

There are profound justice-based problems with this approach, however. As possessors of human dignity, every person deserves to be treated with respect (Outka, 1974). Further, similar patients should be treated similarly (Aristotle, 1953), rendering case-by-case resource-based decision-making inherently problematic. If society as a whole were to determine that patients with a certain condition or prognosis should not be offered a specific therapy, that would ensure standardization of treatment. But if practice standards vary hospital to hospital—or physician to physician—then it is quite likely that essentially equivalent patients would receive substantially different levels of treatment.

Conclusion

Given the highly personal and qualitative nature of the enterprise, ethical deliberations do not lend themselves to linear algorithms and neatly wrapped solutions. While the approach documented here does not guarantee a universally accepted solution to ethical dilemmas, it does represent a structured and comprehensive response. By incorporating elements of several methods of ethical analysis—and by attempting to balance both inductive and deductive approaches—this approach allows an ethical dilemma to be identified, clarified, and analyzed from multiple perspectives. And in situations where resolution is not forthcoming, intermediate steps provide practical guidance while additional information is acquired and further discussions pursued.

Summary Points

- While there are well-documented differences of opinion among clinical ethicists on specific issues, the approach taken in addressing these issues is quite uniform.
- The first step in addressing a supposedly ethical dilemma is to confirm that it is not actually biotechnical, communicative, or relational in nature.
- "Good ethics begin with good facts," and thus all existing information needs to be reviewed and additional relevant information acquired.

- Rather than examining an ethical dilemma from the perspective of a particular paradigm (e.g., principlism), it is more effective to take a broad-ranging approach that takes into account rights, duties, consequences, virtues, and analogous cases.
- Often there is no good solution to an ethical dilemma, and the most one can hope for is to identify the "least bad" option.
- In the absence of immediate resolution, it is wise to temporize as far as possible, as further information or subsequent developments may shed light on the matter.
- In the search for resolution, it is important to avoid options that are clearly bad, impractical solutions, limited options, and rationing at the bedside.

References

Ahronheim, J. C., Moreno, J. D., & Zuckerman, C. (2005). *Ethics in clinical practice* (2nd ed.). Sudbury, MA: Jones and Bartlett.

American Medical Association. (2016). Code of medical ethics, annotated current opinions (p. v.). Chicago: American Medical Association.

Aristotle. (1953). *The Nicomachean ethics* (J. A. K. Thomson, Ed.). London: Allen & Unwin.

Arnlov, J., Ingelsson, E., Sundstrom, J., & Lind, L. (2010). Impact of body mass index and the metabolic syndrome on the risk of cardiovascular disease and death in middle-aged men. *Circulation, 121*(2), 230–236. doi:CIRCULATIONAHA.109.887521 [pii]10.1161/CIRCULATIONAHA.109.887521

Arras, J. D. (1991). Getting down to cases: The revival of casuistry in bioethics. *J Med Philos, 16*(1), 29–51.

Beauchamp, T. L., & Childress, J. F. (2009). *Principles of biomedical ethics* (6th ed.). New York: Oxford University Press.

Berlinger, N., Jennings, B., Wolf, S. M. (2013). *The Hastings Center guidelines for decisions on life-sustaining treatment and care near the end of life* (rev. and expanded 2nd ed.). Oxford: Oxford University Press.

Brody, H. (1989). Transparency: Informed consent in primary care. *Hastings Cent Rep, 19*(5), 5–9.

Buchanan, A. (2004). Mental capacity, legal competence and consent to treatment. *J R Soc Med, 97*(9), 415–420. doi:10.1258/jrsm.97.9.415

Buchanan, A. E., & Brock, D. W. (1989). *Deciding for others: The ethics of surrogate decisionmaking.* New York: Cambridge University Press.

Callahan, D. (1996). Ethics without abstraction: Squaring the circle. *J Med Ethics, 22*(2), 69–71.

Canterbury v. Spence (1972).

Cassel, C. K., & Guest, J. A. (2012). Choosing wisely: Helping physicians and patients make smart decisions about their care. *JAMA, 307*(17), 1801–1802. doi:jama.2012.476

Charon, R. (2006). *Narrative medicine: Honoring the stories of illness.* Oxford; New York: Oxford University Press.

Cruzan v. Director, Missouri Department of Health, 497 261 (S.Ct. 1990).

Curlin, F. A., Lawrence, R. E., Chin, M. H., & Lantos, J. D. (2007). Religion, conscience, and controversial clinical practices. *N Engl J Med, 356*(6), 593–600. doi:356/6/593

Dewey, J. (1991). *How we think.* Buffalo, NY: Prometheus Books.

Dewey, J. (2004). *Reconstruction in philosophy.* Mineola, NY: Dover.

Dorr Goold, S., & Lipkin, M. Jr. (1999). The doctor-patient relationship: Challenges, opportunities, and strategies. *J Gen Intern Med, 14*(Suppl. 1), S26–S33.

Doukas, D. J. (1992). The design and use of the bioethics consultation form. *Theor Med, 13*(1), 5–14.

Doukas, D. J., & McCullough, L. B. (1991). The values history. The evaluation of the patient's values and advance directives. *J Fam Pract, 32*(2), 145–153.

Dubler, N. N., & Liebman, C. B. (2004). *Bioethics mediation: A guide to shaping shared solutions.* New York: United Hospital Fund of New York.

DuBose, E. R., Hamel, R. P., O'Connell, L. J., & Park Ridge Center. (1994). *A matter of principles? Ferment in U.S. bioethics.* Valley Forge, PA: Trinity Press International.

DuVal, G., Sartorius, L., Clarridge, B., Gensler, G., & Danis, M. (2001). What triggers requests for ethics consultations? *J Med Ethics, 27*(Suppl. 1), i24–29.

Eckles, R. E., Meslin, E. M., Gaffney, M., & Helft, P. R. (2005). Medical ethics education: Where are we? Where should we be going? A review. *Acad Med, 80*(12), 1143–1152.

Engelhardt, H. T. (2012). A skeptical reassessment of bioethics. In H. T. Engelhardt (Ed.), *Bioethics critically reconsidered* (pp. 1–30). New York: Springer.

Faden, R. R., Beauchamp, T. L., & King, N. M. P. (1986). *A history and theory of informed consent.* New York: Oxford University Press.

Fagerlin, A., Ditto, P. H., Danks, J. H., Houts, R. M., & Smucker, W. D. (2001). Projection in surrogate decisions about life-sustaining medical treatments. *Health Psychol, 20*(3), 166–175.

Feinberg, J. (1973). *Social philosophy.* Englewood Cliffs, NJ: Prentice-Hall.

Fetters, M. D., & Brody, H. (1999). The epidemiology of bioethics. *J Clin Ethics, 10*(2), 107–115.

Finnerty, J. J., Pinkerton, J. V., Moreno, J., & Ferguson, J. E., 2nd. (2000). Ethical theory and principles: Do they have any relevance to problems arising in everyday practice? *Am J Obstet Gynecol, 183*(2), 301–306. doi:S0002-9378(00)04848-1

Fins, J. J. (1996). From indifference to goodness. *J Relig Health, 35*(3), 245–254.

Fins, J. J., Bacchetta, M. D., & Miller, F. G. (1997). Clinical pragmatism: A method of moral problem solving. *Kennedy Inst Ethics J, 7*(2), 129–145.

Fisher, R., Ury, W., & Patton, B. (1997). *Getting to yes: Negotiating an agreement without giving in* (2nd ed.). London: Arrow Business Books.

Fletcher, J. C., & Boyle, R. (1997). *Introduction to clinical ethics* (2nd ed.). Frederick, MD: University Publishing Group.

Forrow, L., Arnold, R. M., & Frader, J. (1991). Teaching clinical ethics in the residency years: Preparing competent professionals. *J Med Philos, 16*(1), 93–112.

Fox, E., & Stocking, C. (1993). Ethics consultants' recommendations for life-prolonging treatment of patients in a persistent vegetative state. *JAMA, 270*(21), 2578–2582.

Freeden, M. (1991). *Rights.* Minneapolis: University of Minnesota Press.

Frei, H. W. (1974). *The eclipse of Biblical narrative: A study in eighteenth and nineteenth century hermeneutics.* New Haven, CT: Yale University Press.

Gert, B., Culver, C. M., & Clouser, K. D. (2006). *Bioethics: A systematic approach* (2nd ed.). New York: Oxford University Press.

Gillon, R. (1994). Medical ethics: Four principles plus attention to scope. *BMJ, 309*(6948), 184–188.

Gorovitz, S. (1986). Baiting bioethics. *Ethics, 96*(2), 356–374.

Grisso, T., & Appelbaum, P. S. (1998). *Assessing competence to consent to treatment: A guide for physicians and other health professionals.* New York: Oxford University Press.

Groopman, J. E. (2007). *How doctors think.* Boston: Houghton Mifflin.

Hare, R. M. (1981). *Moral thinking: Its levels, method, and point.* Oxford; New York: Clarendon Press.

Health Insurance Portability and Accountability Act, Pub. L. No. 104-191, 110 Stat. 1936 (1996).

Hogan, C., Lunney, J., Gabel, J., & Lynn, J. (2001). Medicare beneficiaries' costs of care in the last year of life. *Health Aff (Millwood), 20*(4), 188–195.

Hunink, M. G. M. (2001). *Decision making in health and medicine: Integrating evidence and values.* New York: Cambridge University Press.

In re Quinlan, 70 10 (N.J. 1976).

Janse, A. J., Gemke, R. J., Uiterwaal, C. S., van der Tweel, I., Kimpen, J. L., & Sinnema, G. (2004). Quality of life: Patients and doctors don't always agree: A meta-analysis. *J Clin Epidemiol, 57*(7), 653–661. doi:10.1016/j.jclinepi.2003.11.013

Jecker, N. S. (1997). Introduction to the methods of bioethics. In N. S. Jecker, A. R. Jonsen, & R. A. Pearlman (Eds.), *Bioethics: An introduction to the history, methods, and practice* (pp. 113–125). Boston: Jones and Bartlett.

Jonsen, A. R., Siegler, M., & Winslade, W. J. (2006). *Clinical ethics: A practical approach to ethical decisions in clinical medicine* (6th ed.). New York: McGraw-Hill.

Jonsen, A. R., Siegler, M., & Winslade, W. J. (2015). *Clinical ethics: A practical approach to ethical decisions in clinical medicine* (8th ed.). New York: McGraw-Hill.

Jonsen, A. R., & Toulmin, S. (1988). *The abuse of casuistry: A history of moral reasoning.* Berkeley: University of California Press.

Kaldjian, L. C., Weir, R. F., & Duffy, T. P. (2005). A clinician's approach to clinical ethical reasoning. *J Gen Intern Med, 20*(3), 306–311. doi:10.1111/j.1525-1497.2005.40204.x

Kant, I. (1998). *Groundwork of the metaphysics of morals.* Cambridge, UK; New York: Cambridge University Press.

Kasman, D. L. (2004). When is medical treatment futile? A guide for students, residents, and physicians. *J Gen Intern Med, 19*(10), 1053–1056. doi:10.1111/j.1525-1497.2004.40134.x

Kelly, S. E., Marshall, P. A., Sanders, L. M., Raffin, T. A., & Koenig, B. A. (1997). Understanding the practice of ethics consultation: Results of an ethnographic multi-site study. *J Clin Ethics, 8*(2), 136–149.

LaPuma, J. (1990). Clinical ethics, mission and vision: Practical wisdom in health care. *Hospital and Health Services Administration, 35,* 321–326.

Levine, C., & Zuckerman, C. (1999). The trouble with families: Toward an ethic of accommodation. *Ann Intern Med, 130*(2), 148–152. doi:199901190-00010

Lo, B. (2009). *Resolving ethical dilemmas: A guide for clinicians* (4th ed.). Philadelphia: Wolters Kluwer Health/Lippincott Williams & Wilkins.

Mathews, B., & Kenny, M. C. (2008). Mandatory reporting legislation in the United States, Canada, and Australia: A cross-jurisdictional review of key features, differences, and issues. *Child Maltreat, 13*(1), 50–63. doi/abs/10.1177/1077559507310613

McCullough, L. B. (1984). Addressing ethical dilemmas: An ethics work-up. *The New Physician, 33.*

McGee, G. (2003). *Pragmatic bioethics* (2nd ed.). Cambridge, MA: MIT Press.

Morreim, E. H. (1991). Gaming the system: Dodging the rules, ruling the dodgers. *Arch Intern Med, 151*(3), 443–447.

Moskop, J. C., Marco, C. A., Larkin, G. L., Geiderman, J. M., & Derse, A. R. (2005). From Hippocrates to HIPAA: Privacy and confidentiality in emergency medicine—Part I: Conceptual, moral, and legal foundations. *Ann Emerg Med, 45*(1), 53–59. doi:S019606440401279X

National Commission for the Protection of Human Subjects of Biomedical and Behavioral Research. (1978). *The Belmont report: Ethical principles and guidelines for the protection of human subjects of research.* Washington, DC: US Government Printing Office.

Organisation for Economic Co-operation and Development. (2014). Coverage for health care. Retrieved from http://dx.doi.org/10.1787/soc_glance-2014-26-en

Orr, R. D., & deLeon, D. M. (2000). The role of the clinical ethicist in conflict resolution. *J Clin Ethics, 11*(1), 21–30.

Orr, R. D., & Shelton, W. (2009). A process and format for clinical ethics consultation. *J Clin Ethics, 20*(1), 79–89.

Outka, G. (1974). Social justice and equal access to health care. *J Relig Ethics, 2*(1), 11–32.

Pellegrino, E. D., & Thomasma, D. C. (1988). *For the patient's good: The restoration of beneficence in health care.* New York: Oxford University Press.

Pellegrino, E. D., & Thomasma, D. C. (1993). *The virtues in medical practice.* New York: Oxford University Press.

Pope, T. M. (2011). Comparing the FHCDA to surrogate decision making laws in other states. *NYSBA Health Law J, 16*(1), 5.

Powderly, K. E. (2003). Ethical issues for risk managers. In F. Kavaler & A. D. Spiegel (Eds.), *Risk management in health care institutions* (2nd ed.). Sudbury, MA: Jones and Bartlett.

Rhodes, R., & Alfandre, D. (2007). A systematic approach to clinical moral reasoning. *J Clin Ethics, 18*(2), 66–70.

Rogers v. Whitaker (High Court of Australia 1992).

Sacks, O. (2006). *The man who mistook his wife for a hat and other clinical tales* (Touchstone ed.). New York: Simon & Schuster.

Saigal, S., Stoskopf, B. L., Feeny, D., Furlong, W., Burrows, E., Rosenbaum, P. L., & Hoult, L. (1999). Differences in preferences for neonatal outcomes among health care professionals, parents, and adolescents. *JAMA, 281*(21), 1991–1997.

Sarbin, T. R. (1986). *Narrative psychology: The storied nature of human conduct.* New York: Praeger.

Savulescu, J. (2006). Conscientious objection in medicine. *BMJ*, *332*(7536), 294–297. doi:332/7536/294

Schiffrin, D., De Fina, A., & Nylund, A. (2010). *Telling stories: Language, narrative, and social life.* Washington, DC: Georgetown University Press.

Schneider, C. E. (2002). The practice of autonomy and the practice of bioethics. *J Clin Ethics*, *13*(1), 72–77.

Scofield, G. R. (1993). Ethics consultation: The least dangerous profession? *Camb Q Healthc Ethics*, *2*(4), 417–426; discussion 426–448.

Searight, H. R., & Gafford, J. (2005). Cultural diversity at the end of life: Issues and guidelines for family physicians. *Am Fam Physician*, *71*(3), 515–522.

Shalit, R. (1997). When we were philosopher kings: The rise of the medical ethicist. *New Repub*, *216*(17), 24–28.

Shalowitz, D. I., Garrett-Mayer, E., & Wendler, D. (2006). The accuracy of surrogate decision makers: A systematic review. *Arch Intern Med*, *166*(5), 493–497. doi:10.1001/archinte.166.5.493

Siegler, M., Pellegrino, E. D., & Singer, P. A. (1990). Clinical medical ethics. *J Clin Ethics*, *1*(1), 5–9.

Smart, J. J. C., & Williams, B. A. O. (1973). *Utilitarianism: For and against.* Cambridge, UK: Cambridge University Press.

Soulier, M. F., Maislen, A., & Beck, J. C. (2010). Status of the psychiatric duty to protect, circa 2006. *J Am Acad Psychiatry Law*, *38*(4), 457–473.

Stiggelbout, A. M., Elstein, A. S., Molewijk, B., Otten, W., & Kievit, J. (2006). Clinical ethical dilemmas: Convergent and divergent views of two scholarly communities. *J Med Ethics*, *32*(7), 381–388. doi.org/10.1136/jme.2005.011791

Sujdak Mackiewicz, B. N. (2016). Good ethics begin with good facts. *Am J Bioeth*, *16*(7), 66–68. doi:10.1080/15265161.2016.1180447

Swensen, S. J., Kaplan, G. S., Meyer, G. S., Nelson, E. C., Hunt, G. C., Pryor, D. B., . . . Chassin, M. R. (2011). Controlling healthcare costs by removing waste: What American doctors can do now. *BMJ Qual Saf*, *20*(6), 534–537. doi:bmjqs.2010.049213

Thomasma, D. C. (1978). Training in medical ethics: An ethical workup. *Forum Med*, *1*(9), 33–36.

Thomasma, D. C. (1983). Beyond medical parentalism and patient autonomy: A model of physician conscience for the physician-patient relationship. *Ann Intern Med*, *98*(2), 243–248.

Turton, F. E., & Snyder, L. (2008). Revision to the American College of Physicians' ethics manual. *Ann Intern Med*, *148*(11), 887–888. doi:148/11/887-a

Veatch, R. M. (2006). Assessing Pellegrino's reconstruction of medical morality. *Am J Bioeth*, *6*(2), 72–75. doi:G06H10V5261872UX

Veatch, R. M. (2009). *Patient, heal thyself: How the new medicine puts the patient in charge.* Oxford; New York: Oxford University Press.

Wardle, L. D. (1993). Protecting the rights of conscience of health care providers. *J Leg Med*, *14*(2), 177–230. doi:10.1080/01947649309510912

Wicclair, M. R. (2008). Is conscientious objection incompatible with a physician's professional obligations? *Theor Med Bioeth*, *29*(3), 171–185. doi:10.1007/s11017-008-9075-z

Ethical Issues in Determining the Plan of Care

3

Advance Care Planning and Surrogate Decision-Making

"It's not very pleasant, though," you may say, "to have death right before one's eyes." To this I would say, firstly, that death ought to be right there before the eyes of a young man just as much as an old one . . . and, secondly, that no one is so very old that it would be quite unnatural for him to hope for one more day. (Seneca, 1969)

In its most essential elements, death is immutable: it is inevitable, universal, and final, despite the human tendency to deny these facts. But in many other respects, death has fundamentally changed over the last 150 years, transitioning from something that was generally quick and unexplained, to something that now is often protracted and artificially deferred. In the developed world, death—at least in terms of its manner, timing, and location—is now often a decision. Most patients who die in the intensive care unit (ICU), for instance, do so after forgoing life-sustaining medical treatment (LSMT) (Sprung et al., 2003). Admittedly, many would have died even if LSMT had been continued, but the fact remains that the terms of one's death are increasingly within the patient's (or physician's) control.

Palliative care clinicians often play a part in these decisions, attending to the "sickest of the sick." ICU patients who receive palliative care consultations, for instance, have longer lengths-of-stay and higher mortality (Hsu-Kim, Friedman, Gracely, & Gasperino, 2015). These patients require expert symptom management, maximal psychosocial support, and wise guidance through complex decisions. Both in anticipation of those decisions—and in making them in real time—palliative care clinicians are integral to ensuring that patients and their families are informed, empowered, and supported. To optimally support patients and their families, clinicians need to understand on what ethical basis treatment decisions are made, the methods and tools available to plan ahead, and the obligations and complexities surrounding prognostication.

Hierarchy of Ethical Decision-Making

Autonomy

As noted previously (p. 5), parentalism was the primary model of decision-making for most of Western medical history, but during the twentieth century in the United States this gradually gave way to autonomy.[1] The word comes from the Greek *autos* (self) and *nomos* (rule or law), referring to the ability of a person to make her own decisions, free of encumbrances.

The appropriate application of this concept is not obvious, however. Some oversimplify it, essentially reducing autonomy to "what the patient wants, the patient gets." This, however, overlooks the distinction noted previously between positive and negative rights (p. 36). The right of self-determination that was codified in seminal court cases (*Cruzan v. Director, Missouri Department of Health*, 1990; *In re Quinlan*, 1976) and now forms the bedrock of American bioethics is based on the negative right to refuse unwanted treatment. Therefore, a patient with sufficient decision-making capacity (DMC) essentially has the right to refuse any treatment, even one that is necessary to sustain her life.

Some have attempted to extend this to a positive right, ranging from the rather mundane (such as patient's demand for antibiotics for a viral infection) to the profound (such as a request for physician-assisted dying or even euthanasia). As noted earlier, a positive right incurs an obligation on another person to provide whatever the first person has a right to, and thus is much more limited in scope. There are relatively few positive rights in American society: education through grade twelve, police protection, fire protection, and military protection. Health care (construed broadly) is not among them, in contrast to nearly every other developed nation (Organisation for Economic Co-operation and Development, 2014). But no nation promises a blanket right to specific treatments, particularly if these are not recommended for one's condition.

Conversely, some have not taken the concept of autonomy far enough, claiming that an autonomous decision must also be "rational." They are not using this term as Kant did (p. 35), to refer to a decision that is free of self-interest and worthy of becoming a universal norm. Rather, they are implicitly claiming that the recommendation of the medical team is "rational," and therefore disagreeing with it would be irrational. This creates a convenient response to requests (or refusals) from patients that conflict with the team's recommendations: if an autonomous choice must be rational, then such a seemingly "irrational" choice cannot be autonomous and thus need not be respected. This represents an invitation to return to the parentalism of a past era, despite the fact that over time it has become clear that physicians are not infallible arbiters of what is rational and what is not.

---

1. This often extreme emphasis on patient autonomy is not shared in other Western countries, or certain cultures within the United States.

A more nuanced understanding of autonomy holds that patients are generally permitted to chart their own course—in the absence of coercion or significant cognitive impairment—regardless of the negative consequences or if their decision deviates from the clinical team's recommendations. In other words, patients are allowed to make "bad choices," as long as these choices reflect their basic values and are not the result of impairment from mental illness, drugs, or other influences (Macauley, 2011).

A healthy and appropriate respect for autonomy, therefore, demands respect for a patient's refusal of treatment as well as her informed consent for treatments that are offered. It does not go so far as to obligate a health care professional to provide a treatment that he feels is not indicated or authorize him to override a patient's refusal of the team's recommendations.

Elements of Informed Consent

As noted earlier (p. 5), over the course of the twentieth century informed consent became a well-established concept in both American jurisprudence and bioethics. To provide informed consent (or refusal) for treatment, three things must exist:

1. The patient must be provided with sufficient information by which to make a decision.
2. The decision be voluntary.
3. The patient must have sufficient DMC to make that particular decision.

The first of these is the responsibility of the medical team, and the manner of providing that information is discussed later. The second underscores the need to protect patients from any coercion, either by friends or family or from clinicians who might feel so strongly that one course of action is preferable that the patient could fear abandonment if she does not concur. Concern for possible coercion should not, however, deter clinicians from offering recommendations, which are an important element in the informed consent process (p. 59).

The third element—that the patient has sufficient DMC—requires significant explication. First, it is important to distinguish between competence and capacity. The former is a legal concept, and thus only a court has the power to declare a patient incompetent. (All adults are presumed to be competent unless declared otherwise.) Competence also is generally an all-or-nothing concept, whereby someone generally is either competent to make decisions or is not.

DMC, on the other hand, is a clinical determination, made by clinicians at the bedside. It is also *decision-dependent*, and thus a patient might have sufficient DMC to make a "low-level" decision but not enough to make a "high-level" one. There are three characteristics that distinguish a high-level from a low-level decision. The first is *gravity*, for a decision where a specific choice could lead to death or permanent impairment understandably requires a higher level of DMC to ensure this truly reflects the patient's wishes. The second is the *complexity* of the decision, as many decisions in medicine are not binary but rather involve multiple variables, time courses, and hypotheticals. The final one is—for lack of a better word—the *unusualness* of the decision. For example, if a patient chooses a treatment plan that only 1% of competent patients would opt for, then logically she is either (literally) exceptional or she is unexceptional and has impaired DMC. This is especially relevant when a patient is declining a procedure that is likely to be beneficial with minimal risk or burden, which suggests that the vast majority of people would consent to it (Roth, Meisel, & Lidz, 1977).

Another way of looking at DMC—which leads to essentially the same conclusion—locates the sliding scale of DMC not in the extent of DMC itself but rather in the *assessed* capacity necessary to make a specific decision. Especially for high-level questions, the team needs to be very sure that the patient has sufficient DMC to make that decision. This requires an increasing margin for error, depending on the gravity (or, by extension, the complexity or unusualness) of the decision (Figure 3.1).

To possess DMC, a patient must be able to perform four distinct tasks (Grisso & Appelbaum, 1998):

1. Communicate a choice.
2. Understand relevant information.
3. Appreciate the consequences of a decision.
4. Manipulate information rationally.

The first should be self-evident: crisply put, it does not really matter whether the patient has the capacity to make a decision if she is unable to express the decision she has

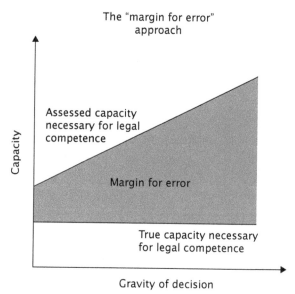

FIGURE 3.1 "Margin for error" approach to assessing DMC, based on the gravity of a decision (Buchanan, 2004)

made. She does not necessarily have to express a decision verbally, as this may be difficult or even impossible in some situations (such as when she is being ventilated through an endotracheal tube). Other means of communication—such as writing, nodding, or gestures—can often be sufficient. To confirm that the patient truly understands the question being asked, it is important to keep the phrasing simple, ask one question at a time, and ideally revisit the same topic from multiple angles to ensure consistency (Ha & Longnecker, 2010).

The second component is the ability to understand the relevant information provided, in terms of risks, benefits, and alternatives of various courses of action. A precondition for the patient understanding relevant information, of course, is that that information be presented to her. This must be done in an understandable manner, because even someone with pristine DMC will not be able to comprehend facts littered with "medicalese" and presented without recognition of the emotional impact the decision may carry.

Rather than providing all of the information at one time in the absence of relevant context—which Aulisio (2016) refers to as the "information dump" approach to autonomy—clinicians should provide the information in stages, allowing time for questions and clarification. Especially when delivering serious or bad news, the "ask-tell-ask" approach ensures that the conversation is a dialogue which respects the patient's questions and concerns (Evans, Tulsky, Back, & Arnold, 2006). Inquiring of the patient as to what her understanding of the information relayed is—ideally in her own words—can help confirm understanding.

Third, the patient must be able to appreciate the consequences of whatever decision she makes. While understanding is primarily cognitive, appreciation is profoundly personal. Rather than merely parroting risks and benefits, to fully appreciate the consequences of a decision the patient must grasp what the likely outcomes would mean *to her*. The clinician could, perhaps, ask "What would happen if you consented to this treatment or refused it?" in order to confirm appreciation of the practical consequences of the decision.

The final requirement for sufficient DMC is that the patient be able to reason from the information to the conclusion. This requires the patient to apply her own values and is not necessarily the same thing as making a "rational" decision in the eyes of an external observer (who may have much different values) or according to the Kantian conception of the categorical imperative (p. 35). Here the clinician might ask the patient why she decided the way she did and what factors played into that decision (Moye & Marson, 2007).

Certain patient groups are at increased risk of having impaired DMC. As one might expect, patients suffering from neurological disease (such as Alzheimer's disease, Parkinson's disease, or traumatic brain injury) or psychiatric conditions (such as schizophrenia or depression) are especially prone, as are patients engaged in substance abuse. Compromised capacity is a particular concern for palliative care, given the gravity and complexity of the decisions involved, as well as a patient's level of illness when she is asked to make them. Forty percent of medical inpatients (Raymont et al., 2004) and hospice patients (Sorger, Rosenfeld, Pessin, Timm, & Cimino, 2007) have impaired DMC increasing to 70% in the final days of life (Silveira, Kim, & Langa, 2010). The situation is even more challenging in the ICU, where up to 90% of patients lack DMC (Ely et al., 2001).

Every clinician (especially those practicing palliative medicine) should possess basic skills in assessing DMC. In most cases, this assessment is informal and ongoing, derived based on interactions with the patient ranging from the official (e.g., whether the patient remembers medical information she has been told) to the casual (e.g., if the patient is able to carry on a coherent social conversation). At one extreme is a patient who evidences absolutely no impairment (whose DMC is unquestioned) and at the other an unconscious patient who obviously lacks DMC.

There is a broad range in the middle, however, and in some cases more formal evaluation is necessary. A common tool that is used—especially when a patient's DMC may be affected by mental illness—is the Folstein Mini Mental Status Exam. While this can be confirmatory for patients at the extreme high or low end of the thirty point scale, it is neither sensitive nor specific for patients in the "gray zone." A score of 19 or less, for instance, is suggestive of (although not definitive for) incapacity, while a score of 23 to 26 or higher suggests (but does not prove) capacity (Marson, Hawkins, McInturff, & Harrell, 1997).

More reliable tools do exist, such as the MacArthur Competency Assessment Tool for Treatment (Grisso & Appelbaum, 1995) or the Assessment of Capacity for Everyday Decisions (Lai et al., 2008). These, however, often require specific training—not to mention significant time—to administer and thus may not be practical for the everyday practice of palliative care.

Much like a primary care physician would not consult cardiology for every heart murmur—or else cardiologists would instantly be overwhelmed by consultations—so also primary teams need not consult experts in DMC to assess every patient who is attempting to make a decision. But when greater DMC (or, at least, greater *evidence* of DMC) is required, expert consultation—generally with a psychiatrist—can be invaluable.

When a patient is determined to lack sufficient DMC to make a decision, the next step—which is often overlooked—is to attempt to restore it. In some cases (such as advanced dementia), this may not be possible. But in certain situations the reason for the compromised DMC may be remediable (such as an electrolyte or metabolic abnormality) or iatrogenic (such as sedation from analgesia). Even patients receiving mechanical ventilation may be able to participate in decision-making if their sedation is lightened. Acknowledging potential reluctance based on a concern that lightening sedation could increase patient suffering—especially for someone on a ventilator—one option is to use the opportunity afforded by a "sedation vacation" (Ackrivo et al., 2016) to engage the patient at a moment of potentially heightened DMC.

When a patient's DMC for a specific decision cannot be restored, one should consider whether there are other important decisions that the patient *does* have sufficient DMC to make. For instance, a patient may have insufficient DMC to refuse LSMT, but she may nevertheless have enough to name a health care agent (which is generally a rather "low-level" decision) (Jefferson et al., 2008). This underscores the fundamental point that just because a patient lacks sufficient DMC to make one decision does not necessarily mean she is incapable of making *all* decisions.

If a patient is unable to make any decisions, the next step is to see if the patient completed a written advance directive (AD) at a time when she did possess DMC. Unfortunately, this document rarely answers all the salient questions. The complexities of ADs are addressed later in this chapter.

Recommendations and Patient Autonomy

A great deal of emphasis has been placed on patient autonomy, such that it may seem like the "holy grail" of Western bioethics. Yet for all of this focus, most patients want more than just a list of options from which to choose. Studies have shown that the most important piece of information a patient uses in making a decision is the physician's recommendation (Scherr et al., 2017). Making such a recommendation has been shown to increase patient satisfaction (Gries, Curtis, Wall, & Engelberg, 2008) and decrease family distress (Vig, Starks, Taylor, Hopley, & Fryer-Edwards, 2007).

To be sure, there are some patients who want "just the facts" (White, Evans, Bautista, Luce, & Lo, 2009). But confirming this is a key element of the informed consent process, in order to tailor not only the information but also the manner of decision-making to the patient's personal values. And even if the patient *does* want a recommendation, that recommendation should be tailored to the individual patient's needs. There are a few "black-and-white" decisions in medicine. Most involve some value judgments about quality of life, duration of life, and associated burden. What may seem to physicians as the "standard of care" often incorporates multiple assumptions about what is important in life and what is not. For this reason, David Eddy (1990) suggests limiting the term "standard" to treatments about which there exists "virtual unanimity among patients about the overall desirability . . . of the outcomes."

So rather than dispensing information and then helping patients interpret it through the lens of one's own goals and values, a physician ideally would identify *the patient's* goals and values in order to determine the manner and extent of information shared. Unless a procedure is truly "standard," a physician could reasonably recommend it to one patient and discourage another from pursuing it, if those patients had different goals. For instance, the first might value life at any cost, while the second might feel that the ability to live independently was key to her quality of life.

If the latter part of the twentieth century was the "era of radical autonomy"—an understandable reaction to a long history of parentalism—the beginning of the twenty-first century saw the pendulum swing back toward the middle. Terms such as "patient-centered care" (Gerteis, 1993) began to proliferate, as professional societies endorsed the concept of "shared decision-making" (Davidson et al., 2007; Thompson et al., 2004). This acknowledges the reality that the physician's experience and perspective are critical in empowering the patient to effectively live out her values. A decision completely deferred to the patient is in no way "shared." That is why the literature on informed consent clearly includes recommendation as a core component of this sacred process (Buchanan & Brock, 1989), and some have even criticized the term "decision-maker" (referring to the patient) as insufficiently acknowledging the shared nature of the process (Aulisio, 2016).

Yet despite the fact that patients seek medical recommendations (Levinson, Kao, Kuby, & Thisted, 2005), physicians vary widely as to how often they actually offer them (Brush, Rasinski, Hall, & Alexander, 2012). In one multicenter study, for instance, physicians refrained from making a recommendation in 47% of cases, including half the time when specifically asked to do so (White, Malvar, Karr, Lo, & Curtis, 2010).

So why are some physicians reluctant to make recommendations? One reason is a misplaced concern over "trampling" the patient's autonomy. The latter concept has become so ingrained in medical practice—especially among younger physicians—that offering a thoughtful recommendation may appear parentalistic. Physicians must recognize, however, that thoughtful recommendations—based, as they should be, on a patient's expressed values—actually enhance (rather than trample on) a patient's right of self-determination. Quill and Brody (1996) thus consider a thoughtful recommendation a critical component of "enhanced autonomy."

Another possible reason for not offering thoughtful recommendations is that these require a nuanced understanding of the patient's goals and values. Obtaining this requires substantial time allocation as well as communication skills. Absent either of these, any recommendation a physician offers may not reflect the patient's goals and values. As a result, it may indeed be parentalistic (based on the physician's own beliefs about what is "best"), and thus his reluctance to offer it may be well-founded.

The final reason for not offering a recommendation is the physician's very human desire to not be "entirely responsible." Especially when a treatment plan turns out not to be successful, the physician may take some comfort in believing that the treatment plan was "the patient's choice," thus absolving the physician of some measure of responsibility for the outcome. Physicians must recognize that there is a broad middle ground between ultimate responsibility (in the form of parentalism) and utter abdication (in the form of presenting the facts in a supposedly "neutral" manner, which is never completely free of implicit bias[2]). There is no way to avoid a sense of responsibility, for it is part of the physician's sacred role to companion the patient along a perilous road, as well as an inherent component of a human interaction.

---

2. For instance, studies have shown that "framing" influences clinical decision-making (Haward, Murphy, & Lorenz, 2008). A patient told that a procedure has a 20% chance of survival is more likely to consent than if she were told it had an 80% chance of death. Less quantitative measures are also influential, as in the difference between describing a mechanical ventilator as "a breathing machine" or "a machine that will force air into your lungs through a tube placed in your throat."

Informed consent is especially challenging in palliative care, given the stakes involved. Many of the decisions patients and families face involve life-sustaining—or potentially curative but heavily burdensome—treatments. The weight of such decisions can be crushing, and their complexity demands the perspective of someone with experience to guide the patient. Recognizing this, a model of "informed assent" has been suggested for situations where the benefit of a possible treatment is quite low—as may be the case for CPR—and does not seem to comport to the patient's expressed values (Curtis, 2007) (p. 382).

Substituted Judgment

From an ethical perspective, a patient should not lose her rights if she becomes incapacitated. To the degree that her goals and values are known, these should be respected in the same way as if she still had DMC. This is precisely the conclusion of the *Quinlan* decision, which asserted a patient's right of privacy that extended to her incapacitated state.

In the absence of a definitive AD to guide treatment, however, someone else—who knows the patient's goals and values—must do so for her. This is a very common occurrence in modern medicine, with >70% of elderly patients in the United States requiring a surrogate at some point (Silveira et al., 2010). Surrogate decision-making is a complex process, including not only *who* the appropriate surrogate is but also *how* that person should make decisions on behalf of the patient. It is not surprising, therefore, that uncertainty about surrogate decision-making is the most common reason for clinical ethics consultation (Sulmasy & Snyder, 2010).

Who Should Decide?

There are three basic types of surrogate decision-makers. The first is a health care *agent* (or proxy), who is someone named by the patient in a Durable Power of Attorney for Health Care (DPA-HC). This is the ideal situation, as the team can be confident that the patient wanted that specific person to make decisions for her (and, hopefully, also discussed goals and values with that person). Unfortunately, with barely one-quarter of Americans having filled out an AD—and barely one-tenth of adults under the age of thirty (Rao, Anderson, Lin, & Laux, 2014)—this is a relatively infrequent occurrence.

A second type of surrogate decision-maker is a *guardian*, who is appointed by the court for a patient who has legally been declared incompetent. At first this may seem to be a higher level of authority as a result of court involvement, but an agent has greater authority by virtue of being named by the patient herself, rather than by an impartial court. Guardianship is generally a very rare occurrence, given the implications of depriving a patient of her legal right to make her own medical decisions. But cases that do involve guardians are still likely to prompt ethical questions, especially when the guardian is not "private" (i.e., someone who knows the patient and accepts the responsibility to make decisions) but rather a public guardian who may have no prior knowledge of the patient. This makes applying substituted judgment extremely difficult.

For the majority of incapacitated patients—who have not named an agent and do not have a guardian—the person tasked with making decisions might simply be called a *surrogate*. To determine who should play this role, most states have a "hierarchy of surrogates" (DeMartino et al., 2017). This typically begins with the patient's spouse and then moves down through adult children, adult siblings, parents, friends, and so on. Most hierarchies are not absolute, recognizing that the highest person in the hierarchy may not be the one who knows the patient's values (or can advocate for them) the best. Typically anyone listed on the hierarchy has the right to challenge the decisions or authority of the person at the top. Ideally such conflicts can be mediated without court involvement, but in intractable situations there is always the option of judicial appeal.

Hierarchies have the advantage of clarity and in many cases grant legal authority to the person who also happens to be the best decision-maker (such as a long-time spouse). Sometimes, however, they can give undue authority to someone who may not know the patient as well as someone lower on the hierarchy or someone acting out of his own goals and values rather than the patient's. Not uncommonly, a patient might share more about her treatment preferences with friends or acquaintances than with close family. Even though hierarchies allow for "challenges," the presumption in favor of the person highest on the list may discourage this from occurring.

The absence of a hierarchy allows the medical team to rely on whomever seems to know the patient's values best. This is not a perfect solution, however. When multiple people are vying to make decisions, it may be unclear who is best equipped to do so. The team might be tempted to "appoint" as surrogate a person who agrees with the team's recommendations (and thus appears the most "rational"). In the face of conflict, petitioning for a guardian—which should be a last resort—may become the norm, thus prolonging decision-making and potentially leading to inappropriate treatment being delivered as the court deliberates.

Ultimately clinicians must work within their state's legal structure, recognizing that both a hierarchy as well as the lack of one carry both benefits and risks.

How a Surrogate Decision-Maker Should Decide

Whoever the surrogate decision-maker is,[3] he is tasked with exercising what is rather unfortunately termed "substituted judgment" on behalf of the patient. At first glance, that term might suggest that the surrogate is supposed to substitute his own judgment for that of the patient. (Indeed, surrogates often rely on their own personal outlook, faith, and intuition in reaching decisions; Boyd et al., 2010.) What the surrogate should actually do, however, is render a decision based on the patient's own values. The operative question to

---

3.   In an attempt to balance ease and clarity, from this point the term "surrogate" is used to refer to any surrogate decision-maker, even if that person has the status of an agent. It should be noted that some states prevent guardians (who are functioning as extensions of the court) from authorizing Do Not Attempt Resuscitation (DNAR) orders or forgoing other LSMT without explicit court permission (Cohen, Wright, Cooney, & Fried, 2015), which is generally not the case for agents or surrogates.

the surrogate, therefore, is not "What do you think we should do?" but rather "What do you think the patient would say about this decision, if [she] could answer for [herself]?" (Curtis & Isaac, 2010).

Surrogates will have varying levels of evidence by which to decide what the patient would have said. Here it is helpful to reference the distinctions made by the New York Supreme Court in the *Conroy* decision (*In re Conroy*, 1985), which identifies three levels of authority/certainty. The "pure subjective" level refers to surrogate decisions based entirely on the patient's own values, as known through prior comments about similar situations or conclusions drawn from more general observations. The "mixed subjective/objective" level applies to situations where expressed personal beliefs and values are not sufficient to generate a decision. Rather, they must be taken in the context of the medical situation and what appears to be in the patient's best interests. When nothing is known of the patient's goals or values, the only recourse is to apply the "pure objective" standard, which focuses entirely on what appears to be in the patient's best interests.

This three-fold division represents a gradual shift from autonomy (based on the patient's goals and values) to beneficence (based on what the surrogate believes to be in the patient's best interests). This may seem to suggest that the pure subjective model is superior and the pure objective model is the least desirable, given the criticisms of the best interest standard noted later (p. 67). But it is important to note that even patients who have named a health care agent may prefer some blend of these two standards, especially in situations that they may not have foreseen where treatment could create significant burden.

While nearly every state allows surrogates to make decisions based on credible reasons why the patient would have chosen a specific course of action, two go further than this. Both New York and Missouri required "clear and convincing" evidence that it was the patient's *actual* wish to forgo LSMT, rather than it merely being probable that the patient would have wished to do so.[4] Both laws have, however, been subsequently modified either by statute (New York) or court decision (Missouri) to allow for more latitude in decision-making (Meisel, 2016).

In practice, it often proves very challenging—if not impossible—for surrogates to determine what the patient would actually have said. Most people have had the experience of someone they felt they knew extremely well completely surprising them by her actions or expressed opinions. Studies have confirmed this, with patients and their agents—not merely surrogates and thus, by definition, having been specifically named by

---

4.   While the *Cruzan* decision (*Cruzan v. Director, Missouri Department of Health*, 1990) is usually cited for its codification of the competent patient's right of refusal, the specific finding was that the Missouri law requiring "clear and convincing evidence" was not unconstitutional. Indeed, it was only the subsequent presentation of evidence (by Nancy's long-time friends, who had previously not associated her with the case, since it used her married name) that led the state of Missouri to drop its appeal, acknowledging that the evidentiary standard had therefore been met.

the patient to make decisions—agreeing about hypothetical treatment decisions only two-thirds of the time. One might surmise that these dyads just had not had the opportunity to discuss the patient's goals and values or specific treatment options (Hines et al., 2001). But even when this is subsequently provided, the rate of concurrence does not improve. In fact, it goes down—although not to a statistically significant degree—underscoring how difficult it is to know with certainty what another person would say or do (Shalowitz, Garrett-Mayer, & Wendler, 2006).

So why are surrogates "wrong" so often (Foo, Lee, & Soh, 2012)? One possibility is that—even though patients' wishes tend to show significant stability over time (Martin & Roberto, 2006)—in specific cases they may shift, perhaps since the last time they discussed them with their surrogates (Wittink et al., 2008). One can certainly imagine a patient saying "I would never want to live like that" but, when faced the choice of impairment or death, choosing the former. Conversely, a patient may experience what is known as "hospitalization" dip, where patients are less likely to want LSMT immediately following a hospitalization, compared with annual reviews prior to it and several months later (Ditto, Jacobson, Smucker, Danks, & Fagerlin, 2006).

Another possibility is that despite the clarifications noted here—and the inherent emphasis of "substituted judgment"—surrogates are making decisions they would make for themselves, rather than what the patient would choose (Marks & Arkes, 2008). Studies have certainly shown that, in addition to their shared experiences with the patient, surrogates also take into consideration their own values and religious beliefs, as well as family consensus about the appropriate course of action (Boyd et al., 2010).

Surrogates may also not be able—or willing—to accept how dire the situation truly is. Studies have shown that surrogates often interpret prognosis too optimistically (Zier, Sottile, Hong, Weissfield, & White, 2012) and may explicitly question the accuracy of the prognosis (Zier et al., 2008). Even when the prognosis is clearly communicated and accepted, nearly one-third of surrogates would choose to continue treatment if there was <1% chance of survival, and 18% would do so even if the physicians said there was "no chance" (Zier et al., 2009).

Whether based on uncertainty, their own beliefs, or overoptimistic interpretation of the data—or some combination of all three—surrogates may opt for more treatment rather than less in order to avoid any possibility of not giving the patient "a chance." This desire to not feel responsible for the patient's death can result in the patient receiving treatment she would never have accepted, if she were able to speak for herself (Schenker et al., 2012). This is particularly true of the proverbial "nephew from Peoria" (Butler, 2013), which refers to a loved one from far away who may not have witnessed a patient's gradual decline and may not fully appreciate the burden of continued medical treatment. An estranged relative may also advocate for aggressive treatment in order to preserve the possibility of reconciliation, prioritizing his own needs over those of the patient.

Despite—or perhaps because of—their tendency to "err on the side of more," surrogates often carry significant doubt with them after having made the decision. Over one-third of surrogates report serious symptoms—including stress and guilt over the decisions they have made—which in some cases can last for years (Wendler & Rid, 2011). In one study, 82% of family members who took part in end-of-life decision-making had subsequent symptoms of posttraumatic stress disorder (Azoulay et al., 2005). These findings cross racial and ethnic boundaries (Braun, Beyth, Ford, & McCullough, 2008).

Recognizing the burden on surrogates, the physician's role cannot be limited to dispensing the facts and ensuring understanding but must also include attention to a surrogate's emotional needs (Schenker et al., 2012). Asking the right question(s), making appropriate recommendations, and using informed assent where appropriate (p. 382) are all useful steps in minimizing the psychological risk of surrogates. Surrogates can also benefit from broad-based emotional and spiritual support from mental health professionals and spiritual care providers (Johnson et al., 2014). Subsequent risk to surrogates also highlights the benefits of hospice enrollment—even at the very end of a patient's life, and perhaps even while hospitalized—as this provides one year of bereavement support for the family.

So how can the process of surrogate decision-making be improved? The first step is to recall the familiar adage that if one asks the wrong question, one will get the wrong answer. In this case, the clinician should avoid asking the surrogate what he thinks the team should do, as this shifts the focus from the patient's goals to the surrogate's.

But even if the clinician focuses on the patient's values, word choice may lead the surrogate to an erroneous conclusion. For instance, the clinician might ask what the patient would "want" in that clinical situation. In the absence of appreciation of the clinical context, this invites a response of "everything" (which is addressed later). But even with sufficient context—and honest recognition of the communicated prognosis—the surrogate can still legitimately respond in terms of what the patient might hope for or aspire to, even if it is not clinically realistic. Framing the question in terms of what the patient would *say* helps shift the conversation away from the patient's potentially unrealistic hopes to what she would actually say—and do—when confronted with treatment questions (Schwarze, Campbell, Cunningham, White, & Arnold, 2016).

Often, however, the surrogate may not be certain what the patient would say. This might reflect genuine humility about how sure someone can be about another person's wishes or a reluctance to authorize forgoing LSMT because of anticipatory grief. In such situations, less factual inquiries—admittedly less precise, though more relational—may yield more accurate "substituted judgment." An example of this might be: "You know the patient and she trusted you to make decisions. What would she want you to do?"

It is also important to note that surrogates may not be doing anything wrong when they deviate from a patient's previously expressed wish. For while medical ethicists tend to emphasize substituted judgment in the "pure subjective" sense of *Conroy* (Luce, 2010), studies have shown more than three-quarters of patients are willing to defer to their surrogate's decision, even if it conflicts with their previously expressed wishes (Covinsky et al., 2000). The likely reason is that patients recognize their inability to foresee precisely what situation they may find themselves in and thus trust their designated decision-makers to make the appropriate decision in real time (Fins, 1999).

Recognizing that most patients would prefer some blend of substituted judgment and best interests, Sulmasy and Snyder (2010) stress *authenticity* in acting based on the patient's expressed goals and values. Avoiding the extremes of "What would your loved one decide?" (substituted judgment) and "What do you think is best for him?" (best interests), the "substituted interests" model is inquisitive and begins with "Tell us about your loved one." The focus shifts from a discrete medical decision to an overall sense of what is most important to the patient, both in the past and in the current situation.

Once ascertained, the patient's goals and values provide a guide for establishing an appropriate plan of care. The concept of appropriateness is key here, as the team is not merely asking the surrogate(s) what the patient would have wanted but rather offering clinically reasonable recommendations based on the patient's goals and values. The final step of the substituted interests approach involves confirming adequate understanding of these, such as by asking, "Knowing your loved one, does our recommendation seem right for him or her? Do you think another plan would be better, given his or her values, preferences, relationships?" (Sulmasy & Snyder, 2010).

By focusing on the patient's values, this model avoids often-impossible questions about what would the patient decide in a specific (and often unforeseen) situation (Hirschman, Kapo, & Karlawish, 2006). It specifically empowers the surrogate to decide differently than they would for themselves, thus respecting the patient's uniqueness and autonomy (Fagerlin, Ditto, Danks, Houts, & Smucker, 2001). This approach also reflects the practical reality that physicians often make decisions by taking patient preferences into consideration, while also considering factors related to best interests and quality of life, especially as patients get older and are dealing with more chronic issues (Torke, Moloney, Siegler, Abalos, & Alexander, 2010).

At the same time, it is important to note that not all patients wish to defer to their surrogate's discretion. The challenge here is to determine whether—in the case of a surrogate deciding contrary to the patient's previously expressed wishes—that particular patient would defer to the surrogate's judgment or not. Recognizing this possibility, it can be helpful to incorporate this question into advance care planning (ACP), by specifically inquiring of patients as to the degree of latitude they would want their surrogate to have.

When Surrogates Disagree

It is not uncommon for potential surrogates to disagree as to what a patient would say if she could choose for herself. The first step in resolving such a conflict is to shift the discussion from who makes the decision to what the decision should be. Especially where there is family strife, the conversation may have devolved into who has control over the situation. Some potential surrogates may strive to be the decision-maker, while others will assiduously avoid this role in order not to bear the weight of having made a major decision.

Often, though, when the focus is reframed on the patient's values and what *she* would have said, surrogates vying for control may turn out to have the same opinion. If so—and this can be identified—the question of who makes that particular decision becomes moot. The medical team can take the group's consensus as informed consent for a particular treatment plan. This is especially important when the decision is to limit LSMT, leaving no one person to carry "the weight of the world" on his shoulders, thus minimizing the risk of psychological consequences noted previously.

If there is disagreement among the potential surrogates as to what treatment course is appropriate, it is important to confirm that they are all answering the correct—and the same—question (i.e., what the *patient* would say, if presented with that clinical situation). Some may be speaking from their own values or needs, rather than applying appropriate substituted judgment (or, more progressively, substituted interests). This is especially common if a potential surrogate's own moral or religious beliefs mandate—or forbid—specific treatments or treatment decisions, such as the withdrawal of LSMT.

If the source of the disagreement remains unclear, it can be helpful to ask the potential surrogates why, specifically, they believe the patient would (or would not) opt for a particular treatment. This may reveal information not shared among all, such as private conversations the patient had with particular individuals. It may also highlight personal biases that potential surrogates may be bringing into the discussion.

When consensus among potential surrogates cannot be achieved, several options remain. One is to continue with the current treatment plan, which generally defaults to a more aggressive course. (Simply put, LSMT can always be withdrawn at a later date; it cannot be subsequently implemented if the patient has already died.) Another is to invite potential surrogates whose views differ from the evolving consensus to withhold objections. This does not require them to endorse the plan but merely to defer to the larger group in a variation on the theme of "informed assent."

Finally, the team may be forced to honor the views that seem to best reflect the patient's values in the absence of consensus. In such cases, the dissenting surrogates may ultimately choose to defer, feeling like they have done as much as they could. Or they may continue to object, even taking the case to court and seeking to be appointed the patient's guardian. This is, of course, their right, and prior to the final determination the court may grant a restraining order to compel ongoing treatment, in order to preserve options. Hopefully, though, the proactive steps noted previously can help prevent this contentious and adversarial context, during which time the patient may be suffering unnecessarily.

Best Interests

When the patient cannot make her own medical decisions and has not completed an AD and no one is available to offer substituted judgment based on her goals and values, the only remaining option is acting in the patient's "best interests." This involves attempting to determine what a "reasonable person" would decide in a similar situation by weighing "the burdens and benefits of treatment to the patient . . . when no clear preferences . . . can be determined" (Kopelman, 2007).

Perhaps the preeminent court case related to this standard is that *Superintendent of Belchertown State School v. Saikewicz* (1977). In this case, a sixty-seven-year-old man with profound cognitive disability was diagnosed with leukemia. Normally this would be treated with chemotherapy, but his physicians recommended against treatment because they did not believe he would be able to understand the need for it. The court concurred, taking into account the potential benefit of treatment as well as the side effects. In doing so, it attempted to "don the mantle of the incompetent" by making a decision in the patient's best interests.

"Best interests" sounds noble and good. After all, what patient would not want others to act in her best interests? Precisely because of this positive connotation, clinicians often speak of doing what is in the patient's best interests, when in fact the predominant value in American bioethics is not beneficence but rather autonomy. Sometimes an action that seems to an external observer like it would be in a patient's best interests is not what the patient would have chosen if she were able to make a decision. For instance, a patient who had a deep love of life—or, conversely, a profound fear of death—might opt for aggressive and burdensome treatment that is unlikely to be effective, which some might view as contrary to her best interests.

So despite the superlative in its name, best interests is the "third-best" of three paradigms for clinical decision-making (after autonomy and substituted judgment). The reason is that it is entirely impersonal, based solely on the assessment of another person as to what would be "best" for a patient, without regard for the patient's values or priorities or lived experience. It is also a very difficult standard to apply. The poor correlation between patients and surrogates in terms of substituted judgment was noted earlier, but the correlation of their respective senses of what is in someone's best interests is actually worse, barely better than a coin flip (Sharma et al., 2011).

The best interest standard applies to two types of patients. The first are those who never had DMC, such as infants or small children (discussed in Section IV) or adults with profound cognitive disability. Decision-making for the former is granted greater latitude, by virtue of the deciders' being the patient's parents. Decisions for the latter are often made by parents who have subsequently become guardians for the now-adult patient, by other relatives, or by public guardians.

The second type of patient for whom best interests is the appropriate paradigm for decision-making are people who currently lack DMC and no one who knows them is available to offer substituted judgment. The latter are commonly referred to as "adult orphans" or "unbefriended patients," and sadly this is not an uncommon situation. Studies suggest that unbefriended patients represent 5% to 10% of ICU deaths (Isaacs & Brody, 2010) and 3% to 4% of long-term care residents (American Bar Association, 2004) in the United States. As suggested by their social isolation, unbefriended patients are often homeless or mentally ill.

The elderly represent a disproportionate percentage of unbefriended patients, in part because they may have had surrogates earlier in their lives, but the "oldest old" (over eighty-five) are often alone now. Even if their surrogates are still alive, they themselves may be hampered by impaired DMC. This problem will only become more prevalent: the US Census Bureau projects that the oldest old will more than triple by 2060, from 5.9 to 18.2 million people (US Census Bureau, 2012).

There are several options for decision-making for unbefriended patients (Connor, Elkin, Lee, Thompson, & Whelan, 2016). The most obvious is pursuing guardianship, although this can be a complex, time-consuming, and often challenging process, given the limited supply of guardians to meet the need. For these reasons, even the American Bar Association deems this an option of last resort (American Bar Association, 1989).

Several alternatives have been proposed. One is that physicians themselves make decisions for these patients, which clearly is already occurring. In one study, three-quarters of physicians reported having made a medical decision within the past month for a patient who lacked DMC and had no available surrogate (Isaacs & Brody, 2010). These were not mundane decisions, either, with one-third of ICU physicians reporting doing so in relation to forgoing LSMT (White, Jonsen, & Lo, 2012).

There are definite advantages to this model. Physicians are clearly able to appreciate the clinical implications of decisions (Volpe & Steinman, 2013). They are also available and involved, already representing part of the ideal "shared decision-making" process. Some states currently grant them broad latitude in decision-making for unbefriended patients (Varma & Wendler, 2007).

At the same time, there are concerns for bias and conflict of interest. For instance, studies have shown that physicians underestimate the quality of life in disabled survivors of critical illness (Janse et al., 2004). Compared to patients, physicians tend to value intervention and biological factors at the expense of psychosocial and spiritual concerns (Jacobs, Burns, & Bennett Jacobs, 2008). There may be financial or professional incentives to either continue treatment (on a fee-for-service model) or forgo it (especially for patients whose care is no longer being reimbursed) (Anstey, Adams, & McGlynn, 2015). And, despite their clinical expertise, physicians are able to predict what their patients want only 50% to 70% of the time (Fischer, Tulsky, Rose, Siminoff, & Arnold, 1998). For all these reasons, in certain states physicians are specifically prohibited from acting as decision-makers (Rai, Siegler, & Lantos, 1999).

Recognizing this complexity, some have suggested that hospital ethics committees be tasked with deciding for unbefriended patients (Pope, 2013; White et al., 2012). Ideally, this would allow a multidisciplinary group—hopefully with patient and family representation—to review the case, thus minimizing the effects of individual biases and potential conflicts of interest. While this model avoids the bureaucratic complexity of court-appointed guardianship, it is also nontransportable and thus would not be able to assist with subsequent medical decisions should the patient survive and be discharged. Such a committee could also be subject to members' own conflicts of interest, with a large proportion presumably being hospital employees (or, at least, those with strong ties to the institution).

Recognizing that neither alternative to guardianship is perfect, some professional societies have recommended seeking out "nontraditional" surrogates (American Geriatrics Society Ethics Committee, 2015). One method involves the use of specially trained volunteers to make decisions for unbefriended patients. This approach recognizes the cumbersome nature of guardianship process, as well as the potential for conflict of interest among hospital staff and ethics committees (Bandy et al., 2014). Another option is a clear decisional pathway for treatment decisions involving unbefriended patients, with increasing levels of oversight based on the complexity and gravity of the decision (Department of Veterans Affairs, 2009).

As is often the case, the truth lies somewhere in the middle. Involving physicians in the decision-making process benefits from their experience and availability, but others need to be involved in order to prevent bias and preserve the fragile "check-and-balance" between autonomy and beneficence. A hospital ethics committee—or some subset of it— that has strong community representation and willingly accepts the weighty responsibility of making potentially life-or-death decisions for vulnerable patients is optimal. This would require institutional buy-in, in terms of accepting that responsibility rather than automatically deferring to the court system, which may involve long waits and impersonal attention. It would also require commitment of resources (in terms of committee member time and training) as well as perhaps legislative approval to allay concerns for liability. Such investment is necessary in order to prevent discrimination, either in the form of insufficient treatment based on quality-of-life biases or conflicts of interest, or defaulting to maximal treatment in the absence of a clear decision-maker who can refuse burdensome treatment on the patient's behalf.

Ultimately, the best response to potential ethical dilemmas regarding unbefriended patients is to prevent them from occurring in the first place. Engaging in a robust ACP process which identifies patient goals and explores relevant foreseeable treatment decisions is invaluable.

Advance Care Planning

While "palliative care" is a broader term than "hospice"—and thus is not exclusively focused on the end of a patient's life—end-of-life (EOL) care is nevertheless a large component of palliative care. This involves not only actually caring for a patient as she approaches death but also preparing for that final stage of life. As the old saying goes, "An ounce of prevention is worth a pound of cure" (Franklin, 1735), and nowhere is this more true than in preparing for the end of one's life.

Before exploring the nuances of ADs, it is critical to note that ACP is much more than completing a piece of paper. It involves thoughtful conversations not only with one's physician but also with family and friends (and especially the person tapped to be one's health care agent). Context is everything in ACP, and unless one's physician and agent appreciate the significance and context of the values and priorities the patient espouses, they will not be able to advocate for the course of action that best reflects the patient's point of view. A patient may be reluctant to engage in those discussions with family—for fear of "weighing them down"—but studies have shown that family members actually welcome these conversations (Janssen, Engelberg, Wouters, & Curtis, 2012), so they will be better able to help their loved one in a time of need, while also reducing their own burden over making subsequent decisions (Shalowitz et al., 2006).

There are a great many benefits to engaging in ACP. Having an AD increases the likelihood that care will reflect one's preferences (Detering, Hancock, Reade, & Silvester, 2010) while also increasing utilization of hospice services (Teno, Gruneir, Schwartz, Nanda, & Wetle, 2007). ACP reduces the probability that the patient will receive high-tech interventions (Silveira et al., 2010) or hospitalization at the end of life (Brinkman-Stoppelenburg, Rietjens, & van der Heide, 2014). There is also emerging data showing ACP reduces the cost of EOL care (Teno et al., 2007), without increasing mortality (Zhang et al., 2009). Conversely, there are clear risks in *not* engaging in ACP: the absence of an AD, for instance, is a barrier to optimal EOL care (Nelson et al., 2006).

ACP also has benefits for surviving loved ones, including positively impacting family assessment of quality of death in ICU (Glavan, Engelberg, Downey, & Curtis, 2008). Stress, anxiety, and depression are also reduced (Detering et al., 2010).

Despite all the reasons to engage in ACP, studies show that relatively few Americans do so. Data varies according to time and nature of the sample, but results range from as few as 5% to up to one-third of Americans having completed an AD (Tillyard, 2007). Several obstacles have been identified, beyond the very human fear of death. For instance, diminished literacy is a risk factor for not having an AD in place (Waite et al., 2013). Preference for greater intensity of care at EOL also reduces the likelihood of ACP (Volandes et al., 2008). Some minority groups are particularly unlikely to engage in ACP, partly due to less knowledge about the elements and benefits of ACP (Kwak & Haley, 2005).

Gradually, ACP is becoming more common (Silveira, Wiitala, & Piette, 2014). Contributing factors include community initiatives (Hammes & Kane, 1998) and long-sought Medicare reimbursement for ACP conversations (Department of Health and Human Services, 2015). Not surprisingly, older patients and those with a history of chronic disease—or a significant current disease burden—are more likely to complete an AD. Nearly three out of four older Americans have completed an AD prior to their death, up from 42% ten years ago (Silveira et al., 2014). Caucasian race, higher education and socioeconomic status, and prior knowledge of ACP and EOL care options are correlated with an increased probability of AD completion (Bullock, 2011; Kwak & Haley, 2005).

The overall numbers appear sobering, but taken in context they may not seem as bad. Countries such as Germany (Evans et al., 2012) and the Netherlands have AD completion rates of less than 10% (van Wijmen, Rurup, Pasman, Kaspers, & Onwuteaka-Philipsen,

2010). A recent study from Canada showed that 86% of people had not even *heard* of ACP (Ipsos-Reid, 2012).

Treatment Directives

The concept of planning ahead in writing for the end of one's life was first proposed in the late 1960s. Luis Kutner coined the term "living will" to describe a document in which a competent patient identifies treatments which she is (and is not) willing to accept if she becomes incapacitated (Kutner, 1969). This proposal came largely as a response to technological innovations that—despite promising initial results (such as CPR, p. 378)—ultimately were determined to offer uncertain benefit. The original boilerplate language of the living will (otherwise known as a terminal care document) went something like this: "If I am terminally ill and there is no reasonable prospect of my recovery, I do not want extraordinary measures to prolong my life but instead prefer measures to ensure my comfort and dignity."

As an acknowledgement that the patient had a right to refuse treatment—and was exercising that right—the original living will was a huge step forward. But however well-intentioned, in terms of guiding specific treatments such a statement was not very helpful. The Medicare Hospice Benefit may define "terminally ill" as having less than six months left to live, but some people completing a living will might have a broader notion in mind (e.g., incurable illness with significant burden over the coming months or years), while others might have a more restricted understanding (e.g., imminently dying). By the same token, what constitutes a "reasonable" prospect of recovery may differ from person to person. For some, *any* chance of recovery is enough to warrant LSMT, while others may feel that, unless recovery is likely, they would not want to endure the potential burdens of LSMT.

Finally, the definition of "extraordinary measures" has changed over time. When first used in the 1950s, mechanical ventilators were considered extraordinary, but now to many they probably seem commonplace. The terminology may invite someone to focus on the intervention itself rather than the context in which it is being considered, which is truly determinative. For instance, mechanically ventilating an otherwise healthy premature baby born at twenty-eight weeks gestation—who has an extremely high probability of unimpaired survival after what will likely be a short period of respiratory support—would hardly seem extraordinary, but the same could not be said for ventilating an extremely elderly patient with advanced emphysema who will likely never be able to breathe independently again.

Ultimately, the most that can be said about the living will with the standard wording is that the patient who signed it did not want everything done, no matter the context or likely outcome. But it does not follow that the patient did not want *anything* done, leaving significant ambiguity in all but the most extreme cases.

Physicians recognize this ambiguity, which explains why in hypothetical scenarios they deviate from the living will two-thirds of the time, favoring other considerations such as prognosis, quality of life, and wishes of family and friends (Hardin & Yusufaly, 2004). As a result, some commentators have proclaimed the living will itself to be "dead" (Fagerlin & Schneider, 2004).

Surrogates, though, still rely on written treatment directives, for in the absence of a formative ACP conversation these may be the only available evidence about what the patient would want (Silveira et al., 2010). This has prompted the development of more specific types of treatment directives, which go beyond "reasonable" probabilities and "extraordinary" measures. Such forms may address specific procedures (such as CPR and intubation) or conditions (e.g., coma with good or bad prognosis, dementia with or without terminal illness) (Emanuel & Emanuel, 1989), or incorporate a values history (Lambert, Gibson, & Nathanson, 1990). They also allow for free-text additions where patients can describe their primary goals, fears, concerns, and so on. Even if the forms cannot foresee every eventuality, the process of completing them—and hopefully discussing the decisions with one's family and friends—may help prepare both the patient and potential surrogates for "in the moment" decisions (Sudore & Fried, 2010).

Even with greater specificity, though, ADs may not be clear and determinative if the context is not sufficiently taken into account. Consider a real-life example: an elderly patient presents to the emergency department in respiratory distress from community-acquired pneumonia. She had previously completed an AD and checked the box for Do Not Intubate (DNI). The medical team, however, strongly believes that she would be able to return to her baseline quality of health—which was generally good—after a short-term intubation while the antibiotics treat the infection.

Her spouse wants her to survive, but he also seeks to respect her wishes. What initially seemed like a rather black-and-white case of respecting patient refusal soon becomes more complex when the husband is asked what the patient understood—at the time she completed the AD—about intubation. He is not certain, but he does recall her referring to a relative who was maintained on mechanical ventilation for several weeks in the ICU before eventually dying. If *that* was what the patient was refusing in her AD, then the document does not reflect an informed refusal of short-term intubation (or perhaps a refusal at all, as this is so different from what she envisioned).

After receiving empathic reassurance that he would not be violating his wife's wishes by consenting to intubation, the husband authorizes it and his wife is indeed ventilated for a few days, and upon returning home—with no decline in her baseline health status—expresses gratitude for the thoughtful interpretation of the "check box" for DNI on her AD.

This example highlights the need for a nuanced and informed process of ACP. For while it is undoubtedly courageous for community groups to sponsor "advance directive fairs" to prompt people to plan ahead, the end result of such events—which often is limited to a written document without thoughtful conversation with one's family and friends, or perspective provided by one's primary care physician—can be at best unhelpful and at worst dangerous, especially when it involves specific treatment directives.

A more thoughtful approach involves focusing on the patient's goals and values, in recognition of the unpredictability of future events. These goals and values could then be *applied* to specific situations as they arise. Recognizing how difficult it is to face one's mortality, several variations on the "one size fits all" terminal care document have been suggested. One involves providing patients with user-friendly tools to empower them to make more informed decisions about specific treatment modalities. Online tools can be especially helpful in providing information and context with which to make complex decisions (University of California, 2012).

Another approach is to engage in "staged" ACP. This recognizes that most young, healthy people need not make a decision at this moment about whether to be intubated or not, and asking them to do so—or even just including that question on a form—may be a disincentive to engaging in ACP at all. The "Respecting Choices" model endorses a staged approach, which begins with young, healthy people naming a health care agent and then offering some thoughts about what they might want in the event of a sudden neurologic injury (which is among the most likely events that would suddenly incapacitate them). As a patient ages and likely accumulates some health problems, more thoughtful conversation takes place about the level of care she wishes to receive (which might include discussion of CPR and intubation). Only as the patient approaches the end of life are specific steps (such as Do Not Attempt Resuscitation orders) actively considered (Gundersen Health System, 2017).

The staged approach underscores the need to revisit whatever ACP was done at an earlier time. Patients age, diseases develop, relationships change. Revisiting a prior AD allows the patient to either confirm that it still accurately reflects her wishes or to modify it accordingly (Hickman, Hammes, Moss, & Tolle, 2005).

A third approach involves shifting the focus from specific treatment decisions to what is important in life. Rather than completing a formal AD, then, a patient might write a letter to her physician or family, stressing what is most important to her as she potentially approaches death (Periyakoil, 2017). This is less threatening than addressing EOL treatment decisions and actually provides more substantive information. It may also prompt heartfelt conversations, which—as stated earlier—are more important than a piece of paper.

When the Patient Is Espousing Different Goals from the AD

The very purpose of a treatment directive is to determine what treatment a patient will (and will not) receive when she lacks sufficient DMC to decide for herself. When the patient is so ill that she is not able to voice any opinion about treatment, the results of the ACP process—which may involve a written AD in addition to direct expressions of goals and values to one's surrogate—are determinative. But on other occasions the patient may be able to express her wishes, which may conflict with those written in the AD. Of course, if she has sufficient DMC, she can override the AD. But assessing DMC is a subjective process (p. 58), and it may be unclear whether the patient has sufficient DMC to override the AD. What should the medical team do in those cases?

One possible scenario is a patient accepting a treatment—at a time of uncertain DMC—that she had previously refused in an AD. This is usually rather straightforward, as long as the treatment is one the medical team feels is reasonable or has even recommended. From a practical point of view, it is hard to imagine a medical team refusing to provide a potentially beneficial treatment that the patient is requesting, based on prior refusal in a written AD. The risk is too great that the patient may truly possess sufficient DMC to override the AD or may have changed her mind since the AD was completed, or—as in the case of the elderly woman who checked the DNI box—did not have a complete grasp of the clinical context when she completed the AD. Given that it is usually wiser, in times of uncertainty, to "do more rather than less" in order to preserve options, the prudent course of action in such cases is to provide the treatment, as the patient currently requests.

In some of these situations one might wonder if the problem may lie less with the patient's uncertain DMC than with the question that was posed to the patient. Admittedly, it is difficult to have a thoughtful conversation about treatment options with a patient in distress. But true informed consent requires that the patient be aware of the proposed plan and its alternatives, appreciate the consequences of her choice, and be able to reason from the question to the answer. When the clinical situation is critical, physicians may not take the time to express all relevant information, and the patient might not be able to process it if she did. Consider the example of a patient in respiratory distress, who is suffering from air hunger that can lead to desperation and extreme suffering. Such patients are often asked by the emergency response team, "Do you want us to put a tube down your throat to help you breathe?"

Given the circumstances, it is quite likely that the patient only hears the part about *help me breathe*. If so, then whatever consent to intubation she might subsequently express is both uninformed and incomplete. To make a thoughtful choice, the patient needs to be assured that her breathlessness will be treated, no matter what course of treatment she opts for. This may involve intubation and other LSMT, or opioids for dyspnea as part of a comfort-directed plan of care. While providing context and explaining both options can be challenging and time-consuming, it is necessary to ensure that the patient's true values are respected.

Viewed in this light, intubating a patient under these circumstances because she "requested it" is not an act of respect for informed consent. Rather, it is providing a partial picture and a limited array of options and then proceeding with an intervention the patient may not want. It also creates additional complexity further down the road, as most patients require significant sedation while on a ventilator. The chance of subsequently restoring the patient's DMC—especially after several days in the ICU—is quite low, and thus the initial conversation where the patient "consented" to intubation might inappropriately influence subsequent decision-making as well.

Here it is imperative to frame the question in simple, understandable terms. An example might be: "I can see you're struggling to breathe, and we will definitely help you with that. One option is to put you on a breathing machine to keep you alive, and the other is to give you medicine to keep you comfortable, which means you will probably die." At least then, if the patient agrees to intubation, there is a stronger sense that it might be driven by the patient's goals and not by suffering and fear.

But what about the converse situation, when a patient is refusing a treatment that ACP evidence suggests she would have wanted to receive? A patient in respiratory distress might *refuse* to be intubated, even though she had previously said she wanted treatment that had a reasonable chance of keeping her alive. Whereas in the earlier case it would have felt wrong to withhold LSMT that the patient was requesting—regardless of her level of DMC—in this case it may feel parentalistic to proceed, given the patient's objections. Yet if the patient is in extremis, it is quite likely that her DMC is compromised, at least to some degree. She may not comprehend the seriousness of her condition and thus fail to appreciate that respect for her refusal would likely lead to her death. She might also *over*estimate the seriousness of her condition and not understand that LSMT could provide significant benefit.

The operative question here is whether she possesses sufficient DMC, for if she does, then her refusal must be respected (*In re Quinlan*, 1976). But if she does not—and thus cannot understand relevant information and grasp the implications of her refusal—then it would be a tragedy to allow a patient to die over a misunderstanding.

Determining whether she has sufficient DMC may be challenging, however, especially in a critical situation. As noted already, DMC is decision-dependent (p. 55), and thus there exists a vast gray area between the extremes of perfectly intact DMC on the one hand and clearly completely absent DMC (i.e., unconsciousness) on the other. The gravity of the decision demands a significant degree of DMC to refuse LSMT.

Several steps can be taken in such a situation. The first is to explore with the patient her reasons for refusing the treatment. DMC sufficient to refuse LSMT requires not only an expression of refusal but also evidence of understanding, appreciation, and reasoning. Reframing the decision from various angles (both positive and negative) can also clarify whether the patient is truly grasping the decision. Referencing the AD directly—and inquiring whether the patient recalls completing it and can articulate her reasons for deviating from it—can be helpful.

One might also review in detail the written AD, to assess the degree of nuance and understanding expressed in it. A handwritten explanation for why a patient was willing to undergo mechanical ventilation would carry far more weight than merely checking the "Intubate" box. If present, friends and family may be able to describe the patient's goals and values and how these might relate to the decision at hand. They might also be able to comment on whether the patient's goals and values had changed since the completion of the document. Here it is important to note that some treatment wishes do tend to remain stable over time, especially in outpatients with serious illness (as opposed to healthy older adults), patients who had engaged in ACP, and those who had made requests to forgo rather than receive treatment (Auriemma et al., 2014).

If uncertainty remains, the physician may be forced to balance the level of confidence in the veracity and stability of the wishes expressed in advance, with the perceived extent of DMC related to the present refusal. Absent confidence that the patient has changed her mind, it may be more prudent to institute LSMT (including intubation), in order to preserve options. This does not commit the patient to ongoing burdensome treatment, of course, given the equivalence of withdrawing and withholding (p. 156). Hopefully more time will yield additional information that will either confirm the original decision or provide justification for a shift in goals.

Proxy Directives

Even with improvements in treatment directive forms and processes, the challenge of how to apply prior statements to specific situations remains. Recognizing this, there has been a subsequent shift of emphasis from treatment directives to *proxy* directives, whereby a specific person is identified as the patient's health care agent. (Some forms combine both treatment and proxy elements; Aging with Dignity, 2015). States began sanctioning the role of the DPA-HC in the 1980s and 1990s, and currently every state has a health care proxy statute as part of its state law (Sabatino, 2010).[5] The advantage of a proxy directive over a treatment directive is that the agent is theoretically able to apply the incapacitated patient's goals and values to specific situations that could not be foreseen in advance (Messinger-Rapport, Baum, & Smith, 2009).

This logically raises the question of who to choose as one's agent and how to best prepare that person to make decisions. As for the first question, some patients assume that the person closest to them (often their spouse) would be the optimal surrogate decision-maker. While it is true that spouse proxies tend to be more accurate in their predictions of patient wishes than patients' children (Parks et al., 2011), there is also risk involved. Asking someone to serve as one's agent is not an honor; it is a responsibility, and one that may require the agent to authorize a course of action that is directly contrary to the agent's personal goals and feelings (as in the case of forgoing LSMT for the person the agent loves most in the world). The alternative is the agent *not* authorizing that course of action, which is all too common and may lead to unnecessary treatment (and suffering) for the patient. In the end, it may be wiser to name someone slightly less intimately involved as one's agent, thus allowing the spouse to be supportive—and attend to his own grief—rather than saddle him with the burden of decision-making.

Whether by following this counsel—or in situations where there is not a spouse—a patient may not be able to identify one person who is clearly the best agent. So rather than choose one potential agent over another, she may be tempted to name "co-agents" (i.e., of equivalent standing rather than one being primary, the next being secondary, etc.). This often occurs when the patient has multiple adult children and does not want to choose between them for fear of showing favoritism.

5. Here it is important to distinguish the DPA-HC from a standard "durable power of attorney," which confers only the authority for financial decision-making.

This, too, can be unwise. An agent is not the person the patient loves most in the world; rather, he should be the person the patient trusts to be able to fulfill an extremely difficult role, without burdening that person too greatly. Naming co-agents simply "kicks the can down the road," creating fertile ground for disagreement and conflict. It is much better to order the agents in terms of priority and to notify them ahead of time of that order and the reason for it so that no one is offended.

Whoever the patient appoints as her agent, it is crucial to ensure that that person is both willing and *able* to perform the responsibilities of a health care agent (Aulisio, 2016). This involves reviewing those responsibilities, clarifying that the agent is willing to make hard decisions if necessary, and also specifying what degree of latitude (if any) the patient would want the agent to use in potentially deviating from a previously agreed-upon plan, given unanticipated clinical situations (Sulmasy et al., 2007). Addressing these topics in advance can help prevent family conflict—which has been associated with decreased surrogate accuracy (Parks et al., 2011)—at the time a decision is necessary.

In addition to empowering the agent with sufficient knowledge about the patient's values to fulfill that role, the patient may also be concerned about the surrogate's well-being, given the increased incidence of anxiety, depression, and posttraumatic stress disorder in that population (p. 65). One way to address this—which patients engaged in ACP should be informed of—is to "forgive" one's agent in advance for not being sure he is doing (or did) the right thing. That very uncertainty drives agents not only to authorize maximal treatment even when the patient likely would not seek it but also saddles them with doubt and grief long into the future. By acknowledging how impossible the role of agent is, expressing gratitude for the agent's willingness to serve, and being clear that all one expects is that the agent do his best, hopefully there will be less psychological impact on the agent. An example of such a sentiment is included in Figure 3.2.

POLST Paradigm

One of the best thing about ADs is that they are so varied and nuanced. They can include treatment specifications and/or naming an agent, with a free text elaboration on personal goals and check boxes for specific authorizations or refusals. However, such nuance also prevents the values and priorities described in them from being applied in real time, especially in emergent situations.

Consider, for example, a paramedic responding to a 911 call and finding a patient unresponsive and in full arrest. Even if—and it is a big *if*—the patient had previously completed an AD and it is available for review, the document may well be several pages long. It could contain vague directives based on the patient's baseline health ("terminal condition") or prognosis with treatment ("no reasonable probability of recovery"), which are unknowable without a thoughtful review of the patient's history and assessment of her current condition. Even if these were possible in real time, they are outside the scope of practice of most first responders.

It is precisely for this reason that first responders are generally instructed to provide maximal treatment, even in the presence of an AD (Sosna, 1998). The document is certainly relevant and important, but it can only be appropriately assessed and implemented

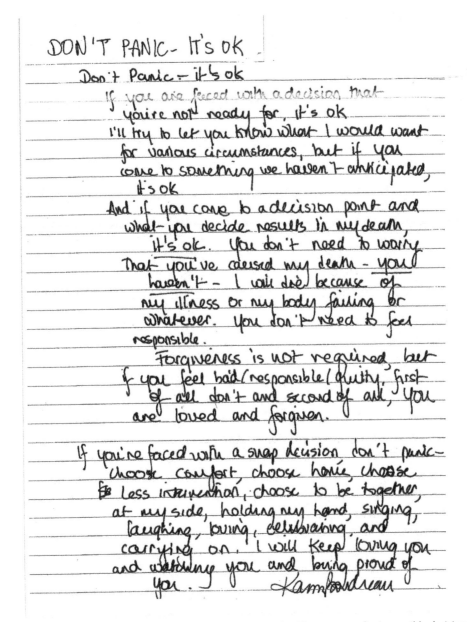

DON'T PANIC- It's OK

Don't Panic — it's ok
If you are faced with a decision that you're not ready for, it's ok
I'll try to let you know what I would want for various circumstances, but if you come to something we haven't anticipated, it's ok
And if you come to a decision point and what you decide results in my death, it's ok. You don't need to worry that you've caused my death — you haven't — I will die because of my illness or my body failing or whatever. You don't need to feel responsible.
Forgiveness is not required, but if you feel bad/responsible/guilty, first of all don't and second of all, you are loved and forgiven.

If you're faced with a snap decision don't panic—choose comfort, choose home, choose less intervention, choose to be together, at my side, holding my hand, singing, laughing, loving, celebrating, and carrying on. I will keep loving you and watching you and being proud of you. Kam Boudreau

FIGURE 3.2 An example of preemptively "forgiving" one's health care agent for impossible decisions he will have to make (Boudreau, 2012)

when the patient's medical history, condition, and prognosis are clarified by a professional such as a physician.

So what should a patient do if she does not wish to receive CPR (or other emergent interventions) and an AD is not a sufficient step to assure this? For a long time, the advice many physicians gave was simply not to call 911, believing that once emergency medical services (EMS) was activated, maximal treatment would have to be provided.[6]

6. This advice would be reasonable if the patient were enrolled in hospice—which can provide necessary symptom management—but otherwise may lead to uncontrolled symptoms as the price paid for avoiding automatic CPR.

While effective at preventing CPR, this approach also deprived patients of potentially beneficial nonresuscitative interventions, such as supplemental oxygen, analgesia, and hospital transport.

Recognizing this dilemma, out-of-hospital Do Not Attempt Resuscitation (DNAR) orders were initiated, which provide clear and explicit instructions to not intervene for a patient who is pulseless and not breathing. These orders, however, were rarely standardized in format and often failed to meet statutory requirements in terms of patient identification and informed consent. Faced with these variables, some EMS squads may adopt an approach of doing more rather than less—in other words, disregarding the out-of-hospital DNAR order too—trusting that the patient's true wishes could be sorted out at the hospital (if the patient survived to that point).

The POLST (Physician Orders for Life Sustaining Treatment) paradigm addresses this dilemma. Developed in Oregon in the 1990s (Tolle, Tilden, Nelson, & Dunn, 1998), this paradigm—which in various states is also known as MOLST ("medical" orders) or COLST ("clinician" orders), or POST and MOST referring to "scope of treatment"—codifies treatment preferences in a standardized clinician order that meets all statutory requirements. As such, it is generally binding on all medical providers, including EMS personnel who are not required to call "medical control" to confirm or review treatment paradigms.[7]

The standard POLST form includes not only a directive about resuscitative interventions in the context of full arrest (i.e., "full code" vs. DNAR) but also orders for situations short of full arrest (Figure 3.3). These include the use of mechanical ventilation, antibiotics, medically administered nutrition and hydration (MANH), and transport to the hospital for any reason other than symptom management. There is also a section for describing treatment goals, which generally offers choices of maximal, comfort only, and a middle ground based on burdens and benefits. Admittedly, on some forms this seems to be something of an afterthought, with the primary emphasis on interventions rather than goals.

Most states require POLST forms to be reviewed on a regular basis, especially when the patient's condition or level of care changes. POLST forms have the added advantage of being "transportable," ideally accompanying the patient from home to hospital to nursing home.

POLST forms seem to be effective. In one study, compared to patients without a POLST form, those who had one were significantly more likely to have treatment preferences beyond CPR specified. Those with a POLST form specifying only comfort measures received fewer medical interventions than those with a traditional DNAR order, reflecting the fact that a DNAR order is only relevant in situations of full arrest (Hickman et al., 2010).

7. In some states the form is merely "permissive," and thus medical professionals "may" follow its instructions but are not bound to (Iowa Healthcare Collaborative, 2017).

At the same time, the POLST is a relatively new innovation. As such, there is still insufficient evidence that completed forms reflect the true goals of the patient or her surrogate (Hickman, Keevern, & Hammes, 2015). Even when the form does reflect the patient's actual goals, physicians may not be sure how to interpret the form and implement appropriate treatments (Mirarchi et al., 2015). There are also reports of the certain aspects

---

HIPAA PERMITS DISCLOSURE OF POLST TO OTHER HEALTH CARE PROVIDERS AS NECESSARY

Physician Orders for Life-Sustaining Treatment (POLST)

Last Name - First Name - Middle Name or Initial

Date of Birth   Last 4 #SSN (optional)

____ ____ ____   ____ ____ ____

FIRST follow these orders, **THEN** contact physician, nurse practitioner or PA-C. The POLST is a set of medical orders intended to guide medical treatment based on a person's current medical condition and goals. Any section not completed implies full treatment for that section. Completing a POLST form is always voluntary. Everyone shall be treated with dignity and respect.

Medical Conditions/Patient Goals:

Agency Info/Sticker

A
Check One

CARDIOPULMONARY RESUSCITATION (CPR): <u>Person has no pulse and is not breathing.</u>
When not in cardiopulmonary arrest, go to part B.

☐ **Attempt Resuscitation/CPR**

☐ **Do Not Attempt Resuscitation/DNAR (Allow Natural Death)**
Choosing DNAR will include appropriate comfort measures.

B
Check One

MEDICAL INTERVENTIONS: <u>Person has pulse and/or is breathing.</u>

☐ **FULL TREATMENT** - primary goal of prolonging life by all medically effective means.
Includes care described below. Use intubation, advanced airway interventions, mechanical ventilation and cardioversion as indicated. **Transfer** to hospital if indicated. Includes intensive care.

☐ **SELECTIVE TREATMENT** - goal of treating medical conditions while avoiding burdensome measures.
Includes care described below. Use medical treatment, IV fluids and cardiac monitor as indicated. Do not intubate. May use less invasive airway support (e.g. CPAP, BiPAP). **Transfer** to hospital if indicated. Avoid intensive care if possible.

☐ **COMFORT-FOCUSED TREATMENT** - primary goal of maximizing comfort.
Relieve pain and suffering with medication by any route as needed. Use oxygen, oral suction and manual treatment of airway obstruction as needed for comfort. **Patient prefers no hospital transfer:** EMS consider contacting medical control to determine if transport is indicated to provide adequate comfort.

Additional Orders: (e.g. dialysis, etc.) _____

C

SIGNATURES: <u>The signatures below verify that these orders are consistent with the patient's medical condition, known preferences and best known information. If signed by a surrogate, the patient must be decisionally incapacitated and the person signing is the legal surrogate.</u>

Discussed with:	PRINT — Physician/ARNP/PA-C Name	Phone Number
☐ Patient ☐ Parent of Minor ☐ Guardian with Health Care Authority ☐ Spouse/Other as authorized by RCW 7.70.065 ☐ Health Care Agent (DPOAHC)	✗ Physician/ARNP/PA-C Signature *(mandatory)*	Date *(mandatory)*
PRINT — Patient or Legal Surrogate Name		Phone Number
✗ Patient or Legal Surrogate Signature *(mandatory)*		Date *(mandatory)*

Person has: ☐ Health Care Directive (living will) ☐ Durable Power of Attorney for Health Care

Encourage all advance care planning documents to accompany POLST

SEND ORIGINAL FORM WITH PERSON WHENEVER TRANSFERRED OR DISCHARGED

Revised 8/2017   Photocopies and faxes of signed POLST forms are legal and valid. May make copies for records.
For more information on POLST visit www.wsma.org/polst.

 WashingtonState Medical Association
Physician Driven Patient Focused

Washington State Department of Health

See back of form for non-emergency preferences ▶

FIGURE 3.3 Sample POLST form (Washington State Medical Association, 2014)

HIPAA PERMITS DISCLOSURE OF POLST TO OTHER HEALTH CARE PROVIDERS AS NECESSARY

Patient and Additional Contact Information (if any)

Patient Name (last, first, middle)	Date of Birth	Phone Number
Name of Guardian, Surrogate or other Contact Person	Relationship	Phone Number

D NON-EMERGENCY MEDICAL TREATMENT PREFERENCES

ANTIBIOTICS:
- ☐ Use antibiotics for prolongation of life.
- ☐ Do not use antibiotics except when needed for symptom management.

MEDICALLY ASSISTED NUTRITION:
Always offer food and liquids by mouth if feasible.
- ☐ No medically assisted nutrition by tube.

- ☐ Trial period of medically assisted nutrition by tube.
  (Goal: _____)
- ☐ Long-term medically assisted nutrition by tube.

ADDITIONAL ORDERS: (e.g. dialysis, blood products, implanted cardiac devices, etc. Attach additional orders if necessary.)

✗ Physician/ARNP/PA-C Signature	Date
✗ Patient or Legal Surrogate Signature	Date

DIRECTIONS FOR HEALTH CARE PROFESSIONALS

Completing POLST

- Completing a POLST form is always voluntary.
- Treatment choices documented on this form should be the result of shared decision-making by an individual or their surrogate and medical provider based on the person's preferences and medical condition.
- POLST must be signed by a physician/ARNP/PA-C and patient, or their surrogate, to be valid. Verbal orders are acceptable with follow-up signature by physician/ARNP/PA-C in accordance with facility/community policy.

Using POLST

Any incomplete section of POLST implies full treatment for that section.

This POLST is valid in all care settings including hospitals until replaced by new physician's orders.

The POLST is a set of medical orders. The most recent POLST replaces all previous orders.

The POLST does not replace an advance directive. An advance directive is encouraged for all competent adults regardless of their health status. An advance directive allows a person to document in detail his/her future health care instructions and/or name a surrogate decision maker to speak on his/her behalf. When available, all documents should be reviewed to ensure consistency, and the forms updated appropriately to resolve any conflicts.

NOTE: A person with capacity may always consent to or refuse medical care or interventions, regardless of information represented on any document, including this one.

SECTIONS A AND B:

- No defibrillator should be used on a person who has chosen "Do Not Attempt Resuscitation."
- When comfort cannot be achieved in the current setting, the person should be transferred to a setting able to provide comfort (e.g., treatment of a hip fracture).
- An IV medication to enhance comfort may be appropriate for a person who has chosen "Comfort-Focused Treatment."
- Treatment of dehydration is a measure which may prolong life. A person who desires IV fluids should indicate "Selective" or "Full Treatment."

SECTION D:

- Oral fluids and nutrition must always be offered if medically feasible.

Reviewing POLST

This POLST should be reviewed periodically whenever:
(1) The person is transferred from one care setting or care level to another, or
(2) There is a substantial change in the person's health status, or
(3) The person's treatment preferences change.

To void this form, draw line through "Physician Orders" and write "VOID" in large letters. Any changes require a new POLST.

Review of this POLST Form

Review Date	Reviewer	Location of Review	Review Outcome
			☐ No Change ☐ Form Voided ☐ New form completed
			☐ No Change ☐ Form Voided ☐ New form completed

SEND ORIGINAL FORM WITH PERSON WHENEVER TRANSFERRED OR DISCHARGED

Photocopies and faxes of signed POLST forms are legal and valid. May make copies for records.   **OVER ▶**
For more information on POLST visit www.wsma.org/polst.

FIGURE 3.3 Continued

of POLST forms—specifically related to antibiotics or MANH—not being followed by medical staff (Hickman et al., 2011).

If nuance is the best and worst thing about an AD, then rigid clarity is the best and worst thing about a POLST, which permits no exceptions to the treatments authorized or withheld. A physician should be very clear that a patient would not want a given procedure under any circumstance before completing a POLST form on her behalf. POLST forms are, therefore, generally reserved for patients with advanced illness (Figure 3.4). A POLST form is clearly not a replacement for an AD, which permits a level of personal expression and nuance not available in a medical order (Moore, Rubin, & Halpern, 2016).

In determining the proper role of each document in ACP, it can be helpful to focus on the word *if*. If in the process of exploring a patient's goals and identifying treatment preferences, the patient uses the word *if*—as in, "If I'm going to die anyway, I don't want CPR"—then that patient needs an AD. But should the patient not use the word *if* in relationship to a procedure—as in, "I never want CPR under any circumstance"—then she needs a POLST as well as an AD.

Despite its documented effectiveness, the POLST paradigm has not been universally embraced, primarily for moral/religious—rather than clinical—reasons. The Catholic Medical Association (CMA), in particular, has expressed several concerns (Brugger et al., 2013). One centers on the lack of any requirement that a patient be terminally ill before having a POLST form completed, since CMA deems such a diagnosis to be a moral requirement for any limitation of LSMT. By considering specific treatments without regard to prognosis or context, the form may not respect the distinction between ordinary (or proportionate) and extraordinary (or disproportionate) treatment (p. 494). This has prompted concerns that the form could be used "as a form of assisted suicide or euthanasia" (Minnesota Catholic Conference, 2013).

In addition, the CMA takes a conservative view of the Ethical and Religious Directives (ERDs) of the Catholic Church, whereby provision of MANH is generally

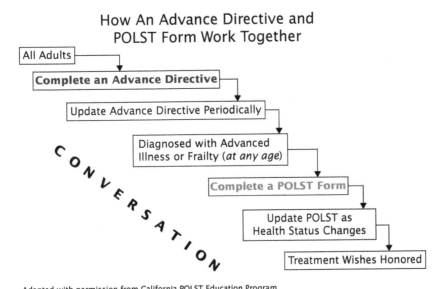

Adapted with permission from California POLST Education Program
©January 2010 Coalition for Compassionate Care of California

FIGURE 3.4 Synergistic roles of the advance directive and POLST form (National POLST Paradigm, 2017)

viewed as an ethical obligation (United States Conference of Catholic Bishops, 2009). The fact that POLST forms specifically authorize the forgoing of MANH even when the patient may not qualify under the exceptions set forth in the ERDs[8] is viewed as problematic, especially since it is a medical order that generally is binding on all medical personnel. Some local Catholic groups have extended their opposition to the POLST to the point of calling into question ACP in general. For example, the Minnesota Catholic Conference (2013) has asserted that "it is difficult to determine in advance whether specific medical treatments will be absolutely necessary or optional."

Based on these concerns, the CMA recommends that Catholic health care facilities—which care for one-sixth of hospitalized patients in the United States (Filteau, 2010)—"not accept POLST forms and decline to participate in the POLST paradigm" (Brugger et al., 2013). This is unfortunate, given the efficacy of the POLST form in preventing unwanted treatments. CMA recommendations to instead rely on surrogate decision-makers are not unreasonable but tend to overlook the inherent ambiguity of the surrogate decision-making process. More than that, reverting back to ADs as the only vehicle for ACP threatens a return to the "don't call 911" days, for patients who do not wish to receive CPR.

In the end, the POLST is a form like any other: full of potential but dependent on proper execution to achieve its aims and avoid abuses. Rather than fight to abolish it, a more thoughtful approach would be to provide spiritual guidance for faithful Catholics as to how to use it appropriately, in light of Church teaching (p. 494). Even if someone who is not imminently dying supposedly "should not" use the form, this does not mean that patients who *are* imminently dying should be deprived of its benefit. And advising Catholic hospitals to not recognize the form runs the risk of discriminating against the many non-Catholic patients who use these facilities.

Prognostication

The role of prognostication in medicine is . . . multifarious. Like prophecy, prognostication affects what people feel, think and do, and what happens as a result. Like prophecy, it addresses issues of meaning and explanation: it seeks order in apparent randomness, good in seeming evil, and hope in inevitable death. The uncertainty and gravity of the future in patients who are suffering from life-threatening illness heighten the need for prognosis, but have on balance militated toward its avoidance. The balance might beneficially be shifted. For although physicians avoid prognostication, they are nevertheless called to it. (Christakis, 1999)

Hippocrates was very clear: physicians have a duty to prognosticate (Hippocrates & Ducachet, 1819). For most of the history of Western medicine, diagnosis, prognosis, and treatment were acknowledged as the three sacred tasks of the physician, with medical

---

8. Specifically, that MANH would not prolong life and where it would be excessively burdensome.

textbooks devoting roughly equal attention to each (Iwashyna & Christakis, 1998). But over the course of the twentieth century—as formerly fatal illnesses such as pneumonia and other infectious diseases began to be cured—prognostication received less attention. With the rise of the "technological imperative" (p. 6), medicine's emphasis came to be on curing and prolonging, not predicting and preparing.

This began to change at the end of century, as it became clear(er) that for all the amazing technological innovations that were available, death was ultimately inevitable. Indeed, as the time course of chronic illness (as well as hospitalization) lengthened, greater emphasis was placed on predicting just how long life could be sustained. With the establishment of the Medicare Hospice Benefit in 1982, prognosis—in this case, death within six months if the disease ran its natural course—for the first time became a factor in satisfying a regulatory requirement.

Prognostication has particular significance in palliative medicine, beyond a specified time frame for admission to hospice. The question is not only whether a patient qualifies for hospice but how to equip the patient to handle the realization that she is dying, as well as to empower her to live fully in whatever time she has left. This impacts long-term dreams and short-term goals, as patients reprioritize in order to make sure they do what is most important to them before they die (or they become too ill to participate in certain activities).

With regard to hospice specifically, the question is not only whether but also *when*. The median time of hospice enrollment is currently only seventeen days and is trending downward. Over one-third of patients are admitted in the last week of life (National Hospice and Palliative Care Organization, 2015). While it is good that these patients received some hospice care, they—and their families—do not benefit nearly as much as they could have if hospice had been presented as an option sooner.

Prognosis is obviously a clinical skill (both in discernment and communication), and it is also an ethical obligation. Respect for autonomy demands that physicians provide patients with relevant information—even if they have not explicitly asked for it—but refrain from burdening them with information they do not want. Prognosis is central to patient empowerment, because a patient cannot make informed decisions that reflect her values unless she understands what the future might bring, to the extent that this is known.

There are three basic components to prognostication: accurately determining a prognosis, communicating it to the patient, and making decisions based on it.

Accuracy

Prognostication is a complex task, and regrettably physicians receive relatively little training in it (Christakis & Iwashyna, 1998). Not surprisingly, then, they are not very good at it, at least in terms of specifics. While physicians are rather adept at determining *whether* a patient is dying or not, they struggle mightily with determining when this will happen (Glare et al., 2003).

This came to public attention through the seminal work of Nicholas Christakis. He and his colleagues identified hospice patients—who, by legal requirement, must have a life expectancy of six months or less—and asked their physicians to predict how long they would live. Then he compared the prediction to reality, ultimately discovering that while some physicians underestimated how long a patient would love, the majority significantly *over*estimated. In fact, on average, physicians overestimated by a factor of 5 how long a patient would live. Put somewhat simplistically, a patient could take her physician's survival prediction, divide by five, and arrive at a reasonable approximation of her life expectancy. Not only that, but physicians would frequently add an "optimistic premium" to their prediction, further distancing the patient from her actual prognosis (Christakis & Iwashyna, 1998).

Certain correlations were identified in the study. Less experienced physicians showed diminished prognostic accuracy, likely due to limited perspective. At the same time, longer duration of the physician-patient relationship led to a greater tendency to overestimate prognosis. From a human standpoint, this is easy to understand: we do not want to think about something bad happening to someone we care about. If nothing else, the study highlighted the extremely human and relational aspect to determining prognosis.

Of note, physicians shared more pessimistic outlooks about their patients with other physicians (Iwashyna & Christakis, 1998). This raises the possibility that they were inappropriately optimistic with patients in order to preserve "hope." Alternatively, they may have been unduly pessimistic—relative to what they really thought—with other professionals in order to obtain certain services (such as hospice) for the patient in question.

This documented unreliability in prognostication has prompted additional research in this area. Palliative care, in particular, has seen an explicit emphasis on empirical research to identify beneficial interventions and provide sufficient context for patients to make decisions (Goldstein & Morrison, 2013). Prognostic tools—such as the Advanced Dementia Prognostic Tool (Mitchell, Miller, Teno, Davis, & Shaffer, 2010) and the Seattle Heart Failure Model (Vakil et al., 2015)—have been developed to guide physicians and minimize individual variation. To make these more accessible in clinical practice, online calculators have been also been developed (Yourman, Lee, Schonberg, Widera, & Smith, 2012).

With the wide variety of conditions that palliative medicine clinicians encounter, it can be difficult to keep up with the latest research on outcomes and prognoses. Clinicians are often forced to rely on the predictions of specialists in the patient's particular disease, who in turn may not be optimally trained in prognostication (or willing to share their honest opinion even if they are). For these and other reasons, palliative care clinicians often rely on functional measures that span disease categories for prognostication. One of the most commonly used is the Palliative Performance Scale (PPS), a modification of the Karnofsky Performance Scale that includes five domains on a scale of 1 to 100 assessed by an observer: ambulation, activity and evidence of disease, self-care, intake, and level of consciousness (Anderson, Downing, Hill, Casorso, & Lerch, 1996). Studies in various contexts have shown that a score of <30 indicates a median survival of less than one week and 30 to 50 a median survival of less than one month (Virik & Glare, 2002). While not predictive with specificity beyond this, the PPS can at least identify those patients at high risk of imminent death.

Not all clinicians are aware of these tools, however. Even if they are, it may still be difficult to recognize and acknowledge that a patient one deeply cares for has a very limited life expectancy. To make such a statement requires an active prediction, and communicating it to the patient sets into motion a complex and deeply felt series of emotional (and practical) events, as the patient and her family come to grips with the prognosis and its implications.

Because of these persistent barriers to prognostication, the "surprise question" is especially helpful. In several studies, physicians were asked of their seriously ill patients, "Would you be surprised if this patient died in the next twelve months?" A reply of "No" identified those patients at significantly higher risk of dying within the next year. Studies have shown utility for patients on dialysis (Moss et al., 2010), with advanced cancer (Moroni et al., 2014), in primary care (Lakin et al., 2016), and with acute surgical conditions (Lilley et al., 2016). Variations of the surprise question have also shown utility in predicting seven-day and thirty-day mortality (Hamano et al., 2015).

The surprise question is not perfect. In one study, 20% of the patients for whom physicians answered "No" survived for more than one year, and 30% of patients for whom physicians answered "Yes" surprised respondents by dying within that time frame (Moroni et al., 2014). While not foolproof, this question can help identify patients at *increased risk* of death, prompting more intensive ACP and perhaps even hospice referral.

Communication

Even when a patient's prognosis is known with some degree of certainty, the question remains of how—or even *if*—to communicate this to her. As noted, for most of the history of Western medicine parentalism was the prevailing model. Physicians not only felt it was permissible to protect patients from "gloomy prognostications" (p. 4), but they felt it was their *duty* to engage in such "beneficent deception." If a patient was going to die, why make her last days especially sad by burdening her with the knowledge that the end of her life was approaching?

Societal expectations and professional codes have shifted over time, such that disclosure is now the norm (Novack et al., 1979). In addition to valuing the truth, communication of prognosis (to the degree that it is understood) is a component of trust within the patient-carer relationship. And from a purely practical point of view, patients need to understand their current condition—and the implication of various choices—in order to make a choice that reflects their values (Randall & Downie, 1999).

Studies have shown that most cancer patients, for instance, want information about their prognosis, whether it is good or bad (Butow, Dowsett, Hagerty, & Tattersall, 2002).

This is not universal, however. In one study, most patients wanted physicians to initiate a conversation about prognosis, while one-quarter wanted physicians to respond only when asked and one-tenth did not wish to discuss survival at all (Hagerty et al., 2004). Certain trends have been observed: women tend to want more information than men do and younger people more than older people (Fallowfield, Jenkins, & Beveridge, 2002).

The first step, then, in communicating prognosis is determining how much a patient really wants to know (Hancock et al., 2007). Open-ended questions that normalize different approaches may be helpful here. For instance, the physician might say, "Some patients in your situation want to know all the data, and others prefer to focus on the big picture. I want to provide information that will be the most helpful to you." This is an especially important preliminary question, because studies have shown that excessive attention to detail may cause patients to lose the "gist" of the overall situation (Fagerlin, Zikmund-Fisher, & Ubel, 2011). Engaging in this process not only shows respect for the patient's autonomy, but it can also serve to deepen the physician-patient relationship (Back & Arnold, 2006a, 2006b).

This is not merely a question of how much information a patient wants to receive but also how she wants to receive it. Some patients opt to "get it all out" at one time, to avoid any subsequent surprises. Others prefer a staged disclosure, allowing time to process what they have been told. Often patients prefer to have loved ones present, both for emotional support as well as to serve as "added memory," in case parts of the conversation are unclear or subsequently forgotten.

Once it is determined how much information the patient wants to know—and how she wants to receive it—the physician can communicate that level of prognosis. This, however, is not as simple as merely conveying information. Whereas the physician possesses the relevant clinical knowledge and is ultimately tasked with offering specific treatments, the patient faces significant challenges. Depending on the time course of her disease, she may have less stamina than she once did. She may be emotionally exhausted from facing her own mortality, with all the concerns (spiritual, relational, financial) that come from that. All of these factors may negatively impact her DMC, thus making assimilating and applying information even more difficult (Randall & Downie, 1999). Not surprisingly, physicians tend to overestimate how much is understood by patients while simultaneously underestimating patients' prognostic needs (Beadle et al., 2004).

Especially when it comes to prognosis, unconscious bias can exert significant influence. As noted earlier (p. 60), framing a decision in terms of probability of survival leads to greater acceptance by patients than framing it in terms of death. Similarly, focusing on available treatments—what medicine can *do*—rather than prognosis can cause false optimism (The, Hak, Koeter, & van Der Wal, 2000). While potentially misleading, nevertheless this is often welcomed by patients, for very real and understandable human reasons. Studies have shown that patients rate their physician more positively when, for instance, they are led to believe chemotherapy is curative, even when it is not (Weeks et al., 2012).

When it comes to communicating prognosis, it is important for physicians to be clear about what they are actually saying, rather than hiding behind vague language. Euphemisms are often used, which could reflect genuine uncertainty as to the patient's prognosis. However, they may also reflect a human desire to not paint oneself into a corner of specific predictions. Among these euphemisms are "exceedingly low chance of success," "immeasurably low chance of working," and even "the odds of this working are close as you can get to zero without actually being zero." These phrases serve the dual purpose of generally communicating pessimism without making any firm prediction that may turn out to be inaccurate.

This is not to say that physicians should follow the lead of doctors on television who boldly proclaim that a patient has, for example, "six weeks to live." Prognostic tools such as the PPS are helpful in providing a median survival, but this is a population-level finding. By definition, a patient with a *median* life expectancy of one week has a fifty-fifty chance of surviving less than a week or more than a week. A representative study showed large individual variation, with 5% of the best prognosis group (expected to live "more than two months") dying in less than two weeks, and 10% of those expected to die in less than two weeks ultimately surviving for two months or more (Gwilliam et al., 2011).

But inability to predict with exactness does not mean that physicians should not provide the information that they do have in a way that is relevant and understandable to the patient. It is important to describe prognosis both in terms of death as well as survival, not being afraid to use "the D-word" (Brayne, 2010). Numerical estimates are helpful, given the ambiguity of some terms that are often used (such as "poor prognosis"). Consistent denominators should be employed, based on the patient's stated goals (Paling, 2003). For instance, if the patient's expressed goal is the ability to return home and live independently, survival alone (which includes patients who are extremely dependent on others) is not the appropriate metric by which to gauge treatments.

Throughout the process of communicating prognosis it is helpful to check in frequently with the patient—such as by employing the Ask-Tell-Ask technique (Evans, Tulsky, Back, & Arnold, 2006)—in order to ensure comprehension. Inviting the patient to rely on loved ones present for information recall may free the patient to react and respond to information in real time. And writing things down (ideally in a legible fashion) can provide reassurance and allow the patient to return to what the physician clearly expressed, rather than relying on her own recollection.

Application

The entire process of ACP depends on a realistic sense of one's prognosis. On the grander level, it is the basis of the "staged advance care planning" process, whereby young, healthy patients—who likely have many years to live—are not asked to focus on treatment decisions but rather on appointing a health care agent (p. 74). Once serious illness is a consideration, palliative care focuses on instilling "prognostic awareness" in patients and families, so that they can make decisions based on a realistic expectation of what the future will likely bring (Chen, Kuo, & Tang, 2017). How can a patient plan for the future, after all, if she has no idea what the future holds or how respective options will impact it?

The accuracy of prognostic information—and the manner in which it is presented—plays an extremely significant role in those decisions. Understandably, terminally ill cancer patients who are unduly optimistic about their survival prospects often request nonbeneficial, aggressive treatment (Weeks et al., 1998). Conversely, inappropriately negative perspectives on prognosis can lead to premature withdrawal (Holloway, Benesch, Burgin, & Zentner, 2005). Early recognition of prognosis is particularly helpful, as ACP conversations prior to the last thirty days of life lead to less aggressive treatment and increased likelihood of hospice enrollment (Mack et al., 2012).

Prognosis also affects the recommendations that physicians make. Depressed patients with a prognosis of days to weeks cannot wait for a selective serotonin reuptake inhibitor (such as Prozac) to work, but they might benefit from a psychostimulant. Certain interventional pain modalities—such as neurolytic nerve blocks—are only appropriate for patients with short life expectancies (Smith & Glare, 2016). And for patients with less than six months to live, statins generally provide no clinical benefit (Kutner et al., 2015) and can be discontinued.

It should be evident by this point that prognostication requires clinical acumen and experience to determine a time frame, as well as advanced communication skills in order to equip the patient with relevant knowledge. In many ways it is a lost art that is being rediscovered, precisely because patients need to understand what their future is likely to look like—in terms of duration and quality—in order to make fundamental decisions. It is precisely for this reason that expert prognostication is an ethical obligation for all clinicians, especially those practicing palliative care.

Summary Points

- Patients do not have the right to any treatment they request, but they do have the right to refuse any treatment they do not want (if they possess sufficient DMC).
- There are three elements of informed consent:
  1. The patient must be provided with sufficient information by which to make a decision.
  2. The decision be voluntary.
  3. The patient must have sufficient DMC to make that particular decision, which requires that the patient be able to
     a. Communicate a choice
     b. Understand relevant information
     c. Appreciate the consequences of a decision
     d. Manipulate information rationally

- Making a thoughtful recommendation, based on the patient's goals and values, is part of the informed consent process and not an infringement on patient autonomy.
- Given the high likelihood that a patient may at some point lose DMC, ACP is critically important. This is not merely a piece of paper; it is a process carried out over time, in consultation with one's physician and in conversation with loved ones.
- If a patient cannot make her own medical decisions, ideally a surrogate decision-maker would do so for her.
- Treatment directives can be ambiguous, and the accuracy of substituted judgment offered by surrogate decision-makers is not very high. This role also increases the risk of negative psychological outcomes.
- Best interests is the "third-best of three" paradigms for decision-making because it is so impersonal, and many patients prefer a blend of their previously stated wishes and what appears to be in their best interests (i.e., "substituted interests").
- When a supposedly incapacitated patient is espousing goals that contrast with her advance directive, generally more treatment is provided, rather than less.
  - If she is requesting more intensive treatment that could be of benefit, it is hard to imagine a clinician refusing the request based on an assessment of her capacity.
  - If she is refusing treatment she once expressed a willingness to receive, temporizing the situation by stabilizing her is often indicated to allow confirmation of her level of DMC.
- A POLST form does not replace an advance directive; rather, it supplements the AD by addressing specific situations where the patient is certain she would want no further treatment.
- Prognostication is an art in which physicians receive relatively little training, and thus survival predictions are often inaccurate (and generally overestimated). Newer tools are available to improve prognostic accuracy.
- Physicians have an ethical obligation to communicate prognosis to the extent the patient seeks it, framed from multiple perspectives to reduce unconscious bias.

References

Ackrivo, J., Horbowicz, K. J., Mordino, J., El Kherba, M., Ellingwood, J., Sloan, K., & Murphy, J. (2016). Successful implementation of an automated sedation vacation process in intensive care units. *Am J Med Qual, 31*(5), 463–469. doi:10.1177/1062860615593340

Aging with Dignity. (2015). Five wishes. Retrieved from https://www.agingwithdignity.org/five-wishes/about-five-wishes

American Bar Association. (1989). *Guardianship: An agenda for reform.* Washington, DC: Commission on the Mentally Disabled and Commission on Legal Problems of the Elderly, American Bar Association.

American Bar Association. (2004). Incapacitated and alone: Healthcare decision making for unbefriended older people. *Hum Rights, 31*(2), 20–23.

American Geriatrics Society Ethics Committee. (2015). American Geriatrics Society care of lesbian, gay, bisexual, and transgender older adults position statement: American Geriatrics Society Ethics Committee. *J Am Geriatr Soc, 63*(3), 423–426. doi:10.1111/jgs.13297

Anderson, F., Downing, G. M., Hill, J., Casorso, L., & Lerch, N. (1996). Palliative Performance Scale (PPS): A new tool. *J Palliat Care, 12*(1), 5–11.

Anstey, M. H., Adams, J. L., & McGlynn, E. A. (2015). Perceptions of the appropriateness of care in California adult intensive care units. *Crit Care, 19,* 51. doi:10.1186/s13054-015-0777-0

Aulisio, M. P. (2016). "So what you want us to do?" Patient's rights, unintended consequences, and the surrogate's role. In S. J. Youngner & R. M. Arnold (Eds.), *The Oxford handbook of ethics at the end of life* (pp. 27–41). New York: Oxford University Press.

Auriemma, C. L., Nguyen, C. A., Bronheim, R., Kent, S., Nadiger, S., Pardo, D., & Halpern, S. D. (2014). Stability of end-of-life preferences: A systematic review of the evidence. *JAMA Intern Med, 174*(7), 1085–1092. doi:10.1001/jamainternmed.2014.1183

Azoulay, E., Pochard, F., Kentish-Barnes, N., Chevret, S., Aboab, J., Adrie, C., . . . Group, F. S. (2005). Risk of post-traumatic stress symptoms in family members of intensive care unit patients. *Am J Respir Crit Care Med, 171*(9), 987–994. doi:10.1164/rccm.200409-1295OC

Back, A. L., & Arnold, R. M. (2006a). Discussing prognosis: "How much do you want to know?" Talking to patients who are prepared for explicit information. *J Clin Oncol, 24*(25), 4209–4213. doi:10.1200/JCO.2006.06.007

Back, A. L., & Arnold, R. M. (2006b). Discussing prognosis: "How much do you want to know?" Talking to patients who do not want information or who are ambivalent. *J Clin Oncol, 24*(25), 4214–4217. doi:10.1200/JCO.2006.06.008

Bandy, R., Sachs, G. A., Montz, K., Inger, L., Bandy, R. W., & Torke, A. M. (2014). Wishard Volunteer Advocates Program: An intervention for at-risk, incapacitated, unbefriended adults. *J Am Geriatr Soc, 62*(11), 2171–2179. doi:10.1111/jgs.13096

Beadle, G. F., Yates, P. M., Najman, J. M., Clavarino, A., Thomson, D., Williams, G., . . . Schlect, D. (2004). Beliefs and practices of patients with advanced cancer: Implications for communication. *Br J Cancer, 91*(2), 254–257. doi:10.1038/sj.bjc.6601950

Boudreau, K. (2012). Don't panic—it's OK. Retrieved from http://theconversationproject.org/wp-content/uploads/2012/08/KarenBoudreauLetter.pdf

Boyd, E. A., Lo, B., Evans, L. R., Malvar, G., Apatira, L., Luce, J. M., & White, D. B. (2010). "It's not just what the doctor tells me:" Factors that influence surrogate decision makers' perceptions of prognosis. *Crit Care Med, 38*(5), 1270–1275. doi:10.1097/CCM.0b013e3181d8a217

Braun, U. K., Beyth, R. J., Ford, M. E., & McCullough, L. B. (2008). Voices of African American, Caucasian, and Hispanic surrogates on the burdens of end-of-life decision making. *J Gen Intern Med, 23*(3), 267–274. doi:10.1007/s11606-007-0487-7

Brayne, S. (2010). *The d-word: Talking about dying: A guide for relatives, friends and carers.* London; New York: Continuum.

Brinkman-Stoppelenburg, A., Rietjens, J. A., & van der Heide, A. (2014). The effects of advance care planning on end-of-life care: A systematic review. *Palliat Med, 28*(8), 1000–1025. doi:10.1177/0269216314526272

Brugger, C., Breschi, L. C., Hart, E. M., Kummer, M., Lane, J. I., Morrow, P. T., . . . Marker, R. L. (2013). The POLST paradigm and form: Facts and analysis. *Linacre Q, 80*(2), 103–138. doi:10.1179/0024363913Z.00000000027

Brush, D. R., Rasinski, K. A., Hall, J. B., & Alexander, G. C. (2012). Recommendations to limit life support: A national survey of critical care physicians. *Am J Respir Crit Care Med, 186*(7), 633–639. doi:10.1164/rccm.201202-0354OC

Buchanan, A. (2004). Mental capacity, legal competence and consent to treatment. *J R Soc Med, 97*(9), 415–420. doi:10.1258/jrsm.97.9.41597/9/415

Buchanan, A. E., & Brock, D. W. (1989). *Deciding for others: The ethics of surrogate decisionmaking.* New York: Cambridge University Press.

Bullock, K. (2011). The influence of culture on end-of-life decision making. *J Soc Work End Life Palliat Care, 7*(1), 83–98. doi:10.1080/15524256.2011.548048

Butler, K. (2013). *Knocking on heaven's door: The path to a better way of death* (1st Scribner hardcover ed.). New York: Scribner.

Butow, P. N., Dowsett, S., Hagerty, R., & Tattersall, M. H. (2002). Communicating prognosis to patients with metastatic disease: What do they really want to know? *Support Care Cancer, 10*(2), 161–168. doi:10.1007/s005200100290

Chen, C. H., Kuo, S. C., & Tang, S. T. (2017). Current status of accurate prognostic awareness in advanced/terminally ill cancer patients: Systematic review and meta-regression analysis. *Palliat Med, 31*(5), 406–418. doi:10.1177/0269216316663976

Christakis, N. A. (1999). *Death foretold: Prophecy and prognosis in medical care.* Chicago: University of Chicago.

Christakis, N. A., & Iwashyna, T. J. (1998). Attitude and self-reported practice regarding prognostication in a national sample of internists. *Arch Intern Med, 158*(21), 2389–2395.

Cohen, A. B., Wright, M. S., Cooney, L. Jr., & Fried, T. (2015). Guardianship and end-of-life decision making. *JAMA Intern Med, 175*(10), 1687–1691. doi:10.1001/jamainternmed.2015.3956

Connor, D. M., Elkin, G. D., Lee, K., Thompson, V., & Whelan, H. (2016). The unbefriended patient: An exercise in ethical clinical reasoning. *J Gen Intern Med, 31*(1), 128–132. doi:10.1007/s11606-015-3522-0

Covinsky, K. E., Fuller, J. D., Yaffe, K., Johnston, C. B., Hamel, M. B., Lynn, J., . . . Phillips, R. S. (2000). Communication and decision making in seriously ill patients: Findings of the SUPPORT project. The Study to Understand Prognoses and Preferences for Outcomes and Risks of Treatments. *J Am Geriatr Soc, 48*(5 Suppl.), S187–S193.

Cruzan v. Director, Missouri Department of Health, 497 261 (S.Ct. 1990).

Curtis, J. R. (2007). Point: The ethics of unilateral "do not resuscitate" orders: The role of "informed assent." *Chest, 132*(3), 748–751; discussion 755–746. doi:10.1378/chest.07-0745

Curtis, J. R., & Isaac, M. (2010). What factors influence a family to support a decision withdrawing life support? In C. S. Deutschman & P. J. Neligan (Eds.), *Evidence-based practice of critical care* (pp. 633–638). Philadelphia, PA: Saunders/Elsevier.

Davidson, J. E., Powers, K., Hedayat, K. M., Tieszen, M., Kon, A. A., Shepard, E., . . Society of Critical Care Medicine American College of Critical Care Medicine Task Force. (2007). Clinical practice guidelines for support of the family in the patient-centered intensive care unit: American College of Critical Care Medicine Task Force 2004–2005. *Crit Care Med, 35*(2), 605–622. doi:10.1097/01.CCM.0000254067.14607.EB

DeMartino, E. S., Dudzinski, D. M., Doyle, C. K., Sperry, B. P., Gregory, S. E., Siegler, M., . . . Kramer, D. B. (2017). Who decides when a patient can't? Statutes on alternate decision makers. *N Engl J Med, 376*(15), 1478–1482. doi:10.1056/NEJMms1611497

Department of Health and Human Services. (2015). MLN matters: Advance care planning as an optional element of an Annual Wellness Visit (AWV). [Press release]. Retrieved from https://www.cms.gov/Outreach-and-Education/Medicare-Learning-Network-MLN/MLNMattersArticles/Downloads/MM9271.pdf

Department of Veterans Affairs. (2009). *Veterans Health Administration handbook.* Washington, DC: Department of Veterans Affairs.

Detering, K. M., Hancock, A. D., Reade, M. C., & Silvester, W. (2010). The impact of advance care planning on end of life care in elderly patients: Randomised controlled trial. *BMJ, 340*, c1345. doi:10.1136/bmj.c1345

Ditto, P. H., Jacobson, J. A., Smucker, W. D., Danks, J. H., & Fagerlin, A. (2006). Context changes choices: A prospective study of the effects of hospitalization on life-sustaining treatment preferences. *Med Decis Making, 26*(4), 313–322. doi:10.1177/0272989X06290494

Eddy, D. M. (1990). Clinical decision making: From theory to practice. Guidelines for policy statements: the explicit approach. *JAMA, 263*(16), 2239–2240, 2243.

Ely, E. W., Margolin, R., Francis, J., May, L., Truman, B., Dittus, R., . . . Inouye, S. K. (2001). Evaluation of delirium in critically ill patients: Validation of the Confusion Assessment Method for the Intensive Care Unit (CAM-ICU). *Crit Care Med, 29*(7), 1370–1379.

Emanuel, L. L., & Emanuel, E. J. (1989). The medical directive. A new comprehensive advance care document. *JAMA, 261*(22), 3288–3293.

Evans, N., Bausewein, C., Menaca, A., Andrew, E. V., Higginson, I. J., Harding, R., . . . Gysels, M. (2012). A critical review of advance directives in Germany: Attitudes, use and healthcare professionals' compliance. *Patient Educ Couns, 87*(3), 277–288. doi:10.1016/j.pec.2011.10.004

Evans, W. G., Tulsky, J. A., Back, A. L., & Arnold, R. M. (2006). Communication at times of transitions: How to help patients cope with loss and re-define hope. *Cancer J, 12*(5), 417–424.

Fagerlin, A., Ditto, P. H., Danks, J. H., Houts, R. M., & Smucker, W. D. (2001). Projection in surrogate decisions about life-sustaining medical treatments. *Health Psychol, 20*(3), 166–175.

Fagerlin, A., & Schneider, C. E. (2004). Enough. The failure of the living will. *Hastings Cent Rep, 34*(2), 30–42.

Fagerlin, A., Zikmund-Fisher, B. J., & Ubel, P. A. (2011). Helping patients decide: Ten steps to better risk communication. *J Natl Cancer Inst, 103*(19), 1436–1443. doi:10.1093/jnci/djr318

Fallowfield, L. J., Jenkins, V. A., & Beveridge, H. A. (2002). Truth may hurt but deceit hurts more: Communication in palliative care. *Palliat Med, 16*(4), 297–303.

Filteau, J. (2010, October 20). Catholic hospitals serve one in six patients in the United States. Retrieved from https://www.ncronline.org/news/catholic-hospitals-serve-one-six-patients-united-states

Fins, J. J. (1999). Commentary: From contract to covenant in advance care planning. *J Law Med Ethics, 27*(1), 46–51.

Fischer, G. S., Tulsky, J. A., Rose, M. R., Siminoff, L. A., & Arnold, R. M. (1998). Patient knowledge and physician predictions of treatment preferences after discussion of advance directives. *J Gen Intern Med, 13*(7), 447–454.

Foo, A. S., Lee, T. W., & Soh, C. R. (2012). Discrepancies in end-of-life decisions between elderly patients and their named surrogates. *Ann Acad Med Singapore, 41*(4), 141–153.

Franklin, B. (1735, February 4). Letter to the editor, *Pennsylvania Gazette.*

Gerteis, M. (1993). *Through the patient's eyes: Understanding and promoting patient-centered care* (1st ed.). San Francisco: Jossey-Bass.

Glare, P., Virik, K., Jones, M., Hudson, M., Eychmuller, S., Simes, J., & Christakis, N. (2003). A systematic review of physicians' survival predictions in terminally ill cancer patients. *BMJ, 327*(7408), 195–198. doi:10.1136/bmj.327.7408.195

Glavan, B. J., Engelberg, R. A., Downey, L., & Curtis, J. R. (2008). Using the medical record to evaluate the quality of end-of-life care in the intensive care unit. *Crit Care Med, 36*(4), 1138–1146. doi:10.1097/CCM.0b013e318168f301

Goldstein, N. E., & Morrison, R. S. (2013). *Evidence-based practice of palliative medicine.* Philadelphia: Elsevier/Saunders.

Gries, C. J., Curtis, J. R., Wall, R. J., & Engelberg, R. A. (2008). Family member satisfaction with end-of-life decision making in the ICU. *Chest, 133*(3), 704–712. doi:10.1378/chest.07-1773

Grisso, T., & Appelbaum, P. S. (1995). The MacArthur Treatment Competence Study. III: Abilities of patients to consent to psychiatric and medical treatments. *Law Hum Behav, 19*(2), 149–174.

Grisso, T., & Appelbaum, P. S. (1998). Abilities related to competence. In T. Grisso & P. S. Appelbaum (Eds.), *Assessing competence to consent to treatment: A guide for physicians and other health professionals* (pp. 31–59). New York: Oxford University Press.

Gundersen Health System. (2017). Respecting choices. Retrieved from http://www.gundersenhealth.org/respecting-choices/

Gwilliam, B., Keeley, V., Todd, C., Gittins, M., Roberts, C., Kelly, L., . . . Stone, P. C. (2011). Development of prognosis in palliative care study (PiPS) predictor models to improve prognostication in advanced cancer: Prospective cohort study. *BMJ, 343*, d4920. doi:10.1136/bmj.d4920

Ha, J. F., & Longnecker, N. (2010). Doctor-patient communication: A review. *Ochsner J, 10*(1), 38–43.

Hagerty, R. G., Butow, P. N., Ellis, P. A., Lobb, E. A., Pendlebury, S., Leighl, N., . . . Tattersall, M. H. (2004). Cancer patient preferences for communication of prognosis in the metastatic setting. *J Clin Oncol, 22*(9), 1721–1730. doi:10.1200/JCO.2004.04.095

Hamano, J., Morita, T., Inoue, S., Ikenaga, M., Matsumoto, Y., Sekine, R., . . . Kinoshita, H. (2015). Surprise questions for survival prediction in patients with advanced cancer: A multicenter prospective cohort study. *Oncologist, 20*(7), 839–844. doi:10.1634/theoncologist.2015-0015

Hammes, B. J., & Kane, R. S. (1998). CPR practices in Wisconsin long-term care facilities. *WMJ, 97*(1), 55–57.

Hancock, K., Clayton, J. M., Parker, S. M., Walder, S., Butow, P. N., Carrick, S., . . . Tattersall, M. H. (2007). Discrepant perceptions about end-of-life communication: A systematic review. *J Pain Symptom Manage, 34*(2), 190–200. doi:10.1016/j.jpainsymman.2006.11.009

Hardin, S. B., & Yusufaly, Y. A. (2004). Difficult end-of-life treatment decisions: Do other factors trump advance directives? *Arch Intern Med, 164*(14), 1531–1533. doi:10.1001/archinte.164.14.1531

Haward, M. F., Murphy, R. O., & Lorenz, J. M. (2008). Message framing and perinatal decisions. *Pediatrics, 122*(1), 109–118. doi:10.1542/peds.2007-0620

Hickman, S. E., Hammes, B. J., Moss, A. H., & Tolle, S. W. (2005). Hope for the future: Achieving the original intent of advance directives. *Hastings Cent Rep, Spec No*, S26–S30.

Hickman, S. E., Keevern, E., & Hammes, B. J. (2015). Use of the physician orders for life-sustaining treatment program in the clinical setting: A systematic review of the literature. *J Am Geriatr Soc, 63*(2), 341–350. doi:10.1111/jgs.13248

Hickman, S. E., Nelson, C. A., Moss, A. H., Tolle, S. W., Perrin, N. A., & Hammes, B. J. (2011). The consistency between treatments provided to nursing facility residents and orders on the physician orders for life-sustaining treatment form. *J Am Geriatr Soc, 59*(11), 2091–2099. doi:10.1111/j.1532-5415.2011.03656.x

Hickman, S. E., Nelson, C. A., Perrin, N. A., Moss, A. H., Hammes, B. J., & Tolle, S. W. (2010). A comparison of methods to communicate treatment preferences in nursing facilities: Traditional practices versus the physician orders for life-sustaining treatment program. *J Am Geriatr Soc, 58*(7), 1241–1248. doi:10.1111/j.1532-5415.2010.02955.x

Hines, S. C., Glover, J. J., Babrow, A. S., Holley, J. L., Badzek, L. A., & Moss, A. H. (2001). Improving advance care planning by accommodating family preferences. *J Palliat Med, 4*(4), 481–489. doi:10.1089/109662101753381629

Hippocrates, & Ducachet, H. W. (1819). *The prognostics and crises of Hippocrates*. New York: J. Eastburn and Co.

Hirschman, K. B., Kapo, J. M., & Karlawish, J. H. (2006). Why doesn't a family member of a person with advanced dementia use a substituted judgment when making a decision for that person? *Am J Geriatr Psychiatry, 14*(8), 659–667. doi:10.1097/01.JGP.0000203179.94036.69

Holloway, R. G., Benesch, C. G., Burgin, W. S., & Zentner, J. B. (2005). Prognosis and decision making in severe stroke. *JAMA, 294*(6), 725–733. doi:10.1001/jama.294.6.725

Hsu-Kim, C., Friedman, T., Gracely, E., & Gasperino, J. (2015). Integrating palliative care into critical care: A quality improvement study. *J Intensive Care Med, 30*(6), 358–364. doi:10.1177/0885066614523923

In re Conroy (N.J. 1985).

In re Quinlan, 70 10 (N.J. 1976).

Iowa Healthcare Collaborative. (2017). IPOST. Retrieved from https://www.ihconline.org/additional-tools/initiatives/ipost/

Ipsos-Reid. (2012). National Ipsos-Reid poll indicates majority of Canadians haven't talked about their wishes for care. Retrieved from http://advancecareplanning.ca/acp-news/national-ipsos-reid-poll-indicates-majority-of-canadians-havent-talked-about-their-wishes-for-care/

Isaacs, E. D., & Brody, R. V. (2010). The unbefriended adult patient: The San Francisco General Hospital approach to ethical dilemmas. *San Francisco Med J., 83*(6), 25–26.

Iwashyna, T. J., & Christakis, N. A. (1998). Attitude and self-reported practice regarding hospice referral in a national sample of internists. *J Palliat Med, 1*(3), 241–248. doi:10.1089/jpm.1998.1.241

Jacobs, L. M., Burns, K., & Bennett Jacobs, B. (2008). Trauma death: Views of the public and trauma professionals on death and dying from injuries. *Arch Surg, 143*(8), 730–735. doi:10.1001/archsurg.143.8.730

Janse, A. J., Gemke, R. J., Uiterwaal, C. S., van der Tweel, I., Kimpen, J. L., & Sinnema, G. (2004). Quality of life: Patients and doctors don't always agree: A meta-analysis. *J Clin Epidemiol, 57*(7), 653–661. doi:10.1016/j.jclinepi.2003.11.013.S0895435604000228

Janssen, D. J., Engelberg, R. A., Wouters, E. F., & Curtis, J. R. (2012). Advance care planning for patients with COPD: Past, present and future. *Patient Educ Couns, 86*(1), 19–24. doi:10.1016/j.pec.2011.01.007

Jefferson, A. L., Lambe, S., Moser, D. J., Byerly, L. K., Ozonoff, A., & Karlawish, J. H. (2008). Decisional capacity for research participation in individuals with mild cognitive impairment. *J Am Geriatr Soc, 56*(7), 1236–1243. doi:10.1111/j.1532-5415.2008.01752.x

Johnson, J. R., Engelberg, R. A., Nielsen, E. L., Kross, E. K., Smith, N. L., Hanada, J. C., . . . Curtis, J. R. (2014). The association of spiritual care providers' activities with family members' satisfaction with care after a death in the ICU. *Crit Care Med, 42*(9), 1991–2000. doi:10.1097/CCM.0000000000000412

Kopelman, L. M. (2007). The best interests standard for incompetent or incapacitated persons of all ages. *J Law Med Ethics*, 35(1), 187–196. doi: JLME123 [pii] 10.1111/j.1748-720X.2007.00123.x

Kutner, J. S., Blatchford, P. J., Taylor, D. H., Jr., Ritchie, C. S., Bull, J. H., Fairclough, D. L., . . . Abernethy, A. P. (2015). Safety and benefit of discontinuing statin therapy in the setting of advanced, life-limiting illness: A randomized clinical trial. *JAMA Intern Med*, 175(5), 691–700. doi:10.1001/jamainternmed.2015.0289

Kutner, L. (1969). Due process of euthanasia: The living will a proposal. *Indiana Law J*, 44.

Kwak, J., & Haley, W. E. (2005). Current research findings on end-of-life decision making among racially or ethnically diverse groups. *Gerontologist*, 45(5), 634–641.

Lai, J. M., Gill, T. M., Cooney, L. M., Bradley, E. H., Hawkins, K. A., & Karlawish, J. H. (2008). Everyday decision making ability in older persons with cognitive impairment. *Am J Geriatr Psychiatry*, 16(8), 693–696. doi:10.1097/JGP.0b013e31816c7b54

Lakin, J. R., Robinson, M. G., Bernacki, R. E., Powers, B. W., Block, S. D., Cunningham, R., & Obermeyer, Z. (2016). Estimating 1-year mortality for high-risk primary care patients using the "surprise" question. *JAMA Intern Med*, 176(12), 1863–1865. doi:10.1001/jamainternmed.2016.5928

Lambert, P., Gibson, J. M., & Nathanson, P. (1990). The values history: An innovation in surrogate medical decision making. *Law Med Health Care*, 18(3), 202–212.

Levinson, W., Kao, A., Kuby, A., & Thisted, R. A. (2005). Not all patients want to participate in decision making: A national study of public preferences. *J Gen Intern Med*, 20(6), 531–535. doi:10.1111/j.1525-1497.2005.04101.x

Lilley, E. J., Gemunden, S. A., Kristo, G., Changoor, N., Scott, J. W., Rickerson, E., . . . Cooper, Z. (2016). Utility of the "surprise" question in predicting survival among older patients with acute surgical conditions. *J Palliat Med*, 20(4), 420–423. doi:10.1089/jpm.2016.0313

Luce, J. M. (2010). End-of-life decision making in the intensive care unit. *Am J Respir Crit Care Med*, 182(1), 6–11. doi:10.1164/rccm.201001-0071CI

Macauley, R. (2011). Patients who make "wrong" choices. *J Palliat Med*, 14(1), 13–16. doi:10.1089/jpm.2010.0318

Mack, J. W., Cronin, A., Keating, N. L., Taback, N., Huskamp, H. A., Malin, J. L., . . . Weeks, J. C. (2012). Associations between end-of-life discussion characteristics and care received near death: A prospective cohort study. *J Clin Oncol*, 30(35), 4387–4395. doi:10.1200/JCO.2012.43.6055

Marks, M. A., & Arkes, H. R. (2008). Patient and surrogate disagreement in end-of-life decisions: Can surrogates accurately predict patients' preferences? *Med Decis Making*, 28(4), 524–531. doi:10.1177/0272989X08315244

Marson, D. C., Hawkins, L., McInturff, B., & Harrell, L. E. (1997). Cognitive models that predict physician judgments of capacity to consent in mild Alzheimer's disease. *J Am Geriatr Soc*, 45(4), 458–464.

Martin, V. C., & Roberto, K. A. (2006). Assessing the stability of values and health care preferences of older adults: A long-term comparison. *J Gerontol Nurs*, 32(11), 23–31; quiz 32–23.

Meisel, A. (2016). Legal issues in death and dying. In S. J. Youngner & R. M. Arnold (Eds.), *The Oxford handbook of ethics at the end of life* (pp. 7–26). New York: Oxford University Press.

Messinger-Rapport, B. J., Baum, E. E., & Smith, M. L. (2009). Advance care planning: Beyond the living will. *Cleve Clin J Med*, 76(5), 276–285. doi:10.3949/ccjm.76a.07002

Minnesota Catholic Conference. (2013). A pastoral statement on physician orders for life-sustaining treatment (POLST). Retrieved from https://www.mncatholic.org/stewards-of-the-gift-of-life/

Mirarchi, F. L., Cammarata, C., Zerkle, S. W., Cooney, T. E., Chenault, J., & Basnak, D. (2015). TRIAD VII: Do prehospital providers understand physician orders for life-sustaining treatment documents? *J Patient Saf*, 11(1), 9–17. doi:10.1097/PTS.0000000000000164

Mitchell, S. L., Miller, S. C., Teno, J. M., Davis, R. B., & Shaffer, M. L. (2010). The advanced dementia prognostic tool: A risk score to estimate survival in nursing home residents with advanced dementia. *J Pain Symptom Manage*, 40(5), 639–651. doi:10.1016/j.jpainsymman.2010.02.014

Moore, K. A., Rubin, E. B., & Halpern, S. D. (2016). The problems with physician orders for life-sustaining treatment. *JAMA*, 315(3), 259–260. doi:10.1001/jama.2015.17362

Moroni, M., Zocchi, D., Bolognesi, D., Abernethy, A., Rondelli, R., Savorani, G., . . . Biasco, G. (2014). The "surprise" question in advanced cancer patients: A prospective study among general practitioners. *Palliat Med*, 28(7), 959–964. doi:10.1177/0269216314526273

Moss, A. H., Lunney, J. R., Culp, S., Auber, M., Kurian, S., Rogers, J., . . . Abraham, J. (2010). Prognostic significance of the "surprise" question in cancer patients. *J Palliat Med*, *13*(7), 837–840. doi:10.1089/jpm.2010.0018

Moye, J., & Marson, D. C. (2007). Assessment of decision making capacity in older adults: An emerging area of practice and research. *J Gerontol B Psychol Sci Soc Sci*, *62*(1), P3–P11.

National Hospice and Palliative Care Organization. (2015). Hospice care in America. Retrieved from https://www.nhpco.org/sites/default/files/public/Statistics_Research/2015_Facts_Figures.pdf

National POLST Paradigm. (2017). POLST and advance directives. Retrieved from http://polst.org/advance-care-planning/polst-and-advance-directives/

Nelson, J. E., Angus, D. C., Weissfeld, L. A., Puntillo, K. A., Danis, M., Deal, D., . . . Cook, D. J. (2006). End-of-life care for the critically ill: A national intensive care unit survey. *Crit Care Med*, *34*(10), 2547–2553. doi: 10.1097/01.CCM.0000239233.63425.1D

Novack, D. H., Plumer, R., Smith, R. L., Ochitill, H., Morrow, G. R., & Bennett, J. M. (1979). Changes in physicians' attitudes toward telling the cancer patient. *JAMA*, *241*(9), 897–900.

Organisation for Economic Co-operation and Development. (2014). Coverage for health care. Retrieved from http://dx.doi.org/10.1787/soc_glance-2014-26-en

Paling, J. (2003). Strategies to help patients understand risks. *BMJ*, *327*(7417), 745–748. doi:10.1136/bmj.327.7417.745

Parks, S. M., Winter, L., Santana, A. J., Parker, B., Diamond, J. J., Rose, M., & Myers, R. E. (2011). Family factors in end-of-life decision making: Family conflict and proxy relationship. *J Palliat Med*, *14*(2), 179–184. doi:10.1089/jpm.2010.0353

Periyakoil, V. S. (2017). Stanford Letter Project. Retrieved from https://med.stanford.edu/letter.html

Pope, T. M. (2013). Making medical decisions for patients without surrogates. *N Engl J Med*, *369*(21), 1976–1978. doi:10.1056/NEJMp1308197

Quill, T. E., & Brody, H. (1996). Physician recommendations and patient autonomy: Finding a balance between physician power and patient choice. *Ann Intern Med*, *125*(9), 763–769.

Rai, A., Siegler, M., & Lantos, J. (1999). The physician as a health care proxy. *Hastings Cent Rep*, *29*(5), 14–19.

Randall, F., & Downie, R. S. (1999). *Palliative care ethics: A companion for all specialties* (2nd ed.). New York: Oxford University Press.

Rao, J. K., Anderson, L. A., Lin, F. C., & Laux, J. P. (2014). Completion of advance directives among U.S. consumers. *Am J Prev Med*, *46*(1), 65–70. doi:10.1016/j.amepre.2013.09.008

Raymont, V., Bingley, W., Buchanan, A., David, A. S., Hayward, P., Wessely, S., & Hotopf, M. (2004). Prevalence of mental incapacity in medical inpatients and associated risk factors: Cross-sectional study. *Lancet*, *364*(9443), 1421–1427. doi:10.1016/S0140-6736(04)17224-3

Roth, L. H., Meisel, A., & Lidz, C. W. (1977). Tests of competency to consent to treatment. *Am J Psychiatry*, *134*(3), 279–284. doi:10.1176/ajp.134.3.279

Sabatino, C. P. (2010). The evolution of health care advance planning law and policy. *Milbank Q*, *88*(2), 211–239. doi:10.1111/j.1468-0009.2010.00596.x

Schenker, Y., Crowley-Matoka, M., Dohan, D., Tiver, G. A., Arnold, R. M., & White, D. B. (2012). I don't want to be the one saying "we should just let him die": Intrapersonal tensions experienced by surrogate decision makers in the ICU. *J Gen Intern Med*, *27*(12), 1657–1665. doi:10.1007/s11606-012-2129-y

Scherr, K. A., Fagerlin, A., Hofer, T., Scherer, L. D., Holmes-Rovner, M., Williamson, L. D., . . . Ubel, P. A. (2017). Physician recommendations trump patient preferences in prostate cancer treatment decisions. *Med Decis Making*, *37*(1), 56–69. doi:10.1177/0272989X16662841

Schwarze, M. L., Campbell, T. C., Cunningham, T. V., White, D. B., & Arnold, R. M. (2016). You can't get what you want: Innovation for end-of-life communication in the intensive care unit. *Am J Respir Crit Care Med*, *193*(1), 14–16. doi:10.1164/rccm.201508-1592OE

Seneca. (1969). *Letters from a Stoic* (R. Campbell, Trans.). Harmondsworth, UK: Penguin.

Shalowitz, D. I., Garrett-Mayer, E., & Wendler, D. (2006). The accuracy of surrogate decision makers: A systematic review. *Arch Intern Med*, *166*(5), 493–497. doi:166/5/493 [pii]10.1001/archinte.166.5.493

Sharma, R. K., Hughes, M. T., Nolan, M. T., Tudor, C., Kub, J., Terry, P. B., & Sulmasy, D. P. (2011). Family understanding of seriously-ill patient preferences for family involvement in healthcare decision making. *J Gen Intern Med*, *26*(8), 881–886. doi:10.1007/s11606-011-1717-6

Silveira, M. J., Kim, S. Y., & Langa, K. M. (2010). Advance directives and outcomes of surrogate decision making before death. *N Engl J Med, 362*(13), 1211–1218. doi:10.1056/NEJMsa0907901

Silveira, M. J., Wiitala, W., & Piette, J. (2014). Advance directive completion by elderly Americans: A decade of change. *J Am Geriatr Soc, 62*(4), 706–710. doi:10.1111/jgs.12736

Smith, A. K., & Glare, P. (2016). Ethical issues in prognosis and prognostication. In S. J. Youngner & R. M. Arnold (Eds.), *The Oxford handbook of ethics at the end of life* (pp. 170–189). New York: Oxford University Press.

Sorger, B. M., Rosenfeld, B., Pessin, H., Timm, A. K., & Cimino, J. (2007). Decision-making capacity in elderly, terminally ill patients with cancer. *Behav Sci Law, 25*(3), 393–404. doi:10.1002/bsl.764

Sosna, D. (1998). Advance directives for emergency medical service workers: The struggle continues. *Bioethics Forum, 14*(1), 33–36.

Sprung, C. L., Cohen, S. L., Sjokvist, P., Baras, M., Bulow, H. H., Hovilehto, S., . . . Ethicus Study Group. (2003). End-of-life practices in European intensive care units: The Ethicus Study. *JAMA, 290*(6), 790–797. doi:10.1001/jama.290.6.790

Sudore, R. L., & Fried, T. R. (2010). Redefining the "planning" in advance care planning: Preparing for end-of-life decision making. *Ann Intern Med, 153*(4), 256–261. doi:10.7326/0003-4819-153-4-201008170-00008

Sulmasy, D. P., Hughes, M. T., Thompson, R. E., Astrow, A. B., Terry, P. B., Kub, J., & Nolan, M. T. (2007). How would terminally ill patients have others make decisions for them in the event of decisional incapacity? A longitudinal study. *J Am Geriatr Soc, 55*(12), 1981–1988. doi:10.1111/j.1532-5415.2007.01473.x

Sulmasy, D. P., & Snyder, L. (2010). Substituted interests and best judgments: An integrated model of surrogate decision making. *JAMA, 304*(17), 1946–1947. doi:10.1001/jama.2010.1595

Superintendent of Belchertown State School v. Saikewicz (Mass. Sup. Jud. Ct. 1977).

Teno, J. M., Gruneir, A., Schwartz, Z., Nanda, A., & Wetle, T. (2007). Association between advance directives and quality of end-of-life care: A national study. *J Am Geriatr Soc, 55*(2), 189–194. doi:10.1111/j.1532-5415.2007.01045.x

The, A. M., Hak, T., Koeter, G., & van Der Wal, G. (2000). Collusion in doctor-patient communication about imminent death: An ethnographic study. *BMJ, 321*(7273), 1376–1381.

Thompson, B. T., Cox, P. N., Antonelli, M., Carlet, J. M., Cassell, J., Hill, N. S., . . . Thijs, L. G. (2004). Challenges in end-of-life care in the ICU: Statement of the 5th International Consensus Conference in Critical Care: Brussels, Belgium, April 2003: Executive summary. *Crit Care Med, 32*(8), 1781–1784.

Tillyard, A. R. (2007). Ethics review: "Living wills" and intensive care—an overview of the American experience. *Crit Care, 11*(4), 219. doi:10.1186/cc5945

Tolle, S. W., Tilden, V. P., Nelson, C. A., & Dunn, P. M. (1998). A prospective study of the efficacy of the physician order form for life-sustaining treatment. *J Am Geriatr Soc, 46*(9), 1097–1102.

Torke, A. M., Moloney, R., Siegler, M., Abalos, A., & Alexander, G. C. (2010). Physicians' views on the importance of patient preferences in surrogate decision making. *J Am Geriatr Soc, 58*(3), 533–538. doi:10.1111/j.1532-5415.2010.02720.x

United States Conference of Catholic Bishops. (2009). *Ethical and religious directives for Catholic health care services* (5th ed.). Washington, DC: USCCB Publishing.

University of California. (2012). Prepare for your care. Retrieved from https://prepareforyourcare.org/page

US Census Bureau. (2012). U.S. Census Bureau projections show a slower growing, older, more diverse nation a half century from now. Retrieved from https://www.census.gov/newsroom/releases/archives/population/cb12-243.html

Vakil, K. P., Roukoz, H., Tung, R., Levy, W. C., Anand, I. S., Shivkumar, K., . . . Tholakanahalli, V. (2015). Mortality prediction using a modified Seattle Heart Failure Model may improve patient selection for ventricular tachycardia ablation. *Am Heart J, 170*(6), 1099–1104. doi:10.1016/j.ahj.2015.09.008

van Wijmen, M. P., Rurup, M. L., Pasman, H. R., Kaspers, P. J., & Onwuteaka-Philipsen, B. D. (2010). Advance directives in the Netherlands: An empirical contribution to the exploration of a cross-cultural perspective on advance directives. *Bioethics, 24*(3), 118–126. doi:10.1111/j.1467-8519.2009.01788.x

Varma, S., & Wendler, D. (2007). Medical decision making for patients without surrogates. *Arch Intern Med, 167*(16), 1711–1715. doi:10.1001/archinte.167.16.1711

Vig, E. K., Starks, H., Taylor, J. S., Hopley, E. K., & Fryer-Edwards, K. (2007). Surviving surrogate decision making: What helps and hampers the experience of making medical decisions for others. *J Gen Intern Med, 22*(9), 1274–1279. doi:10.1007/s11606-007-0252-y

Virik, K., & Glare, P. (2002). Validation of the palliative performance scale for inpatients admitted to a palliative care unit in Sydney, Australia. *J Pain Symptom Manage, 23*(6), 455–457.

Volandes, A. E., Paasche-Orlow, M., Gillick, M. R., Cook, E. F., Shaykevich, S., Abbo, E. D., & Lehmann, L. (2008). Health literacy not race predicts end-of-life care preferences. *J Palliat Med, 11*(5), 754–762. doi:10.1089/jpm.2007.0224

Volpe, R., & Steinman, D. (2013). Peeking inside the black box: One institution's experience developing policy for unrepresented patients. *Hamline Law Rev, 36*, 265–274.

Waite, K. R., Federman, A. D., McCarthy, D. M., Sudore, R., Curtis, L. M., Baker, D. W., . . . Paasche-Orlow, M. K. (2013). Literacy and race as risk factors for low rates of advance directives in older adults. *J Am Geriatr Soc, 61*(3), 403–406. doi:10.1111/jgs.12134

Washington State Medical Association. (2014). Sample POLST form. Retrieved from https://wsma.org/doc_library/ForPatients/EndOfLifeResources/POLST/POLST_Master_final_2014.pdf

Weeks, J. C., Catalano, P. J., Cronin, A., Finkelman, M. D., Mack, J. W., Keating, N. L., & Schrag, D. (2012). Patients' expectations about effects of chemotherapy for advanced cancer. *N Engl J Med, 367*(17), 1616–1625. doi:10.1056/NEJMoa1204410

Weeks, J. C., Cook, E. F., O'Day, S. J., Peterson, L. M., Wenger, N., Reding, D., . . . Phillips, R. S. (1998). Relationship between cancer patients' predictions of prognosis and their treatment preferences. *JAMA, 279*(21), 1709–1714.

Wendler, D., & Rid, A. (2011). Systematic review: The effect on surrogates of making treatment decisions for others. *Ann Intern Med, 154*(5), 336–346. doi:10.7326/0003-4819-154-5-201103010-00008

White, D. B., Evans, L. R., Bautista, C. A., Luce, J. M., & Lo, B. (2009). Are physicians' recommendations to limit life support beneficial or burdensome? Bringing empirical data to the debate. *Am J Respir Crit Care Med, 180*(4), 320–325. doi:10.1164/rccm.200811-1776OC

White, D. B., Jonsen, A., & Lo, B. (2012). Ethical challenge: When clinicians act as surrogates for unrepresented patients. *Am J Crit Care, 21*(3), 202–207. doi:10.4037/AJCC2012514

White, D. B., Malvar, G., Karr, J., Lo, B., & Curtis, J. R. (2010). Expanding the paradigm of the physician's role in surrogate decision making: An empirically derived framework. *Crit Care Med, 38*(3), 743–750. doi:10.1097/CCM.0b013e3181c58842

Wittink, M. N., Morales, K. H., Meoni, L. A., Ford, D. E., Wang, N. Y., Klag, M. J., & Gallo, J. J. (2008). Stability of preferences for end-of-life treatment after 3 years of follow-up: The Johns Hopkins Precursors Study. *Arch Intern Med, 168*(19), 2125–2130. doi:10.1001/archinte.168.19.2125

Yourman, L. C., Lee, S. J., Schonberg, M. A., Widera, E. W., & Smith, A. K. (2012). Prognostic indices for older adults: A systematic review. *JAMA, 307*(2), 182–192. doi:10.1001/jama.2011.1966

Zhang, B., Wright, A. A., Huskamp, H. A., Nilsson, M. E., Maciejewski, M. L., Earle, C. C., . . . Prigerson, H. G. (2009). Health care costs in the last week of life: Associations with end-of-life conversations. *Arch Intern Med, 169*(5), 480–488. doi:10.1001/archinternmed.2008.587

Zier, L. S., Burack, J. H., Micco, G., Chipman, A. K., Frank, J. A., Luce, J. M., & White, D. B. (2008). Doubt and belief in physicians' ability to prognosticate during critical illness: The perspective of surrogate decision makers. *Crit Care Med, 36*(8), 2341–2347. doi:10.1097/CCM.0b013e318180ddf9

Zier, L. S., Burack, J. H., Micco, G., Chipman, A. K., Frank, J. A., & White, D. B. (2009). Surrogate decision makers' responses to physicians' predictions of medical futility. *Chest, 136*(1), 110–117. doi:10.1378/chest.08-2753

Zier, L. S., Sottile, P. D., Hong, S. Y., Weissfield, L. A., & White, D. B. (2012). Surrogate decision makers' interpretation of prognostic information: A mixed-methods study. *Ann Intern Med, 156*(5), 360–366. doi:10.7326/0003-4819-156-5-201203060-00008

4

Specific Ethical Issues at the End of Life

Determining Code Status

Case Study

An eighty-one-year-old man with a history of coronary artery disease and chronic obstructive pulmonary disease is admitted to the hospital for community-acquired pneumonia. He lives at home with his wife and is a very active retiree, playing golf regularly and enjoying seeing his grandchildren. He has not completed an advance directive.

The internal medicine intern is called down to the emergency room to admit the patient. It is a very busy night, with several unstable patients on the medical ward. This hospitalization should be rather straightforward, likely involving only a few days of intravenous antibiotics and a very good prognosis. Before leaving to tend to the patients on the ward, the intern is required to document the code status of her new admission. She's not sure, however, of the best way to go about it.

As noted in the previous chapter, advance care planning (ACP) is a core component of palliative care. By establishing and communicating prognosis (p. 84), a palliative care clinician can help a patient devise a treatment plan that reflects his own values as well as clinical reality, thereby empowering the patient to live out however much time he has left on his own terms. As is often said in the hospice and palliative care world, "Palliative care: It's about how you *live*" (Colby, 2006; emphasis added).

The staged approach to ACP (p. 74) begins with the naming of a health care agent and perhaps some preliminary exploration of appropriate treatments in the context of sudden and catastrophic injury. The next stage includes decisions related to overall goals of care—with specific references to burden and intensity—documented in a treatment directive. The final stage includes the use of limitation of treatment orders to ensure that the patient does not receive interventions that are unlikely to benefit him and may well cause harm (Gundersen Health System, 2017).

For patients sick enough to be admitted to the hospital, resuscitation-related decisions take on immediate and greater significance. Every inpatient must have a "code status," so that the team responding to an acute clinical deterioration understands what treatments should be provided. The default—in the absence of a decision by the patient to forgo life-sustaining medical treatment (LSMT) or (much more rarely) a physician's determination that such treatment would not provide benefit (see chapter 14)—is that a patient is "full code," meaning all relevant interventions will be used in the context of respiratory or hemodynamic instability or arrest. At the other extreme is "comfort measures only," where life-sustaining interventions—particularly those that entail significant burden, such as CPR and intubation—are forgone. Between these two extremes, however, is a vast gray area that requires significant nuance to effectively navigate (Vanpee & Swine, 2004).

Being hospitalized ideally presents an opportunity reevaluate the patient's treatment plan in light of his established goals. Some time may have passed since these were last examined, and thus review and clarification may be necessary. Even if the last goals of care discussion was relatively recent, the health event that precipitated hospitalization may indicate that some of the patient's goals are no longer achievable, leading to modification of the existing advance directive.

Unfortunately, often upon admission to the hospital the discussion with the medical team—frequently a resident working under extreme time pressure—is not very nuanced. In some cases, the patient is merely assumed to be "full code," based on assumptions about his overall goals. While sometimes this may be justified—as in the case of an otherwise healthy young adult who is admitted for minor orthopedic surgery—in other circumstances it could reflect an unwillingness to have a difficult conversation. It could also reflect an *inability* to have such a conversation, in which many physicians receive inadequate training (Knauft, Nielsen, Engelberg, Patrick, & Curtis, 2005). Failure to address code status can lead to a treatment plan that is incongruous with goals of care, which has been shown to increase family stress, anxiety, and decisional regret, potentially leading to subsequent depressive symptoms (Weiner & Essis, 2006).

Code status conversations are not the unique domain of palliative care clinicians. All physicians should possess generalist palliative care skills (Quill & Abernethy, 2013), which include the ability to identify goals of care and formulate a consonant treatment plan. By virtue of their training in prognostication and communication, though, palliative care clinicians are especially well-suited to facilitating conversations about goals of care and formulating a treatment plan that accords with them.

Often, though, palliative care clinicians are not involved early on in the hospital course, because a palliative care need has yet to be identified. (As is often said in palliative care circles, "It's always too early until it's too late"; Byock, 2012). When palliative care is eventually consulted, it is frequently to "get the DNR" for a patient whose prognosis is poor and is requesting a treatment plan that the primary team feels is inappropriately aggressive (Billings, 2012). Such a request from the primary team may reflect a misunderstanding of what palliative care really is, such as falsely equating it with hospice or—even worse—with "giving up" (Gawande, 2010). It may also reflect the primary team's discomfort in engaging in difficult conversations or honoring a treatment plan that appears inappropriate, even though it may be consistent with the patient's goals.

Several ethical issues are related to the determination of code status, including the terminology used, the approach used to determining this status (including the role of "modified codes"), and the potential modification of code status in unique contexts, such as the operating room (OR).

Terminology

Prior to the patients' rights movements of the 1970s, there was an assumption that patients would receive any treatment that could potentially prolong their lives, including CPR, which had shown great promise in early studies in the context of the OR (Kouwenhoven, Jude, & Knickerbocker, 1960). As it became clear, though, that CPR in other hospital settings—and particularly outside the hospital—was not as effective (Schneider, Nelson, & Brown, 1993), the American Medical Association (AMA) began to recommend that it be withheld from certain patients. "Resuscitation in these circumstances," the AMA concluded, "may represent a positive violation of an individual's right to die with dignity" ("Standards for Cardiopulmonary Resuscitation (CPR) and Emergency Cardiac Care (ECC)," 1974).

Given CPR's unique status—by virtue of its emergent nature—as the one medical intervention that every patient would receive unless he refused it, there needed to be some way to identify patients who would not receive it. Consequently, the first Do Not Resuscitate (DNR) orders began to be implemented around this time (Rabkin, Gillerman, and Rice, 1976). At first, though, clinicians were not even sure they were actually legal (Margolick, 1982). This led to surreptitious documentation—often in the form of symbols such as purple dots on charts of patients who were not to receive CPR—and, not surprisingly, to "shocking procedural abuses" (Sullivan, 1984).

Gradually the practice of withholding CPR became widely accepted and the methodology became standardized, such that "DNR" entered the common lexicon. Over time, though, the deficiencies of the term have become clear. Most obviously, an order to not perform "resuscitation" seems to imply that, were it not for the order, resuscitation would have been achievable. But as has become all too clear, CPR is ineffective in achieving its primary goal—not only survival to discharge from the hospital but even return of spontaneous circulation—most of the time. The term DNR, therefore, may itself perpetuate a misunderstanding that CPR is more effective than it actually is.

For this reason, some have suggested using the term Do Not Attempt Resuscitation (DNAR) instead (Sokol, 2009). This emphasizes that the most medicine can promise is to *attempt* resuscitation, with the end result dependent on a wide range of variables such as the response time, the skills of the first responder, and so on (Pitcher, Smith, Nolan, & Soar, 2009). This makes DNAR a preferable term and the one generally used in this textbook.

DNAR is far from perfect, however, being just as negative as DNR by defining code status with reference to what will *not* be done, rather than what will be. The negative emphasis of the term may therefore give a distorted impression of the team's dedication to the patient and his well-being. With the need to confirm the plan with the patient at increasingly frequent hand-offs from one team to another, the perpetual reiteration of what will not be done for a patient who is DNR/DNAR could justifiably lead a patient to wonder what, if anything, *will* be done (Anderson, Chase, Pantilat, Tulsky, & Auerbach, 2011; Anderson, Pantilat, et al., 2011).

DNAR—like DNR—is also open to inappropriate inferences (Burns, Edwards, Johnson, Cassem, & Truog, 2003; Ehlenbach & Curtis, 2011). Since patients receiving a comfort-directed plan of care are obviously DNAR, staff might make false assumptions about the overall goals of any patient with a DNAR order (Truog, 2011). For instance, studies have shown that for patients with a DNAR order physicians are less likely to use standard treatment for acute heart failure (Chen, Sosnov, Lessard, & Goldberg, 2008), nurses are less likely to perform certain interventions (Henneman, Baird, Bellamy, Faber, & Oye, 1994), and admission to the intensive care unit (ICU) is more often denied (Cohen, Lisker, Eichorn, Multz, & Silver, 2009). Several recently-publicized examples of this so-called "DNR creep" reveal that physicians may assume that a patient who is DNAR does not want life-sustaining measures beyond CPR, such as intravenous fluids or supplemental oxygen (Billings & Block, 2013; Fink, 2013). At the same time, a few recent studies have suggested some improvement in clinicians' understanding of DNAR, with provision of equivalent care to patients regardless of their code status (Saager et al., 2011).

One reason for these misunderstandings may lie in the multiple meanings of the term "resuscitation," which does not necessarily refer to CPR following cardiac arrest. It may also, for instance, refer to the "fluid resuscitation" of a profoundly dehydrated patient (Perel, Roberts, & Ker, 2013). Another reason may be that aside from chest compressions, modalities used in response to cardiac arrest are also used in other contexts. Many clinicians consider powerful medications such as atropine and epinephrine to be "resuscitative"—and they are certainly used in response to certain forms of cardiac arrest—but they are also used to counteract chemical exposures and treat severe allergic reactions. A patient who requests to be DNAR because he understands the poor outcomes following cardiac arrest might well wish to receive epinephrine for an anaphylactic reaction to medication.

Rather than intrinsically associating certain medications or interventions with CPR, it is better to view DNAR orders contextually. By definition, CPR "is used in cases of cardiac arrest or apparent cardiac death" (Martin, 2010). A patient with a DNAR order should not, therefore, receive further interventions in the event of a cardiac arrest. But as long as a patient has a pulse, the fact that he is DNAR should have no impact on the treatment plan. To be sure, a DNAR order may reflect an overall emphasis on comfort, but it could also signify that a patient has elected not to receive a particularly high-burden/low-benefit intervention, while still wishing to receive other interventions for which the balance of benefits and burdens is more favorable (Macauley, 2014).

Misunderstandings about what DNAR means—and what it does not—can have a significant impact on clinical care. Patients (or their families) may be reluctant to consent to a DNAR order out of concern that the medical team may not "try as hard" in treating the patient. In response, clinicians—particularly those who work in palliative care and are well aware of the burden/benefit balance of CPR—are often known to say that "DNR doesn't mean 'do not respond'" (Fins, 2006). Given the studies noted previously, though, perhaps it would be more honest to say that DNR—or DNAR—*should not* mean that but sometimes does.

Improvements to DNAR orders have been suggested. One is the greater detail and portability afforded by the Physician Orders for Life Sustaining Treatment (POLST) paradigm (p. 78). Another proposed option is to move beyond the rigid parameters of current DNAR order forms to a goal-directed approach (Truog, Waisel, & Burns, 1999). Precisely because CPR has varying rates of success depending on the patient's condition and the clinical context, goal-directed DNAR orders permit some latitude to the medical team to provide or withhold CPR depending on the clinical situation. After all, CPR itself is never a patient's goal but rather a necessary means to possibly achieving what he is truly hoping for (such as survival or discharge from the hospital). A goal-directed DNAR permits physicians to administer CPR when it is likely to achieve the patient's goal (such as in the case of an intraoperative arrest, which carries a high rate of recovery) but withhold it when it is not likely to (as in the case of a catastrophic stroke).

While this approach would ideally better respect a patient's wishes, it is not without drawbacks. It requires an extremely nuanced conversation with the patient, going far beyond whether he is willing to accept CPR to explore overall goals and values. This conversation needs to be documented in a narrative fashion, exceeding the scope of checkboxes on DNAR and POLST forms. The degree to which this descriptive summary can be understood and applied in the current medical world of frequent hand-offs between teams is unclear. For all these reasons, many consider the goal-directed approach to be an unachievable ideal, best reserved for situations where context is critical.

Others, though, argue that the terms DNR/DNAR cannot be resuscitated, and a different term should be used: "Allow Natural Death" (AND; Cohen, 2004). Studies have shown that it is more palatable to both professionals as well as laypeople, probably by virtue of its less negative emphasis (Venneman, Narnor-Harris, Perish, & Hamilton, 2008). Rather than focusing on what will be withheld from the patient, AND conjures an image of noninterference and perhaps even peaceful death. In so doing, it attempts to describe a broader overall goal of care, far beyond the modality-specific nature of DNR or DNAR.

While intuitively more attractive, AND is also imprecise and even potentially misleading. The word "natural" may conjure images of comfort and companionship without the burden of technology, but it is important to note that much of high-quality end-of-life care is unnatural (Chessa, 2004). After all, benzodiazepines for anxiety and opioids for pain—both scientific creations—are mainstays of modern palliative care. In many ways, palliative care is dedicated to *not* allowing patients to die "naturally," if that means crying out in pain or gasping for breath (Macauley, 2014).

DNR and AND are both well-intentioned terms but are also potentially misleading and thus should be avoided. While DNAR is far from perfect—especially with its negative emphasis—it avoids implying that resuscitation is always achievable and can be very helpful when properly understood as applying only to situations of full arrest. Ultimately, no abbreviation is sufficient to encapsulate a patient's hopes and dreams, and no term should bear that responsibility. A few letters on a patient's chart or armband can never replace a thoughtful conversation, appropriately documented, that should guide treatment, especially at the end of life.

Before moving on, one other term that deserves some degree of clarification is "comfort care." This term has several strengths, such as its focus on the positive—rather than emphasizing what treatments will be forgone—and its affirmation that patients will always be cared for, no matter what their goals are (Fine, 2007). It is a helpful reminder that "doing nothing" is never an option, nor is "giving up."

It is, however, also subject to considerable misunderstanding. Some interpret it broadly, to mean that while no burdensome or "uncomfortable" procedures should be performed, low-burden interventions directed at life prolongation are acceptable. Alternatively, one might interpret it narrowly to mean that *only* interventions directed at comfort should be used. LSMT of minimal burden would be consistent with the broader understanding of "comfort care" but not with the narrower one.

This can lead to unfortunate misunderstandings. Imagine, for instance, a patient in the ICU with a very low probability of recovery. After extensive explanation and ongoing emotional support, the family authorizes a shift to "comfort care," which they take to mean that no more burdensome interventions will be used (i.e., the broad definition). A DNAR order is entered into the chart, as CPR is clearly not a part of "comfort care" by any definition. But the team, working on the narrower definition, also withdraws nonburdensome modalities that are not comfort-directed, such as antibiotics and insulin. The following morning the family is irate that the team has "given up" on the patient, revealing that when they had all agreed on "comfort care," they were working under very different definitions.

The term "comfort measures only" is an improvement over the more general "comfort care" (Do, 2014). This makes clear that the narrower understanding is intended, with the sole focus being comfort. But with greater acceptance the term has come to be known by its abbreviation—CMO—which has some overlap with DNAR. To be sure, a patient who is CMO will also be DNAR, but the converse is not necessarily true, for the reasons noted previously. This once again highlights the pitfalls of attempting to condense complex patient goals into a handful of letters.

How to Determine Code Status

Respect for the patient requires the physician to explore the patient's end-of-life preferences with him. Code status represents these preferences and communicates them to others. Once a patient experiences cardiac arrest, there is no time to discuss what treatments should or should not be provided, and thus whatever conversations (and documentation) have taken place up until that point will determine the medical team's response. Properly determining a patient's code status is, therefore, an ethical obligation.

Unfortunately, this conversation is often bypassed, either due to time constraints, physician discomfort, or failure to recognize its importance. When it does take place, it may occur in a perfunctory way that perverts—rather than respects—the patient's autonomy. Rather than exploring the patient's goals and how they relate to code status, a clinician may focus entirely on resuscitative procedures and attempt to express the relevant question in lay terminology. For example, she might ask the patient, "If your heart were to stop, do you want us to restart it?"

This is extremely misleading, though, as it presumes that the patient's heart *could* be restarted, which is far from certain. Given the rosy depiction of CPR outcomes in popular media (Diem, Lantos, & Tulsky, 1996), the patient may assume that the probability of success is much higher than it actually is. There is also no discussion of the burden and complications that can be associated with CPR. Finally, the end point of the discussion appears to be return of spontaneous circulation, whereas the patient may have other goals—such as survival to hospital discharge or the ability to return to independent living—that are preeminent. For all these reasons, such a question is likely to elicit a positive response from the patient but not necessarily one that accurately reflects his underlying goals.

An alternative to oversimplification is excessive detail in the form of a long list of potential interventions (Roeland et al., 2014), leading to what might be called a "dim sum approach" to code status. In situations short of full arrest, a patient could be offered a wide swath of treatments, including cardioversion, pressors, dialysis, intubation, and so on. But if patients generally do not understand the likely outcomes of CPR, they are far less likely to understand the clinical implications and results of these even less familiar procedures. Left to their own devices, such a range of patient choices often leads to so-called "modified" or "partial" codes, whereby a patient receives "some, but not all, of the discrete elements of cardiopulmonary resuscitation" (Berger, 2003).

Such codes are relatively rare—representing less than 10% of limitation of treatment orders (Dumot et al., 2001)—but the outcomes are worse than for typical CPR (Marik & Craft, 1997). A likely reason is that the patient-formulated treatment plan may be clinically nonsensical. For instance, authorizing all treatments except chest compressions could lead to the administration of intravenous medication to a pulseless patient, without the chest compressions required to circulate those medications. Perhaps the most common nonsensical plan is refusing intubation—which is usually required during or after CPR to maintain adequate oxygenation and ventilation—while accepting CPR itself, perhaps based on an inappropriate inference that mechanical ventilation is more burdensome and less effective than CPR.[1]

Admittedly, there are rare instances when partial codes may be clinically reasonable, such as malignant arrhythmias after myocardial infarction, which can respond to cardioversion without the need for intubation (Berger, 2003). But in most cases partial codes stem from a combination of physician reluctance to engage in a thoughtful exploration of patient goals (which are generally ill-served by partial codes) and some degree of patient misunderstanding related to specific procedures. As such, this approach may represent abandonment, leaving the patient and his family to choose between modalities that they do not comprehend.

On the opposite end of the spectrum of offering a patient whatever he wants (even if it is inappropriate) is *not* providing what he requests (even though he expects to receive it). An example of this is a patient who is not likely to benefit from CPR yet steadfastly requests it. Rather than going through the work of exploring his goals in light of the requested treatment (as discussed in the following section), the medical team may simply "go through the motions" of a code, in order to fulfill the letter—though not the spirit—of the law. Known as a "slow code," "show code," or "Hollywood code," this generally involves strolling to the bedside in response to an emergent page and, once there, tapping lightly on the chest rather than performing compressions in a manner necessary to maintain blood flow.

Defenders of the practice argue that its intention is to avoid unnecessary suffering by sparing the patient potential harm without sufficient chance of benefit (Morrow, Plunkitt, & Basta, 1999). Some patients or families simply cannot bring themselves to consent to DNAR status, as this suggests that they would be "giving up." A slow code provides them the reassurance (or, at least, the appearance) that they did everything they could for the patient and enables the medical team to avoid inflicting suffering.

There are several serious problems with the slow code, though. First and foremost, it is inherently deceptive. The patient thinks he knows what treatments will and will not be provided, but the medical team intends something very different. This, in turn, has significant effects on the physician-patient relationship, which is based on trust. If the team is not willing to abide by its promise to provide CPR in the context of cardiac arrest, what other promises might they also be willing to break?

The slow code is also inherently parentalistic. The patient and/or family has expressed what their goals and values are, but the medical team is superimposing their own values

---

1. It should be noted that the converse of this order—refusing CPR while accepting intubation—can be quite a reasonable plan and one that is often suggested in the course of a code status discussion.

in withholding a requested treatment. Certainly, the team is free to disagree with the patient or family's conclusion, but such a disagreement should be openly acknowledged and worked through. If unresolvable, ultimately either the team should invoke a non-beneficial treatment (NBT) policy and openly withhold CPR (see chapter 14), or defer to the patient or family's wishes. The latter is both respectful and humble, acknowledging that different people have different values and that the medical team may not be "right" in their belief that CPR should not be offered.

As in many apparently ethical dilemmas, the problem here may primarily be one of communication. In such an emotional context—where the burden on surrogate decision-makers is high, especially related to forgoing LSMT—expecting the patient or family to clearly refuse CPR may be unrealistic. Rather than resorting to a slow code, the team might approach the discussion from the point of view of informed assent (p. 382), thus sparing the family the burden of guilt and the patient the burden of NBT.

But what if enhanced communication and honest sharing does not resolve the issue? The broader question of how to approach patients who "want everything" is addressed in the following section, but with regard to CPR specifically, there exists an ethically acceptable variant of the slow code. In a recent provocative commentary, Lantos and Meadow (2011) suggest "resuscitating" the slow code in the form of a short-lived, largely symbolic gesture that will assure the family that no stone has been left unturned. The "symbolic" nature of the intervention is admittedly troublesome, risking deception by prompting the family to draw erroneous conclusions. It is also rather haughty, as the medical team is so certain that CPR will not be effective that they are unwilling to even give it a chance.

But the short-lived aspect of this modern twist on the slow code is relevant and defensible. There is no clear-cut minimum time requirement for CPR to be continued before being deemed ineffective in the face of continued pulselessness. There exists wide variation, with longer codes generally provided to patients with a better prognosis who seem to have a remediable problem, if circulation is maintained until it can be corrected. By the same reasoning, it would seem appropriate to perform what might be called a "fast" or "tailored" code in situations where the preintervention probability of success is quite low (as in cases where teams might otherwise be tempted to perform a slow code).

In a fast code, CPR is performed effectively not merely symbolically—and appropriate next steps (such as medication administration) are taken according to the Advanced Cardiac Life Support protocol. But there is no reason to continue to attempt resuscitation when it has become obvious that it will be ineffective, at which point it provides only additional suffering. By performing a fast code, the team shows respect for the family's values as well as humility as they accept the possibility that (despite their dire predictions) it might be effective, after all, if administered appropriately.

Whether planned in advance or not, fast codes often occur when family members witness resuscitative efforts. Traditionally, the family was ushered from the room when a patient arrested to permit the medical team to concentrate on the resuscitation and to spare the family unnecessary suffering. But it is now becoming more common to offer the family the option of being present during CPR. Studies have shown broad family acceptance of this practice (Meyers et al., 2000), which hopefully would provide families with a more tangible sense of "having tried everything" to save their loved one (Compton et al., 2011). (A side benefit for the patient, of course, is not being subjected to prolonged resuscitative efforts.)

This practice has not been universally accepted, out of concerns for increased psychological harm to families as well as potential negative impact on the efficacy of witnessed resuscitative efforts (McClenathan, Torrington, & Uyehara, 2002). A recent randomized clinical trial, however, found that families who witnessed CPR had a *lower* incidence of posttraumatic stress disorder–related symptoms, anxiety, and depression, and their presence did not negatively impact resuscitative efforts (Jabre et al., 2013).

One characteristic that the "default full code," the "dim sum code," and the "slow/fast code" all share is that they are based on what the patient says he wants his code status to be. A more enlightened approach is for the physician to recommend to the patient what his code status *should* be. This may at first seem just as parentalistic as the "slow code," and it would be if the recommended code status were based on the physician's external estimate of the patient's quality of life, or the physician's own values. But when the recommendation is a reflection of the *patient's* expressed values, it is actually a sign of respect for autonomy, and a rather profound one at that.

Such an approach assumes, of course, that the physician has appropriately identified what the patient's goals are. These take time and skill to elicit, especially at a pivotal time in the patient's life (such as inpatient admission). But the methods put forth for determining overall goals of care (Bernacki, Block, & American College of Physicians High Value Care Task Force, 2014) are also relevant here. If the physician can elicit the patient's goals, fears, minimum level of function, willing trade-offs, and ideal degree of family involvement, these can be translated—in light of the clinical situation and likely outcomes of various interventions—into a code status. So rather than starting the discussion with code status, this should actually be the conclusion of a longer conversation that begins with the patient's goals.

Once these goals and values have been elicited, the physician can then offer a code status recommendation based on them. For example, the physician might say, "Based on what you've told me about your goals, I don't believe that CPR will help you get where you want to go, and might make things worse. For that reason, I don't think we should do that to you."

The strength and specificity of the recommendation largely depend on the physician's certainty about whether a given intervention will meet the patient's expressed needs. If it clearly will not—as in the case of CPR for a patient with oxygen-dependent chronic obstructive pulmonary disease who wishes to return home to independent living (Stapleton, Ehlenbach, Deyo, & Curtis, 2014)—the "informed assent" approach (p. 382) can be used. If there is some ambiguity, the recommendation can be framed in more open-ended terms, inviting the patient into deeper conversation about likely outcomes, to the degree the patient wishes.

The recommendation is not a dictate; the patient must be given an opportunity to clarify, disagree, and amend the proposed treatment plan. After all, the physician might have misunderstood what the patient was saying, rendering the recommendation inconsistent with the patient's goals. Or, perhaps, the logical and appropriate conclusion drawn from the patient's expressed goals is not acceptable to the patient. He might, for example, have expressed a desire to die peacefully and avoid burdensome treatments that are unlikely to benefit him, but being declared "DNR" feels to him like "giving up." This dilemma is often more emotional than cognitive, and the proper response is not amending the code status but rather exploring the patient's fears and concerns and assuring him that any treatment that is beneficial would still be used.

There are clearly drawbacks to this approach. It is quite time-consuming and requires significant communication skills. It also places the physician in a position of greater responsibility, at least compared to the overly deferential "dim sum" approach, for which the patient or surrogate bears total responsibility (as well as significant emotional and cognitive burden). But if shared decision-making is truly the ideal (p. 59), there is no more appropriate—or important—context for this to occur than mutually determining a code status that best meets the patient's goals and needs. Viewed in that light, this approach shows much greater respect for the patient's autonomy than assuming he wants something he may not want, or inundating him with information that he can neither process nor apply.

Code Status in the Operating Room

The OR context adds additional complexity to code status discussions because of several unique aspects of this environment. First, CPR is more likely to be effective in the OR, where the equivalent of a code team is constantly monitoring the patient, ready to intervene at a second's notice. (Indeed, the preliminary studies on CPR—which were so optimistic—took place in the operative environment; Kouwenhoven, Jude, & Knickerbocker, 1960). Second, many of the interventions commonly used in the OR—such as pressors and chronotropes—are also part of the standard response to a code, thus blurring the line between what is "resuscitative" (in the CPR sense) and what is not. Third, the very act of surgery makes cardiac arrest more likely, for such an invasive procedure always makes a patient more unstable before ultimately (hopefully) fulfilling its goal of improved health. Anesthesia can cause significant hemodynamic instability as well. Fourth, surgery—especially one requiring general anesthesia—is a very invasive intervention that carries with it great risk and entails at least some degree of suffering, and thus refusing CPR may seem inconsistent with the overall goals of care.

For all these reasons, DNAR orders—once they came to be accepted in the 1970s—initially were routinely suspended in the OR. As of 1991, for instance, 81% of anesthesiology programs reported automatically rescinding DNAR orders in the OR (Franklin & Rothenberg, 1992). After all, why would a patient consent to surgery but not allow the team to address anticipated complications of that surgery, especially with relatively good outcomes from potential CPR?

Gradually, however, this stance was reconsidered. Operations were being performed on sicker patients, such that even in the OR outcome statistics from CPR were rather sobering. It also became increasingly apparent that some patients wanted to give themselves every opportunity to survive, but if they "died" then they did not want "heroic measures."[2] Professional societies took note of this, with the American Society of Anesthesiologists acknowledging that routinely rescinding DNAR orders in the OR "may not sufficiently address a patient's rights to self-determination in a responsible and ethical manner" (American Society of Anesthesiologists, 2001). The American College of Surgeons (1994) and the Association of Operating Room Nurses (Eckberg, 1998) also came to reject automatic suspension of DNAR orders in the OR.

This does not, however, necessarily mean that a patient's pre-existing DNAR should remain in place. For the reasons noted previously, CPR may make sense in the OR in a way that it does not in other contexts. For instance, a well-informed patient might seek an out-of-hospital DNAR order, recognizing the exceedingly poor outcomes associated with CPR in that context. But that same patient might accept CPR in the hospital—and especially in the OR—in light of the improved outcomes in those environments.

Refusing CPR might also sufficiently alter the probability of successful surgery such that the surgeon declines to proceed if the patient insists on a DNAR order. To be clear, a surgeon should respect a patient's refusal of CPR, but she is not obligated to proceed with surgery under that restriction. Imagine, for example, a surgery that carries a high likelihood of cardiac arrest (and a commensurately high likelihood of successful resuscitation in that event). A surgeon could in good conscience offer the procedure if the patient were full code but decline to proceed if the patient requested to remain DNAR, since an arrest under those circumstances would be fatal rather than remediable.

Given these complexities, the appropriate response to a patient with a DNAR order who is considering surgery is a "required reconsideration" of the order (Cohen & Cohen, 1992). The patient should be made aware of the degree of increased likelihood of cardiac arrest due to surgery, as well as the likely outcomes should that occur. He should also be informed whether surgery with a DNAR order is an option, or if maintaining his refusal of CPR would negate that possibility.

At that point the patient has three options: keep the DNAR in place (which might preempt surgery), revert to full code, or temporarily suspend the DNAR. The last of these is a reasonable middle ground, as it makes an exception for the unique environment of the OR while reverting back to the previous DNAR status once outside this context. This, however, raises the practical question of how long to suspend the DNAR. Many operative procedures carry increased risk for cardiac or hemodynamic instability beyond the OR itself, into the perioperative period. It would, therefore, be reasonable to place a time limit

---

2. These terms are placed in quotation marks because they are commonly used but clinically imprecise or inaccurate. A patient is only considered "dead" if he has *irreversible* cessation of cardiorespiratory function, and thus a patient who arrests in the OR is not necessarily dead in the clinical sense. Similarly, "heroic measures" is a subjective term, and one might argue that much of surgery is far more heroic than closed chest compressions (i.e., CPR).

on the reversion to DNAR—perhaps on the order of six to twenty-four hours—in order to permit the team to address foreseen complications that are likely remediable.

Up to this point, the discussion has assumed a procedure-directed limitation of treatment, in the form of a DNAR order. But this situation highlights the benefits of a goal-directed limitation of treatment order (p. 105), which would permit the team to respond proportionately to the patient's expressed goals. The reason, after all, for suspending the DNAR order is that the patient's goals might be achieved through CPR in the OR, where they likely would not have been through CPR in other contexts. However, an intraoperative cardiac arrest could stem from a catastrophic complication that makes meaningful recovery (as the patient himself defines it) extremely unlikely. In such a case, even though the patient might have agreed to rescind or suspend the DNAR order during surgery, it may not be appropriate to administer CPR. If the team was able to provide treatments that were likely to achieve the patient's goals but withhold those that were not, this would ideally respect the patient's values.

The challenges of goal-directed DNAR orders were noted earlier and perhaps are even more relevant in the surgical context. It is not uncommon, for instance, for one anesthesiologist to seek informed consent from a patient the evening before surgery and another to anesthetize the patient the following day. Communicating the essence of a goals of care conversation from the first anesthesiologist to the second—with the decision of whether to initiate CPR hinging on the accuracy of understanding of the attending anesthesiologist at the time—can certainly be a challenge. But the rewards for doing so—in terms of applying the patient's goals to a complex situation—are equally great.

Return to the Case

The intern has watched her supervising residents handle "code status discussions" very efficiently, essentially asking the patient if he wanted to receive CPR if his heart were to stop. But she has done additional reading in palliative care—and has seen the infrequency with which CPR is effective in patients like this one—so she takes a more nuanced approach.

She begins not with code status but with goals. She asks the patient what he is most hoping for and most afraid of. She explores what minimum level of functioning he would be willing to accept and what trade-offs he would be able to tolerate. His wife is present for the conversation, and he stresses that he wants her involved in all decision-making as well.

The intern gradually forms a sense of the patient's goals: ideally to maintain his current quality of life but willing to undergo some degree of burden and decreased function if that is the only way to survive. He does express a deep sense of peace, however, that he has lived life on his own terms and wants to "go out on his own terms" too. He does not want any "heroic measures," especially ones that might leave him dependent on others.

Based on that conversation, the intern feels that intensive treatments such as intubation and ICU care would be appropriate for the patient but that CPR might not be. She is not certain enough about this to take an "informed assent" approach, but she does communicate her impression to him: "From what you've told me, I'm not sure if CPR would be best for you, in the unlikely event your heart were to stop."

"Why would you think that?" the patient asks, inquisitively. After the long conversation about his goals, a level of trust has developed between them.

The intern explains a bit more about CPR, noting the difference between television and the real world. She also promises that if he declines CPR, it does not mean he will not get all the other treatments that could help him achieve his goals.

The patient is not sure what to do at that point, so the intern suggests that he be "full code" for the time being, but after he has had some time to think about it, they can discuss it further. He is grateful for this, and she not only places a full code order in his chart, she also makes a point of returning to meet with him and his wife the following day to continue the conversation.

Patients Who Want "Everything"
Case Study

A seventy-six-year-old man with multiple medical problems—hypertension, coronary artery disease, chronic obstructive pulmonary disease, and chronic kidney disease—is admitted to the ICU with sepsis. He does not have an advance directive and was reluctant to see his doctor, let alone talk about what he wanted should his health decline.

Recognizing the patient's very poor prognosis, the medical team engages in the thoughtful approach outlined in the previous section. Through conversation with the family—since the patient lacks decision-making capacity (DMC)—the team identifies the patient's goals and fears, his functional needs, and the trade-offs he is willing to make. It seems clear to the team that he would not want the aggressive treatment he is receiving—especially with the low probability of benefit—and they recommend to the family that he be made DNAR and that consideration be given to forgoing intubation as well.

To the team's surprise, the family is adamant that "everything be done." They remain resolute in this demand, even when the team identifies how this is incompatible with the goals they have just identified.

It is ethically concerning when physicians either assume that a patient is full code or offer choices absent crucial context, such as inquiring whether a patient wants his heart restarted if it happens to stop beating. But posing sensitive questions about personal goals and recommending a plan of treatment is no guarantee of reaching a universally accepted code status. Indeed, it is not uncommon for patients—even when invited into a thoughtful and informed conversation—to blankly state that they "want everything."

This should not be taken literally, of course. With so many modalities in its arsenal, no patient truly wants everything medicine has to offer, as the burden of that would be overwhelming. In fact, "everything" can mean a great many things, depending on what is motivating the patient or family to make that request. Such a request could reflect emotional concerns about being abandoned or ignored, a lack of understanding of the seriousness of one's condition, a sense of spiritual obligation to prolong life as long as possible, or family or social pressures to accept—or even demand—maximal treatment. Given such a wide range of potential meanings, Quill, Arnold, and Back (2009) rightly observe, "Physicians must not assume that 'everything' means any and all invasive treatments unless they have explored what the patient is trying to express with the request." The first step, then, is to determine what exactly the patient means by "everything." Often the unspoken addendum is "[everything] that might help me achieve my goals," which naturally raises the question of what those goals are and what likelihood of benefit would justify the associated burdens. Absent those nuances, the patient would seem to be requesting any treatment that has the remotest chance of providing some manner of benefit. If so, CPR (despite its documented shortcomings) would fall under that rubric.

Here it is helpful to seek additional clarification, framed not in all-or-nothing terms but rather in relation to the patient's goals and his willingness to endure suffering in order to achieve them (Bernacki et al., 2014). His request may certainly stem from rather unique goals that most patients would not share, but it also could involve misperception about what treatments "everything" would entail and their probability of benefit. The request may also stem from a concern that any limitation of treatment may cause the team to be less vigilant in the care they provide (Beach & Morrison, 2002), which could be a legitimate concern (p. 104).

There may also be emotional reasons for the request. For instance, the patient might be experiencing grief over his declining health and be unprepared to admit what that means for him (Kübler-Ross, 1969). This may provoke existential distress, perhaps calling into question religious or spiritual beliefs that he had long derived comfort from (Phelps et al., 2009). Alternatively, he might fear abandonment, unsure if the team might still care about him if he declined certain treatments (Quill & Cassel, 1995). A question such as "What are you most concerned about/scared of?" can help identify driving concerns (Quill, 2000).

There may also be social reasons for his request. He may fear leaving his family vulnerable and grieving and thus seek any possibility of benefit irrespective of burden. His family could be encouraging him to continue to "fight," unable to recognize (as the patient may already have) that certain treatments are highly unlikely to benefit him. Sensitive probing—such as by asking "How is your family handling your illness?"—may be helpful here (King & Quill, 2006).

After identifying what underlying goals/fears/concerns are driving the patient to request "everything," the team can propose a treatment plan with specific reference to these. This is a "second order" application of the recommendation approach described previously, with deeper exploration occasioned by the request for treatment the team feels to be excessive. Quill et al. (2009) suggest verifying proper understanding of overarching goals in this way: "Given what we know about your illness and what I have learned about your priorities, it sounds like you would prefer the following balance of burdens and benefits in your treatment."

If the patient concurs—reflecting that the team has understood the patient correctly—the team can then offer recommendations based on those goals. Often, despite an explicit request for maximal treatment, the patient's goals may actually suggest a more balanced treatment plan. This should include an affirmation of what *will* be done for the patient as well as what will be forgone due to excessive burden or unlikelihood of benefit.

A nonmaximal treatment plan—even if accurately reflecting the patient's goals—may nevertheless provoke a strong response. The patient may not comprehend that certain treatments (such as CPR) are unlikely to benefit him. Alternatively, he may recognize this but be burdened by the implications for his future and his mortality. Emotional support is critical here, as are communication tools and memory aids that can assist in explicitly linking the patient's expressed goals to the recommended treatment plan (Pollak et al., 2007).

Upon receiving such support, the patient may accept the recommended treatment plan, thus leading to consensus. He may, however, persist in his request for "everything." At this point the physician could go back through the prior steps, attempting to identify sources of misunderstanding and providing additional clarification. If the patient is resolute in his request, one option is a time-limited trial (TLT), which is discussed in detail in the next section. This represents something of a middle ground between blanket acceptance of the patient's request on the one hand and unilateral withholding on the other.

In some cases, the patient may either decline the TLT—in favor of indefinite application of the requested interventions—or maintain his request for maximal treatment after the conclusion of the TLT. One option in such a case is to enact institutional mechanisms related to potentially nonbeneficial treatment, which is examined in detail in chapter 14. A less extreme alternative is to revisit the conversation at a later time, hoping that the patient may have changed his mind during the interval, perhaps because of additional reflection or in response to intervening events.

If the thoughtful steps noted here were taken at the outset, however, frequent revisiting tends not to produce a different outcome and may cause the patient and family to feel badgered. The end result is that they become more entrenched in their position, and the physician-patient relationship suffers.

Some have argued that in such situations—particularly those that reflect maladaptive coping—it is appropriate to engage in what has been termed "palliative parentalism" (Roeland et al., 2014). Always a last resort, it is only considered when the patient or family is requesting a treatment plan that is clearly contrary to the patient's expressed values. Roeland et al. have proposed a specific algorithm that initially is consistent with the approach presented here (Figure 4.1).

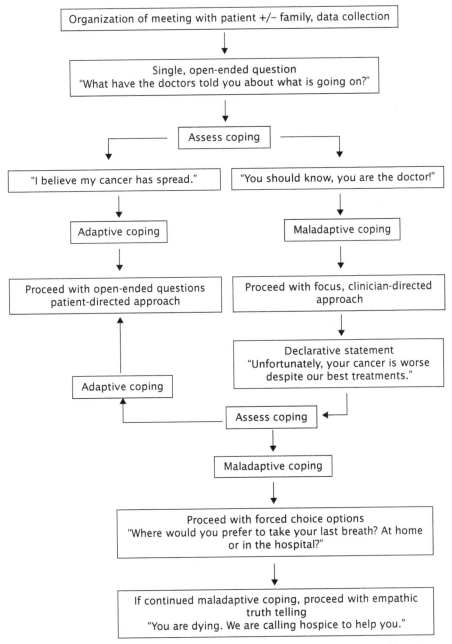

FIGURE 4.1 "Palliative paternalism" in response to requests that are not consonant with patient goals (Roeland, 2014)

The motivation for this approach is clear: a desire to not see the patient and family suffer unnecessarily. The stakes, though, are extremely high, and if the patient and family are unable to accept the "empathic truth telling" of the final stage, there may be a very emotional confrontation. From a purely practical standpoint, it is hard to imagine a patient or family in that situation accepting hospice care, let alone benefitting from it. As such, this approach has the potential to worsen—rather than relieve—suffering in some cases.

When the request for maximal treatment comes from a surrogate decision-maker—and there is a strong sense that the patient himself would not have wanted it—palliative parentalism may be an appropriate option. This would not represent the physician inserting her own values into the discussion as much as acting for the patient's well-being in the context of inaccurate substituted judgment.

But in situations when the patient himself is requesting maximal treatment, Quill et al. (2009) are correct that it is appropriate to provide that treatment, even if it is exceedingly unlikely to be effective. Doing so shows respect for the patient's wishes—which have been discussed in a very open and nuanced way—and also humility on the part of the team, who recognize that merely because the patient's values differ from their own does not make his values "wrong." Rather than continually revisiting this decision, the team can extend an open invitation to the patient that they are always open to further conversation, but only if the patient wishes to pursue it.

Admittedly, some members of the team—especially those who did not participate in (or may not even be aware of) the previous discussions—may experience moral distress (p. 514) at what they perceive to be unnecessary suffering. It is important to communicate to them all the steps that were taken to try to resolve the disagreement with the patient and the rationale for accommodating the patient's request. Some members of the team may not be able, in good conscience, to continue to care for the patient. This should be respected, as long as it does not negatively impact patient care.

Ultimately, when it comes time to administer requested treatments that the team wishes they did not have to provide, a "fast code" is certainly reasonable, whether discontinued by the team or with permission of the family (who may wish to be present). As Quill et al. (2009) write, "This allows the patient and family to know that 'everything possible' was done but avoids having staff go through the futile ordeal of prolonged CPR with no prospect of recovery."

Time-Limited Trials

As noted, one potential response to patients who are requesting potentially inappropriate treatment is a TLT. This approach involves instituting a treatment with a clearly defined time frame, at which point its utility would be reconsidered. Ideally, before initiating the TLT, the hoped-for outcomes would be delineated, as well as the implications of not achieving these. Some have therefore characterized the TLT as "provisional intensive care" (Giannini et al., 2008).

The TLT has received increasing attention as a useful approach to take with a family that is debating whether to initiate burdensome LSMT (Quill & Holloway, 2011), especially mechanical ventilation (Holloway, Benesch, Burgin, & Zentner, 2005; Quill et al., 2009) and enteric feeding (Dy, 2006; Stroud, Duncan, Nightingale, & British Society of Gastroenterology, 2003). For while there is no ethical or legal distinction between withdrawing and withholding (p. 156), there is clearly an emotional difference. In contrast to authorizing LSMT with no clear end-point, a TLT can help families feel that they have tried everything reasonable to help their loved one, while giving a clear time frame when the initial authorization should be reconsidered in light of subsequent developments. Some have argued that it may also assist families in abiding by religious proscriptions on actively discontinuing LSMT (Ravitsky, 2005).

Rather than a blanket acceptance of a request for potentially nonbeneficial treatment—or an authoritarian refusal of it—the TLT creates a middle ground where the family's wishes are respected while also recognizing the low likelihood of meaningful benefit. The time afforded by a limited trial may permit the family to come to grips with the reality of the situation and also build trust with the team as a shift of goals is considered. In the meantime, additional supportive resources can be marshaled and the patient closely monitored for any signs of improvement (Kirschner et al., 2011).

In order to be effective, a TLT needs to have clearly defined limits, during which there is a reasonable probability of either acquiring additional relevant information about the patient's condition or the family assimilating information in such a way as to authorize a shift in goals. Often both are considerations, but the time frame may depend on which is the most relevant. For instance, it would not make sense to institute a twenty-four-hour TLT for mechanical ventilation, as failure to improve over this time frame rarely signals a worsened prognosis. By the same token, in other cases a two-week TLT may be too long—as in the case of severe stroke without recovery of consciousness—as the seminal prognostic interval is much shorter than that (Goodman, Kasner, & Park, 2013).

A TLT is, of course, not binding. At its conclusion a family could certainly continue to request LSMT, even if the clearly delineated treatment goals were not met. There are many reasons for this, including a subjective perception that the patient is indeed improving or a recognition that while they thought they might "come to peace" with forgoing LSMT, this has not occurred.

In such a situation, it is impractical—and counterproductive—to attempt to "enforce" the terms of the TLT. Instead, the team should take a step back and confirm what the family's understanding of the patient's condition and prognosis are. This involves re-engaging the family in terms of the patient's goals and what (if anything) might be leading them to believe that the patient is now improving.

The family's responses to these sensitive queries will help determine next steps. If the family still feels it is "too soon," another TLT could be initiated. In the meantime, the option of Do Not Escalate Treatment (DNET) order (as discussed in the next section) could be raised. If the family is emotionally unable to authorize forgoing LSMT—and the team decides certain forms of LSMT (such as CPR) will not help the patient achieve his goals—an "informed assent" approach (p. 382) could be used. In the most extreme situations, where the team determines that the family is requesting nonbeneficial treatment and all attempts at mediation have failed, the algorithm set forth in chapter 14 could be used. In the vast majority of cases, however, more moderate steps will prove effective.

In addition to showing humility—in terms of admitting the possibility that the patient could exceed the prognosis the team has offered—the medical team should also recognize that time "moves differently" in the hospital. This is particularly true in the ICU, where patients are actively treated twenty-four hours a day. Especially in the early days following ICU admission, the treatment can be very labor-intensive, with the placement of an endotracheal tube, intravenous and intrarterial lines, and other invasive procedures. Further, the ICU team has only known the patient in his critically ill state, which may bear little resemblance to his previous level of health, especially if a catastrophic event (whether traumatic like a motor vehicle accident or nontraumatic such as a massive stroke) has occurred.

It is not uncommon for ICU teams—especially when the patient's prognosis is extremely poor—to feel like intensive treatment has been going on too long and that they are "torturing" the patient (Badger, 2005). An ethics consult addressing unreasonable treatment requests may be requested within the first few days. That may certainly seem like a long time to the team caring for the patient, as they perform invasive procedures on someone who their medical knowledge tells them is extremely unlikely to benefit. But to the family—who loves the patient and knew him in his healthier state (which he might have experienced up until a few days earlier)—any discussion of a shift of goals might seem premature at best and uncaring at worst. A reluctance to even consider such a suggestion is not a sign of incomprehension or pathological denial but rather a normal human response to an abrupt change in a loved one's condition. In that respect, it is often the ICU team's perception of time that is distorted, rather than the family's.

Especially in such a foreign and overwhelming environment as the ICU, it may take more than a few days for a family to appreciate the significance of what this means for their formerly healthy loved one. In how they relay information and in the plans they recommend to the family, the medical team would do well to recognize how time moves much slower for them than for the family, due to these very different backgrounds and real-time experiences.

No Escalation of Treatment

Another middle ground between blanket acceptance and patent refusal of requests for potentially nonbeneficial treatment is a DNET order (Jacobsen & Billings, 2015), which is also referred to as a No Escalation of Care order (Morgan, Varas, Pedroza, & Almoosa, 2014). Rather than withholding a specific treatment—as a DNAR or Do Not Intubate (DNI) order would do—a DNET order generally indicates that current LSMT will not be escalated, and no new forms of LSMT will be initiated. Examples might include not instituting antibiotics or adding vasopressors for low blood pressure.

There are several advantages to DNET orders. Recognizing the long-term psychological impact of surrogate decision-making—especially related to forgoing LSMT (p. 65)—this approach could lessen the psychological burden by "absolving" the decision-maker of ultimate responsibility (Seymour, 2000). The surrogate may be left with a stronger sense that the disease ended the patient's life—as standard treatment continued—rather than death resulting from her decision to forgo LSMT.

As in the case of a TLT, the more gradual time course (compared to withdrawing treatment already in place) may help the family come to terms with the patient's impending death (Duggleby & Berry, 2005; Vig, Starks, Taylor, Hopley, & Fryer-Edwards, 2007) and have an opportunity to grieve, which not surprisingly improves satisfaction rates with end-of-life care (Gerstel, Engelberg, Koepsell, & Curtis, 2008). A DNET order may also pave the way for subsequent withdrawal of treatment already in use, as occurred in the majority of cases in one study of DNET orders (Morgan et al., 2014). Given all these advantages, it is not surprising that 30% of ICU patients in a recent study had a DNET order in place (Morgan et al., 2014).

At the same time, DNET orders have significant drawbacks. In the first place, they can be very imprecise. To add a vasopressor for a patient who is not already receiving that class of medication would clearly constitute "escalation," but what about adding a second vasopressor to a patient already receiving one? Increasing ventilation pressures might seem to be escalation—as it would be a reaction to lack of sufficient response to current settings—but what about "dialing up the oxygen," if only temporarily, which could be required by a transient event like a mucous plug? Is stopping and then restarting a medication considered an "escalation" or merely a "resumption"?

These examples highlight the drawbacks of using an acronym in place of a goal-directed plan of care (Curtis & White, 2008). More than merely a semantic difference, this can have profound implications for palliative medicine because of its unintended consequences. For instance, initiation—or upward titration, if already in use—of symptomatic treatment (such as opioids for pain) might be considered by some to be an escalation. A DNET order would seem to preempt this, even though it is entirely consistent with the underlying goal of that order (i.e., minimizing unnecessary suffering).

Ultimately, a DNET order should be recognized as something of an artifice. It functions as an accommodation for patients and families who—despite the purported ethical and moral equivalence—still find a salient difference between withdrawing and withholding LSMT.[3] While not misleading in the same way a "slow code" is, it is also not nearly as clear as other "Do Not" orders (such as DNAR or DNI) are. Essentially, a DNET order represents patient/family permission for physicians to use their own

---

3. Whether this represents "cognitive bias" on the patient's part (Curtis & Rubenfeld, 2014) or an indication of how physicians and ethicists are out of touch with reality (Dickenson, 2000) is a matter of perspective.

discretion as to what constitutes an "escalation" and what does not, based on what seems consistent with the overall plan of care. Even defenders of the practice admit this: "The guiding principle of no escalation is established by the surrogate (or patient), but the physician typically holds the knowledge of what treatments are to be forgone" (Jacobsen & Billings, 2015).

This seems a necessary component of DNET orders, which are designed to spare families from having to make specific limitation of treatment decisions that they are not yet prepared to make. (A notable exception is situations involving moral or religious beliefs that mandate the continuation—but not necessarily escalation—of certain treatments; Thompson, 2014). When such orders are used following a thoughtful discussion of patient goals as a temporizing measure to allow the patient or family to grips with the reality of a situation, they can be quite useful. But when DNET orders are used as a shortcut to *avoid* having tense and complex conversations with families about what goals are achievable, then their imprecision may ultimately lead to harm. As Curtis and Rubenfeld (2014) rightly observe, "Such an approach should be a reluctant, negotiated settlement rather than a frequently used strategy."

Return to the Case

> In response to the family's demand that "everything" be done for the patient, rather than becoming argumentative the team steps back and asks what the family means by that term. Family members express an expectation that anything that could conceivably help the patient—irrespective of burden—be used, to make sure that he has every chance to survive.
>
> "He's a real fighter," the patient's wife says.
>
> The team attempts to reframe the discussion in terms of the patient's goals—to absolve the family of any potential guilt over not advocating for maximal treatment—and explore the emotional struggles that the family may be experiencing. After reclarifying the patient's goals, the team summarizes them for the family in terms of seeking a positive balance of benefit and burden and respecting the patient's historic aversion to medical care in general.
>
> The family agrees that this is how the patient has lived his life but continues to demand "everything."
>
> Rather than taking a confrontational approach, the team recognizes that while it is clear to them that the patient will not survive, the family is gradually adapting to recent developments in the patient's condition. The team therefore suggests a TLT of intensive care, with maximal treatment (including CPR, if necessary) for the first seventy-two hours, at which point they will meet again to revisit the patient's situation.
>
> Over that period of time the patient's condition worsens slightly, but the team respects the family's privacy and does not attempt to pressure them into changing

the patient's treatment plan. At the seventy-two-hour mark, another meeting is held, at which time the family seems to better appreciate the seriousness of the patient's condition. While still not prepared to authorize forgoing LSMT, they are amenable to the team's suggestion of a DNET order. While the team did not go into specific detail about what was involved in this, they do feel comfortable entering a DNAR order on the chart, with an understanding that significant increases in level of treatment (such as initiation of dialysis) would not occur.

The patient's condition continues to deteriorate, and approximately two days later the family asked how much longer this might go on. With that implicit invitation, the team reviews the patient's condition, prognosis, and treatment options, and the decision is made—likely made more palatable by the prior DNET order—to withdraw mechanical ventilation, after which the patient dies peacefully surrounded by his family.

Overriding Patient Refusal
Case Study

A seventy-eight-year-old man is admitted to the ICU following a partial colectomy for diverticulitis. He has had a complicated postoperative course, remaining intubated and requiring pressors to support his blood pressure. He has no advance directive and the surgery was performed based on "emergency consent," as he lacked DMC at the time.

His prognosis is guarded, but the nursing staff is concerned that his wishes are not being taken seriously. He seems very anxious and continually pulls on the endotracheal tube, like he is trying to remove it.

On rounds on postoperative day 3, the medical student assigned to the patient asks the rest of the team, "But what about this gentleman's autonomy? Doesn't he have the right to say no?"

The preceding section addressed one side of a potential disagreement between physician and patient, namely, a patient who wants everything while the physician feels certain interventions are not indicated. The opposite situation is also quite common: a physician believing a patient would benefit from an intervention but the patient refuses.

At first, this may seem like a straightforward issue, given the well-established (though fairly recent) right of patients with sufficient DMC to refuse any treatment, including one that is life-sustaining (*In re Quinlan*, 1976). In this case, the patient is unable to speak, but his actions certainly seem to indicate he wants the endotracheal tube removed. Shouldn't he have the right to refuse this treatment?

This question, however, is not as simple as it might appear. The patient could be reacting to the discomfort of an indwelling endotracheal tube without full appreciation of the implications of his decision. The operative question, therefore, is not whether the patient wants the tube out—the answer to which appears obvious—but rather whether he would prefer to live with the tube in or have it removed and subsequently die.

As noted, a patient must possess sufficient DMC to refuse LSMT (p. 58), and since DMC is decision-dependent—and forgoing the treatment in question is likely to lead to the patient's death—a greater degree of DMC is required to refuse it. This is particularly relevant because the patient's DMC may be compromised for several reasons. In the first place, he is critically ill, or else he would not be in the ICU. Simply being in the ICU for a period of time can cause delirium (Misak, 2005), affecting the majority of intubated elderly patients in that environment (Ely et al., 2004). Also, he is likely receiving medications (such as sedatives) that can impair DMC.

As with any situation involving potentially impaired DMC, the first step is to assess the patient's level of capacity. This can be very difficult for an intubated patient who is unable to speak. Lip-reading can be very challenging for the medical team (not to mention the patient, who is struggling to be understood). Interpreters can be helpful (Meltzer, Gallagher, Suppes, & Fins, 2012), and message boards have shown some success, though with limited ability to communicate novel utterances. Some newer communication modalities have shown promise but are not universally available (Ten Hoorn, Elbers, Girbes, & Tuinman, 2016).

If DMC is felt to be impaired, the next step is to attempt to restore (or at least maximize) it. Often, however, this is not possible, and as long as the patient remains intubated communication will continue to be a challenge. The next step is to turn to an advance directive or surrogate decision-maker for guidance. Often, however, the former does not exist and the latter is not readily available, leaving the team with an objecting patient and no way to determine with certainty whether he really wants treatment discontinued, given the likely consequences.

Prior to the dawn of the era of "radical autonomy," the solution to this dilemma seemed clear: continue treatment. Indeed, before the right of treatment refusal was fully codified, the typical response to refusal of treatment—even when there was no reason to doubt the patient's DMC—was a psychiatric consultation, because a desire to no longer live was presumed to result from some form of mental illness (p. 8).

Over time, though, the pendulum has swung to the other extreme, equating any refusal of treatment with an invocation of the sacred right of autonomy. This emphasis on patient autonomy is sometimes taken too far, though, overlooking the complexities noted previously. This could potentially lead to precipitous forgoing of treatment and the unnecessary loss of life, which may violate—rather than respect—the patient's actual goals.

Therefore, unless an advance directive or appropriate substituted judgment supports forgoing treatment, a nonverbal expression of refusal of treatment—especially in a context where DMC is likely to be impaired—is not sufficient evidence to forgo that treatment. Confronted with such an expression, the team should "err on the side of life" by stabilizing the patient, in order to preserve options. Additional time may yield greater prognostic certainty as well as provide further opportunities for maximizing DMC. If the patient remains consistent in his refusal of treatment, this may reflect a truly autonomous refusal. The treatment can then be withdrawn based on the ethical equivalence of withdrawing and withholding (p. 156).

This may at first appear to a betrayal of patient autonomy and a return to the paternalism of old. But here it is important to distinguish between "hard" and "soft" paternalism. The former involves overriding an autonomous decision on the part of the patient (Feinberg, 1971) and (as noted earlier) is legally and ethically unacceptable. Soft paternalism, on the other hand, allows restricting certain conduct "when that conduct is substantially nonvoluntary or when temporary intervention is necessary to establish whether it is voluntary or not" (Feinberg, 1984). A patient with delirium is not capable of making autonomous decisions, and thus overriding his refusal is not a violation of his "autonomy" in the hard sense. Rather, it is a temporizing measure to permit the acquisition of additional information, in order to be sure of what the patient's actual goals are.

Even granting this distinction, paternalism of any sort is viewed negatively in a culture that prizes human freedom. We allow people to make "bad" decisions based on faulty reasoning, especially when the alternative is coercion and conformity. But there are limits to this, not only when that decision puts other people at risk but also when it places only the decider in danger. Even the most ardent "antipaternalists" are willing to endorse certain actions that override a compromised person's decisions, such as stopping a visibly inebriated driver from getting behind the wheel of a car. Dworkin (1972) has gone so far as to assert that a rational person would ascribe to soft paternalism as a "social insurance policy" to protect himself from harm at times of irrationality or incapacity.

Two caveats are important here. The first is that while many patients in situations like this lack sufficient DMC to refuse LSMT, not all do. Concerns about impaired DMC could lead to an unjustified blanket overriding of patient refusal, especially given the medical impetus to do everything possible to save a patient's life. A patient's refusal of treatment should *always* be taken seriously, and if it is overridden there needs to be clear justification for doing so, beyond an appeal to what the team feels is in the patient's "best interests."

Second, even if a patient is deemed to lack sufficient DMC to refuse LSMT, this does not necessarily mean that the team should administer that treatment over the patient's objections. Depending on the situation, compulsory treatment could further exacerbate the patient's suffering and sense of helplessness such that the burden of the treatment—administered involuntarily—exceeds its benefit. This is especially true in less acute settings, where the consequences of forgoing treatment are less severe and the burden of imposed treatment greater.

For instance, a patient with impaired DMC might be refusing an ongoing treatment known to have beneficial effects (e.g., oral hypertensives for high blood pressure or oral anticoagulants to mitigate the risk of blood clots from atrial fibrillation). Forgoing the treatment might not have immediate consequences—thus lowering the gravity of the decision and the proportionate level of DMC required to make it—but it could have significant impact over time.

The burden of compulsory treatment is profound, however. This impacts the patient's placement—for it is hard to imagine compelling treatment in a home setting—as well as his sense of control over his life. Such treatment may not even be logistically possible, especially with oral medications that often have to be taken multiple times a day over a prolonged period of time. Since clinical ethics has to be practical (p. 42), there is little point in debating whether or not something can be done, if ultimately it is not an achievable goal.

In some cases, then, the question of whether a patient possesses sufficient DMC to refuse a specific medication may be moot. For if he does possess it, he has the right to refuse, as overriding his refusal would be an example of hard parentalism. But even if his DMC falls short of the required level, is it really appropriate—not to mention compassionate—to force him to swallow pills every day in order to reduce the risk of potential complications?

Palliative care clinicians may not often confront the issue of refusal of recommended non-life-sustaining treatment. Indeed, one of the primary tasks of palliative care clinicians is to winnow down medications whose benefits no longer outweigh their burdens, given the patient's prognosis (Kutner et al., 2015). One area where refusal of treatment can present an ethical dilemma to palliative care clinicians involves symptomatic treatment, such as opioids, which is addressed in detail elsewhere (p. 214). But it is nevertheless crucial for palliative care clinicians to appreciate the ethical nuances surrounding refusal of treatment, in both critical and outpatient settings.

Return to the Case

In response to the medical student's question about the patient's right of autonomy, the physician begins by validating his concerns.

"It's really hard to see someone struggle like that," the physician says. "And it's never pleasant to have to put someone in restraints."

The physician goes on to explain that refusing LSMT requires a significant degree of DMC, and there are several reasons why this patient likely does not possess that: critical illness, several days in the ICU, age. She acknowledges that it is very hard to assess DMC in an intubated patient who cannot speak.

The physician then puts forth a thoughtful plan: optimize treatment for any delirium that may be present, continue to reassure the patient in understandable terms that the team is dedicated to honoring his wishes, and continue to monitor the patient's responses to determine if they are consistent over time.

The physician also informs the student that the patient's family (who live on the other side of the country) will be arriving soon and hopefully will be able to give a fuller picture of the patient's goals and values, for up to that point the team had been working on the assumption that the patient—if he had DMC—would want all the treatment they were providing.

The medical student was not aware of the attempts to reach the patient's family and is reassured by the thoughtful approach being taken.

Summary Points

- Code status (which is usually an abbreviation of letters) should reflect—but does not fully encapsulate—a patient's goals of care.
- Rather than asking a patient what he wants his code status to be, physicians should recommend a code status that reflects the patient's goals (after determining what those goals are).
- DNR is an inadequate term because it implies that resuscitation is possible (if attempted), and AND overlooks the "unnatural" interventions that are a core component of palliative care. DNAR is, therefore, the preferable (though still imperfect) terminology for withholding further interventions in the event of cardiac arrest.
- A DNAR order should not be automatically rescinded in the OR; rather, there should be a "required consideration" as to whether it should remain in place or be temporarily suspended (and, if so, for how long).
- When a patient says he wants "everything," this can mean many different things. Instead of immediately acceding to this request, further exploration is necessary to clarify the patient's understanding and reason for the request.
- If the patient remains resolute in his request for maximal treatment—even when it seems to conflict with his stated goals—it is generally better to honor this request so as to safeguard the physician–patient relationship, with the offer of revisiting this decision at a later time.
- Requested treatment could be instituted as a TLT, at the conclusion of which the patient's condition and prognosis could be reassessed in light of his goals.
- An intermediate position between maximal treatment and forgoing LSMT is a DNET order, which admittedly is imprecise but can relieve the family of significant burden and spare the patient additional suffering.
- If the family is demanding maximal treatment that the team feels conflicts with the patient's goals, this may reflect inappropriate substituted judgment and does not incur the same level of ethical obligation.

- A patient with intact DMC has the right to refuse any treatment, even one that is life sustaining. But for a patient whose DMC is uncertain, it may be wiser to continue treatment until DMC can be maximized or further details about the patient's goals obtained, in order to preserve options.

References

American College of Surgeons. (1994). Statement of the American College of Surgeons on advance directives by patients: "Do not resuscitate" in the operating room. *Bull Am Coll of Surg, 79*(9), 29.

American Society of Anesthesiologists. (2001). Ethical guidelines for the anesthesia care of patients with do-not-resuscitate orders or other directives that limit treatment. Retrieved from http://www.asahq.org/~/media/Sites/ASAHQ/Files/Public/Resources/standards-guidelines/ethical-guidelines-for-the-anesthesia-care-of-patients.pdf

Anderson, W. G., Chase, R., Pantilat, S. Z., Tulsky, J. A., & Auerbach, A. D. (2011). Code status discussions between attending hospitalist physicians and medical patients at hospital admission. *J Gen Intern Med, 26*(4), 359–366. doi:10.1007/s11606-010-1568-6

Anderson, W. G., Pantilat, S. Z., Meltzer, D., Schnipper, J., Kaboli, P., Wetterneck, T. B., . . . Auerbach, A. D. (2011). Code status discussions at hospital admission are not associated with patient and surrogate satisfaction with hospital care: Results from the multicenter hospitalist study. *Am J Hosp Palliat Care, 28*(2), 102–108. doi:10.1177/1049909110374352

Badger, J. M. (2005). A descriptive study of coping strategies used by medical intensive care unit nurses during transitions from cure- to comfort-oriented care. *Heart Lung, 34*(1), 63–68. doi:10.1016/j.hrtlng.2004.08.005

Beach, M. C., & Morrison, R. S. (2002). The effect of do-not-resuscitate orders on physician decision-making. *J Am Geriatr Soc, 50*(12), 2057–2061.

Berger, J. T. (2003). Ethical challenges of partial do-not-resuscitate (DNR) orders: Placing DNR orders in the context of a life-threatening conditions care plan. *Arch Intern Med, 163*(19), 2270–2275. doi:10.1001/archinte.163.19.2270

Bernacki, R. E., Block, S. D., & American College of Physicians High Value Care Task Force. (2014). Communication about serious illness care goals: A review and synthesis of best practices. *JAMA Intern Med, 174*(12), 1994–2003. doi:10.1001/jamainternmed.2014.5271

Billings, J. A. (2012). Getting the DNR. *J Palliat Med, 15*(12), 1288–1290. doi:10.1089/jpm.2012.9544

Billings, J. A., & Block, S. D. (2013). The demise of the Liverpool Care Pathway? A cautionary tale for palliative care. *J Palliat Med, 16*(12), 1492–1495. doi:10.1089/jpm.2013.0493

Burns, J. P., Edwards, J., Johnson, J., Cassem, N. H., & Truog, R. D. (2003). Do-not-resuscitate order after 25 years. *Crit Care Med, 31*(5), 1543–1550. doi:10.1097/01.CCM.0000064743.44696.49

Byock, I. (2012). *The best care possible: A physician's quest to transform care through the end of life.* New York: Avery.

Chen, J. L., Sosnov, J., Lessard, D., & Goldberg, R. J. (2008). Impact of do-not-resuscitation orders on quality of care performance measures in patients hospitalized with acute heart failure. *Am Heart J, 156*(1), 78–84. doi:10.1016/j.ahj.2008.01.030

Chessa F. (2004). "Allow natural death"—not so fast. *Hastings Cent Rep, 34*, 49.

Cohen, C. B., & Cohen, P. J. (1992). Required reconsideration of "do-not-resuscitate" orders in the operating room and certain other treatment settings. *Law Med Health Care, 20*(4), 354–363.

Cohen, R. I., Lisker, G. N., Eichorn, A., Multz, A. S., & Silver, A. (2009). The impact of do-not-resuscitate order on triage decisions to a medical intensive care unit. *J Crit Care, 24*(2), 311–315. doi:10.1016/j.jcrc.2008.01.007

Cohen, R. W. (2004). A tale of two conversations. *Hastings Cent Rep, 34*, 49.

Colby, W. H. (2006). *Unplugged: Reclaiming our right to die in America.* New York: American Management Association.

Compton, S., Levy, P., Griffin, M., Waselewsky, D., Mango, L., & Zalenski, R. (2011). Family-witnessed resuscitation: Bereavement outcomes in an urban environment. *J Palliat Med, 14*(6), 715–721. doi:10.1089/jpm.2010.0463

Curtis, J. R., & Rubenfeld, G. D. (2014). "No escalation of treatment" as a routine strategy for decision-making in the ICU: Con. *Intensive Care Med, 40*(9), 1374–1376. doi:10.1007/s00134-014-3421-6

Curtis, J. R., & White, D. B. (2008). Practical guidance for evidence-based ICU family conferences. *Chest, 134*(4), 835–843. doi:10.1378/chest.08-0235

Dickenson, D. L. (2000). Are medical ethicists out of touch? Practitioner attitudes in the US and UK towards decisions at the end of life. *J Med Ethics, 26*(4), 254–260.

Diem, S. J., Lantos, J. D., & Tulsky, J. A. (1996). Cardiopulmonary resuscitation on television: Miracles and misinformation. *N Engl J Med, 334*(24), 1578–1582. doi:10.1056/NEJM199606133342406

Do, D. T. (2014). Comfort measures only and the value of an informal curriculum. *J Palliat Med, 17*(2), 129–130. doi:10.1089/jpm.2013.0515

Dumot, J. A., Burval, D. J., Sprung, J., Waters, J. H., Mraovic, B., Karafa, M. T., . . . Bourke, D. L. (2001). Outcome of adult cardiopulmonary resuscitations at a tertiary referral center including results of "limited" resuscitations. *Arch Intern Med, 161*(14), 1751–1758.

Duggleby, W., & Berry, P. (2005). Transitions and shifting goals of care for palliative patients and their families. *Clin J Oncol Nurs, 9*(4), 425–428. doi:10.1188/05.CJON.425-428

Dworkin, G. (1972). Parentalism. *The Monist, 56*, 64–84.

Dy, S. M. (2006). Enteral and parenteral nutrition in terminally ill cancer patients: A review of the literature. *Am J Hosp Palliat Care, 23*(5), 369–377. doi:10.1177/1049909106292167

Eckberg, E. (1998). The continuing ethical dilemma of the do-not-resuscitate order. *AORN J, 67*(4), 783–787, 789–790.

Ehlenbach, W. J., & Curtis, J. R. (2011). The meaning of do-not-resuscitation orders: A need for clarity. *Crit Care Med, 39*(1), 193–194. doi:10.1097/CCM.0b013e318202e7d4

Ely, E. W., Shintani, A., Truman, B., Speroff, T., Gordon, S. M., Harrell, F. E. Jr., . . . Dittus, R. S. (2004). Delirium as a predictor of mortality in mechanically ventilated patients in the intensive care unit. *JAMA, 291*(14), 1753–1762. doi:10.1001/jama.291.14.1753

Feinberg, J. (1971). Legal parentalism. *Can J Philos, 1*, 105–124.

Feinberg, J. (1984). *Harm to self: The moral limits of the criminal law.* New York: Oxford University Press.

Fine, R. L. (2007). Language matters: "Sometimes we withdraw treatment but we never withdraw care." *J Palliat Med, 10*(6), 1239–1240. doi:10.1089/jpm.2007.0114

Fink, S. (2013). *Five days at Memorial: Life and death in a storm-ravaged hospital* (1st ed.). New York: Crown.

Fins, J. (2006). *A palliative ethic of care: Clinical wisdom at life's end.* Sudbury, MA: Jones and Bartlett.

Franklin, C. M., & Rothenberg, D. M. (1992). Do-not-resuscitate orders in the presurgical patient. *J Clin Anesth, 4*(3), 181–184.

Gawande, A. (2010, August 2). Letting go. *The New Yorker.*

Gerstel, E., Engelberg, R. A., Koepsell, T., & Curtis, J. R. (2008). Duration of withdrawal of life support in the intensive care unit and association with family satisfaction. *Am J Respir Crit Care Med, 178*(8), 798–804. doi:10.1164/rccm.200711-1617OC

Giannini, A., Messeri, A., Aprile, A., Casalone, C., Jankovic, M., Scarani, R., . . . Viafora, C. (2008). End-of-life decisions in pediatric intensive care. Recommendations of the Italian Society of Neonatal and Pediatric Anesthesia and Intensive Care (SARNePI). *Paediatr Anaesth, 18*(11), 1089–1095. doi:10.1111/j.1460-9592.2008.02777.x

Goodman, D., Kasner, S. E., & Park, S. (2013). Predicting early awakening from coma after intracerebral hemorrhage. *Front Neurol, 4*, 162. doi:10.3389/fneur.2013.00162

Grisso, T., & Appelbaum, P. S. (1998). *Assessing competence to consent to treatment: A guide for physicians and other health professionals.* New York: Oxford University Press.

Gundersen Health System. (2017). Respecting choices. Retrieved from http://www.gundersenhealth.org/respecting-choices

Henneman, E. A., Baird, B., Bellamy, P. E., Faber, L. L., & Oye, R. K. (1994). Effect of do-not-resuscitate orders on the nursing care of critically ill patients. *Am J Crit Care, 3*(6), 467–472.

Holloway, R. G., Benesch, C. G., Burgin, W. S., & Zentner, J. B. (2005). Prognosis and decision making in severe stroke. *JAMA, 294*(6), 725–733. doi:10.1001/jama.294.6.725

In re Quinlan, 70 10 (N.J. 1976).

Jacobsen, J., & Billings, A. (2015). Easing the burden of surrogate decision making: The role of a do-not-escalate-treatment order. *J Palliat Med, 18*(3), 306–309. doi:10.1089/jpm.2014.0295

Jabre, P., Belpomme, V., Azoulay, E., Jacob, L., Bertrand, L., Lapostolle, F., . . . Adnet, F. (2013). Family presence during cardiopulmonary resuscitation. *N Engl J Med, 368*(11), 1008–1018. doi:10.1056/NEJMoa1203366

King, D. A., & Quill, T. (2006). Working with families in palliative care: One size does not fit all. *J Palliat Med, 9*(3), 704–715. doi:10.1089/jpm.2006.9.704

Kirschner, K. L., Kerkhoff, T. R., Butt, L., Yamada, R., Battaglia, C. C., Wu, J., . . . Bahr, E. (2011). "I don't want to live this way, doc. Please take me off the ventilator and let me die." *PM R, 3*(10), 968–975. doi:10.1016/j.pmrj.2011.09.001

Kouwenhoven, W. B., Jude, J. R., & Knickerbocker, G. G. (1960). Closed-chest cardiac massage. *JAMA, 173*, 1064–1067.

Knauft, E., Nielsen, E. L., Engelberg, R. A., Patrick, D. L., & Curtis, J. R. (2005). Barriers and facilitators to end-of-life care communication for patients with COPD. *Chest, 127*(6), 2188–2196. doi: 10.1378/chest.127.6.2188

Kübler-Ross, E. (1969). *On death and dying.* New York: Macmillan.

Kutner, J. S., Blatchford, P. J., Taylor, D. H., Jr., Ritchie, C. S., Bull, J. H., Fairclough, D. L., . . . Abernethy, A. P. (2015). Safety and benefit of discontinuing statin therapy in the setting of advanced, life-limiting illness: A randomized clinical trial. *JAMA Intern Med, 175*(5), 691–700. doi:10.1001/jamainternmed.2015.0289

Lantos, J. D., & Meadow, W. L. (2011). Should the "slow code" be resuscitated? *Am J Bioeth, 11*(11), 8–12. doi:10.1080/15265161.2011.603793

Macauley, R. (2014). You keep using that term. *J Palliat Med, 17*(7), 747–748. doi:10.1089/jpm.2014.0059

Margolick, D. (1982, June 20). Hospital is investigated on life-support policy. *New York Times.* Retrieved from http://www.nytimes.com/1982/06/20/nyregion/hospital-is-investigated-on-life-support-policy.html

Marik, P. E., & Craft, M. (1997). An outcomes analysis of in-hospital cardiopulmonary resuscitation: The futility rationale for do not resuscitate orders. *J Crit Care, 12*(3), 142–146.

Martin, E. A. (Ed.). (2010). *Concise colour medical dictionary* (5th ed.). Oxford: Oxford University Press.

McClenathan, B. M., Torrington, K. G., & Uyehara, C. F. (2002). Family member presence during cardiopulmonary resuscitation: A survey of US and international critical care professionals. *Chest, 122*(6), 2204–2211.

Meltzer, E. C., Gallagher, J. J., Suppes, A., & Fins, J. J. (2012). Lip-reading and the ventilated patient. *Crit Care Med, 40*(5), 1529–1531. doi:10.1097/CCM.0b013e318241e56c

Meyers, T. A., Eichhorn, D. J., Guzzetta, C. E., Clark, A. P., Klein, J. D., Taliaferro, E., & Calvin, A. (2000). Family presence during invasive procedures and resuscitation. *Am J Nurs, 100*(2), 32–42; quiz 43.

Misak, C. (2005). ICU psychosis and patient autonomy: Some thoughts from the inside. *J Med Philos, 30*(4), 411–430. doi:10.1080/03605310591008603

Morgan, C. K., Varas, G. M., Pedroza, C., & Almoosa, K. F. (2014). Defining the practice of "no escalation of care" in the ICU. *Crit Care Med, 42*(2), 357–361. doi:10.1097/CCM.0b013e3182a276c9

Morrow, M. F., Plunkitt, K., & Basta, L. L. (1999). Ethical issues in the management of geriatric cardiac patients—A "slow code" is suggested in response to a critical situation involving a patient with multiple medical problems. *Am J Geriatr Cardiol, 8*(4), 184–185.

Perel, P., Roberts, I., & Ker, K. (2013). Colloids versus crystalloids for fluid resuscitation in critically ill patients. *Cochrane Database Syst Rev, 2*, CD000567. doi:10.1002/14651858.CD000567.pub6

Phelps, A. C., Maciejewski, P. K., Nilsson, M., Balboni, T. A., Wright, A. A., Paulk, M. E., . . . Prigerson, H. G. (2009). Religious coping and use of intensive life-prolonging care near death in patients with advanced cancer. *JAMA, 301*(11), 1140–1147. doi:10.1001/jama.2009.341

Pitcher, D., Smith, G., Nolan, J., & Soar, J. (2009). The death of DNR. Training is needed to dispel confusion around DNAR. *BMJ, 338*, b2021. doi: 10.1136/bmj.b2021

Pollak, K. I., Arnold, R. M., Jeffreys, A. S., Alexander, S. C., Olsen, M. K., Abernethy, A. P., . . . Tulsky, J. A. (2007). Oncologist communication about emotion during visits with patients with advanced cancer. *J Clin Oncol, 25*(36), 5748–5752. doi:10.1200/JCO.2007.12.4180

Quill, T. E. (2000). Perspectives on care at the close of life: Initiating end-of-life discussions with seriously ill patients: Addressing the "elephant in the room." *JAMA, 284*(19), 2502–2507.

Quill, T. E., & Abernethy, A. P. (2013). Generalist plus specialist palliative care—creating a more sustainable model. *N Engl J Med, 368*(13), 1173–1175. doi:10.1056/NEJMp1215620

Quill, T. E., Arnold, R., & Back, A. L. (2009). Discussing treatment preferences with patients who want "everything." *Ann Intern Med, 151*(5), 345–349.

Quill, T. E., & Cassel, C. K. (1995). Nonabandonment: A central obligation for physicians. *Ann Intern Med, 122*(5), 368–374.

Quill, T. E., & Holloway, R. (2011). Time-limited trials near the end of life. *JAMA, 306*(13), 1483–1484. doi:10.1001/jama.2011.1413

Rabkin, M. T., Gillerman, G., & Rice, N. R. (1976). Orders not to resuscitate. *N Engl J Med, 295*(7), 364–366. doi:10.1056/NEJM197608122950705

Ravitsky, V. (2005). Timers on ventilators. *BMJ, 330*(7488), 415–417. doi:10.1136/bmj.330.7488.415

Roeland, E., Cain, J., Onderdonk, C., Kerr, K., Mitchell, W., & Thornberry, K. (2014). When open-ended questions don't work: The role of palliative parentalism in difficult medical decisions. *J Palliat Med, 17*(4), 415–420. doi:10.1089/jpm.2013.0408

Saager, L., Kurz, A., Deogaonkar, A., You, J., Mascha, E. J., Jahan, A., . . . Turan, A. (2011). Pre-existing do-not-resuscitate orders are not associated with increased postoperative morbidity at 30 days in surgical patients. *Crit Care Med, 39*(5), 1036–1041. doi:10.1097/CCM.0b013e31820eb4fc

Schneider, A. P. 2nd, Nelson, D. J., & Brown, D. D. (1993). In-hospital cardiopulmonary resuscitation: A 30-year review. *J Am Board Fam Pract, 6*(2), 91–101.

Seymour, J. E. (2000). Negotiating natural death in intensive care. *Soc Sci Med, 51*(8), 1241–1252.

Sokol, D. K. (2009). The death of DNR. *BMJ, 338*, b1723. doi:10.1136/bmj.b1723

Standards for cardiopulmonary resuscitation (CPR) and emergency cardiac care (ECC). (1974). *JAMA, 227*(7 Suppl.), 864–868.

Stapleton, R. D., Ehlenbach, W. J., Deyo, R. A., & Curtis, J. R. (2014). Long-term outcomes after in-hospital CPR in older adults with chronic illness. *Chest, 146*(5), 1214–1225. doi:10.1378/chest.13-2110

Stroud, M., Duncan, H., Nightingale, J., & British Society of Gastroenterology. (2003). Guidelines for enteral feeding in adult hospital patients. *Gut, 52*(Suppl. 7), vii1–vii12.

Sullivan, R. (1984, March 24). Queens hospital accused of denial of care. *New York Times*, p. A17.

Ten Hoorn, S., Elbers, P. W., Girbes, A. R., & Tuinman, P. R. (2016). Communicating with conscious and mechanically ventilated critically ill patients: A systematic review. *Crit Care, 20*(1), 333. doi:10.1186/s13054-016-1483-2

Thompson, D. R. (2014). "No escalation of treatment" as a routine strategy for decision-making in the ICU: Pro. *Intensive Care Med, 40*(9), 1372–1373. doi:10.1007/s00134-014-3422-5

Truog, R. D. (2011). Do-not-resuscitate orders in evolution: Matching medical interventions with patient goals. *Crit Care Med, 39*(5), 1213–1214. doi:10.1097/CCM.0b013e31821488b4

Truog, R. D., Waisel, D. B., & Burns, J. P. (1999). DNR in the OR: A goal-directed approach. *Anesthesiology, 90*(1), 289–295.

Vanpee, D., & Swine, C. (2004). Scale of levels of care versus DNR orders. *J Med Ethics, 30*(4), 351–352.

Venneman, S. S., Narnor-Harris, P., Perish, M., & Hamilton, M. (2008). "Allow natural death" versus "do not resuscitate": Three words that can change a life. *J Med Ethics, 34*, 2–6.

Vig, E. K., Starks, H., Taylor, J. S., Hopley, E. K., & Fryer-Edwards, K. (2007). Surviving surrogate decision-making: What helps and hampers the experience of making medical decisions for others. *J Gen Intern Med, 22*(9), 1274–1279. doi:10.1007/s11606-007-0252-y

Weiner, B. K., & Essis, F. M. (2006). Patient preferences regarding spine surgical decision making. *Spine (Phila Pa 1976), 31*(24), 2857–2860. doi: 10.1097/01.brs.0000245840.42669.f1

Death and Dying

5

The "Right to Die"

One of the most common misconceptions about palliative care is that it is only about dying. Granted, hospice care in the United States is reserved for patients with a life expectancy of six months or less, but palliative care is appropriate for any patient facing life-limiting illness. It is quite possible that a palliative care team could follow a patient for years through successive stages of illness. In its quest to help a patient maximize quality of life and formulate a treatment plan based on her goals, a palliative care consultation might well recommend maximal treatment—up to and including CPR—if that reflects the patient's values. It is also possible that a patient might "graduate" from palliative care, if she is ultimately cured of a disease that previously threatened her life.

Yet while palliative care is not *only* about dying, it certainly includes dying: planning for it, minimizing suffering through it, and supporting a family after it. As such, one of the fundamental ethical questions in the practice of palliative care is whether or not a patient has "the right to die." But in order to answer this question, one must first clarify what is meant by having a right to something.

As noted earlier, there are essentially two types of rights (Feinberg, 1973). A negative right is one of noninterference, according to which others cannot stand in the way of a person's obtaining something. This right is clearly expressed in the Fourteenth Amendment to the Constitution, which bars the government from depriving a person of "life, liberty, or property" without due process of law.

A positive right, on the other hand, is a right of entitlement, which necessarily incurs an obligation on the part of another (often the government) to help a person obtain that to which she has a right, if she is unable to do so on her own. Because positive rights are so broad, there are relatively few in American society: education through grade twelve, police protection, fire protection, and military protection are among them. Notably absent on this list is the universal right to health care, which every member nation of the Organisation for Economic Co-operation and Development—with the exception of the United States and Mexico—provides (Organisation for Economic Co-operation and Development, 2014).

The current discussion about the "right to die" pertains to a positive right to assisted or hastened death, in the form of physician-assisted dying (PAD) or euthanasia. This is not because the negative right to die—in the form of a patient's right to refuse life-sustaining medical treatment (LSMT)[1]—is unimportant but rather because it is universally acknowledged (and thus not ethically contentious). This was not the case, however, in the 1970s, when the right to die began to be hotly debated in American society. Back then, advocates for expanding a patient's rights in this area went to great lengths to emphasize that they were *only* talking about the negative right. Recognizing the broad societal consensus that active euthanasia was morally wrong (for reasons that are explored later), defenders of a patient's right to refuse LSMT—which was then called "passive euthanasia"—centered on distinguishing this practice from active euthanasia, so as to avoid "guilt by association."

As we will see, the pendulum has now swung back to the other side, with active methods being the focus of the debate and the distinction that was emphasized in order to justify "passive" methods now being questioned in order to potentially justify active ones.

Gradual Acceptance of a Right to Die

The middle of the twentieth century witnessed an explosion of medical technology, including antibiotics, mechanical ventilators, and dialysis machines. Suddenly it was possible to prolong the lives of patients who in an earlier era would certainly have died. But just because it is possible to do something does not mean that one *should* do it, which is the classic distinction between the science of medicine and the art of ethics.

Technological innovation logically raised the question of whether there was a "right to die." To appreciate what that term meant at the outset of the US societal debate in the 1970s—and what it has come to refer to now—it is helpful to lay out treatment plans on something of a spectrum (Figure 5.1). On one side is focus on curative treatment, which is not ethically contentious as autonomy and beneficence are in perfect alignment. But as soon as the goal (of both the patient and her medical team) ceases to be life prolongation, there is a broad range of treatment plans that may result in—or even ultimately cause, with increasing levels of intention and physician involvement—the patient's death. This end of the spectrum is open to significant interpretation, and the degree of specificity one applies to it will largely determine one's ethical position on certain practices.

Curative	Forgoing	Intensive	PAD	Active
treatment	LSMT	symptom management		euthanasia

FIGURE 5.1 Spectrum of treatment goals

1. Life-sustaining medical therapies are those that are known or strongly believed to extend survival, such as assisted ventilation, medically administered nutrition and hydration, renal replacement therapy (i.e., dialysis), vasoactive infusions, implanted electronic cardiac devices, as well as transfusions, oxygen, antibiotics, and insulin.

Forgoing LSMT

When the right to die debate began in earnest in the 1970s, essentially any treatment that did not prioritize survival was considered a form of "euthanasia" (Figure 5.2). Two general categories of euthanasia were frequently discussed (Randall & Downie, 1999): active and passive. Active euthanasia involved an external step taken either by the patient herself (in the form of "assisted dying") or by another person (generally the physician, as in the case of lethal injection). Active euthanasia can be further subdivided into voluntary, nonvoluntary, and involuntary forms, depending on whether the patient requested it, expressed no preference, or refused it. The second type of euthanasia was passive, which referred to forgoing LSMT that ultimately resulted in the death of a patient from her underlying disease. Today this would be called either "limiting treatment" or "allowing to die" and is discussed in detail in the following chapter.

	Euthanasia			
	Passive	**Double effect**		**Active**
Curative treatment	Forgoing LSMT	Intensive symptom management	PAD	Active euthanasia

FIGURE 5.2 Broad conception of "euthanasia" at the outset of the right to die debate in the United States

In between these two resides intensive symptom management that *could* hasten the patient's death. This merits thoughtful examination because it too was once deemed ethically suspect.[2] Indeed, it is the root of the opiophobia that has resulted in many painful deaths.

While euthanasia literally means "good death," the term carries an extremely negative connotation in American society. Attempts to justify all forms of euthanasia had failed before (as detailed in the discussion of active euthanasia), so the only recourse for establishing a patient's right to refuse LSMT (i.e., passive euthanasia) was to claim that this differed in some meaningful way from active euthanasia. If it did not, then the societal approbation directed at the latter would also apply to the former. Without this clear line between passive and active, substantive discussion about forgoing LSMT would never have occurred. As Meisel (2016) writes, "The keystone of the consensus about end-of-life decision making that evolved from the 1970s to the 1990s was that there is a clear, bright line between passively hastening death and actively hastening death."

---

2. It is critical to stress that intensive symptom management only *potentially*—and rarely—hastens death. In point of fact, optimal pain management can often prolong life. This topic is explored in detail in chapter 7.

The distinction between hastening a patient's death and refraining from intervening to save a patient's life might seem obvious. However, the active/passive distinction is not as crisp as it first appears. In many situations, so-called passive euthanasia doesn't seem "passive" at all. Withdrawing LSMT requires an action on the part of the medical team, whether in the form of writing an order to discontinue a treatment or physically removing an intervention (such as an endotracheal tube). By the same token, withholding LSMT involves an active decision to not intervene. One might go so far as to assert that each time one treatment is provided, this represents a decision not to use any number of alternative treatments. Rachels (1975) therefore claims that "for any purpose of moral assessment, [the decision to let a patient die] is a type of action nonetheless."

If the active/passive distinction does not hold, what then can set forgoing LSMT apart from active euthanasia? Some have argued that the true distinction is one of causality: when forgoing LSMT, the physician's action does not cause the patient's death; rather, the underlying disease does. After all, refraining from intubating a healthy patient will not cause her death, which will only ensue if the patient is in respiratory failure. In philosophical terms, forgoing LSMT is a necessary but not sufficient cause of the latter patient's death, whereas active euthanasia is both a necessary and sufficient cause for a patient not dependent on LSMT (Fins, 2006). As Callahan (1996) observes, "Only dying people will die when life support is removed, not those of us who are healthy."

While this is factually true, it does not directly answer the question of whether the physician is ethically culpable for his conduct in not intervening to prevent the patient's death (Meisel, 2016). To illustrate this point, Rachels (1975) puts forth what has become a famous hypothetical case in medical ethics. Suppose a person stands to inherit a great deal of money if something should happen to his six-year-old cousin. In order to get the money, the man plans to drown the child in the bathtub and then claim that it was an accident. This would obviously be a case of murder and, therefore, clearly wrong.

But further suppose that when the man enters the bathroom to drown the child, he discovers that the child has fallen and hit his head and is now face down in the water. The man watches as the child dies, although he could easily have prevented the death by removing the child from the bath. Is the man any less morally culpable, Rachels (1975) asks, for standing by while the child drowns "of natural causes," when he could so easily have helped him?

Rachels (1975) claims that if there really were a difference between killing and letting die—as is posited by defenders of passive euthanasia—then watching the child die should be less objectionable than having physically drowned him. But since passively standing by and watching the child die is morally reprehensible in its own right, then the distinction fails. As such, active and passive euthanasia succeed or fail together: if one is acceptable then so is the other, and if one is ethically impermissible, so too is the other.

Rachels' (1975) argument can be critiqued on several grounds. First, from a crisply legal perspective, there exists a distinction between killing a person—which is universally illegal—and declining to offer assistance to a person at risk of harm or death, which is a legal requirement in only a minority of states (Volokh, 2009). However, while this may be a compelling legal argument, it does not make the man's actions in the latter scenario *ethically* acceptable.

Yet even if one grants that there is no moral difference between letting die and killing in Rachels' hypothetical scenario, this does not mean that there is *never* a moral difference (Randall & Downie, 2006). The real problem is with his reasoning by analogy, in attempting to extend conclusions relevant to a healthy boy in a bathtub to a patient who requires LSMT in order to survive. These contexts are fundamentally different and thus generate divergent conclusions.

One proposed difference between Rachels' hypothetical scenario and that of a patient dependent on LSMT is that the patient was going to die anyway. Thus failure to act results in death only because of the patient's disease process. This is not a compelling criticism, however, because the boy in the bathtub also was suffering from a medical condition—in this case, unconsciousness secondary to trauma—that prevented him from obtaining the oxygen he needed to survive. To be sure, this is a much milder medical condition than, for instance, multisystem organ failure in the intensive care unit (ICU). But as soon as one says that forgoing LSMT is acceptable as long as a disease is "serious enough," it introduces an external value judgment that potentially limits a patient's freedom to choose.

The more relevant distinction between Rachels' example and forgoing LSMT is the fact that the patient does not want to receive the treatment in question. One presumes that the six-year-old boy would have wanted to be saved from drowning, and thus the uncle's actions—whether actively drowning or refraining from saving—deprive the boy of the life he wanted to lead. By contrast, a physician who withholds or withdraws LSMT based on patient refusal is respecting the patient's right to not have things done to her. Just because a child drowning in a bathtub would want to be saved does not mean every patient with a life-threatening condition would, too.

Should there be any doubt of this, it might help to carry Rachels' argument to its logical conclusion. If not providing a patient with LSMT is as wrong as watching a child drown in a bathtub, then all patients would have to receive every treatment (including CPR) that could conceivably benefit them. Honoring DNAR orders would become morally equivalent to murder. The technological imperative would no longer be a clinical tendency that bioethics attempts to keep in check but rather a *moral* imperative that bioethics should defend and propagate, with the end result being maximal treatment for all patients whether they want it or not (Gert, Culver, & Clouser, 1998).

Clearly this situation would be absurd and destructive, subjecting patients to extensive burdensome and unwanted treatment. But Rachels' provocative argument does force defenders of so-called passive euthanasia to articulate an ethical defense of the practice, rather than simply assuming it is acceptable. That ethical defense lies not in the "passivity" of forgoing LSMT or the underlying condition of the patient, but in the right of privacy of competent patients (sometimes exercised by their surrogates) to refuse procedures done to their bodies.

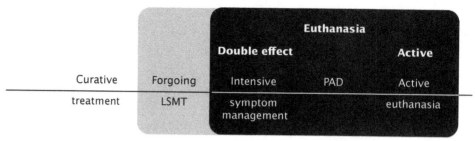

FIGURE 5.3 Narrowing conception of euthanasia, with societal acceptance of "letting die"

This was the conclusion of the first major US court to affirm the right to refuse LSMT (*In re Quinlan*, 1976). When Karen Ann Quinlan's parents requested discontinuation of her ventilator, the hospital initially refused, considering it a violation of medical ethics. Even when the New Jersey Supreme Court mandated extubation, Karen Ann's physician was reluctant, considering this akin to murder. Clearly not appreciating the distinction between active and passive euthanasia, he weaned the ventilator, and to many people's surprise she was able to breathe on her own. She remained in a vegetative state until her death from pneumonia ten years later.

That same year California passed the first law empowering patients to refuse LSMT (California Natural Death Act, 1976). In following years both professional statements (President's Commission for the Study of Ethical Problems in Medicine and Biomedical and Behavioral Research, 1983) and practical guidelines (The Hastings Center, 1987) supported this right.

Thus untethered from the approbation of active euthanasia, cultural acceptance of the right to refuse LSMT grew swiftly (Truog et al., 2008). Over the next few years courts affirmed the right of patients to forgo chemotherapy (*Superintendent of Belchertown State School v. Saikewicz*, 1977) and of conscious patients to refuse ventilatory support (*Satz v. Perlmutter*, 1980). Medically administered nutrition and hydration (MANH) continued to be an issue even after physicians who had discontinued it were acquitted in a criminal case (*Barber v. Superior Court*, 1983), until it was definitively resolved by the US Supreme Court (*Cruzan v. Director, Missouri Department of Health*, 1990).

As refusal of LSMT came to be known as "letting die," the term "passive euthanasia" faded from public discourse. The prior link to euthanasia was effectively severed (Figure 5.3).

Intensive Symptom Management

Having established precedent for a patient's right to forgo LSMT, the next topic to be addressed in relationship to the right to die was a patient's right to receive symptomatic treatment that could (hypothetically) hasten her death. No one dared claim that this was a "passive" process, for it involved the administration of medications with significant side effects. As such, it expanded beyond the patient's negative right to noninterference and encompassed a positive claim to symptomatic relief, even at the risk of hastened death.

Given the link between medication administration and (potential) death, some viewed this as closely related—if not equivalent—to active euthanasia. Indeed, some have even termed the practice "double effect euthanasia" (Vaux, 1989) or (referring to a distorted form of the practice) "slow euthanasia" (Billings & Block, 1996).

Once again, defenders of the practice strove to distinguish it from active euthanasia. The primary distinction lies in the purpose of the action: unlike PAD or active euthanasia (whose purpose is the death of the patient) intensive symptom management focuses on the patient's comfort while also recognizing the risks involved. More nuanced justification of the practice rests upon the Rule of Double Effect, which is discussed in detail later (p. 209).

As was the case with "letting die," intensive symptom management at the end of life also came to be well accepted over time (AMA Council on Ethical and Judicial Affairs, 1992; Foley, 1997; Pellegrino, 1992; President's Commission for the Study of Ethical Problems in Medicine and Biomedical and Behavioral Research, 1983; The Hastings Center, 1987). It was also eventually endorsed by the US Supreme Court, in a case that ostensibly was considering the legality of PAD: "It is widely recognized that the provision of pain medication is ethically and professionally acceptable even when the treatment may hasten the patient's death if the medication is intended to alleviate pain and severe discomfort, not to cause death" (*Vacco v. Quill*, 1997).

Like limitation of LSMT before it, intensive symptom management was effectively distinguished from euthanasia, which continued to be rejected by physicians, ethicists, and the courts (Figure 5.4).

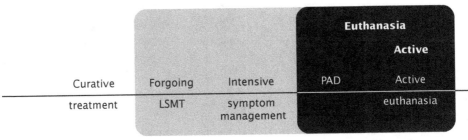

FIGURE 5.4 Narrowing conception of euthanasia, with societal acceptance of intensive symptom management

Physician-Assisted Dying

By this point the term "euthanasia" had become much narrower in scope, with forgoing LSMT and intensive symptom management now distinguished from it and generally accepted by society. There now arose a fork in the road. One path led to continued progression toward methods of hastened death that were indisputably purposeful, including active euthanasia itself. The other was content with the gains made and focused exclusively on palliative care, "which intends neither to hasten nor postpone death" (World Health Organization, 2002).

The latter path was based on concern that further progression toward euthanasia was unwise. This could be due to moral reservations about actions clearly intended to hasten death—sometimes based on religious or spiritual convictions—or a sense of professional obligation. The Hippocratic Oath, after all, puts it quite clearly: "I will not give a lethal drug to anyone if I am asked, nor will I advise such a plan" (Hippocrates, 1959). There was also a very practical concern: with each step toward active euthanasia, the distinction lessened between it and the interventions that society had previously come to endorse. If that distinction ultimately dissolved, previous gains might be lost.

The issue of PAD is comprehensively explored in chapter 8. But suffice it to say here that if one were to reject PAD on ethical grounds, the conversation about whether to continue to further extend the right to die would cease. For those who consider PAD and euthanasia to be ethically equivalent (Kass, 1992), rejection of PAD is equivalent to rejection of active euthanasia. And for those who draw distinctions between the two practices, PAD is certainly more ethically palatable than active euthanasia.[3] Therefore, if PAD fails the ethical litmus test, active euthanasia certainly would as well.

But if one were to approve of PAD at least in certain instances (Figure 5.5), this necessarily raises the question about whether the distinctions drawn between it and

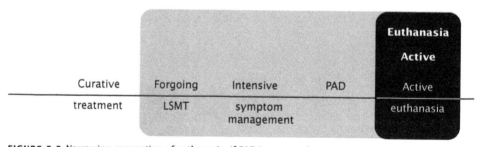

FIGURE 5.5 Narrowing conception of euthanasia, if PAD is accepted

3. Relevant differences include the fact that informed consent for PAD appears assured by the patient's self-administration, and the physician does not administer the lethal dose.

euthanasia are of sufficient ethical importance to render a different conclusion about the latter. Some advocates of PAD argue that there is precious little difference between it and active euthanasia (Dworkin, Frey, & Bok, 1998). Indeed, Canada's recently legalized "medically assisted dying," a term that refers to both PAD as well as active euthanasia (Bill C-14, 2016). Such assertions of equivalence attempt to extend the evolving societal acceptance of the former to envelope the latter (which would have been unfathomable at the outset of the right to die debate). If this equivalence is accepted, then all the respective versions of the right to die—ranging from forgoing LSMT to active euthanasia, once thought to be clearly distinct—would either stand together or fall as one.

This brings us to an in-depth discussion of euthanasia, the moral approbation of which necessitated the nuanced analysis of forgoing LSMT, intensive symptom management, and PAD in the first place.

Euthanasia

On one level, it may seem unusual to include "euthanasia" in a textbook of the ethics of *palliative care*, given that palliative care by definition excludes active hastening of death (Randall & Downie, 1999). Strictly speaking, the concept of euthanasia is more appropriate for a textbook related to the ethics at the end of life, since euthanasia intends to end the patient's life. But since palliative care clinicians attend to terminally ill patients—as well as those whose suffering may make them request actively hastened death—the question of euthanasia not uncommonly arises. Indeed, euthanasia and PAD are the most commonly discussed ethical issues in palliative care journals (Hermsen & ten Have, 2001). Clinicians therefore need to understand—and be able to articulate—why euthanasia is not part of palliative care or part of ethical medical care as a whole. Absent a reasoned critique of euthanasia, it could become incorporated into the more common and much less precise term "the right to die" or equated with the ethically defensible practices already discussed, thereby tainting them.

So why shouldn't palliative care clinicians actively—and intentionally—hasten a patient's death? After all, palliative care is focused on respecting patient rights and doing everything in its power to alleviate suffering. For the vast majority of patients suffering from terminal illness, transdisciplinary palliative care can effectively alleviate suffering and help assure what that patient considers a "good death." But what of the important minority of patients whose suffering cannot be alleviated, despite every good effort? Such patients may turn to their trusted palliative care clinician—who has walked with them every step of the way and who understands what makes life worth living for them (or, at least, once did)—and specifically request to be "put out of their misery." Does not the duty of compassion, which is so firmly rooted within palliative care, obligate the clinician to assist that patient in hastening her own death?

To effectively answer this question, the historical evolution of euthanasia—both in terms of what it referred to and who effected it—needs to be traced.

Historicolegal Evolution

While carrying a distinctly negative connotation in modern Western society, eutha-nasia—like some other now-rejected practices, such as infanticide (p. 305)—was once generally accepted. Literally coming from the words "good" and "death" in Greek, it was widely practiced in the ancient world (Amundsen, 1978), even though the Hippocratic Oath condemned it (Dowbiggin, 2003).

With the rise of Christianity, however, euthanasia fell into disfavor. Thomas Aquinas ultimately put forth a detailed critique of suicide, which has been applied to voluntary euthanasia and continues to influence Christian theology. He cited several reasons why suicide is contrary to God's will, including that it violates one's duty to oneself (as well as the natural inclination of self-perpetuation), injures the commu-nity that the individual was a part of, and fails to recognize that life is a divine gift, belonging to God alone (Aquinas & Gilby, 1969). While certain commentators still defended taking a life (even voluntarily), by the Middle Ages this practice was almost universally rejected (Manning, 1998).

The term "euthanasia" was first used in English for actively hastened death by Thomas More in his novel *Utopia*:

> Should life become unbearable for these incurables the magistrates and priests do not hesitate to prescribe euthanasia. . . . When the sick have been persuaded of this, they end their lives willingly either by starvation or drugs, that dissolve their lives without any sensation of death. Still, the Utopians do not do away with anyone without his permission, nor lessen any of their duties to him. (More & Turner, 1984)

Voluntariness is clearly part of More's concept of euthanasia, but there is no explicit ref-erence to medical professionals playing a role.

The participation of the physician was explored by Francis Bacon. He felt that physicians had an obligation to "not only restore the health, but to mitigate pain and dolours; and not only when such mitigation may conduce to recovery, but when it may serve a fair and easy passage" (Bacon, 1924). While Bacon also used the term "eutha-nasia," he was referring to an easy, painless death, not the active hastening of death.

Others took the discussion further. Some English and continental philosophers—such as John Donne and David Hume—argued in favor of the right to end one's own life (Fye, 1978). Anglo-American common law, however, wholeheartedly rejected the prac-tice (Cushing, 1977).

With the coming of the Enlightenment (and related questioning of religious princi-ples), this moral consensus dissolved. But other ethical matters received greater attention than suicide, and before this concept could be fully explored—let alone implemented—the Great Awakening of the mid-eighteenth century began. As religious devotion grew, the moral prohibition on suicide returned, with widespread adoption of state laws banning assisted suicide beginning with New York in 1828. There was, however, greater mercy shown toward those who did take their own lives, with widespread repeal of anti-suicide laws, which mandated forfeiture of assets (Dowbiggin, 2003).

At around the same time, sedatives and analgesics—such as ether, chloroform, and morphine—were being increasingly used to ease a patient's dying (Warren, 1848). Recognizing that these could, at very high doses, hasten death, some advocated for their use in this way. One of the first was Samuel Williams:

> In all cases of hopeless and painful illness, it should be the recognized duty of the medical attendant, whenever so desired by the patient, to administer chloroform or such other anaesthetic . . . so as to destroy consciousness at once, and put the sufferer to a quick and painless death. (Williams, 1872)

Such proposals were met with stiff opposition from professional societies such as the American Medical Association, which asserted that such practice would force "the physician [to] don the robes of an executioner" ("The Moral Side of Euthanasia," 1885). This was just the first of many times that advocates of active euthanasia came forward and made arguments, only to see professional groups—or social forces—repel their advances, only to have the same seesaw battle resume when enough time had passed (or circumstances had changed).

The next iteration of the cycle occurred at the beginning of the twentieth century when Charles Eliot Norton, a noted Harvard professor, advocated for voluntary active euthanasia (Emanuel, 1994). This led to the first proposed legislation legalizing euthanasia, which failed in 1905 in Ohio as did similar legislation in Iowa. Soon thereafter other issues—such as World War I and the Great Depression—took center stage, rendering the debate about euthanasia temporarily moot.

The issue of euthanasia returned to public debate in the 1930s. The conversation went so far that the Voluntary Euthanasia Society was founded in Britain in 1935 ("Voluntary Euthanasia," 1935) and the Euthanasia Society of America in 1938. The House of Lords considered (and ultimately rejected) a euthanasia bill in 1936. A similar bill was introduced into the US Senate that same year but was not voted on (Hilliard, 2000). Yet again the debate was truncated by pressing world events, this time in the form of World War II. The subsequent revelation of abuses of prisoners by Nazi physicians prompted greater caution about so-called "mercy killing."

The ebb and flow continued in the following decade, which saw a resurgence of conversation on the topic (Kamisar, 1958; Williams, 1957). This prompted the House of Lords to reconsider legalizing euthanasia in 1969, only to again reject it. It was against this backdrop of solid opposition to active euthanasia that the focus of the right to die movement shifted toward more "passive" methods, with great pains taken to distinguish them from active euthanasia (p. 143). Thus the American Hospital Association's Patient Bill of Rights (1973), the California Natural Death Act (1976), and the *Quinlan* decision

(*In re Quinlan*, 1976) all focused on the right to refuse LSMT, rather than having death actively hastened.

What had repeatedly been rejected in Great Britain and the United States found a more favorable reception in the Netherlands. The "Postma case" brought the practice to public notice in 1973, when a Dutch physician ended the life of her ailing mother (at the mother's request). The physician was found guilty of murder but only received a short, suspended sentence. The court concluded that a physician is not always obligated to keep a patient—who is experiencing extreme suffering—alive (Rietjens, van der Maas, Onwuteaka-Philipsen, van Delden, & van der Heide, 2009).

Having allowed that euthanasia might sometimes be acceptable, much discussion ensued about what circumstances would justify the practice. The Dutch Supreme Court addressed the issue for the first time in 1984 in the *Schoonheim* case, acquitting a physician who performed euthanasia because it was a situation "of necessity" (Griffiths, Bood, & Weyers, 1998).

That same year the Royal Dutch Medical Society published guidelines about how physicians ought to respond to a request for euthanasia (Central Board of the Royal Dutch Medical Association, 1984), which have been modified several times since. The following year a State Commission completed its report on euthanasia, which was defined as "intentionally terminating another person's life at the person's request." The Commission outlined the conditions in which it was deemed acceptable, which were later incorporated into the Euthanasia Act:

- Patient's request is voluntary and well-considered.
- Patient's suffering is unbearable and hopeless.
- Patient is fully informed.
- There are no reasonable alternatives.
- A second opinion should be obtained.
- Termination of life should be performed with due medical care and attention (de Haan, 2002).

The system moved beyond recommendations in the 1990s, when the Ministry of Justice established a formal reporting procedure which—if completed and the requirements met—would shield physicians from prosecution. This prompted widespread reporting (van der Maas et al., 1996) and commentary (Angell, 1996) on the practice, as it became more commonly used. When the Euthanasia Act was finally passed in 2002, it was legalizing a practice already in use.

A handful of countries have followed suit. Belgium legalized both PAD and euthanasia in 2002, for adults and emancipated minors who were experiencing "constant and unbearable physical or mental suffering that cannot be alleviated," but need not be terminally ill (Chambre des Représentants de Belgique, 2002). Luxembourg legalized PAD and euthanasia in 2008 for patients with a "grave and incurable condition" who had made repeated requests (Watson, 2009).

Children can also be eligible for euthanasia. The Netherlands permits euthanasia for children age twelve and older with their parents' consent and also has a specific protocol for infants (p. 326). Prompting much international debate, Belgium subsequently expanded its law in 2014 to apply to minors of any age (again, with their parents' consent) (Siegel, Sisti, & Caplan, 2014).

Canada—after many preliminary explorations and court stays—passed a law in 2016 that applies to adults who suffer from a "grievous and irremediable medical condition." As noted, the law permits a physician to provide such a patient with a substance that causes death, either administered by the physician or by the patient herself (Bill C-14, 2016).

Active euthanasia was not realistically considered in the United States, and thus most of the attention related to hastened death centered on PAD (Quill, 1991). This was logical, given that PAD is the next logical extension of the right to die (Figure 5.4), and the societal approbation of active euthanasia remained strong.[4] A comparison of the countries where euthanasia has not only been extensively debated but also legalized (the Netherlands, in particular) suggests a reason for this. In contrast to the United States—which continues to espouse relatively strong religious beliefs, especially in the deep South—the Netherlands has a deep and hallowed history in natural law (Grotius et al., 1682). Over three-quarters of the Dutch population consider religion "unimportant," whereas only one-third of Americans do (Gallup, 2009). This might represent a partial explanation for Canada joining the select group of nations having legalized euthanasia, given its significantly decreased religiosity compared with the United States (Gallup, 2003).

Even though the focus of philosophical and legislative debate in the United States remains PAD, the topic of euthanasia is still relevant, as palliative care clinicians should be able to articulate the reasons why it is not part of the current ethical discussion. They should also appreciate the consequences for reintroducing it into the debate, especially if the proposed justification is its asserted equivalence to other forms of the right to die, which could have profound implications for the practice of palliative care.

Ethical
Arguments For

The two primary arguments in favor of euthanasia are the same as those for PAD and are discussed more fully in chapter 8. The first is autonomy, according to which patients have the right to determine their own course of action. Applied to euthanasia, this is a significant extension of the right to die, going beyond the negative right of noninterference to a positive right to assistance in achieving one's goal (in this case, the ending of one's life).

---

4. There were a few exceptions, however. One was a seminal (and anonymous) editorial in *JAMA* by a physician who described performing nonvoluntary euthanasia on a patient ("It's over, Debbie," 1988). Published surveys also revealed physicians did, on occasion, actively hasten death (Asch, 1996; Back, Wallace, Starks, & Pearlman, 1996).

The aforementioned argument about rights is especially applicable here (p. 36). Negative rights are broad and well-defended in Western society; positive rights, by contrast, are few because they incur an obligation on the part of others (in this case physicians, who have sufficient skills and access to the means to accomplish euthanasia). It is well-established that a patient's positive right to obtain sought-after treatment is not absolute. For instance, patients do not have the right to treatments that either are not clinically indicated or which an individual physician has a moral objection to. The American Medical Association (2016) clearly states that "respecting patient autonomy does not mean that patients should receive specific interventions simply because they (or their surrogates) request them." By the same reasoning, patients cannot claim a right to active euthanasia, which has historically been rejected by the medical profession (Hippocrates, 1959).

The second argument in favor of euthanasia is based on compassion for those who are suffering. This is a precondition in every country where it is legal, which require that the patient's condition be "grievous and irremediable" (Canada), "grave and incurable" (Luxembourg), "unbearable and hopeless" (the Netherlands), or "unbearable physical or mental suffering that cannot be alleviated" (Belgium). Why should a patient be forced to live a life of such agony, when medical means are readily available to definitely end such suffering?

The standard retort to this argument is that other modalities are available to treat such suffering, up to and including intensive symptom management that risks hastened death, or even continuous sedation to unconsciousness. The defender of euthanasia would reply that such means unnecessarily delay the inevitable. As such, these "lesser steps" are really more of a salve for the physician's conscience than appropriate treatment for the patient's suffering. Even PAD—which shares the same primary goal as euthanasia—could be viewed as insufficient, as it requires the patient to be able to "self-administer" (which some patients lack the physical ability to do) and also involves both waiting and some uncertainty of outcome.[5] All of these limitations would be eliminated with an intravenous dose of a lethal drug.

This actually leads into a third argument in favor of active euthanasia, namely, that it is not substantially different from other end-of-life treatments, such as forgoing LSMT, intensive symptom management, and PAD. Thus equating euthanasia with these now-accepted[6] practices—while extolling the advantages of euthanasia in terms of rapidity and efficacy—is an implicit attempt to pull the "blanket of acceptability" that now covers these other practices onto euthanasia. The evolution of thinking in end-of-life decision-making thus comes full circle, with a shift in focus from decoupling to equating. Whereas the original argument was based on the assumption that euthanasia was unacceptable and

---

5. Given the rare complications and failures of PAD, as documented in Oregon (Oregon Health Authority, 2017).

6. It should be noted that PAD falls far short of the consensus attached to forgoing LSMT and intensive symptom management, but as noted earlier, if PAD is not deemed acceptable, there would be no reason to explore whether euthanasia might be.

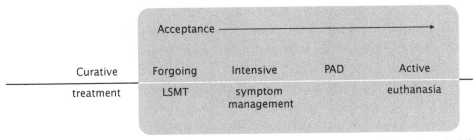

FIGURE 5.6 Extension of societal embrace of other forms of the right to die to include euthanasia (left to right)

sought to justify other interventions by distinguishing them from euthanasia, this line of argument seeks to re-link these concepts in order to associate the acceptance of these other activities with active euthanasia itself. Put more colloquially, the original claim was *Euthanasia is wrong, but these other actions are not euthanasia so maybe they are okay.* By contrast, the newer one is *Those other actions are not so different from euthanasia, so if they are okay, maybe euthanasia is too* (Figure 5.6).

There are really only two responses to this line of argument. One is to admit that the distinction between euthanasia and these other practices is faint and the original linking may have been correct after all. In that respect, this strategy is not without risk in that it essentially weighs the relatively recent societal acceptance of these other practices against the longstanding and broad-ranging cultural rejection of euthanasia. By grouping all the practices together, one is forced to either accept them all or reject them all. In the case of the latter, the attempt to justify such a controversial practice may cast a shadow of doubt over generally accepted practices and set end-of-life care back decades (Figure 5.7).

The alternative, of course, is to maintain the distinction between euthanasia and these other practices, thus allowing one to reject the former but accept the latter. This is the approach taken in this textbook, which is admittedly easier to accomplish because PAD is also called into question. But even if PAD were accepted, the line can

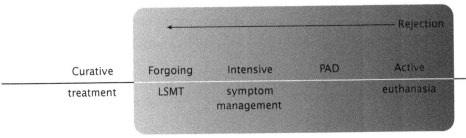

FIGURE 5.7 Extension of societal rejection of euthanasia to include other forms of the right to die (right to left)

still be held against embracing euthanasia, given PAD's "safety measure" of requiring self-administration, thus ostensibly ensuring voluntariness on the part of the patient and providing some measure of distance between the physician and the act of hastening death.

The reason for drawing a line between euthanasia and these other forms of the right to die is not only practical, in terms of the implications that acceptance of euthanasia would have on end-of-life care as a whole. It also stems from an observation about human nature. Those who advocate for extending the right to die further and further—up to and including euthanasia—seem to feel that physicians will generally do the right thing if given the opportunity (and provided with common-sense safeguards).

There is, however, a long and well-documented history of human beings initially being motivated by compassion, and ultimately—either through an inappropriate extension of that compassion, or perhaps from having taken a less noble turn along the way—committing acts that are ethically indefensible, if only in retrospect. The names Nuremberg, Beecher, and Tuskegee (p. 7) should be proof enough of this.

It is not enough to trust in the good intentions of physicians, especially when vulnerable patients are at risk. To draw the line of the right to die before one reaches euthanasia does not require one to be a pessimist, but merely a realist about what happens when such power is bestowed on fallible persons whose initially good intentions could lead to dire outcomes.

Arguments Against

There are several arguments against euthanasia. One is from the professional standpoint, given the longstanding prohibition on it throughout the history of Western medicine. Admittedly, that prohibition was not always honored even in the age of Hippocrates, and nowadays the oath that bears his name is rarely used because it harbors antiquated clinical notions (such as how to treat kidney stones) and ethical admonitions against legal practices (such as terminating pregnancy). Even so, there is no more central facet to the practice of medicine than that physicians should not act with the intention of ending a patient's life (Gaylin, Kass, Pellegrino, & Siegler, 1988). And given the implications for palliative care, in particular—which has already been tainted with accusations of acting as "death panels" (p. 510) and actively hastening death (when it does not)—the consequences of even *appearing* to endorse euthanasia would be profound.

There are also very practical arguments against euthanasia. Physicians have been shown to underestimate a patient's quality of life (Saigal et al., 1996), potentially leading to a willingness to engage in euthanasia that might seem to stem from compassion, but might actually result from bias. The power imbalance between clinicians and patients heightens this concern.

Another criticism of euthanasia is the so-called "slippery slope" argument, for even if the initial requirements placed on euthanasia upon legalization are ethically accept-able, over time these may ease and broaden. For instance, even though the law in the Netherlands requires that the patient's request for euthanasia be "voluntary and well-considered," 0.4% *of all deaths* in the Netherlands are "the result of the ending of life without an explicit request by the patient" (van der Heide et al., 2007). The reported jus-tification is that those patients were terminally ill and had lost their capacity for decision-making, thus rendering this nonvoluntary—rather than involuntary—euthanasia. This may reflect a Dutch cultural bias whereby "an individual patient's suffering outweighs the obligation to obey the law in these difficult cases" (Quill & Greenlaw, 2008).

But even that degree of suffering—which is required for euthanasia according to Dutch law—was noted by only 30% of physicians in cases of nonvoluntary euthanasia. In the other cases, factors more susceptible to bias—such as low quality of life, relatives' in-ability to cope, and no prospect for improvement—were the justification (van der Maas, van Delden, & Pijnenborg, 1992).

This slide down the slippery slope is not unique to the Netherlands. In Belgium, for instance, euthanasia is now an option for children of any age, and advocates are campaigning to also include demented patients, as long as they expressed a wish for eutha-nasia at some point in the past (Aviv, 2015). Required reporting—which was established to monitor usage and assure quality control—has also become more haphazard. A recent study revealed that only half of euthanasia cases in the Flanders region were reported to the Federal Control and Evaluation Commission, as required by law (Smets et al., 2010).

As with PAD (p. 225), acceptance of euthanasia could have a deleterious impact on the care of patients who do not wish it. For most of the history of Western medicine, a physician's sole tasks were to help a patient live longer and live better. The latter was specifically expanded in the second half of the twentieth century to include dying more comfortably and according to one's goals. But if "die sooner" were added to that list, the complexity of the physician-patient relationship would increase, potentially leading to concerns that a physician was suggesting hastened death or might carry it out even absent the patient's specific request. This would especially apply to those with disabilities, who could fear that the same "quality of life" concerns that drove Dutch physicians to perform nonvoluntary euthanasia would be applied to them.

Last, while the modern world of vast medical technology might make euthanasia seem more of a logical consideration, in point of fact that world—and the modern sensibilities that accompany it—make euthanasia unnecessary. Patients dependent on LSMT have the right to refuse it. Patients in extreme pain have the right to intensive treatment, even at the risk of hastened death. Patients at the end of life whose suffering is intolerable have the option of continuous sedation to unconsciousness (chapter 9). And currently one-sixth of the US population live in states where PAD is legal. Even those for whom none of these are options still have the choice to voluntarily stop eating and drinking (VSED).

The standard retort to this litany of other options is *Why wait, and why risk?* Why wait for a patient to dehydrate to death from VSED, or for a patient to gradually stop breathing from PAD? Why run the risk of a complication or "treatment failure" from PAD, as reported in roughly 1% of cases in Oregon (Oregon Health Authority, 2017)? Why engage in the "façade" of watching a patient under continuous deep sedation finally expire, thus exacerbating the suffering of family?

These are all very real concerns, but they are also the necessary price for ensuring that a patient really did want her death hastened and that her physician is not morally responsible for that death. Voluntariness for any action that risks hastening death—and especially one that would specifically cause death, immediately and reliably—is absolutely essential, in order to prevent the quality of life estimations that are so unreliable and start the tumble down the slippery slope. While some aspects of the Hippocratic Oath are outdated, the mandate to not actively hasten death remains a bright line that physicians must not cross.

Viewed in this light, hastening one's death *should* be hard, because of the stakes involved. In the meantime, the moral obligation to optimally manage symptoms remains. And the end result is maintaining the crucial distinction between active euthanasia and ethically acceptable versions of the right to die.

Voluntarily Stopping Eating and Drinking

Up to this point, the discussion of the right to die has focused on medical interventions: which can be declined and which a patient has the right to. For patients whose quality of life is so poor that they no longer wish to live, forgoing LSMT[7] is ethically permissible. If a patient is *not* dependent on LSMT and lives in a state where PAD is legal, this is also an option (albeit one which raises profound ethical concerns, as discussed in chapter 8.) But what if a patient is not dependent on LSMT, and PAD is not available in the state where she resides (or it violates her personal beliefs)? Is that patient "condemned" to live out her life, until an infection (which would not be treated) or some other complication finally ends it?

One option that is available to any patient is VSED, which is also known as voluntary refusal of food and fluids, terminal dehydration, and voluntary death by dehydration (Pope & Anderson, 2011), as well as more incendiary terms like "voluntary palliated starvation" (Savulescu, 2014). Referring to the decision by a patient with decision-making capacity choosing to hasten her death, it is distinct from a patient who is physically unable to eat or who has lost her appetite due to advanced disease. It also differs from refusal of

---

7.   This includes refusing MANH, which is addressed in detail later.

MANH in that it is entirely non-technical and does not require the involvement of—or even discussion with—a physician.

Before analyzing the ethics of VSED, it is important to appreciate the practicalities.

Clinical

The human body can survive for extended periods without nutrition and also with minimal amounts of hydration. To achieve its goal, therefore, VSED requires absolutely forgoing oral intake (especially liquids). Even a few sips here and there—or sucking on ice chips to lessen the sensation of dry mouth—can significantly prolong life.

Absolutely no intake of fluids leads to hypovolemia and then to uremia as the kidneys have insufficient fluids to filter. This causes the patient to become drowsy and eventually comatose. Rather than causing suffering, such dehydration can actually ameliorate suffering by depressing level of consciousness. If the patient is not receiving any fluids by mouth, the median time to death is approximately one week, although up to one-fifth of patients could survive two weeks or more (Bolt, Hagens, Willems, & Onwuteaka-Philipsen, 2015).

Since the patient is also not receiving nutrition, she will also enter a state of ketosis, burning fat instead of glucose for energy. The significance for end-of-life care is that ketosis causes the release of endorphins and reduces the perception of hunger (Winter, 2000). It is also postulated to have an analgesic effect, thereby also protective against suffering (Masino & Ruskin, 2013).

It is important to note these clinical realities, not only so that patients understand that VSED does not worsen suffering—quite the opposite, in many cases—but also to distinguish it from the emotionally-charged concept of "starvation." Some have gone so far as to argue that dehydration is the "natural" way to die (McCue, 1995), as historically patients approaching the end of life would either not be able—or, alternatively, not want—to drink, thus leading to dehydration. The most important take-home point is that VSED is not uncomfortable as long as symptoms (including dry mouth through the use of moist swabs) are adequately treated (Bernat, Gert, & Mogielnicki, 1993; Brody, Campbell, Faber-Langendoen, & Ogle, 1997; Printz, 1992; Quill, Lo, & Brock, 1997).

Perhaps the most compelling data illustrating this comes from an Oregon study of hospice patients who, by definition, had a life expectancy of six months or less. Some chose to avail themselves of PAD—as Oregon was the first state to legalize it—while others chose to hasten their deaths through VSED. Nurses caring for these patients reported less suffering and greater peacefulness among the patients who engaged in VSED, as well as less emotional distress and greater acceptance among those patients' family members (Ganzini et al., 2003). Obviously, this was not a randomized controlled trial (p. 452), as the choice of VSED or PAD (or neither) was up to the patients themselves. As such, it should not be taken as a "prescription" for terminally ill patients to engage in VSED, but rather an observation that if a patient chooses to pursue VSED, the end result is the opposite of the increased suffering some might expect.

In addition to the potential benefits of VSED, there are also drawbacks to continuing to eat and drink. Hunger and thirst are generally part of the dying process, but patients often feel an "obligation" to continue to eat and drink, based on the expectations and encouragement of their families. In those situations, patients frequently suffer abdominal discomfort and nausea (Hui, Dev, & Bruera, 2015). Overhydration also causes increased secretions, which can negatively impact respiratory status and cause added burden in the form of diarrhea and frequent urination, often leading to skin irritation and breakdown.

VSED is rather common. In a recent study, nearly half of family physician respondents reported having cared for a patient who hastened her death in this manner. These patients tended to be over eighty and suffering from severe disease (most commonly cancer), with significant dependence on others (Bolt, Hagens, Willems, & Onwuteaka-Philipsen, 2015). In states where PAD is not legal, VSED represents the only manner of hastening death available to patients who are not dependent on LSMT.

Ethical

As a manner of hastening death, VSED offers many ethical advantages. It would seem a logical extension of the right to refuse medical treatment, based on the right of privacy. Informed consent is not a concern, as it requires ongoing consent (at least at the outset, before dehydration becomes so significant as to affect consciousness). It does not require the participation of a physician, nor the ability to ingest a lethal amount of a drug (as in the case of PAD). VSED is not illegal (Pope & West, 2014), making it a reasonable alternative for patients who either do not qualify for PAD or live in a state where that practice is illegal (Muller, 2012). While for some the prolonged course can be agonizing, for others it provides valuable opportunities for closure.

For all these reasons, some view VSED as a "simple solution" (Savulescu, 2014) to the question of hastened death, which "avoids moral controversy altogether" (Bernat et al., 1993). Studies have shown it is widely accepted among hospice workers, who believe patients should be apprised of this option and continue to be cared for if they opt for it (Harvath et al., 2004).

VSED is not entirely uncontroversial, however. Like PAD—but unlike forgoing LSMT or intensive pain management—its purpose is to hasten death. As such, some consider it akin to suicide, including Justice Scalia in his dissent in the *Cruzan* decision where he said that "starving oneself to death is no different from putting a gun to one's temple as far as the common-law definition of suicide is concerned" (*Cruzan v. Director, Missouri Department of Health*). Concerns have also been expressed about potential discrimination against patients with disabilities (Peace, 2013), or conflation of VSED with starvation through medical neglect. Others have warned against "subtle coercion" in the form of not continuing to offer food and drink to a patient who had previously expressed a wish to pursue VSED (Quill et al., 1997). Finally, some argue that food and drink are basic human care—akin to cleaning a patient after she has soiled herself—and thus are distinct from *medically administered* nutrition and hydration, which the patient clearly has the right to refuse (*Cruzan v. Director, Missouri, Department of Health*, 1990).

There are thoughtful responses to all of these critiques. Voluntariness must, of course, be safeguarded and food and drink continued to be offered in a thoughtful and respectful fashion. But this is the extent of one's ethical obligation, for even if food and drink are part of basic human care—rather than "medical care"—it is the provider's responsibility to *offer* the food and drink, not the patient's obligation to ingest it.

Ultimately, the most compelling ethical argument in favor of respecting a patient's right to VSED is to envision what *not* respecting that right would look like. Would health care professionals have an obligation to intervene if a patient chose not to eat and drink? Would a nasogastric tube be inserted, requiring a patient to be physically restrained to prevent her from pulling it out? Would a gastrostomy tube be placed—thereby incurring the risks of an invasive procedure—which is more secure but still depends on a patient allowing it to be used, or at least not ripping it out?

Unlike other interventions that can be provided on a time-limited basis over incapacitated objection until the need for them is past (p. 123), there will never be a time when a patient is not "dependent" on nutrition and hydration. Whatever interventions are instituted—to be clear, over *capacitated* objection—would therefore have to be maintained until the patient died of a medical complication or ultimately acquiesced to authority. Thus, even if one harbors ethical reservations about VSED, the alternatives to respecting a patient's choice in this area are far more distasteful.

So how should a clinician respond to a patient's inquiry about (or stated intention to pursue) VSED? As always, a request for hastened death—whether through VSED or any other means—should prompt an exploration for the reasons for the request and whether any of these are remediable. If the patient is experiencing intolerable symptoms, these should be addressed. If a patient is feeling like she is losing control of her life, all attempts should be made to restore as much control as possible.

If no remediable causes for the request are identified, the clinician should make sure the patient understands what is involved in the process of VSED, as well as the alternative options. But if the patient is resolute, there is little that can—or should—be done to stop her. The palliative care clinician is better off respecting the decision, and trusting that time will determine whether the patient is truly committed to VSED.

As noted, VSED ensures informed consent because it is not a "one-moment-in-time" refusal of food and drink but rather an ongoing refusal over a period of time. To avoid any risk of "subtle coercion" to continue with VSED, food and drink should continue to be available to the patient, in case she changes her mind at some point along the way. Indeed, it is not uncommon for a patient to proclaim her intention to stop eating and drinking but change her mind when presented with her favorite pie, right out of the oven.

This recommendation to continue to offer food and drink is not entirely uncontroversial, however. Some believe this disrespects the patient's wishes and even go so far as to term it "battery."[8] A more modest claim might be one of coercion, with the sight and smell of food eliciting physiologic responses that exacerbate hunger, thus making it harder for the patient to achieve her stated goal (Pope & Anderson, 2011).

While it may be inappropriate to repeatedly present the patient with food after consistent and clearly voluntary refusals, to proclaim such an action as "battery" or even "coercion" seems to take the matter too far. A patient who proclaims an initial intent to pursue VSED may not be so resolute as to bring it to completion. For many, eating is one of the great pleasures of life, and being presented with a favorite dish or meal might tilt the balance of benefits and burdens. If nothing else, it represents an expression of caring—and hope for continued life—from a loved one. Indeed, overstated concern for "battery" might lead to the very form of "subtle coercion" to *continue* forgoing nutrition and hydration that critics of VSED have cited (Quill et al., 1997).

The truth would seem to reside somewhere in the middle, between expressions of human caring in the form of food and drink on the one hand and potentially manipulative steps to impede the patient from reaching her stated goal on the other. The palliative care clinician must therefore walk a fine line. At times he might be called upon to help the patient understand why her family is struggling to respect her decision and searching for ways to show they love her. In other situations his task is to help the family see that the patient has made a thoughtful and informed decision and is not suffering.

Relationship of Withdrawing and Withholding

As noted earlier, there is a clear and substantial difference between letting die (i.e., forgoing LSMT) and actively hastening death through euthanasia. Not all forgoing is the same though. There are actually two distinct forms: not instituting a treatment (withholding) and stopping a treatment already in use (withdrawing).

Withholding is clearly ethically permissible, based on the right of privacy noted previously (p. 8). If it were not, then a patient would be ethically obligated to receive every treatment that could potentially prolong her life (which, given the vast arsenal of modern medicine, is a humbling prospect). DNAR orders would be unethical, and not intubating a dying patient to fleetingly prolong her life would be tantamount to murder. The entire patients' rights movement of the 1970s onward would crumble.

One of the fundamental mantras of clinical ethics is that "there is no ethical distinction between withdrawing and withholding life-sustaining treatment" (American Medical Association, 2016). If true—and withholding is ethically permissible—then

---

8. The legal definition of this term is quite broad and does not require direct person-to-person contact (*Fisher v. Carrousel Motor Hotel, Inc.*, 1967).

withdrawing also would be.[9] But is withdrawing a treatment already in use ethically equivalent to forgoing that treatment in the first place?

In some older studies, as many as one-quarter of physicians surveyed have disputed this equivalence, feeling that withdrawing is more ethically troublesome than withholding (Faber-Langendoen, 1994). Nurses—with the exception of those who work in specialties that are frequently called upon to withdraw LSMT (such as critical care)—frequently believe that withholding is ethically distinct from (and, indeed, superior to) withdrawing treatment (Solomon et al., 2005).

A common argument for the "nonequivalence" of withholding and withdrawing asserts that the former is passive, while the latter is active. After all, extubating a patient requires turning off a ventilator or removing an endotracheal tube, whereas not intubating a patient requires no action at all. However, as noted earlier (p. 138), the choice to institute one set of treatments—including those focused on comfort, in lieu of mechanical ventilation—involves the active choice *not* to institute a wide range of alternatives. Withholding LSMT is, therefore, not as "passive" as it first appears.

Nor is withdrawing the only "active" response to treatments already in place. Few treatments continue independently and indefinitely; rather, they require frequent monitoring and modifying (such as to ventilator settings based on the patient's evolving respiratory requirements). Deeming withdrawing to be unethical would seem to compel a patient to accept increased ventilator settings, replaced central lines to prevent infection, and modified dialysis settings based on blood chemistries. Viewed in this light, maintaining treatment already in place is just as "active" as withdrawing it, and the patient's right of autonomy should apply equally to both.

Another argument that has been cited in favor of nonequivalence is the *prima facie* claim that a patient already receiving a treatment has to continue receiving that treatment, which takes precedence over another patient's claim to initiate that treatment (Sulmasy & Sugarman, 1994). But here the context is critical: such an assertion of nonequivalence only pertains to a treatment a patient desires—and might be withdrawn in a situation of exceedingly scarce resources—not one she is refusing. The argument, therefore, does not question the applicability of the right of privacy to all forms of refusal of treatment but rather the competing claims of patients in a triage situation.

A common clinical example may serve to eradicate any remaining doubt about the equivalence of withdrawing and withholding. Suppose a patient presents to the emergency department in extremis and is thus not able to participate in decision-making. The physicians are unsure whether intensive treatment will be successful, but as they are not able to determine the patient's goals, they proceed with treatment and hope for the best. Suppose, further, that the patient's condition worsens despite the treatment she is receiving, such that it becomes clear that she will die. Or, alternatively, her advance directive

---

9. This is precisely the reason that "forgoing" is used throughout this textbook to refer to both withdrawing and withholding.

subsequently becomes available—or family members offer substituted judgment on her behalf—and it turns out that she would not have wanted any of the treatments she has received but rather to die in peace.

It certainly seems unjust to compel the patient to receive unwanted treatments simply because the medical team was not aware of her objections when it initiated them (Wilkinson & Savulescu, 2014). Treatments already in use represent the same intrusion of one's bodily integrity as those which the patient had a right to demand withheld initially—if she had been able—and thus are equally covered by the right of privacy. Claiming that withdrawing is somehow ethically more questionable than withholding therefore "condemns" the patient to continuing to receive every treatment she is currently receiving, without regard for burden, prognosis, or values.

Recognizing this, there has evolved a strong ethical and legal consensus in favor of the equivalence of withdrawing and withholding.[10] This was the clear conclusion of the President's Commission (1983), and courts have consistently recognized this as well: "Whether necessary treatment is withheld at the outset or withdrawn later on, the consequence—the patient's death—is the same" (*In re Conroy*, 1985).

So if there is such a clear ethical and legal consensus—specific religious requirements notwithstanding—why do some still believe that withdrawing is somehow different than withholding (Wilkinson & Savulescu, 2014)? One reason is the "status quo bias" (Samuelson & Zeckhauser, 1988), which may lead some clinicians to conclude that it is worse to stop something that is already in use (Christakis & Asch, 1993). There are also clinical differences between the two practices, with studies showing that patients from whom LSMT is withdrawn are more certain to die and do so more quickly (Sprung et al., 2003). Withholding—in the form of denying ICU admission—plays a larger role in critical care than withdrawing, primarily out of concern for resource allocation (Strauss, LoGerfo, Yeltatzie, Temkin, & Hudson, 1986).[11] It is important to recognize that these reasons stem from personal biases or clinical differences, not ethical distinctions.

Ultimately, though, the reason some people think the two practices are different is not based on ethical argument but rather emotional response. Discontinuing a treatment that is currently keeping a patient alive *feels* different—both to clinicians and to family members—than choosing not to institute that treatment in the first place. There are several reasons for this. First, treatments that are not instituted are less tangible. They are, ultimately, hypothetical proposals that the team or the family chose not to act on, thus leaving the deciders with less concrete regret. They are also less momentous—or memorable—in the sense that there are hundreds or even thousands of treatments that

---

10. It should also be noted that some religious traditions (such as Orthodox Judaism) draw a line between withholding a treatment and doing anything "active" to cease a treatment already in use (Kunin, 2011). Various solutions have been suggested to the dilemma of a patient receiving treatment he does not want, even including time-limited ventilators that at least offer the appearance of not doing anything "active" to withdraw treatment.

11. For precisely the reasons Sulmasy and Sugarman (1994) note, many ICU physicians are reluctant to withdraw potentially beneficial treatment out of justice concerns (Sprung et al. 2008).

could potentially be provided to a given patient, but nearly all are rejected for a wide variety of reasons, such as propriety, availability, safety, or patient refusal. It is much clearer that stopping the ventilator which is oxygenating a patient will impact her duration of life than going down the long list of all the other potential therapies that were never reasonably considered and were uncertain to have benefitted the patient even if initiated.

Finally—and perhaps most importantly for clinicians—the physical act of withdrawing a treatment can be extremely tactile. In some cases, this may be accomplished by simply writing an order (e.g., "discontinue antibiotics"). But often in the case of LSMT, the treatments in question require some physical manipulation of a device in close proximity to the patient to discontinue them. It may not be the physician who actually performs that task, but for a ventilator to be withdrawn someone has to manually turn it off. To be sure, the patient has the ethical and legal right to have that treatment discontinued, but that does not prevent the clinician from feeling some degree of responsibility—or even culpability—for having done so. Thus Meisel (2005) concludes:

> It may be simple to conclude that there is no morally significant difference between withdrawing and withholding treatment, but those who withdraw treatment may have substantially greater ethical or psychological qualms about doing so than they do about withholding the same treatment.

Rather than denying that clinicians (or surrogates) experience a distinction between withdrawing and withholding, it is better to admit that such a distinction exists while also clarifying that it is emotional in nature, not ethical. The ethical equivalence of the two types of forgoing is well established and should provide some comfort to clinicians or surrogates who feel like they might be doing something "wrong." Honestly acknowledging the emotional burden that the clinician may experience can deepen conversation and allow for expressions of empathy and support. Reframing the discussion to focus on the patient's goals—and right to refuse treatments whose burdens outweigh the benefits, whether under consideration or already implemented—can also provide reassurance.

It may also be helpful to note that while withdrawing may be more difficult from an emotional perspective, it may be superior from a clinical perspective (Levin & Sprung, 2005). Withdrawing a treatment that ultimately proves to be ineffective at least gave that treatment the chance to work. Upon discontinuation, the team and the family can take some consolation in the knowledge that they "gave it a try."

By contrast, if one were to act on the belief that somehow withdrawing was worse—or at least more difficult—than withholding, there might be a temptation to not initiate a potentially beneficial treatment, for fear that it could not later be stopped. Indeed, one of the reasons that ethicists repeat the mantra of equivalence so often is to counteract the formerly prevalent notion among physicians that once a patient is receiving LSMT—such as mechanical ventilation—it cannot be discontinued. Even today, some physicians may be reluctant to intubate a patient because "once the tube goes in, it's hard to remove it." It may, admittedly, be "hard," but in an emotional sense rather than an ethical one. Failure to recognize this distinction may lead to substandard care by not giving patients the opportunity they are seeking to survive.

Physicians, therefore, should not be reluctant to offer a trial of LSMT, recognizing that it can subsequently be discontinued if it is not achieving its intended goal. But before proceeding, surrogates should be informed that this may make an already emotionally fraught situation even more difficult. If it was hard to consider not intubating a loved one in respiratory failure, it will likely be even harder to ultimately decide to extubate, when the proximity and tangibility of that action are so much greater. There will be a natural human inclination to defer the decision to withdraw LSMT, perhaps in the hope of an unexpected improvement, a "miracle" (p. 490) or the patient dying despite maximal treatment, thus sparing the surrogate the burden of having made a definitive decision (p. 65).

Not making a decision to stop a treatment is, however, practically equivalent to a decision to continue it (once again highlighting the artificial distinction between "passive" and "active" steps in relationship to forgoing LSMT). This is precisely the reason why instituting LSMT on a time-limited basis to allow for reevaluation can be so helpful (p. 118). It also highlights the need to maintain open lines of communication with the patient's family, offering ongoing emotional support while continuing to evaluate subsequent decisions in light of the patient's goals, which are determinative for withdrawing treatment as well as withholding it.

Summary Points

- Active euthanasia is not a component of palliative care, which "intends neither to hasten nor postpone death" (World Health Organization, 2002).
- The societal approbation of active euthanasia in the United States prompted the right to die movement to distinguish other forms of (potentially) hastened death from this practice.
- Gradually, forgoing LSMT—which used to be called "passive euthanasia"—came to be accepted, as did intensive symptom management at the end of life (which only potentially could hasten death and might well prolong life). This established the "negative" right to die (i.e., without interference) but not a "positive" right.
- Having achieved this acceptance, some attempted to extend the right to die to include actively hastening death, while others opted to focus exclusively on palliative care.
- If one rejects PAD (which is addressed in detail in chapter 8), then there is no reason to seriously consider active euthanasia. But if PAD—which is now legal in several states—is deemed acceptable, this naturally raises the question of whether active euthanasia is, too.
- Arguments in favor of active euthanasia include patient autonomy, compassion, and questioning the distinction between it and other forms of the right to die, in an attempt to extend the societal acceptance of those other forms to active euthanasia.

If this argument were accepted, either all forms of the right to die would be ethically permissible, or they would all fall together.

- Compelling arguments against active euthanasia include professionalism, personal bias, slippery slope, harm to the physician-patient relationship, and lack of necessity.
- For patients who are not dependent on life-sustaining medical treatment, voluntarily stopping eating and drinking is always an option. This practice need not cause suffering and entails less ethical complexity.
- There is no ethical or legal distinction between withdrawing and withholding, but the former may be both clinical superior and emotionally taxing on families and staff.

References

American Medical Association. (2016). *Code of medical ethics.* Chicago: American Medical Association.

AMA Council on Ethical and Judicial Affairs. (1992). Decisions near the end of life. *JAMA, 267*(16), 2229–2233.

Amundsen, D. W. (1978). The physician's obligation to prolong life: A medical duty without classical roots. *Hastings Cent Rep, 8*(4), 23–30.

Angell, M. (1996). Euthanasia in the Netherlands—good news or bad? *N Engl J Med, 335*(22), 1676–1678. doi:10.1056/NEJM199611283352209

Aquinas, T., & Gilby, T. (1969). *Summa theologiae.* Garden City, NY: Image Books.

Asch, D. A. (1996). The role of critical care nurses in euthanasia and assisted suicide. *N Engl J Med, 334*(21), 1374–1379. doi:10.1056/NEJM199605233342106

Aviv, R. (2015, June 22). The death treatment. *The New Yorker.*

Back, A. L., Wallace, J. I., Starks, H. E., & Pearlman, R. A. (1996). Physician-assisted suicide and euthanasia in Washington State: Patient requests and physician responses. *JAMA, 275*(12), 919–925.

Bacon, F. (1924). *New Atlantis.* New York: Oxford University Press.

Barber v. Superior Court, 147 Cal. Ap. 3d 1006, 15 Cal. Rptr. 484 (1983).

Bernat, J. L., Gert, B., & Mogielnicki, R. P. (1993). Patient refusal of hydration and nutrition: An alternative to physician-assisted suicide or voluntary active euthanasia. *Arch Intern Med, 153*(24), 2723–2728.

Bill C-14, An act to amend the Criminal Code and to make related amendments to other acts (medical assistance in dying). Passed June 16, 2016. Retrieved from http://www.parl.ca/DocumentViewer/en/42-1/bill/C-14/royal-assent

Billings, J. A., & Block, S. D. (1996). Slow euthanasia. *J Palliat Care, 12*(4), 21–30.

Bolt, E. E., Hagens, M., Willems, D., & Onwuteaka-Philipsen, B. D. (2015). Primary care patients hastening death by voluntarily stopping eating and drinking. *Ann Fam Med, 13*(5), 421–428. doi:10.1370/afm.1814

Brody, H., Campbell, M. L., Faber-Langendoen, K., & Ogle, K. S. (1997). Withdrawing intensive life-sustaining treatment—recommendations for compassionate clinical management. *N Engl J Med, 336*(9), 652–657. doi:10.1056/NEJM199702273360910

Callahan, D. (1996, April 11). Physician-assisted suicide: Opening the poor to moral mischief. *Newsday.*

Central Board of the Royal Dutch Medical Association. (1984). Vision on euthanasia. *Medisch Contact, 39,* 990–997.

Chambre des Représentants de Belgique. (2002). Project de loi relatif à l'euthanasie: Doc 501488/001. Brussels: Chambre des Représentants de Belgique.

Christakis, N. A., & Asch, D. A. (1993). Biases in how physicians choose to withdraw life support. *Lancet, 342*(8872), 642–646.

Cruzan v. Director, Missouri Department of Health, 497 261 (S.Ct. 1990).

Cushing, J. (Ed.). (1977). *The earliest acts and laws of the colony of Rhode Island and providence plantations 1647–1719.* Wilmington, DE: M. Glazier.

de Haan, J. (2002). The new Dutch law on euthanasia. *Med Law Rev, 10*(1), 57–75.

Dowbiggin, I. R. (2003). *A merciful end: The euthanasia movement in modern America*. Oxford; New York: Oxford University Press.

Dworkin, G., Frey, R. G., & Bok, S. (1998). *Euthanasia and physician-assisted suicide*. Cambridge; New York: Cambridge University Press.

Emanuel, E. J. (1994). The history of euthanasia debates in the United States and Britain. *Ann Intern Med, 121*(10), 793–802.

Faber-Langendoen, K. (1994). The clinical management of dying patients receiving mechanical ventilation: A survey of physician practice. *Chest, 106*(3), 880–888.

Feinberg, J. (1973). *Social philosophy*. Englewood Cliffs, N.J.: Prentice-Hall.

Fins, J. (2006). *A palliative ethic of care: Clinical wisdom at life's end*. Sudbury, MA: Jones and Bartlett.

Fisher v. Carrousel Motor Hotel, Inc. (1967). (424 S.W.2d 627, 629-30 (Tex. 1967).

Foley, K. M. (1997). Competent care for the dying instead of physician-assisted suicide. *N Engl J Med, 336*(1), 54–58. doi:10.1056/NEJM199701023360109.

Fye, W. B. (1978). Active euthanasia: An historical survey of its conceptual origins and introduction into medical thought. *Bull Hist Med, 52*(4), 492–502.

Gallup. (2003). Worlds apart: Religion in Canada, Britain, U.S. Retrieved from http://www.gallup.com/poll/9016/worlds-apart-religion-canada-britain-us.aspx

Gallup. (2009). Religiosity highest in world's poorest nations. Retrieved from http://www.gallup.com/poll/142727/religiosity-highest-world-poorest-nations.aspx

Ganzini, L., Goy, E. R., Miller, L. L., Harvath, T. A., Jackson, A., & Delorit, M. A. (2003). Nurses' experiences with hospice patients who refuse food and fluids to hasten death. *N Engl J Med, 349*(4), 359–365. doi:10.1056/NEJMsa035086

Gaylin, W., Kass, L. R., Pellegrino, E. D., & Siegler, M. (1988). "Doctors must not kill". *JAMA, 259*(14), 2139–2140.

Gert, B., Culver, C. M., & Clouser, K. D. (1998). An alternative to physician-assisted suicide. In M. P. Battin, R. Rhodes, & A. Silvers (Eds.), *Physician assisted suicide: Expanding the debate* (pp. 182–202). New York: Routledge.

Griffiths, J., Bood, A., & Weyers, H. (1998). *Euthanasia and law in the Netherlands*. Amsterdam: Amsterdam University Press.

Grotius, H., Evats, W., Cross, T., Bassett, T., Smith, R., White, M., . . . Birmingham Law Society. (1682). *The most excellent Hugo Grotius, his three books treating of the rights of war & peace: In the first is handled, Whether any war be just. In the second is shewed, the causes of war, both just and unjust. In the third is declared, what in war is lawful, that is, unpunishable. With the annotations digested into the body of every chapter*. London: M. W.

Harvath, T. A., Miller, L. L., Goy, E., Jackson, A., Delorit, M., & Ganzini, L. (2004). Voluntary refusal of food and fluids: Attitudes of Oregon hospice nurses and social workers. *Int J Palliat Nurs, 10*(5), 236–241; discussion 242–233. doi:10.12968/ijpn.2004.10.5.13072

The Hastings Center. (1987). *Guidelines on the termination of life sustaining treatment and the care of the dying*. Bloomington: Indiana University Press.

Hermsen, M. A., & ten Have, H. A. (2001). Moral problems in palliative care journals. *Palliat Med, 15*(5), 425–431.

Hilliard, B. (2000). The moral and legal status of physician-assisted death: Quality of life and the patient-physician relationship. *Issues Integr Studies, 18*, 45–63.

Hippocrates. (1959). *The art* (Vol. 2). Cambridge, MA: Harvard University Press.

Hui, D., Dev, R., & Bruera, E. (2015). The last days of life: Symptom burden and impact on nutrition and hydration in cancer patients. *Curr Opin Support Palliat Care, 9*(4), 346–354. doi:10.1097/SPC.0000000000000171

Humphry, D. (2005). Chronology of euthanasia and right-to-die events during the 20th century and into the millennium. Retrieved from https://libertytothecaptives.net/chronology_of_euthanasia.html

In re Conroy, 98 N.J. 321, 486 A.2d 1209 (1985).

In re Quinlan, 70 N.J. 10, 355 A.2d 647 (NJ 1976).

It's over, Debbie. (1988). *JAMA, 259*(2), 272.

Kamisar, Y. (1958). Some non-religious views against proposed "mercy killing" legislation. *Minn Law Rev, 42*, 969–1042.

Kass, L. R. (1992). "I will give no deadly drug." Why doctors must not kill. *Bull Am Coll Surg, 77*(3), 6–17.

Kunin, J. (2011). Caring for the terminally ill: Halachic approaches to withholding and withdrawing therapy. Retrieved from http://www.medethics.org.il/articles/JME/JMEM9/JMEM.9.2.asp

Levin, P. D., & Sprung, C. L. (2005). Withdrawing and withholding life-sustaining therapies are not the same. *Crit Care, 9*(3), 230–232. doi:10.1186/cc3487

Manning, M. (1998). *Euthanasia and physician-assisted suicide: Killing or caring?* New York: Paulist Press.

Masino, S. A., & Ruskin, D. N. (2013). Ketogenic diets and pain. *J Child Neurol, 28*(8), 993–1001. doi:10.1177/0883073813487595

McCue, J. D. (1995). The naturalness of dying. *JAMA, 273*(13), 1039–1043.

Meisel, A. (2005). Ethics and law: Physician-assisted dying. *J Palliat Med, 8*(3), 609–621. doi:10.1089/jpm.2005.8.609

Meisel, A. (2016). Legal issues in death and dying: How rights and autonomy have shaped clinical practice. In S. J. Youngner & R. M. Arnold (Eds.), *The Oxford handbook of ethics at the end of life* (pp. 7–26). New York: Oxford University Press.

More, T., & Turner, P. (1984). *Utopia.* London; New York: Penguin Books.

Muller, D. (2012). Physician-assisted death is illegal in most states, so my patient made another choice. *Health Aff (Millwood), 31*(10), 2343–2346. doi:10.1377/hlthaff.2011.0833

Natural Death Act, 7. (1976). California Health and Safety Code § 7185-95, 1 Stat.

Oregon Health Authority. (2017). Death with Dignity Act: 2016 data summary. Retrieved from http://www.oregon.gov/oha/PH/PROVIDERPARTNERRESOURCES/EVALUATIONRESEARCH/DEATHWITHDIGNITYACT/Documents/year19.pdf

Organisation for Economic Co-operation and Development. (2014). Coverage for health care. Retrieved from http://dx.doi.org/10.1787/soc_glance-2014-26-en

Peace, W. J. (2013). A peaceful death or a risk to people with disabilities? Retrieved from http://www.thehastingscenter.org/a-peaceful-death-or-a-risk-to-people-with-disabilities/

Pellegrino, E. D. (1992). Doctors must not kill. *J Clin Ethics, 3*, 95–102.

Pope, T., & Anderson, L. (2011). Voluntarily stopping eating and drinking: A legal treatment option at the end of life. *Widener Law Rev, 17*(2), 363–427.

Pope, T. M., & West, A. (2014). Legal briefing: Voluntarily stopping eating and drinking. *J Clin Ethics, 25*(1), 68–80.

President's Commission for the Study of Ethical Problems in Medicine and Biomedical and Behavioral Research. (1983). *Deciding to forego life-sustaining treatment: A report on the ethical, medical, and legal issues in treatment decisions.* Washington, DC: U.S. Government Printing Office.

Printz, L. A. (1992). Terminal dehydration, a compassionate treatment. *Arch Intern Med, 152*(4), 697–700.

Quill, T. E. (1991). Death and dignity. A case of individualized decision making. *N Engl J Med, 324*(10), 691–694. doi:10.1056/NEJM199103073241010

Quill, T.E., and Greenlaw, J. (2008). Physician-assisted death. In M. Crowley (Ed.), *From birth to death and bench to clinic: The Hastings Center bioethics briefing book for journalists, policymakers, and campaigns* (pp. 137–142). Garrison, NY: The Hastings Center.

Quill, T. E., Lo, B., & Brock, D. W. (1997). Palliative options of last resort: A comparison of voluntarily stopping eating and drinking, terminal sedation, physician-assisted suicide, and voluntary active euthanasia. *JAMA, 278*(23), 2099–2104.

Rachels, J. (1975). Active and passive euthanasia. *N Engl J Med, 292*(2), 78–80. doi:10.1056/NEJM197501092920206

Randall, F., & Downie, R. S. (1999). *Palliative care ethics: A companion for all specialties* (2nd ed.). New York: Oxford University Press.

Randall, F., & Downie, R. S. (2006). *The philosophy of palliative care: Critique and reconstruction.* Oxford; New York: Oxford University Press.

Rietjens, J. A., van der Maas, P. J., Onwuteaka-Philipsen, B. D., van Delden, J. J., & van der Heide, A. (2009). Two decades of research on euthanasia from the Netherlands: What have we learnt and what questions remain? *J Bioeth Inq, 6*(3), 271–283. doi:10.1007/s11673-009-9172-3

Saigal, S., Feeny, D., Rosenbaum, P., Furlong, W., Burrows, E., & Stoskopf, B. (1996). Self-perceived health status and health-related quality of life of extremely low-birth-weight infants at adolescence. *JAMA, 276*(6), 453–459.

Samuelson, W., & Zeckhauser, R. (1988). Status quo bias refers to an irrational or inappropriate preference for the status quo: Status quo bias in decision making. *J Risk Uncertainty, 1,* 7–59.

Satz v. Perlmutter, 362 So. 2d 160 (Fla. Dist. Ct. App. 1978), *aff'd* 379 So. 2d 359 (Fla. 1980).

Savulescu, J. (2014). A simple solution to the puzzles of end of life? Voluntary palliated starvation. *J Med Ethics, 40*(2), 110–113. doi:10.1136/medethics-2013-101379

Siegel, A. M., Sisti, D. A., & Caplan, A. L. (2014). Pediatric euthanasia in Belgium: Disturbing developments. *JAMA, 311*(19), 1963–1964. doi:10.1001/jama.2014.4257

Smets, T., Bilsen, J., Cohen, J., Rurup, M. L., Mortier, F., & Deliens, L. (2010). Reporting of euthanasia in medical practice in Flanders, Belgium: Cross sectional analysis of reported and unreported cases. *BMJ, 341,* c5174. doi:10.1136/bmj.c5174

Solomon, M. Z., Sellers, D. E., Heller, K. S., Dokken, D. L., Levetown, M., Rushton, C., . . . Fleischman, A. R. (2005). New and lingering controversies in pediatric end-of-life care. *Pediatrics, 116*(4), 872–883. doi:10.1542/peds.2004-0905

Sprung, C. L., Cohen, S. L., Sjokvist, P., Baras, M., Bulow, H. H., Hovilehto, S., . . . Ethicus Study Group. (2003). End-of-life practices in European intensive care units: The Ethicus study. *JAMA, 290*(6), 790–797. doi:10.1001/jama.290.6.790

Strauss, M. J., LoGerfo, J. P., Yeltatzie, J. A., Temkin, N., & Hudson, L. D. (1986). Rationing of intensive care unit services. An everyday occurrence. *JAMA, 255*(9), 1143–1146.

Sulmasy, D. P., & Sugarman, J. (1994). Are withholding and withdrawing therapy always morally equivalent? *J Med Ethics, 20*(4), 218–222; discussion 223–214.

Superintendent of Belchertown State School v. Saikewicz, 370 N.E.2d 417, 373 Mass. 728 (1977).

The Hastings Center. (1987). *Guidelines on the termination of life sustaining treatment and the care of the dying.* Bloomington: Indiana University Press.

The moral side of euthanasia (Editorial). (1885). *JAMA, 5,* 382–383.

Truog, R. D., Campbell, M. L., Curtis, J. R., Haas, C. E., Luce, J. M., Rubenfeld, G. D., . . . American Academy of Critical Care Medicine. (2008). Recommendations for end-of-life care in the intensive care unit: A consensus statement by the American College [corrected] of Critical Care Medicine. *Crit Care Med, 36*(3), 953–963. doi:10.1097/CCM.0B013E3181659096

Vacco v. Quill. (1997). U.S. 521 793.

van der Heide, A., Onwuteaka-Philipsen, B. D., Rurup, M. L., Buiting, H. M., van Delden, J. J., Hanssen-de Wolf, J. E., . . . van der Wal, G. (2007). End-of-life practices in the Netherlands under the Euthanasia Act. *N Engl J Med, 356*(19), 1957–1965. doi:10.1056/NEJMsa071143

van der Maas, P. J., van Delden, J. J., & Pijnenborg, L. (1992). Euthanasia and other medical decisions concerning the end of life: An investigation performed upon request of the Commission of Inquiry into the Medical Practice concerning Euthanasia. *Health Policy, 21*(1–2), vi–x, 1–262.

van der Maas, P. J., van der Wal, G., Haverkate, I., de Graaff, C. L., Kester, J. G., Onwuteaka-Philipsen, B. D., . . . Willems, D. L. (1996). Euthanasia, physician-assisted suicide, and other medical practices involving the end of life in the Netherlands, 1990–1995. *N Engl J Med, 335*(22), 1699–1705. doi:10.1056/NEJM199611283352227

Vaux, K. L. (1989). Mercy, murder, & morality: Perspectives on euthanasia. The theological ethics of euthanasia. *Hastings Cent Rep, 19*(1 Suppl.), 19–22.

Volokh, E. (2009). Duty to rescue/report statutes. Retrieved from http://volokh.com/2009/11/03/duty-to-rescuereport-statutes/

Voluntary euthanasia: The new society states its case (Editorial). (1935). *BMJ, 2,* 1168–1169.

Warren, J. C. (1848). *Etherization.* Boston: W. D. Ticknor & Company.

Watson, R. (2009). Luxembourg is to allow euthanasia from 1 April. *BMJ, 338,* b1248. doi:10.1136/bmj.b1248

Wilkinson, D., & Savulescu, J. (2014). A costly separation between withdrawing and withholding treatment in intensive care. *Bioethics, 28*(3), 127–137. doi:10.1111/j.1467-8519.2012.01981.x

Williams, G. L. (1957). *The sanctity of life and the criminal law* (1st ed.). New York: Knopf.

Williams, S. D. (1872). *Euthanasia.* London: Williams and Norgate.

Winter, S. M. (2000). Terminal nutrition: Framing the debate for the withdrawal of nutritional support in terminally ill patients. *Am J Med, 109*(9), 723–726.

World Health Organization. (2002). WHO definition of palliative care. Retrieved from www.who.int/cancer/palliative/definition/en/

6

Forgoing Life-Sustaining Medical Treatment

Up until the early twentieth century, relatively few forms of life-sustaining medical treatment (LSMT) existed, and people generally died precipitously (such as from untreatable infectious disease) or for unspecified reasons (such as from undiagnosed cancer) (p. 13). Over the course of the century, however—thanks to the development of antibiotics, mechanical ventilation, dialysis, and advanced cardiac life support—it became possible to sustain patients for long periods of time. Initially patients were not asked whether they wanted to be sustained; the presumption was that someone, given the choice between living and dying, would always choose the former.

As the "era of radical autonomy" dawned—with precedent-setting court cases (*In re Quinlan*, 1976) and legislative accomplishments (California Natural Death Act, 1976)—patients with sufficient decision-making capacity (DMC) were acknowledged to have the right to refuse any medical treatment, including one that is life sustaining. Whether because their preceding quality of life was so poor, the treatment so burdensome, or the likelihood recovery so remote, a substantial percentage of patients who now die do so as a result of refusing some form of LSMT. This is especially true in the intensive care unit (ICU), where up to 90% of deaths involve forgoing LSMT (Prendergast & Luce, 1997).

For patients with single organ failure—such as a patient with end stage renal disease (ESRD) on dialysis—there may only be one life-sustaining modality to limit. But for patients on several life-sustaining modalities—such as a patient in the ICU with multisystem organ failure—there are multiple options. When responding to requests to forgo LSMT, physicians tend to withdraw interventions that are costly, scarce, or invasive or are likely to lead to rapid death once removed (Asch & Christakis, 1996). One multi-institutional study, for instance, found that the most common sequence started with vasopressors, antibiotics, and enteral feedings, only then moving on to mechanical ventilation (Faber-Langendoen, 1996). But there is no "magic formula" for forgoing

LSMT, as each modality should be viewed in light of its respective benefits and burdens. Each modality also comes with its own particular ethical considerations, which need to be explored in detail.

Respiratory

Respiratory support is a frequent consideration in discussions about forgoing LSMT. Most critically ill patients require it, even if only for a brief period of time. The fact that it may only be for a brief period is significant because once the patient is no longer dependent on mechanical ventilation, only more protracted—and often ethically contentious—options may remain, such as forgoing medically administered nutrition and hydration (MANH). This period has, therefore, been termed the "window of opportunity" (p. 317), and surrogate decision-makers should be made aware of the time-limited nature of some of the options available to them in such a situation.

In addition to being potentially time-limited, the decision to forgo mechanical ventilation is also complex because it is generally made by a surrogate decision-maker. In most cases, patients who are compassionately extubated are so ill—or under sufficient sedation[1]—that they are unable to participate in the decision to do so (Smedira et al. 1990).

Called by some "terminal extubation," the term "compassionate extubation" is preferable because it both recognizes the focus on comfort, as well as avoids giving the impression that the purpose of extubation is to end the patient's life. Quite the contrary, some patients who are compassionately extubated with the full expectation that they will die quickly defy expectations and survive for extended periods of time. In one study the median time from extubation to death was 35 minutes, but the range was 1 to 890 minutes (Chan et al., 2004). In another study, 11% of "terminally weaned" patients ultimately left the hospital (Carlson, Campbell, & Frank, 1996). Not surprisingly, clinicians are "very confident" of their survival predictions in only a minority of cases (Billings, 2012).

The clinical standard for compassionate extubation involves three types of medications. Opioids are standard treatment for dyspnea and benzodiazepines for anxiety. Rather than waiting for the patient to suffer and then respond, the medical team generally boluses the patient—so-called anticipatory dosing (Truog et al., 2001)—before extubation, as well as providing liberal prn ("as needed") orders to respond promptly to any signs of distress. Lastly, antisialogogues are often given to minimize secretions, thus preventing the so-called "death rattle" (Brody et al. 1997) which occurs in approximately one-third of patients after extubation and can be quite distressing to families (Wee, Coleman, Hillier, & Holgate, 2006).

---

1. This is particularly true of invasive ventilation (whereby an endotracheal tube is inserted into the patient's trachea). Noninvasive positive pressure ventilation—such as bilevel positive airway pressure—does not require sedation and a patient may be still able to make his own decisions.

Despite many clinical guidelines for compassionate extubation, practice varies widely, with clinicians varying up to ten-fold in the doses of medication they typically administer (Hall & Rocker, 2000). In an attempt to walk the fine line between providing too little medication (and thus worsening suffering) and too much medication (and thus potentially hastening death[2]), greater emphasis is often placed on avoiding the latter. Billings (2012), for instance, asserts that "minimization of opioid and sedative doses receives greater emphasis than minimization of suffering." The end result is reports of patients gasping for air or becoming cyanotic while still conscious (Perkin & Resnik, 2002).

Even absent visible signs of distress, patients may nevertheless be suffering following extubation. Studies have shown that those who are unable to report dyspnea may still experience it at the end of life (Campbell, Templin, & Walch, 2009). This further highlights the obligation of the clinical team to effectively prevent suffering at the end of life, whether visible or not.

Another form of suffering may also come into play: the family's. This is especially true in cases of dyspnea, where some palliative medicine clinicians may feel pressure from the family to "get this over quickly" (Keizer, 2004). Here clinicians must recognize that it is appropriate to use opioids to treat a patient's dyspnea but not a family's anxiety or grief. There are other ways of tending to the family's emotional needs—such as empathetic listening, counseling, and spiritual support—that are clinical and ethically superior.

Beyond the ethical requirement to effectively prevent patient suffering related to compassionate extubation—and to make the patient or surrogate are aware of any time-limited nature of life-sustaining mechanical ventilation, so that they can make relevant treatment decisions within the "window of opportunity"—there may not initially appear to be a great deal of ethical complexity to that decision. This is clearly an invasive intervention which—unlike MANH, for instance—does not require any clarification as to whether it is a "medical treatment." However, there are two specific situations where the ethical complexity of withdrawal of mechanical ventilation is increased: those involving an alert patient and those involving a patient whose neuromuscular blockade has yet to wear off.[3]

---

2. It is imperative to note that opioids do not always hasten death; in point of fact, they often prolong life when used appropriately (p. 213).

3. Two other ethical issues that may arise related to respiratory support are addressed elsewhere: the relevance of prior refusal of mechanical ventilation to a situation where only short term support may be necessary to restore the patient to his baseline health (p. 73) and apparent rejection of continued mechanical ventilation by a patient with uncertain DMC (p. 123). Another ethical issue that may arise is whether to proceed from endotracheal intubation to a more comfortable and stable tracheostomy, to permit long-term ventilation. This is quite analogous to the shift from a nasogastric to gastrostomy tube for long-term administration of nutrition and hydration, and thus many of the principles discussed later would also apply to this situation.

Compassionate Extubation of the Alert Patient
Case Study

A fifty-seven-year-old man with amyotrophic lateral sclerosis (also known as Lou Gehrig's disease) has had worsening respiratory status over several years. His level of support has gradually increased, moving from intermittent bilevel positive airway pressure (BiPAP) to continuous BiPAP and ultimately to invasive mechanical ventilation through a tracheostomy. His quality of life has also been declining, despite optimal palliative care support. He has decided to discontinue mechanical ventilation, with the full realization that this will lead to his death.

In preparation for compassionate extubation, the team reviews the standard approach of bolus dosing of opioids and benzodiazepines, followed by thoughtful upward titration of doses to treat symptoms that emerge. Unlike many patients approaching terminal extubation, this gentleman is cognitively intact and is extremely concerned about suffering while waiting for the medications to take effect. He asks the team if he can be preemptively sedated in order to avoid any risk of this.

The majority of patients who are compassionately extubated have a significantly depressed level of consciousness, by virtue of either the underlying disease process (which necessitated mechanical ventilation in the first place) or sedation necessary to address the discomfort of an indwelling endotracheal tube. Some, however, may be quite awake and not require significant sedation. This is often true for those with isolated neurologic disease.

In these situations, the largely *reactive* approach to compassionate extubation noted previously may lead to unnecessary suffering. For even if a bolus of opioids is given prior to extubation, there is no way to know for sure what the appropriate dose is—as the effects are dependent on many factors, including the patient's tolerance to the medication (p. 207)—and thus how much suffering the patient will experience. Liberal *prn* dosing allows prompt response to suffering that is already occurring, but it does not prevent suffering in the first place (which is always more efficient for the physician, not to mention more pleasant for the patient). In many situations the team is forced to "play catch-up" by reacting to suffering once it has already occurred.

Terminal extubation of the alert patient (TEAP; Billings, 2011)—has garnered increasing attention, given the increased risk of the patient suffering in the last moments of life while the medical team plays catch-up. This can also take a toll on family members forced to watch their loved one suffer, as well as on physicians who may feel that they have not done enough to protect their patient from unnecessary distress. Historically, the medical literature has provided scant guidance for physicians in this predicament, "especially at the feeling level" (Edwards & Tolle, 1992).

Concern for respiratory depression—which is often overstated in relationship to opioids (p. 213)—may be a legitimate concern here. In contrast to patients who are so critically ill as to have a depressed level of consciousness, the alert patient may be able to breathe independently after extubation, depending on his underlying disease process. Some have therefore expressed concern that even an opioid-tolerant patient may experience some degree of respiratory depression from additional dosing. This could prove to be the crucial difference between being able to breathe independently or not (Truog, Arnold, & Rockoff, 1991).

Others, however, consider the obligation to prevent suffering to be a moral imperative. They argue that alert patients should be given significant sedation to prevent suffering from occurring (Schneiderman & Spragg, 1988). Billings (2012) writes:

> Any potentially conscious and imminently dying patient who is undergoing withdrawal of ventilator support and hence faces the extreme distress of respiratory failure should be offered preemptive high doses of opioids and sedatives for anesthesia, or at least deep sedation to assure comfort, regardless of concerns about suppressing respiratory drive.

Framed in this way, some argue that the central question is misdirected: rather than asking whether it is morally justifiable to sedate a patient before ventilator withdrawal—recognizing the risk of hastened death—perhaps we should really be asking ourselves whether it is morally justifiable *not* to sedate the patient (Schneiderman, 1991).

As usual, a one-size-fits-all approach is insufficient. The fact that a patient about to be extubated is alert is certainly relevant, but so are several other aspects of the patient's condition. One is the likelihood that sedation will cause clinically significant respiratory depression, given the often beneficial effects of opioids on life expectancy (p. 213). A patient with a very high opioid tolerance is less likely to experience such depression, thus allowing more aggressive preemptive dosing.

Another relevant aspect is the likelihood of spontaneous respiration (and, ultimately, continued survival) after ventilator withdrawal. A patient such as the one discussed in this section—who requires mechanical ventilation because of progressive respiratory failure—will not be able to breathe independently and sustain life. A different patient with failure of a different organ system (including primary lung disease), on the other hand, could conceivably surpass expectations and survive for some time following removal of respiratory support.

Taking a balanced approach to the issue of TEAP, sedation should be used judiciously in an alert patient who is generally opioid-naïve and who could conceivably survive following extubation. By contrast, "preemptive high doses of opioids and sedatives" would be indicated for opioid-tolerant patients who are likely to suffer with only standard dosing and are not expected to survive even without whatever respiratory depression might be caused by opioids (Edwards & Ueno, 1991).

This discussion of the role of sedatives in treating (and preventing) suffering related to compassionate extubation largely assumes that they effectively accomplish this goal; however, this is not entirely certain. There have been recent case reports of anxiety and panic in patients undergoing general anesthesia (Ghoneim et al., 2009) as well as new evidence of brain activity in patients in so-called "vegetative" states (Monti et al., 2010).

Recognizing this, Billings (2011) goes so far as to say that "a case can be made that all non-brain-dead patients dying a respiratory death may experience dyspnea and anxiety, even though they may be unable to communicate it." If so, the central question of this section—*Is it morally justifiable to not sedate a patient prior to compassionate extubation?*—may miss the mark. One might better ask whether it is *clinically sufficient* to sedate such a patient.

The appropriate moral of this story is not that sedation is of unclear benefit—thus diminishing the obligation to provide it—but rather that one cannot be sure precisely what a sedated patient is truly experiencing. It is possible that the patient is suffering more than previously realized, despite sedation. (Perhaps, then, the discussion should be extended to include not only preemptive sedation but even general anesthesia, depending on the relevant factors noted previously.) By contrast, there is ample—and disturbing—evidence of just how much a nonsedated alert patient may suffer following compassionate extubation, if the physicians merely react to symptoms as they arise.

In the end, all one can do is act in good faith and with compassion within the limits of available knowledge and be prepared to modify beliefs and practices based on whatever evidence subsequently becomes available.

Return to the Case

> The patient was not opioid-naïve, but he has only been receiving low-dose opioids for dyspnea. The team feels like there is substantial risk of respiratory depression from increased opioid dosing, while also recognizing that this is clinically irrelevant because his neuromuscular disease will prevent him from breathing on his own, irrespective of whatever medications he is receiving. (Indeed, it is this very disease that necessitated mechanical ventilation in the first place.)
>
> After the patient has had the opportunity to say whatever he needs to say to his family and friends, he is heavily sedated prior to compassionate extubation. As expected, he does not breathe after the mechanical ventilator is stopped, and he does not appear to be suffering in any way.

Compassionate Extubation of the Paralyzed Patient
Case Study

> A forty-three-year-old man sustained severe head trauma following a motor vehicle accident nearly two weeks ago. Increased intracranial pressure led the patient to "buck the vent" (i.e., "ventilator dyssynchrony"), for which a neuromuscular blocker

was administered to facilitate adequate ventilation. His condition did not improve, however, and his family eventually decided he would not want to continue with aggressive treatment.

The infusion of the neuromuscular blocker was stopped, but its effects will continue for some time until it is fully metabolized. The medical team wants to defer compassionate extubation until paralysis has abated in order to avoid any risk of "causing" the patient's death. The family, though—after having made such a heart-wrenching decision—cannot bear to wait any longer.

Neuromuscular blockers (also known as "paralytics") are sometimes used to optimize mechanical ventilation, especially when a patient's intrinsic respiratory effort is not synchronous with—and thus impedes—the actions of the ventilator (Stewart et al., 1998). At the end of the twentieth century, they were used in the majority of ventilated patients in ICUs (Merriman, 1981). Surveys of physicians during that period revealed that in a minority of cases patients received neuromuscular blockers immediately preceding compassionate extubation, either as part of their therapeutic regimen or even in preparation for extubation itself (Faber-Langendoen, 1994). The rationale was that the patient would therefore not struggle or gasp, sparing the family and others in attendance additional emotional suffering (Rushton & Terry, 1995).

Over time, though, the negative side effects of neuromuscular blockade—including development of prolonged ICU-acquired weakness as well as the risk of patient awareness during paralysis—have led to decreased use (Warr, Thiboutot, Rose, Mehta, & Burry, 2011). A more recent study showed that less than one in seven ICU patients are chemically paralyzed (Arroliga et al., 2005).

From an ethical perspective, it is clearly impermissible to *initiate* paralytics prior to extubation (Schneiderman & Spragg, 1988). Such medications have no analgesic effects—a fact, sadly, not recognized by all physicians (Loper, Butler, Nessly, & Wild, 1989)—and thus do nothing to minimize suffering. While a paralyzed patient may appear at peace—thus providing illusory comfort to the family—he is simply unable (by virtue of being paralyzed) to communicate the degree of distress he is experiencing (Brody, Campbell, Faber-Langendoen, & Ogle, 1997). Indeed, he is unable to communicate at all, thus eliminating the possibility of any meaningful interaction (let alone survival) following extubation. This is precisely why sedatives are always administered *before* paralytics: to eliminate the frightening possibility that the patient could be awake, alert, and paralyzed. Thus the old saying: "Sedatives are for the patient, and paralytics are for the physician" (i.e., to keep the patient comfortable and to optimize ventilation, respectively).

Precisely because paralytics do not lessen—and, indeed, could exacerbate—a patient's suffering, their use at the end of life cannot be justified by the Rule of Double Effect (p. 209). Simply put, initiating paralysis prior to extubation is an act of euthanasia (p. 143) done to prevent others' emotional distress while risking magnifying the patient's own (Larcher et al., 2015).

The relevant ethical question here is whether, for a patient who is *already receiving* paralytics for clinical indications, compassionate extubation must be delayed until the effects of those paralytics wear off. In certain cases significant time may be required for this to occur, with paralysis sometimes continuing for a matter of weeks (Partridge, Abrams, Bazemore, & Rubin, 1990). In cases of long-term use of paralytics, their effects may also be resistant to reversal agents (Segredo et al., 1992).

Several arguments have been proposed to support continuing ventilation until the patient is no longer paralyzed, echoing the arguments against initiating neuromuscular blockade prior to extubation. One is that extubating before paralysis has worn off increases the likelihood of suffering, given the challenges in assessing symptoms while a patient is experiencing neuromuscular blockade. Another is the impossibility of meaningful interaction with loved ones after extubation. The third objection involves the inherent uncertainty of how long a patient—absent the influence of paralytics—would survive after compassionate extubation, given that some patients exceed expectations. The effects of neuromuscular blockers, of course, make this is a physiological impossibility. For this reason, some have argued extubation before resolution of preexisting neuromuscular blockade is equivalent to killing (Sottile, 1995).

While effective in avoiding any possibility of euthanasia, the conservative approach of waiting for all paralytic effects to wear off creates two significant problems. One involves allocation of scarce resources, as continued intensive care—which is required to provide mechanical ventilation that is in turn necessitated by the neuromuscular blockade still in effect—would be required for an indeterminate amount of time. To take up a precious ICU bed for someone who does not wish to continue aggressive treatment may have negative effects on other patients, who could be deprived of the care that they need to survive.

Continued treatment could also have significant negative impact on the patient's loved ones, who have finally come to the gut-wrenching conclusion that the patient is not going to survive and that he would not want to continue to receive such burdensome treatment. Had paralytics not been required to facilitate ventilation, the next steps would have been clear. The patient would have been provided with appropriate comfort-directed medications and the endotracheal tube removed, with the family at his bedside providing comfort to him and to one another as he died. But if one were to take the "safe route" and defer extubation for the hours, days, or even weeks required for paralysis to abate, this could inflict deep emotional suffering on the family, as they wait for the team to finally "let him go."

Recognizing the significant drawbacks of waiting for neuromuscular blockade to wear off, some have advocated waiting "no more than two to three hours" after discontinuation of paralytics and then administering large doses of sedatives and opioids prior to compassionate extubation (Brody et al., 1997). While providing a crisp guide for action, this seems a rather arbitrary cut-off which fails to take into account the ethical and clinical concerns noted earlier.

Truog, Burns, Mitchell, Johnson, and Robinson (2000) put forth a more broad-based approach that provides practical guidance in addressing this situation. They begin by countering some of the objections to compassionate extubation in the context of paralytics. With regard to the difficulty in assessing and appropriate treating symptoms, they note that anesthesiologists, in particular, are frequently tasked with ensuring patient comfort in the context of neuromuscular blockade. Indeed, surgical patients under general anesthesia are routinely paralyzed, requiring nuanced assessment of comfort absent many of the usual indicators. Thus while symptom management can be challenging in the context of neuromuscular blockade, it is not impossible, as long as sufficiently experienced clinicians are available.

Truog et al. (2000) also acknowledge the impossibility of meaningful interaction in the presence of neuromuscular blockade. For patients who might reasonably be expected to have such interaction in the absence of that blockade, deferring compassionate extubation until paralysis has worn off is a reasonable consideration. But for patients who are so ill—or enduring such a high symptom burden—that this would not be possible even absent paralytics, waiting for the latter's effects to abate provides no practical benefit.

Finally, Truog et al. (2000) address the possibility of survival without mechanical ventilation. Recognizing the inherent uncertainty in such predictions, there are nevertheless situations of at least *substantial*—if not absolute—certainty that a patient will not be able to survive off the ventilator. These may be appropriate for extubation before paralytics have fully worn off, while cases of significant uncertainty would not be.

Thus while acknowledging that "as a general rule . . . neuromuscular function should be restored before the life support is withdrawn," Truog et al. (2000) posit an important exception to that rule, namely,

> when death is expected to be both rapid and certain after the removal of the
> ventilator and when the burdens to the patient and family of waiting for the
> neuromuscular blockade to diminish to a reversible level exceed the benefits
> of allowing better assessment of the patient's comfort and the possibility of
> interaction with loved ones.

This argument is compelling, for it acknowledges both the inherent uncertainty of clinical predictions as well as the relatively rare but extremely real emotional suffering that could be inflicted on a family by waiting an indefinite period of time before doing what they know is right for the patient.

The dictum that patients who are "chemically paralyzed" should not be compassionately extubated is, therefore, not absolute. It is, however, generally reliable and should be taken as the norm absent exceptional circumstances and expertise in complex symptom management.

Return to the Case

After the family requested a shift of goals to comfort, the paralytics currently in use were immediately discontinued. All efforts were made to reverse their effects, but since they had been in use for a prolonged period, their duration of action was uncertain. The family is given the option of waiting for these effects to wear off, but they are exhausted and understandably eager for "this nightmare to be over."

The team discusses the clinical situation, and there is consensus that the patient is so critically ill that even if the paralytics are given time to wear off, the probability of spontaneous respiration—let alone meaningful interaction with his family—is negligible. The obligation to prevent additional family suffering is felt to be primary, and the patient is compassionately extubated after providing substantial symptomatic pretreatment (which is necessary given the challenges in accurately assessing his degree of suffering).

The family feels that he died very comfortably because he showed no evidence of distress, but the team knows that this is not a reliable indicator. The team takes comfort, however, in knowing that they treated any potential symptoms aggressively and proactively and closely monitored him for any indications of distress.

Cardiac

Case Study

An eighty-nine-year-old man has worsening dementia. He lacks DMC, and at this point cannot even recognize his family. His advance directive explicitly states that if he were to reach such a state, he would not want life-sustaining medical treatment. He currently lives in a nursing home and requires few medications and in his present condition could survive for several years.

Six years earlier—before the onset of dementia—he had a pacemaker/defibrillator inserted for sick sinus syndrome. Recognizing that this could likely prolong a life the patient would not want to live, his family requests that this be deactivated. The cardiologist, however, is reluctant to do so, believing that the device is now a part of the patient and—given that the patient is pacemaker-dependent—deactivating it is equivalent to active euthanasia.

An ethics consultation is requested.

The right of patients with sufficient DMC to refuse LSMT is well-established in ethics and the law. While initially applied (in the *Quinlan* case) to mechanical ventilation, the most common application is cardiac in the form of Do Not Attempt Resuscitation orders in the event of a cardiac arrest. This includes not only chest compressions but also forms of advanced cardiac life support (Jacobs et al., 2010), including medications as well as external defibrillation. A patient—or his surrogate, if he lacks DMC—clearly has the right to refuse the implantation of a cardiovascular implantable electronic device (CIED), whether an implantable cardioverter-defibrillator (ICD) or a pacemaker, or a combination of the two. But if the patient previously consented to the CIED—and it is now implanted in his body—does he subsequently have the right to have it deactivated?

This is an increasingly common dilemma, as clinical indications for CIEDs are expanding (Goldberger & Lampert, 2006) and more and more patients are having them implanted (Hammill et al., 2010). At some later point, though, these devices may no longer be beneficial and can actually be burdensome. In the final weeks of life, for instance, 20% of patients with ICDs receive shocks which can be quite painful (Ahmad, Bloomstein, Roelke, Bernstein, & Parsonnet, 2000), diminishing patients' quality of life (Schron et al., 2002) and burdening both them and their family members (Goldstein, Lampert, Bradley, Lynn, & Krumholz, 2004). Patients who may not be imminently dying—but whose quality of life is so poor that they do not wish it artificially prolonged in the event of a life-threatening arrhythmia—may also request deactivation of their pacemakers.

It should not come as a surprise—given the documented discomfort of other specialists in discussing end-of-life (EOL) decisions (p. 183 and p. 394)—that cardiologists report unease in discussing deactivation of such devices (Goldstein, Bradley, Zeidman, Mehta, & Morrison, 2009). The end result is that deactivation is rarely discussed, not only as part of the informed consent process for device insertion but also as the end of life approaches (Goldstein et al., 2004).

The standard teaching of modern bioethics is that there is no ethical or legal difference between withdrawing and withholding (p. 156). The cardiological application of this maxim is affirmed in a recent consensus statement (Lampert et al., 2010), which clearly states that withdrawal of CIED therapy is ethically and legally equivalent to refusing it in the first place. The statement goes on to assert that neither pacemaker nor ICD deactivation is equivalent to either physician-assisted dying (PAD) or euthanasia. In both PAD and euthanasia, the clinician's intention is to effect the patient's death, whereas in CIED deactivation the intention is to withdraw a burdensome treatment (Rhymes, McCullough, Luchi, Teasdale, & Wilson, 2000). In addition, the cause of death in the former two instances is the intervention itself, whereas in CIED deactivation the patient's underlying cardiac disease ultimately leads to his death (Zellner, Aulisio, & Lewis, 2009).

Yet even though a professional consensus statement exists, that does not mean that every cardiologist agrees with it. Of the two types of CIEDs, deactivation of an ICD provokes less controversy (Berger, 2005; Goldstein et al., 2004; Lewis et al., 2006; Mueller, Hook, & Hayes, 2003). Unlike a pacemaker, this form of CIED plays no ongoing role in maintaining heart function, and when it does activate the resultant shocks can be extremely painful. For a terminally ill patient, an ICD may prolong the process of dying while also increasing the symptom burden. A patient who is not terminally ill may also request ICD deactivation based on the physical, emotional, and spiritual burdens of his current quality of life, as well as other considerations (such as financial and the impact on family) of artificially prolonged life.

Unanimity is lacking, however, with regard to deactivating pacemakers. Several reasons have been given for objecting to the practice. The first is clinical, with critics asserting that—unlike an ICD—the pacemaker incurs negligible burden. Rather than sparing a patient unpleasant symptoms, in some cases deactivation of a pacemaker can actually worsen heart failure–related symptoms (Braun, Hagen, Hatfield, & Wyse, 1999).

Even conceding the latter point, the former overlooks the prevailing reason for requesting pacemaker deactivation: not the direct burden of the intervention but the poor quality of life that the intervention is sustaining. Patients are not required to "prove" direct burden when they refuse other LSMTs, such as MANH. Neither should they be required to do so in relation to a pacemaker.

Critics of pacemaker deactivation point to another distinction between the two types of CIEDs: whereas ICD function is episodic, a pacemaker functions continuously. Deactivating an ICD means that a patient will subsequently die for want of defibrillation when an arrhythmia eventually occurs, but deactivating a pacemaker on which a patient is dependent necessarily leads to the patient's death, often in very short order. This explains why, in a recent survey, one in ten clinicians who care for patients with CIEDs viewed deactivation of a pacemaker in a pacemaker-dependent patient as a form of euthanasia or PAD (Mueller, Jenkins, Bramstedt, & Hayes, 2008).

The mere fact that a pacemaker functions *continuously* to sustain the dependent patient does not, however, mean that there is an obligation to maintain its use. After all, mechanical ventilation is a continuous life-sustaining procedure, and there is no debate about the patient's right to refuse it (Sulmasy, 2008).

One might respond that unlike a ventilator—which in most cases is used for relatively short periods of time—a pacemaker is a longstanding treatment that can be effective for years or even decades. Once again, though, the fact that a treatment is *longstanding* in nature does not mean it cannnot be limited. As noted in the following section, a significant percentage of patients with ESRD choose to discontinue dialysis—which they may have been dependent on for years or even decades—prior to death.

Acknowledging this, critics of pacemaker deactivation have drawn a further distinction among continuous therapies: some are "regulative" (in that they coax the body back into its normal, healthy status) while others are "constitutive" (thus taking over a function the body formerly was able to provide). Whereas an ICD is a regulative therapy, a pacemaker essentially takes over the role of the sinoatrial node in prompting the heart to beat. As a constitutive therapy there may exist an increased ethical obligation to maintain—or, at the very least, not discontinue—its use.

Once again, though, counterexamples quickly come to mind. Extracorporeal membrane oxygenation (ECMO) takes over the role previously played by healthy lungs and dialysis the role once played by non-functioning kidneys. Both, therefore, are constitutive, yet clearly permissible to withdraw or withhold at the patient's discretion.

A further distinction could be drawn between different types of constitutive therapies: some are substitutes for lost functions (e.g., ECMO or dialysis), whereas others represent actual *replacements* for those functions (e.g., a transplanted kidney or prosthetic heart valve). While the former can clearly be withdrawn, the latter are viewed by some as becoming "part of the patient." Some have gone so far as to term these "biofixtures," emphasizing their indwelling nature (Paola & Walker, 2000). Just as one would never consider surgically removing a prosthetic heart valve upon patient request, so—the argument goes—one should not take steps to deactivate a pacemaker. As Sulmasy (2008) writes, "The more a technology can be classified as a replacement therapy, the greater the case for judging that its discontinuation would constitute an immoral act of killing."

However, there are relevant differences between a prosthetic heart valve and a pacemaker. Unlike the heart valve, the pacemaker is dependent on external support, in the form of a battery that requires regular replacement, as well as ongoing maintenance and monitoring (Sulmasy, 2008). These are generally not characteristics one associates with "parts of a patient" but rather technologies which serve a specific purpose. It is therefore possible to distinguish between replacement therapies that are truly part of a patient—and would continue to function independent of any external support—and therapies that integrate into the patient's functioning but still require ongoing monitoring and maintenance. The former should not be removed, but the latter constitute medical intervention that the patient has the right to refuse.

Ultimately, the most profound difference between an ICD and a pacemaker (especially in a pacemaker-dependent patient) may be an emotional one. Deactivating an ICD—or, for that matter, a pacemaker in a patient who is not dependent on it—does not immediately lead to the patient's death. A patient could conceivably live for a prolonged period until dying for wont of these devices, until an arrhythmia ultimately causes his death.

But for a patient who is pacemaker-dependent, deactivation of the device leads directly and promptly to the patient's death. Understandably, this can lead the physician to *feel* responsible for that death. And on some level she is, at least from a causal perspective. Were it not for the physician's actions, the pacemaker would still be working and the patient would still be alive.

She is not *morally* responsible for it, however, because only a patient with serious heart disease would die for the absence of a pacemaker. (Just as only a patient with pulmonary failure would die for lack of a ventilator.) On a moral level, the physician is not causing the patient's death but rather acting out of respect for patient autonomy, in deactivating a device that is not truly "part of the patient" and which the patient has every right to be free of.

However reassuring this philosophical justification of pacemaker deactivation may be, the proximity of deactivation and death—in terms of both time and space (for the clinician or technician must be physically present to deactivate the device)—can be very trying for the physician. The forgoing of other life-sustaining modalities rarely leads to death with such certainty and rapidity. And while a physician could derive some comfort from "liberating" a patient from a burdensome treatment such as dialysis or mechanical ventilation, the burden of a pacemaker is largely invisible. For all these reasons, a physician may be unwilling to perform the deactivation.

Generally, when a physician is faced with a request that is morally objectionable to her—whether cardiac or otherwise—she is not required to accommodate it (American Medical Association, 2010–2011). (Exceptions may exist where that physician is the only person qualified to perform the procedure, and thus refusing to do so essentially prevents the patient from obtaining the treatment he is seeking.) The consensus statement recognizes this right of conscience, concluding that "a clinician cannot be compelled to carry out an ethically and legally permissible procedure (i.e., CIED deactivation) that s/he personally views in conflict with his/her personal values" (Lampert et al., 2010).

The statement goes on to set forth a series of steps the physician should take in such a situation. She should express her reservations in a respectful fashion and in such a way so as to not increase the patient's distress. Ideally, the physician should refer the patient to another physician who is willing to provide the treatment (AMA Council on Ethical and Judicial Affairs, 2007).

As always, "an ounce of prevention is worth a pound of cure." Rather than having to confront the question of CIED deactivation when the patient requests it, this should be incorporated into the informed consent process for CIED insertion, and advance care planning (ACP) as a whole. At the very least, this would let patients know that CIED deactivation is an option, which many do not realize (at least with regard to pacemakers) (Goldstein et al., 2008). This would also allow patients to clarify under what circumstances they might request CIED deactivation and also permit physicians who are uncomfortable doing so to inform patients that they would not be able to provide this service.

Such a discussion is relevant not only to subsequent CIED deactivation but also to the question of whether to accept a CIED in the first place. For many patients considering pacemaker placement, in particular, the choice seems almost commonsensical: if one's heart is not beating effectively, why *not* insert a painless device to ensure a regular and healthy rhythm? These patients may, however, be focusing on the current problem and not be looking ahead to what might occur in the future, which is relevant given the long lifespan of pacemakers and the changes in one's health that can occur over that period.

If a patient knew that his physician was not willing to deactivate a pacemaker on which he might subsequently become dependent—and there were no other physicians willing to do so nearby—this could impact the decision to proceed with pacemaker insertion in the first place. This is precisely the point made so poignantly in Katy Butler's story of her father, who suffered for years in a state that he never wanted, as a pacemaker kept him alive and no physician in his area was willing to deactivate it (Butler, 2013).

If physicians can refuse such a request based on a right of conscience, patients definitely have the right to know that this is what awaits them before making a major medical decision. And given the general consensus regarding the ethical acceptability of pacemaker deactivation, physicians caring for patients at the end of their lives—or what they *hope* is the end of their lives—have an obligation to advocate for these patients by educating their colleagues on the ethical nuances of this topic and ideally identifying physicians who can provide a service that patients have a right to receive.

Return to the Case

The ethics consultant begins by listening to the cardiologist's concerns: that the pacemaker is not causing any "harm," that it is now part of the patient (and deactivating it would be akin to "ripping out" the patient's prosthetic aortic valve), and that deactivating it would feel like she was killing her patient.

The consultant thoughtfully addresses each of these concerns. He begins by noting the patient's worsening quality of life (which he clearly never wanted for himself). He goes on to distinguish between something that functions independently and in perpetuity within a patient (like a heart valve) and one that requires monitoring, modification, and even battery replacement to continue to function. He spends most of his time, though, on the emotional reservations that the cardiologist has, recognizing this not as moral obstinacy but evidence of the cardiologist's care for the patient and high professional standards.

The consultant tries to identify a solution that simultaneously honors the patient's wishes and respects the cardiologist's beliefs, which have not been swayed by the conversation. Citing the consensus statement on this topic, the consultant suggests seeking a second opinion from another cardiologist who does not share the first's moral reservations. Unlike an ICD—which may be actively inflicting suffering, thus creating more time pressure—the pacemaker itself is not currently a burden to the patient, and a slight delay in deactivation is acceptable to the family.

Ultimately another cardiologist is identified, who recognizes the right of the patient (through his surrogate decision-makers) to refuse treatment. She deactivates the pacemaker at the patient's home, and the patient dies comfortably, with his family at his side.

Renal

Case Study

An eighty-two-year old man has dealt with chronic kidney disease for many years and has finally progressed to ESRD, for which dialysis is indicated. His quality of life is still quite good: he lives in an assisted living facility and sees family and friends frequently. He is not excited about the thought of dialysis but would like to prolong his life if it remains at its current level.

He thinks this seems like an appropriate time to do some advance care planning, and thus a palliative care consultation is requested. To his surprise, dialysis is not as obvious a choice for him as he first imagined.

Up until the mid-twentieth century, kidney failure inevitably led to death. However, after the invention of dialysis—a form of renal replacement therapy (RRT)—patients with ESRD were able to survive for extended periods of time. Access to hemodialysis initially was extremely limited, leading to challenging and controversial allocation of resources decisions (Alexander, 1962). Now, however, there are various forms of RRT—including peritoneal dialysis and home hemodialysis—which are readily available and universally covered by Medicare. The primary ethical issue related to RRT, therefore, is not one of resource allocation as much as informed decision-making and the appropriateness of RRT.

At first the question of *whether* to institute RRT seems rather obvious—yes, in order to survive—as does the question of *when*—at the point when one's kidney function is no longer sufficient to sustain life. But both of these are actually rather complex questions, given the burdens of RRT as well as the uncertain benefit in specific populations. Due to this complexity, palliative care consultation may be requested. In some ways, this consultation bears striking resemblance to its role in other disease processes: treating unrecognized symptoms, clarifying prognosis, optimizing communication, and identifying the choices that are often obscured by blanket assumptions. In this context, however, palliative care consultation must also take into account the specific nuances of ESRD, which are often not recognized.

Palliative care views treatment decisions in light of the respective benefits and burdens of that treatment. And the burden of RRT is significant: nearly half of patients experience a reduction in satisfaction with life scores after dialysis initiation, with scores remaining stable without improvement over time (Da Silva-Gane et al., 2012). Many patients with ESRD—including younger patients—suffer significant frailty and disability (Johansen et al., 2007). The majority of patients on chronic dialysis experience fatigue, pain, muscle cramps, difficulty with sleep, and sexual dysfunction (Abdel-Kader, Unruh, & Weisbord, 2009), which are often untreated or potentially not even recognized. One-quarter of patients suffer from depression, which independently increases the risk of death (Kimmel et al., 2000). Overall, symptom burden in ESRD is equivalent to that of cancer (Murtagh, Cohen, & Germain, 2007), underscoring the need to provide not only guidance related to treatment choices but also optimal management of the symptoms that may arise because of those choices (O'Connor & Corcoran, 2012).

Counterbalancing the burdens of RRT is the anticipated benefit: prolonged life. In some populations, however, this is not certain to be the case. Specific groups of patients— such as those over eighty years of age with ESRD—survive just as long with conservative management as with RRT (Verberne et al., 2016) and with fewer complications (Da Silva-Gane et al., 2012).

But even if RRT did convey a survival advantage for a specific patient, this needs to be weighed against the diminution in quality of life. For patients whose primary goal is survival—especially those under eighty and without significant comorbidities—RRT is a very reasonable option. But for others who are seeking some balance of quantity and quality of life, it may not be the best choice. In addition to the symptoms noted previously, the burden of receiving regular dialysis—and attending to frequent complications—is significant. Among older patients over the age of seventy, for instance, those who elected dialysis spent approximately half of their days-survived either receiving dialysis or in the hospital, compared to those conservatively managed who spent less than 5% of their days-survived in those contexts (Carson, Juszczak, Davenport, & Burns, 2009). It not difficult to understand, therefore, why up to 20% of patients already receiving RRT choose to stop it prior to death.

Therefore, the decision about whether to initiate—or continue with—dialysis is not so simple as it might initially seem, and here the same steps noted earlier with regard to ACP (p. 70) are applicable. Having been diagnosed with kidney disease, a patient needs to understand the risks and benefits of RRT. He also needs to grasp his prognosis with and without potential forms of therapy, absent which it is impossible to make informed treatment decisions that accurately reflect his personal values.

Recent data, however, suggests that patients with ESRD have unrealistic expectations about their expected disease course and appropriate treatment options. For instance, the majority of patients in one study had a life expectancy of five years or less, but only 6% of them grasped this fact. In contrast, nearly two-thirds of patients overestimated their prognosis (Wachterman et al., 2013).

One of the reasons that a patient may not appreciate his prognosis is he might not have been informed of it. In that same study, three out of five nephrologists refused to provide an estimate of prognosis to a patient, even if requested by the patient (Wachterman et al., 2013). This could reflect a lack of confidence in establishing prognosis (p. 84), as well as the complex condition of many patients with ESRD (who often suffer from multiple comorbidities). Alternatively, nephrologists may feel that it is the primary care physician's responsibility to "bring it all together" and estimate prognosis from a broader perspective.

The implications of this lack of prognostic awareness should not be underestimated. The majority of patients in that study said that, if they were seriously ill, they would prefer care focused on improving quality of life over quantity. Consistent with this, less than 10% of patients with a more realistic sense of their prognosis preferred care focused on life extension. But among patients with an (over-)optimistic sense of their prognosis, nearly half preferred it (Wachterman et al., 2013).

Beyond specifically addressing prognosis, nephrologists traditionally have not engaged patients about EOL care. For instance, less than one-third of patients with ESRD report discussing CPR or mechanical ventilation with their nephrologist (Janssen et al., 2013), and less than one in ten discuss EOL or palliative care (Davison, 2010). Beyond a lack of adequate training, this can reflect systems-level barriers to optimal ACP, including fragmented care from multiple providers, unclear locus of responsibility for ACP, and lack of active collaboration and communication between providers (O'Hare et al., 2016).

Recently there has been increasing attention on the role of nephrologists in palliative and EOL care. Professional recommendations have affirmed that screening for depression, assessment of DMC, identification of prognostic indicators, participation in ACP, and ultimately EOL care are all part of nephrology care (Renal Physicians Association, 2010). Prognostic tools are more readily available, based on the Charlson morbidity score (Hemmelgarn, Manns, Quan, & Ghali, 2003), functional status, and the "surprise question" (Moss et al., 2008) (p. 87). These have identified populations with an especially poor prognosis, including patients over seventy-five years of age as well as those with high comorbidity scores, marked functional impairment, and severe chronic malnutrition. Prognostic models incorporating these variables have been devised (Cohen, Ruthazer, Moss, & Germain, 2010), and online calculators estimating disease progression are available (Tangri et al., 2016).

This deeper understanding of prognosis translates into the ability to engage in more substantive ACP, which studies have shown may contribute to a more peaceful death (Singer et al., 1995). Initiation of RRT should not be the default response to evolving ESRD; rather, it should be an option presented to patients in the context of a clear understanding of risks and benefits (Renal Physicians Association, 2010). Indeed, more and more patients are electing not to initiate dialysis (Murtagh et al., 2007), based on greater understanding of what it entails and—hopefully—a more realistic sense of their prognoses.

In considering whether to forgo RRT, a patient needs to understand what this means for him. As noted, conservative management does not necessarily lead to a shorter life expectancy, depending on the patient's age and comorbidities. He may have sufficient (though significantly diminished) renal function that would permit survival for a period of time.

Once kidney function essentially ceases—such as in the case of a patient who has received RRT for some time and then chooses to discontinue it—mean survival is six to eight days, with a wide range of up to 100 days for those who may have some residual kidney function (Moss, 1995). Uremia generally leads to decreased level of consciousness, but this in no way negates the responsibility to provide optimal symptom management

(Schmidt & Moss, 2014). So while there may be some uncertainty as to the precise duration of life after discontinuing RRT, life expectancy can be framed "on the order of days" in most cases, and clinicians can assure the patient that his suffering will be optimally and effectively addressed.

If a patient does elect to initiate RRT, it should not be considered an indefinite intervention, thereby creating a "new normal" for the patient. Instead, RRT should be viewed as a time-limited trial (TLT, p. 118) to assess its impact on quality of life. Like any other TLT, its net benefit should be revisited at the end of the established time period (perhaps six months), at which point it can be continued for another discrete period of time—when it will again be reevaluated—or withheld based on a lack of net benefit. Approaching RRT in this way avoids continuing indefinitely "by default" and also spares the patient the burden of bringing up the possibility of discontinuing it or of arbitrarily deciding when it should end.

These are obviously not easy conversations to have, and only a minority of nephrologists feel equipped to facilitate them (Davison, Jhangri, Holley, & Moss, 2006). Nephrology fellows receive relatively little training in this area, leading to significant discomfort providing this aspect of care (Combs et al., 2015). This is particularly concerning given the need for "generalist" palliative care (Quill & Abernethy, 2013) for the increasing numbers of patients—especially the elderly—suffering from ESRD (Kurella, Covinsky, Collins, & Chertow, 2007).

Fortunately, recent initiatives (such as Nephrotalk) have focused on equipping nephrologists with the necessary communication skills to carry on such nuanced discussions (Schell, Green, Tulsky, & Arnold, 2013). This is particularly crucial since many patients with ESRD—while usually seeing other physicians for their various comorbidities—view their nephrologist as their "primary" physician, based on the regularity and centrality of RRT in their lives. This places the nephrologist in a unique and sacred position, ideally poised to guide the patient through difficult decisions and continue to care for him no matter what he ultimately decides.

Return to the Case

The nephrologist—fresh off a Nephrotalk seminar—begins by learning more about the patient's background and personal values. She then asks the patient what he understands about his condition and the available treatment options. The patient responds that dialysis seems like the logical next step, given the orderly progression of his kidney disease and the fact that he "isn't ready to die."

The nephrologist responds that dialysis is certainly an option but should be considered only on a trial basis to assess how much it is helping the patient and how much of a burden it may present. She notes that many patients of a similar age who opt for dialysis end up spending a great deal of time in the renal clinic or hospital.

"I certainly don't want that," says the patient. "But is there really any choice?"

The nephrologist informs the patient that dialysis has not been shown to prolong life in patients his age with renal failure. There is no way to know for certain whether he—as an individual patient—would live longer with or without dialysis, but given his goals and values, she recommends that he not pursue dialysis at the present time. She also reassures him that that decision could be revisited at any point.

In light of the information provided, the patient opts to defer dialysis for the present and focus on conservative management. The nephrologist schedules him to come back and see her in two weeks to answer any further questions that might come up in subsequent conversations with his family. Before he leaves the office, she asks if it would be okay if they talked about other health issues that might come up in the future, like who should make decisions for him should he lose the ability to make them for himself.

Nutrition and Hydration

People who wish to eat and drink have an ethical right to do so. This is not medical treatment but rather basic human care. The only potential caveat is for patients with sufficiently significant dysphagia that oral consumption presents a risk of aspiration. This should prompt an overall discussion of risks and benefits of oral intake, with some patients choosing to forgo it in order to prolong life. Other patients, however, take such pleasure in eating and drinking that they are willing to accept the risk of aspiration. Once again, this is a values-based decision that requires understanding of the risks and benefits and support in making a decision that reflects one's underlying values.

By the same token, patients can also choose *not* to eat or drink, which is an ethically acceptable manner of hastening one's death (p. 152). Ethical complexity rises when the decision to forgo eating and drinking was made previously, and now the patient lacks DMC (and often, especially in the case of severe dementia, also requires assistance in eating). The specific case of advance refusal of spoon-feeding is addressed elsewhere (p. 399).

When a patient cannot eat and drink, MANH is an option. This can be administered via either an enteral route (i.e., through the gastrointestinal tract) or a parenteral route (i.e., intravenously). The goal of each is to provide sufficient nutrition and hydration to sustain life and optimize function, but each raises its own set of potential risks and burdens.

MANH may appear to blur the line between the basic human care of providing food and drink on the one hand and a medical intervention on the other. This is especially true of enteral administration, which at first glance resembles eating and drinking (except that the mouth and esophagus are bypassed). Even the term used for the device that permits infusion of nutrition and hydration into the gastrointestinal tract—a "feeding tube"—reinforces this connection to eating and drinking.

This connection evokes two strong sentiments. The first is the emotional resonance of food and drink, which are fundamental ways that human beings show concern and affection for each other. A baby is utterly dependent on his parents to provide nourishment. People bring chicken soup to a friend who is ill. When a friend gets married or graduates from medical school, a banquet is thrown in her honor. Withholding such sustenance from a patient who is unable to eat or drink may therefore give the impression of abandoning that person in a time of need and is especially resonant in cultures that place particular emphasis on sharing meals together (Blank, 2011).

The second sentiment is the strong emotional reaction provoked by the thought of dying for lack of food and water. Anyone who has thoughtfully contemplated the plight of victims of famine—or merely skipped breakfast—may have a literally visceral reaction to the notion of hunger. The possibility that a loved one might "starve" to death is abhorrent, especially when the solution seems rather obvious and burden-free (i.e., instilling nutrition and hydration directly into the patient's stomach, via artificial means).

Given this deep symbolism, it is not surprising that the first major court case about refusal of LSMT (*In re Quinlan*, 1976) specifically focused on withdrawal of mechanical ventilation but did not address MANH. Karen Ann Quinlan's family never considered forgoing the latter, in large part because of their religious beliefs. The landmark court case involving MANH did not come until a decade and a half later (*Cruzan v. Director, Missouri Department of Health*, 1990), when another young woman in a persistent vegetative state—which is better termed unresponsive wakefulness syndrome (p. 405)—was breathing independently, and thus there was no ventilator to withdraw.

Recognizing that she did not want to continue to live in such a condition—and that MANH was the only LSMT she was receiving—Nancy Cruzan's parents requested discontinuation of the gastrostomy tube. The state of Missouri opposed this, however, arguing that a "feeding tube" did not constitute medical treatment (which could be limited) but rather basic human care. When the lower court ruled in the state's favor, the Cruzans appealed to the US Supreme Court, which found that a competent person has "a constitutionally protected right to refuse lifesaving hydration and nutrition" (*Cruzan v. Director, Missouri Department of Health*, 1990). Justice O'Connor's concurring opinion clearly states that

> artificial feeding cannot readily be distinguished from other forms of medical treatment. Whether or not the techniques used to pass food and water into the patient's alimentary tract are termed "medical treatment," it is clear they all involve some degree of intrusion and restraint.

Since that time, it has become quite common for patients to forgo MANH at the end of life (Martins Pereira, Pasman, van der Heide, van Delden, & Onwuteaka-Philipsen, 2015). Often patients are not dependent on any other forms of LSMT, and thus it provides the only "exit ramp" from a life they no longer wish to live. Interestingly, despite this relative frequency, there are few good studies in palliative care patients of the decision-making process and outcomes of forgoing MANH (Good, Richard, Syrmis, Jenkins-Marsh, & Stephens, 2014).

A patient's decision regarding MANH is also associated with placement. Most patients with advanced cancer who remain at home do not receive MANH, while most in facilities do (Dalal & Bruera, 2004). The causation here could be bidirectional: MANH is more likely to be recommended to patients in facilities, where it can more easily be administered (especially in intravenous form). By contrast, patients who have made a conscious choice to forgo MANH might well refuse other LSMTs and prioritize time at home among family and friends.

In discussing the option of forgoing either form of MANH—especially enteral—it is important to directly address the two emotional connotations noted previously. The symbolic significance of eating and drinking stems largely from the pleasure derived and the social context of shared meals. Preparing a meal for someone and subsequently eating it with them is a sacred and communal act which bears scant resemblance to MANH, where nutrition and hydration are received in isolation and without any of the related pleasure. So rather than conflating these two very different experiences—such as by using the term "feeding tube" to describe the method for delivering enteral MANH—it is more accurate (and helpful) to refer to artificial nutrition and hydration delivered via a gastrostomy tube, thereby emphasizing clinically efficacy without falsely imputing emotional significance.

With regard to the emotionally charged concept of "starvation," it is important to clarify what really happens when MANH is forgone. Absence of nutrition does not rapidly lead to death; indeed, a person can survive for weeks or longer without nutrition. The cause of death from forgoing MANH is dehydration. The distinction here is significant, not only for avoiding the provocative connotations of "starvation" but also for clarifying the experience of the patient.

Absolutely no intake of fluids—by either parenteral or enteral means—leads to hypovolemia and then to uremia as the kidneys have insufficient fluids to filter. This leads to a depression of level of consciousness—similar to that seen in patients with renal failure who withdraw RRT—leading the patient to become drowsy and eventually comatose. Rather than causing suffering, this can actually ameliorate suffering by depressing level of consciousness. If the patient is not receiving any fluids by mouth, the median time to death is approximately one week, although up to one-fifth of patients could survive two weeks or more (Bolt, Hagens, Willems, & Onwuteaka-Philipsen, 2015).

Since the patient is probably not receiving nutrition either, he will also enter a state of ketosis, burning fat instead of glucose for energy. The significance for EOL care is that ketosis is postulated to have an analgesic effect, thus protective against suffering (Masino & Ruskin, 2013). The combination of uremia and ketosis may help explain the decreased suffering experienced by patients who voluntarily stop eating and drinking as a means of hastening their deaths (Ganzini et al., 2003).

The time line noted here pertains to receiving absolutely no hydration, and ketosis only takes effect when no glucose is available to fuel the body. This is important to note, because even a small amount of hydration—including sips of water, or just the "carrier liquid" of intravenous medications—can sustain life for a prolonged period. Similarly, even a small amount of dextrose can prevent the onset of ketosis and its potential analgesic effects. The instinct of some physicians to continue intravenous fluids (which often contain dextrose) at the end of life—even at a very low "keep vein open" rate—to maintain intravenous access in case of an emergency can, therefore, be quite deleterious. Rather than acting as a safeguard against suffering, such a plan could actually exacerbate it by delaying uremia and preventing ketosis.

Up to this point, the decision about MANH has been portrayed as one of quality versus quantity of life. But it is important to note that there are certain situations where MANH does not even confer a survival benefit. Among hospitalized patients with multisystem organ failure and acute renal failure, for instance, MANH is associated with decreased survival (Borum et al., 2000). The case of MANH in the context of dementia-related dysphagia is addressed elsewhere (p. 401).

Beyond these observations about MANH in general, specific aspects of both enteral and parenteral MANH are relevant to making informed decisions about whether to pursue these interventions.

Enteral
Case Study

A seventy-eight-year-old patient is involved in a motor vehicle accident, sustaining significant head trauma. He is intubated and transferred to the ICU, where a nasogastric (NG) tube is placed to provide nutrition, according to clinical protocol.

Prior to the accident he lived at home with his wife of nearly fifty years and enjoyed gardening and dining out with friends. He has always valued his independence, and previously expressed that he would never want to live in a nursing home. He did not complete an advance directive (AD).

His family believes he "deserves a chance," so maximal treatment is provided and eventually he is extubated. His neurologic status does not significantly change, however. He does not speak and cannot eat or drink. It is remotely possible this could improve over time, but at this point he no longer requires hospital-level care. To be transferred to a nursing home, however, he would need a permanent feeding tube inserted.

His family is very concerned that this is not the manner of life he would have found acceptable, but they want to do what is right for him and above all prevent suffering. A palliative care consultation is requested.

There are two ways to administer enteral nutrition and hydration: via temporary means generally through the nose (i.e., an NG tube) or via more permanent means through a tube implanted either surgically or endoscopically through the abdominal wall into the stomach (or, less frequently, into the small intestine). An NG tube is commonly used in time-limited situations, such as in ICUs following major trauma or surgery, when a patient is expected to ultimately regain the ability to eat or drink. Though simple to insert, an NG tube also entails risks (related to becoming dislodged and leading to aspiration) as well as burden (as it can be quite uncomfortable).

Two ethical issues arise in the use of NG tubes. The first is whether an incapacitated patient's prior statements about MANH apply to them. Many AD forms include a section that allows a patient to refuse a "feeding tube," generally without specifying whether this is a short-term NG tube or a more permanent gastrostomy tube. (Some forms helpfully offer a third option of a "trial period" of a feeding tube, which likely refers to an NG tube.) Some consider a patient having checked that box to be a refusal of all MANH, including time-limited use of an NG tube such as following major surgery or trauma.

Here it is important to explore the *context* of the patient's prior refusal of MANH. Did the patient have any personal experience with an NG or gastrostomy tube that might have led him to make such a declaration? If not, what did he anticipate as the clinical situation where a feeding tube might be recommended? It is quite possible the patient may have envisioned a feeding tube in the context of a progressive and untreatable illness, such as dementia. If so, dependence on a feeding tube would coincide with a loss of what made live worth living for him (such as independence and the ability to partake in pleasurable activities). Refusal of MANH may, therefore, have appeared to be his only "exit ramp" from a life he did not want to continue living.

Such a refusal would certainly apply to a gastrostomy tube in preparation for permanent nursing home placement but not necessarily to temporary use of an NG tube. Once again, rather than going by the "letter" of the document, it is important to inquire as to the "spirit of the AD." This typically involves thoughtful conversations with the patient's family and friends, to determine what his overall goals were and the degree to which an NG tube either comports or conflicts with these. In short, then, the fact that the patient checked off that box on his AD is relevant information, but it is not determinative and requires greater exploration of the context the patient anticipated when he filled out the form.[4]

In addition to prior (apparent) refusal of an NG tube, the other ethical issue related to its use is contemporaneous expressions of refusal of either placement or maintaining of the tube. It is not uncommon for patients to pull at the tube or motion for it to be removed. This is not difficult to understand, given that inserting it usually elicits a gag reflex, and even once in place it represents a noxious stimulus to the patient's posterior

---

4. In this respect, the situation is analogous to a patient who checked off a box for "Do Not Intubate," never anticipating that mechanical ventilation might only be required for a short period of time (p. 73).

oropharynx. Some have, therefore, interpreted expressions of refusal as indications that the tube should be removed, out of respect for the patient's autonomy.

Once again, though, context is everything. To be sure, a patient with sufficient DMC has the right to refuse any form of treatment (including MANH). But while some patients who require an NG tube have sufficient DMC to decide whether to accept it, many are critically ill and their DMC is compromised by a combination of their illness and the medications (including analgesics and sedatives) that they are receiving. As such, they may be reacting to an unpleasant sensation without full appreciation that forgoing the tube will severely compromise—and perhaps prevent—their recovery. In that respect, this situation is analogous to that of an intubated patient motioning for the endotracheal tube to be removed (p. 123).

The appropriate response to expressions of refusal, therefore, is a thoughtful evaluation of the patient's current level of DMC, as well as a review of his prior statements related to MANH. Unless there is confidence that the patient truly would not want an NG tube even for a brief period, a trial of its use is justified. This not only offers the opportunity to see if the patient's condition improves but also keeps open the possibility of subsequently being able to engage the patient in conversation about his goals. Given the importance of adequate nutrition in the healing process—and the superiority of enteral nutrition over parenteral (Seres, Valcarcel, & Guillaume, 2013)—this can be seen as a temporizing measure, preserving options until the patient is (hopefully) able to make informed choices for himself.

At the same time, the practical implications of ongoing use of an NG tube must be acknowledged, especially outside the ICU context. It may represent the start of a cascade of other interventions, with increased risk of aspiration necessitating the use of pulse oximetry and restraints required to prevent the patient from dislodging the tube. This combination is sometimes referred to as "Weissman's Triad" (Weissman, 2013) and significantly restricts the patient's freedom and movement. As such, it should only be a very temporary intervention and one undertaken thoughtfully and not as an automatic response to any situation where a patient is unable to eat or drink.

When longer term nutrition is required—and especially prior to discharge from the hospital to skilled nursing facilities, which generally do not accept patients with NG tubes—a gastrostomy tube can be placed. This may at first appear to be a logical extension of the nasogastric tube. Technically, inserting it is not a complex procedure. After the initial healing process, it is much more comfortable than an NG tube and also firmly embedded and thus not as susceptible to accidental dislodging. Providing nutrition and hydration by such means may appear to be a low-burden intervention with undeniable benefit.

Proceeding with gastrostomy tube placement is an ethically complex step, however. Potential complications include infection, irritation, overhydration, diarrhea, and secondary aspiration (Taboada, Palma, & Shand, 2010). In addition, the benefit in terms of survival is not as obvious as it might originally seem, such as in cases of advanced dementia (p. 401) or critically ill hospitalized patients with cirrhosis and chronic obstructive pulmonary disease (Borum et al., 2000). And even if a patient will likely survive longer as a result of having a gastrostomy tube, for some "survival" is not the hoped-for benefit, as in cases where a patient's quality of life is so poor that any LSMT—including MANH—merely prolongs the burden of existence.

Another ethical complexity is that while an incapacitated patient who previously refused a feeding tube might be willing to accept a trial of NG feeds, this would not extend to a gastrostomy tube. Just as the shift from an endotracheal tube to a tracheostomy represents a logical division between short- and long-term treatment, so also does the shift from an NG to a gastrostomy tube. The shift in context is important, and thus additional exploration of the patient's goals, values, and expressed wishes is required before automatically "upgrading" from an NG to a gastrostomy tube.

The third reason why inserting a gastrostomy tube is ethically complex relates to ultimately discontinuing its use. Unlike an NG tube—which is perpetually uncomfortable, susceptible to dislodging, and often requires physical restraints to maintain—a longstanding gastrostomy tube provokes little direct suffering. The burden of such a tube comes from the complications of the treatment it makes possible (such as overhydration at the end of life) or simply the perpetuation of a life that the patient no longer wants to live. As such, one cannot simply justify its discontinuation by appealing to the discomfort and restrictions of its continuing use.

In addition, there may be legal complexity to withdrawing it.[5] As noted earlier (p. 185), the US Supreme Court has determined that patients have the right to refuse MANH, like any other medical treatment (*Cruzan v. Director, Missouri Department of Health*, 1991). But that same decision reaffirmed the right of states to require a higher level of evidence (which is "clear and convincing") before this is done: "Missouri may legitimately seek to safeguard the personal element of this choice through the imposition of heightened evidentiary requirements."[6] This is precisely the reason why some states' AD forms include a provision allowing the patient to authorize his agent to make decisions specifically related to MANH, thereby fulfilling the higher evidentiary standard (Vermont Ethics Network, 2016).

Discontinuing use of a gastrostomy tube may also appear to conflict with certain religious traditions. The Ethical and Religious Directives of the Roman Catholic Church, for instance, assert that "in principle, there is an obligation to provide patients with food and water, including medically assisted nutrition and hydration for those who cannot take food orally" (United States Conference of Catholic Bishops, 2009). This directive is

---

5. "Withdrawing" does not necessarily refer to removing the tube but rather simply no longer using it to administer nutrition and hydration.

6. This is precisely what happened for Nancy Cruzan: there was initially insufficient evidence of her wishes to meet the standard set by Missouri law, but as a result of the publicity related to her Supreme Court case, additional witnesses came forward. Their testimony ultimately fulfilled the original standard, leading to discontinuation of MANH.

not, however, as monolithic as it first appears, which should prompt further exploration of the context in which it was issued and the degree to which this applies to the clinical situation being considered (p. 73).

Thus, while perhaps initially appearing rather straightforward, enteral MANH is quite ethically complex. Rather than being the automatic response to a patient who cannot eat or drink, this step should be thoughtfully considered in light of the patient's goals and prognosis. Depending on the context, it may be appropriate to initiate NG feedings on a trial basis, in order to give the patient the chance to recover (or, at least, regain sufficient DMC in order to decide for himself). The family's understanding of the implications of *not* providing MANH should also be explored, in order to identify any misconceptions related to suffering or starvation.

If extended MANH is required to sustain life, a gastrostomy tube—although certainly less uncomfortable and restrictive than an NG tube—should not be the automatic response. Before proceeding with this step, the potential legal and religious implications of its insertion should be reviewed with the patient and family. The reason for proceeding to a gastrostomy tube should also be clarified: is it being done merely to facilitate transfer to a long-term care facility or because it reflects the goals of the patient? If the former, one should explore whether the patient would seek not only the gastrostomy tube but also the manner and quality of life that comes with it.

One should not assume that dependence on MANH necessarily means decreased cognition, awareness, or the possibility of an adequate quality of life. Patients with neuromuscular disease where cognition remains largely intact—such as amyotrophic lateral sclerosis—can live for long periods thanks to MANH (Silani, Kasarskis, & Yanagisawa, 1998). And for patients who espouse a *vitalistic* sense that any life is better than no life, MANH is effective in sustaining life even in the absence of awareness (Multi-Society Task Force on PVS, 1994).

In practice, the placement of a gastrostomy tube is often entirely open-ended, with the expectation that it will continue to be used indefinitely, over which time the focus on the patient's goals may be lost. However, it is much more appropriate to consider the tube as a "time-limited trial" (p. 118) in order to estimate the patient's overall quality of life and whether his goals are being achieved.

During all of these conversations, the team should avoid using terms with misleading and emotional connotations (such as "feeding tube") and frame decisions not only in terms of the modality being considered but more so in terms of the overall quality of life this will make possible for the patient, in light of his goals. The ramifications of discontinuing use of the gastrostomy tube—especially as they might relate to a patient or family's perception of suffering or even "starvation"—should be explored.

Throughout these discussions, it is important to recognize that not deciding to forgo a treatment is equivalent to deciding—if only by default—to continue it. While the relatively lower burdens of a gastrostomy tube (compared to a mechanical ventilator, for instance) diminish the time pressure to decide, over a longer period the burdens of continued treatment may accrue.

Return to the Case

The palliative care consultant begins by sitting down with the family and asking what they understand about the current situation. They convey a very accurate sense of the patient's current condition and prognosis. When asked about the decisions they are currently facing, they describe the issue of a "permanent feeding tube" as more of a requirement than a question.

"There's not much of a choice, is there?" his daughter says.

The palliative care consultant tries to reframe the discussion in light of the patient's goals and prognosis. Using less emotionally resonant language, she notes that a percutaneous endoscopic gastrostomy tube is less uncomfortable and more stable than a NG tube. But she goes on to note that the need for it reflects the patient's inability to eat and drink, as well as the need for ongoing care in a nursing home setting.

When the family states emphatically that he would not want that, the consultant raises the option of forgoing MANH.

"So we'd just sit by and watch him starve?" his family asks in disbelief.

The consultant acknowledges their concern but quickly goes on to describe what would happen if the NG tube were removed without proceeding to gastrostomy tube placement. She describes the burdens that would be avoided, including restraining his hands and the pain and complications of an invasive procedure. She reassures them that he would not suffer, explaining what happens over the course of dehydration. There are also complications associated with a gastrostomy tube, including increased secretions, diarrhea, and—most of all—a life he would not have wanted to live.

Over the course of several conversations, many questions are answered, and the family comes to consensus that the patient would have refused the gastrostomy tube (as they had come to call it) if he could speak for himself. The NG tube is removed, and the patient is discharged to home on hospice care, dying peacefully approximately one week later.

Parenteral
Case Study

A fifty-seven-year-old man is dying of metastatic colon cancer. Based on functional measures, his life expectancy is on the order of weeks to months. Through a combination of progressive disease and the effects of opioids on his bowel function, he is unable to tolerate enteral feeds. He previously received a brief course of total parenteral nutrition (TPN) after the initial tumor was discovered and subsequently resected, and he inquires about resuming TPN now, in light of his inability to eat and drink without severe nausea and vomiting.

The clinical team is wondering if he appreciates the gravity of his diagnosis and whether TPN makes sense in terms of his overall goals of care. A palliative care consultation is requested.

Enteral nutrition is superior in many ways to parenteral nutrition. The gastrointestinal tract is able to extract what it needs and maintain better homeostatic balance compared to an intravenous infusion of a solution that is estimated to meet the body's needs and requires regular monitoring and modification. TPN carries with it many complications, including increased risk of bloodstream infections (Kritchevsky et al., 2008), refeeding syndrome (Mehanna, Moledina, & Travis, 2008), hypoglycemia (Petrov & Zagainov, 2007), hepatic dysfunction (Grau et al., 2007), Wernicke's encephalopathy (Mattioli et al., 1988), and all of the complications normally associated with central venous catheters (Kornbau, Lee, Hughes, & Firstenberg, 2015). There are also significant financial costs incurred by having to monitor and modify the intravenous solution and then formulate it (Richards & Irving, 1996). Finally, there are emotional and personal costs borne by the patient and family related to administering the solution and caring for a patient at home with higher tech needs (Sayers, Lloyd, & Gabe, 2006), since nursing homes generally do not administer TPN.

Yet while enteral MANH is highly preferable, there are some situations when it is not clinically feasible. Examples include extreme mucosal irritation, blockage, or significant absence of the gastrointestinal tract (such as in the case of short bowel syndrome). In those cases, TPN provides the only method for providing life-sustaining nutrition and hydration.

The choice exists, of course, to forgo MANH entirely. In some ways, it is emotionally and culturally easier to forgo *parenteral* MANH, given that it lacks the resonance of "tube feedings." It is indisputably a medical intervention, and a highly burdensome one at that. Concerns may still exist regarding starvation and suffering, but the same clarifications noted previously in relationship to enteral MANH are even more applicable here. MANH is also ineffective in preventing some symptoms that may be of concern to patients and families, such as thirst (Musgrave, Bartal, & Opstad, 1995).

The pivotal questions with relation to TPN, therefore, are why the patient requires it and whether there is reason to be believe the patient at some point will no longer do so. Clearly, situations where enteral nutrition and hydration are temporarily impossible lend themselves to the use of TPN as a "bridge" to resumption of enteral feedings. These include patients whose gastrointestinal tract is temporarily compromised due to obstruction or inflammation, such as patients undergoing radiation therapy or with tumors that impede flow through the gut (Bozzetti et al., 2009). In such situations, TPN represents a life-saving measure until enteral feedings can be resumed (or, conversely, it becomes absolutely clear that they will never be resumed).

In other situations, though, TPN could be characterized as a "bridge to nowhere." When there is no reasonable expectation of restoring the patient's ability to tolerate enteral nutrition—such as extreme situations where a patient literally lacks sufficient intestinal mucosa to absorb vital nutrients—the patient will be permanently dependent on TPN for survival. As noted, the medical, practical, financial, and personal impacts of TPN are significant, especially over prolonged periods.

There may certainly be situations where TPN nevertheless makes sense. If a patient wants to survive long enough to have a specific experience—such as seeing a grandchild graduate from high school or attending a child's wedding—then TPN may be the only way to make this possible. In such situations, the rationale for implementing TPN (and the anticipated plan for cessation after the anticipated event) should be discussed in advance.

Absent such a discrete event the patient is literally "living for," implementing TPN without hope of restoration of enteral feeding creates the intensely difficult situation of requiring the patient to decide when to discontinue its use. Each day becomes a decision, albeit an implicit one. In this respect it is not intrinsically different from other ongoing LSMT, such as RRT. Here, again, instituting TPN as a TLT can help frame the expected benefits and burdens—the latter of which may be greater than expected—and provide clear waypoints for reevaluation of the treatment plan.

One context where TPN has specifically been shown to *not* be helpful—and thus not even merit a TLT—is at the end of life. Here the burdens clearly outweigh the benefits, as the requirement of an indwelling line, the need for frequent monitoring, and the simple matter of distracting from more profound priorities (in anticipation of death) represent significant drawbacks. Conversely, expected benefits are unlikely to result. At such a point—where the body's metabolic needs are lessening and long-term sustenance is not a consideration—parenteral nutrition provides no clear benefit.

Nor does parenteral hydration, which is easier to administer and logically would seem to prolong life (at least in terms of preventing dehydration). Excellent studies, however, have shown that parenteral hydration in the last week of life does not improve symptoms, quality of life, or survival (Bruera et al., 2013). In situations where a patient approaching the end of life is unable to eat or drink, it is preferable both from a medical and personal point of view to classify lack of thirst and appetite as normal symptoms of this phase of life, rather than medical problems that demand treatment. Instead of attempting to bypass them—thus incurring greater burden—it is generally wiser to accept them and focus on issues of greater meaning, such as optimizing comfort and attending to important relationships.

Return to the Case

The palliative care team's first response to the patient's inquiry is to validate it: it makes perfect sense to inquire about TPN, given that it was previously effective in a somewhat similar situation.

"Things are a bit different now, though," the team informs the patient.

Rather than TPN serving as a bridge to resumed enteral nutrition—as it was before—this time TPN would have to continue for the rest of the patient's life. As such, it is less of a bridge than a destination, and one that the patient may not be seeking.

Using this image as a jumping-off point, the team inquires as to what the patient's goals are in the time he has left. They are trying to determine whether his priority is to extend life—which at this point TPN could help achieve—or to maximize quality, in which case TPN could cause undue complications and prevent him from achieving some of his goals (such as returning home).

The patient notes that his daughter is expecting her third child in just over a month, and he would very much like to survive to meet his new grandson. After reviewing the risks and burdens associated with TPN, the team recommends instituting it on a time-limited basis, in order to help the patient achieve his goal.

A plan is formulated to revisit the appropriateness of treatment after the birth of his grandson. The team also notes that if the patient were to begin the active dying process before that time, TPN would no longer be prolonging his life and would only incur additional burden. He appreciates that and authorizes its discontinuation in that situation, which he hopes will not come to pass before the anticipated birth.

Summary Points

- Respiratory
  - Mechanical ventilation is a medical treatment that can be forgone—either withheld or withdrawn—like any other.
  - One ethically complex aspect of mechanical ventilation is the compassionate extubation of the alert patient, given concerns for unnecessary suffering. Preemptive analgesic dosing is imperative, and strong consideration should be given to sedation prior to extubation, particularly if there is high confidence that the patient will not be able to breathe independently.
  - Another ethically complex issue is the compassionate extubation of patients receiving paralytics. Generally this should wait until neuromuscular blockade has worn off but can be acceptable in exceptional cases where the patient is clearly unable to breathe independently, has minimal opportunity for meaningful interaction, and whose family would be burdened by additional waiting.

- Cardiac
  - Deactivating implantable cardiac defibrillators is not contentious, given the burden incurred and the lack of immediate effects of deactivation.
  - Some cardiologists are reluctant to deactivate pacemakers—especially in patients dependent on them—given the lack of obvious burden, as well as the temporal and physical proximity to the patient's death. A recent consensus statement affirms the ethicality of deactivation, and if a cardiologist is unwilling to do so, she should refer the patient to one who is willing. Potential deactivation should also be a part of ACP related to potential pacemaker insertion.
- Renal
  - RRT incurs significant burden and may not provide a survival benefit in certain populations.
  - Rather than being the default response to ESRD, RRT should be an option presented with full explanation of the risks and benefits, as part of the broader process of ACP. If instituted, it should be as a TLT to allow for thoughtful reevaluation after an appropriate period of time.
- Medically administered nutrition and hydration
  - MANH provokes strong emotional responses, due to the resonance of eating and drinking and concern for abandonment and "starvation" in their absence. It is important to clarify that forgoing MANH does not entail suffering and to avoid emotionally charged terms (like "feeding tube") by using accurate terminology (such as "gastrostomy tube").
  - An NG tube is burdensome and susceptible to complications but represents a potentially valuable temporary measure in situations where a patient cannot eat or drink. Previous refusals of a "feeding tube" may or may not be relevant to short-term NG placement.
  - Progressing from an NG tube to a permanent gastrostomy tube should not be a default action or one driven only by placement concerns (as nursing homes generally do not accept patients with NG tubes). Such a step should reflect a patient's goals, and patients and their surrogates should be aware of potentially added legal complexity in discontinuing use of a gastrostomy tube.
  - Parenteral MANH carries with it a greater degree of burden and complexity. It can be an invaluable "bridge" to resumed enteral nutrition, but in situations where this will never again be possible, parenteral MANH should be reserved for situations where it can sustain the patient to reach a discrete personal goal.
  - MANH of either type is nonbeneficial at the very end of life, and may entail significant burden.

References

Abdel-Kader, K., Unruh, M. L., & Weisbord, S. D. (2009). Symptom burden, depression, and quality of life in chronic and end-stage kidney disease. *Clin J Am Soc Nephrol*, 4(6), 1057–1064. doi:10.2215/CJN.00430109

Ahmad, M., Bloomstein, L., Roelke, M., Bernstein, A. D., & Parsonnet, V. (2000). Patients' attitudes toward implanted defibrillator shocks. *Pacing Clin Electrophysiol, 23*(6), 934–938.

Alexander, S. (1962). They decide who lives, who dies. *Life, 53*(19), 102–124.

AMA Council on Ethical and Judicial Affairs. (2007). Physician objection to treatment and individual patient discrimination: CEJA Report 6-A-07. Chicago: AMA Press.

American Medical Association. (2010–2011). *Code of medical ethics, annotated current opinions* (1076-3996). Chicago: American Medical Association.

Arroliga, A., Frutos-Vivar, F., Hall, J., Esteban, A., Apezteguia, C., Soto, L., . . . International Mechanical Ventilation Study Group. (2005). Use of sedatives and neuromuscular blockers in a cohort of patients receiving mechanical ventilation. *Chest, 128*(2), 496–506. doi:10.1378/chest.128.2.496

Asch, D. A., & Christakis, N. A. (1996). Why do physicians prefer to withdraw some forms of life support over others? Intrinsic attributes of life-sustaining treatments are associated with physicians' preferences. *Med Care, 34*(2), 103–111.

Berger, J. T. (2005). The ethics of deactivating implanted cardioverter defibrillators. *Ann Intern Med, 142*(8), 631–634.

Billings, J. A. (2011). Terminal extubation of the alert patient. *J Palliat Med, 14*(7), 800–801. doi:10.1089/jpm.2011.9676

Billings, J. A. (2012). Humane terminal extubation reconsidered: The role for preemptive analgesia and sedation. *Crit Care Med, 40*(2), 625–630. doi:10.1097/CCM.0b013e318228235d

Blank, R. H. (2011). End-of-life decision making across cultures. *J Law Med Ethics, 39*(2), 201–214. doi:10.1111/j.1748-720X.2011.00589.x

Bolt, E. E., Hagens, M., Willems, D., & Onwuteaka-Philipsen, B. D. (2015). Primary care patients hastening death by voluntarily stopping eating and drinking. *Ann Fam Med, 13*(5), 421–428. doi:10.1370/afm.1814

Borum, M. L., Lynn, J., Zhong, Z., Roth, K., Connors, A. F. Jr., Desbiens, N. A., . . . Dawson, N. V. (2000). The effect of nutritional supplementation on survival in seriously ill hospitalized adults: an evaluation of the SUPPORT data. Study to Understand Prognoses and Preferences for Outcomes and Risks of Treatments. *J Am Geriatr Soc, 48*(5 Suppl.), S33–S38.

Bozzetti, F., Arends, J., Lundholm, K., Micklewright, A., Zurcher, G., Muscaritoli, M., & ESPEN. (2009). ESPEN guidelines on parenteral nutrition: Non-surgical oncology. *Clin Nutr, 28*(4), 445–454. doi:10.1016/j.clnu.2009.04.011

Braun, T. C., Hagen, N. A., Hatfield, R. E., & Wyse, D. G. (1999). Cardiac pacemakers and implantable defibrillators in terminal care. *J Pain Symptom Manage, 18*(2), 126–131.

Brody, H., Campbell, M. L., Faber-Langendoen, K., & Ogle, K. S. (1997). Withdrawing intensive life-sustaining treatment—recommendations for compassionate clinical management. *N Engl J Med, 336*(9), 652–657. doi:10.1056/NEJM199702273360910

Bruera, E., Hui, D., Dalal, S., Torres-Vigil, I., Trumble, J., Roosth, J., . . . Tarleton, K. (2013). Parenteral hydration in patients with advanced cancer: A multicenter, double-blind, placebo-controlled randomized trial. *J Clin Oncol, 31*(1), 111–118. doi:10.1200/JCO.2012.44.6518

Butler, K. (2013). *Knocking on heaven's door: The path to a better way of death* (1st Scribner hardcover ed.). New York: Scribner.

Campbell, M. L., Templin, T., & Walch, J. (2009). Patients who are near death are frequently unable to self-report dyspnea. *J Palliat Med, 12*(10): 881–884. doi:10.1089/jpm.2009.0082

Carlson, R. W., Campbell, M. L., & Frank, R. R. (1996). Life support: The debate continues. *Chest, 109*(3), 852–853.

Carson, R. C., Juszczak, M., Davenport, A., & Burns, A. (2009). Is maximum conservative management an equivalent treatment option to dialysis for elderly patients with significant comorbid disease? *Clin J Am Soc Nephrol, 4*(10), 1611–1619. doi:10.2215/CJN.00510109

Chan, J. D., et al. (2004). Narcotic and benzodiazepine use after withdrawal of life support: association with time to death? *Chest, 126*(1): 286–293. doi:10.1378/chest.126.1.286.

Cohen, L. M., Ruthazer, R., Moss, A. H., & Germain, M. J. (2010). Predicting six-month mortality for patients who are on maintenance hemodialysis. *Clin J Am Soc Nephrol, 5*(1), 72–79. doi:10.2215/CJN.03860609

Combs, S. A., Culp, S., Matlock, D. D., Kutner, J. S., Holley, J. L., & Moss, A. H. (2015). Update on end-of-life care training during nephrology fellowship: A cross-sectional national survey of fellows. *Am J Kidney Dis, 65*(2), 233–239. doi:10.1053/j.ajkd.2014.07.018

Cruzan v. Director, Missouri Department of Health, 497 261 (S.Ct. 1990).

Da Silva-Gane, M., Wellsted, D., Greenshields, H., Norton, S., Chandna, S. M., & Farrington, K. (2012). Quality of life and survival in patients with advanced kidney failure managed conservatively or by dialysis. *Clin J Am Soc Nephrol*, 7(12), 2002–2009. doi:10.2215/CJN.01130112

Dalal, S., & Bruera, E. (2004). Dehydration in cancer patients: To treat or not to treat. *J Support Oncol*, 2(6), 467–479, 483.

Davison, S. N. (2010). End-of-life care preferences and needs: Perceptions of patients with chronic kidney disease. *Clin J Am Soc Nephrol*, 5(2), 195–204. doi:10.2215/CJN.05960809

Davison, S. N., Jhangri, G. S., Holley, J. L., & Moss, A. H. (2006). Nephrologists' reported preparedness for end-of-life decision-making. *Clin J Am Soc Nephrol*, 1(6), 1256–1262. doi:10.2215/CJN.02040606

Edwards, M. J., & Tolle, S. W. (1992). Disconnecting a ventilator at the request of a patient who knows he will then die: The doctor's anguish. *Ann Intern Med*, 117(3), 254–256.

Edwards, B. S., & Ueno, W. M. (1991). Sedation before ventilator withdrawal. *J Med Ethics*,2(2):118–122; discussion 122-30.

Faber-Langendoen, K. (1994). The clinical management of dying patients receiving mechanical ventilation: A survey of physician practice. *Chest*, 106(3), 880–888.

Faber-Langendoen, K. (1996). A multi-institutional study of care given to patients dying in hospitals: Ethical and practice implications. *Arch Intern Med*, 156(18), 2130–2136.

Ganzini, L., Goy, E. R., Miller, L. L., Harvath, T. A., Jackson, A., & Delorit, M. A. (2003). Nurses' experiences with hospice patients who refuse food and fluids to hasten death. *N Engl J Med*, 349(4), 359–365. doi:10.1056/NEJMsa035086

Ghoneim, M. M., et al. (2009). Awareness during anesthesia: risk factors, causes and sequelae: a review of reported cases in the literature. *Anesth Analg*,108(2): 527–535. doi:108/2/527 [pii]

Goldberger, Z., & Lampert, R. (2006). Implantable cardioverter-defibrillators: Expanding indications and technologies. *JAMA*, 295(7), 809–818. doi:10.1001/jama.295.7.809

Goldstein, N., Bradley, E., Zeidman, J., Mehta, D., & Morrison, R. S. (2009). Barriers to conversations about deactivation of implantable defibrillators in seriously ill patients: Results of a nationwide survey comparing cardiology specialists to primary care physicians. *J Am Coll Cardiol*, 54(4), 371–373. doi:10.1016/j.jacc.2009.04.030

Goldstein, N. E., Lampert, R., Bradley, E., Lynn, J., & Krumholz, H. M. (2004). Management of implantable cardioverter defibrillators in end-of-life care. *Ann Intern Med*, 141(11), 835–838.

Goldstein, N. E., Mehta, D., Siddiqui, S., Teitelbaum, E., Zeidman, J., Singson, M., . . . Morrison, R. S. (2008). "That's like an act of suicide": Patients' attitudes toward deactivation of implantable defibrillators. *J Gen Intern Med*, 23(Suppl. 1), 7–12. doi:10.1007/s11606-007-0239-8

Good, P., Richard, R., Syrmis, W., Jenkins-Marsh, S., & Stephens, J. (2014). Medically assisted nutrition for adult palliative care patients. *Cochrane Database Syst Rev*(4), CD006274. doi:10.1002/14651858.CD006274.pub3

Grau, T., Bonet, A., Rubio, M., Mateo, D., Farre, M., Acosta, J. A., . . . Metabolism of the Spanish Society of Critical Care. (2007). Liver dysfunction associated with artificial nutrition in critically ill patients. *Crit Care*, 11(1), R10. doi:10.1186/cc5670

Hall, R. I., &Rocker, G. M. (2000). End-of-life care in the ICU: Treatments provided when life support was or was not withdrawn. *Chest*,118(5):1424–1430.

Hammill, S. C., Kremers, M. S., Stevenson, L. W., Heidenreich, P. A., Lang, C. M., Curtis, J. P., . . . Brindis, R. G. (2010). Review of the registry's fourth year, incorporating lead data and pediatric ICD procedures, and use as a national performance measure. *Heart Rhythm*, 7(9), 1340–1345. doi:10.1016/j.hrthm.2010.07.015

Hemmelgarn, B. R., Manns, B. J., Quan, H., & Ghali, W. A. (2003). Adapting the Charlson Comorbidity Index for use in patients with ESRD. *Am J Kidney Dis*, 42(1), 125–132.

In re Quinlan, 70 10 (N.J. 1976).

Jacobs, I., Sunde, K., Deakin, C. D., Hazinski, M. F., Kerber, R. E., Koster, R. W., . . . Defibrillation Chapter Collaborators. (2010). Part 6: Defibrillation: 2010 International Consensus on Cardiopulmonary Resuscitation and Emergency Cardiovascular Care Science with Treatment Recommendations. *Circulation*, 122(16 Suppl. 2), S325–S337. doi:10.1161/CIRCULATIONAHA.110.971010

Janssen, D. J., Spruit, M. A., Schols, J. M., van der Sande, F. M., Frenken, L. A., & Wouters, E. F. (2013). Insight into advance care planning for patients on dialysis. *J Pain Symptom Manage, 45*(1), 104–113. doi:10.1016/j.jpainsymman.2012.01.010

Johansen, K. L., Chertow, G. M., Jin, C., & Kutner, N. G. (2007). Significance of frailty among dialysis patients. *J Am Soc Nephrol, 18*(11), 2960–2967.

Keizer, G. (2004). *Help : The original human dilemma* (1st ed.). San Francisco: HarperSanFrancisco.

Kimmel, P. L., Peterson, R. A., Weihs, K. L., Simmens, S. J., Alleyne, S., Cruz, I., & Veis, J. H. (2000). Multiple measurements of depression predict mortality in a longitudinal study of chronic hemodialysis outpatients. *Kidney Int, 57*(5), 2093–2098. doi:10.1046/j.1523-1755.2000.00059.x

Kornbau, C., Lee, K. C., Hughes, G. D., & Firstenberg, M. S. (2015). Central line complications. *Int J Crit Illn Inj Sci, 5*(3), 170–178. doi:10.4103/2229-5151.164940

Kritchevsky, S. B., Braun, B. I., Kusek, L., Wong, E. S., Solomon, S. L., Parry, M. F., . . . Indicators in Infection Control Study Group. (2008). The impact of hospital practice on central venous catheter associated bloodstream infection rates at the patient and unit level: A multicenter study. *Am J Med Qual, 23*(1), 24–38. doi:10.1177/1062860607310918

Kurella, M., Covinsky, K. E., Collins, A. J., & Chertow, G. M. (2007). Octogenarians and nonagenarians starting dialysis in the United States. *Ann Intern Med, 146*(3), 177–183.

Lampert, R., Hayes, D. L., Annas, G. J., Farley, M. A., Goldstein, N. E., Hamilton, R. M., . . . Palliative Nurses Association. (2010). HRS Expert Consensus Statement on the Management of Cardiovascular Implantable Electronic Devices (CIEDs) in patients nearing end of life or requesting withdrawal of therapy. *Heart Rhythm, 7*(7), 1008–1026. doi:10.1016/j.hrthm.2010.04.033

Larcher, V., et al. (2015). Making decisions to limit treatment in life-limiting and life-threatening conditions in children: a framework for practice. *Arch Dis Child, 100*(Suppl 2): s3–23. doi:10.1136/archdischild-2014-306666.

Lewis, W. R., Luebke, D. L., Johnson, N. J., Harrington, M. D., Costantini, O., & Aulisio, M. P. (2006). Withdrawing implantable defibrillator shock therapy in terminally ill patients. *Am J Med, 119*(10), 892–896. doi:10.1016/j.amjmed.2006.01.017

Loper, K. A., Butler, S., Nessly, M., & Wild, L. (1989). Paralyzed with pain: The need for education. *Pain, 37*(3), 315–316.

Martins Pereira, S., Pasman, H. R., van der Heide, A., van Delden, J. J., & Onwuteaka-Philipsen, B. D. (2015). Old age and forgoing treatment: A nationwide mortality follow-back study in the Netherlands. *J Med Ethics, 41*(9), 766–770. doi:10.1136/medethics-2014-102367

Masino, S. A., & Ruskin, D. N. (2013). Ketogenic diets and pain. *J Child Neurol, 28*(8), 993–1001. doi:10.1177/0883073813487595

Mattioli, S., Miglioli, M., Montagna, P., Lerro, M. F., Pilotti, V., & Gozzetti, G. (1988). Wernicke's encephalopathy during total parenteral nutrition: Observation in one case. *JPEN J Parenter Enteral Nutr, 12*(6), 626–627. doi:10.1177/0148607188012006626

Mehanna, H. M., Moledina, J., & Travis, J. (2008). Refeeding syndrome: What it is, and how to prevent and treat it. *BMJ, 336*(7659), 1495–1498. doi:10.1136/bmj.a301

Merriman, H. M. (1981). The techniques used to sedate ventilated patients: A survey of methods used in 34 ICUs in Great Britain. *Intensive Care Med, 7*(5), 217–224.

Monti, M. M., et al. (2010). Willful modulation of brain activity in disorders of consciousness. *N Engl J Med, 362*(7): 579–589. doi:NEJMoa0905370 [pii]

Moss, A. H. (1995). To use dialysis appropriately: The emerging consensus on patient selection guidelines. *Adv Ren Replace Ther, 2*(2), 175–183.

Moss, A. H., Ganjoo, J., Sharma, S., Gansor, J., Senft, S., Weaner, B., . . . Schmidt, R. (2008). Utility of the "surprise" question to identify dialysis patients with high mortality. *Clin J Am Soc Nephrol, 3*(5), 1379–1384. doi:10.2215/CJN.00940208

Mueller, P. S., Hook, C. C., & Hayes, D. L. (2003). Ethical analysis of withdrawal of pacemaker or implantable cardioverter-defibrillator support at the end of life. *Mayo Clin Proc, 78*(8), 959–963. doi:10.4065/78.8.959

Mueller, P. S., Jenkins, S. M., Bramstedt, K. A., & Hayes, D. L. (2008). Deactivating implanted cardiac devices in terminally ill patients: Practices and attitudes. *Pacing Clin Electrophysiol, 31*(5), 560–568. doi:10.1111/j.1540-8159.2008.01041.x

Multi-Society Task Force on PVS. (1994). Medical aspects of the persistent vegetative state (2). *N Engl J Med, 330*(22), 1572–1579. doi:10.1056/NEJM199406023302206

Murtagh F., Cohen L.M., & Germain M.J. (2007). Dialysis discontinuation: quo vadis? *Adv Chronic Kidney Dis 14*(4), 379–401.

Murtagh, F. E., Marsh, J. E., Donohoe, P., Ekbal, N. J., Sheerin, N. S., & Harris, F. E. (2007). Dialysis or not? A comparative survival study of patients over 75 years with chronic kidney disease stage 5. *Nephrol Dial Transplant, 22*(7), 1955–1962. doi:10.1093/ndt/gfm153

Musgrave, C. F., Bartal, N., & Opstad, J. (1995). The sensation of thirst in dying patients receiving IV hydration. *J Palliat Care, 11*(4), 17–21.

Natural Death Act, 7, California Health and Safety Code § 7185-95, 1 Stat. (1976).

O'Connor, N. R., & Corcoran, A. M. (2012). End-stage renal disease: Symptom management and advance care planning. *Am Fam Physician, 85*(7), 705–710.

O'Hare, A. M., Szarka, J., McFarland, L. V., Taylor, J. S., Sudore, R. L., Trivedi, R., . . . Vig, E. K. (2016). Provider perspectives on advance care planning for patients with kidney disease: Whose job is it anyway? *Clin J Am Soc Nephrol, 11*(5), 855–866. doi:10.2215/CJN.11351015

Paola, F. A., & Walker, R. M. (2000). Deactivating the implantable cardioverter-defibrillator: A biofixture analysis. *South Med J, 93*(1), 20–23.

Partridge, B. L., Abrams, J. H., Bazemore, C., & Rubin, R. (1990). Prolonged neuromuscular blockade after long-term infusion of vecuronium bromide in the intensive care unit. *Crit Care Med, 18*(10), 1177–1179.

Perkin R. M., & Resnik D.B. (2002). The agony of agonal respiration: is the last gasp necessary? *J Med Ethics, 28*(3), 164–169.

Petrov, M. S., & Zagainov, V. E. (2007). Influence of enteral versus parenteral nutrition on blood glucose control in acute pancreatitis: A systematic review. *Clin Nutr, 26*(5), 514–523. doi:10.1016/j.clnu.2007.04.009

Prendergast, T. J., &Luce, J. M (1997). Increasing incidence of withholding and withdrawal of life support from the critically ill. *Am J Respir Crit Care Med, 155*(1):15–20. doi:10.1164/ajrccm.155.1.9001282

Quill, T. E., & Abernethy, A. P. (2013). Generalist plus specialist palliative care—creating a more sustainable model. *N Engl J Med, 368*(13), 1173–1175. doi:10.1056/NEJMp1215620

Renal Physicians Association Clinical Practice Guideline. (2010). Shared Decision-Making in the Appropriate Initiation of and Withdrawal from Dialysis, 2nd ed.

Rhymes, J. A., McCullough, L. B., Luchi, R. J., Teasdale, T. A., & Wilson, N. (2000). Withdrawing very low-burden interventions in chronically ill patients. *JAMA, 283*(8), 1061–1063.

Richards, D. M., & Irving, M. H. (1996). Cost-utility analysis of home parenteral nutrition. *Br J Surg, 83*(9), 1226–1229.

Rushton, C. H., & Terry, P. B. (1995). Neuromuscular blockade and ventilator withdrawal: Ethical controversies. *Am J Crit Care, 4*(2), 112–115.

Sayers, G. M., Lloyd, D. A., & Gabe, S. M. (2006). Parenteral nutrition: Ethical and legal considerations. *Postgrad Med J, 82*(964), 79–83. doi:10.1136/pgmj.2005.037127

Schell, J. O., Green, J. A., Tulsky, J. A., & Arnold, R. M. (2013). Communication skills training for dialysis decision-making and end-of-life care in nephrology. *Clin J Am Soc Nephrol, 8*(4), 675–680. doi:10.2215/CJN.05220512

Schmidt, R. J., & Moss, A. H. (2014). Dying on dialysis: The case for a dignified withdrawal. *Clin J Am Soc Nephrol, 9*(1), 174–180. doi:10.2215/CJN.05730513

Schneiderman, L. J. (1991). Is it morally justifiable not to sedate this patient before ventilator withdrawal? *Journal of Clinical Ethics, 2*, 129–130.

Schneiderman, L. J., & Spragg, R. G. (1988). Ethical decisions in discontinuing mechanical ventilation. *N Engl J Med, 318*(15), 984–988. doi:10.1056/NEJM198804143181509

Schron, E. B., Exner, D. V., Yao, Q., Jenkins, L. S., Steinberg, J. S., Cook, J. R., . . . Powell, J. (2002). Quality of life in the antiarrhythmics versus implantable defibrillators trial: Impact of therapy and influence of adverse symptoms and defibrillator shocks. *Circulation, 105*(5), 589–594.

Segredo, V., Caldwell, J. E., Matthay, M. A., Sharma, M. L., Gruenke, L. D., & Miller, R. D. (1992). Persistent paralysis in critically ill patients after long-term administration of vecuronium. *N Engl J Med, 327*(8), 524–528. doi:10.1056/NEJM199208203270804

Seres, D. S., Valcarcel, M., & Guillaume, A. (2013). Advantages of enteral nutrition over parenteral nutrition. *Therap Adv Gastroenterol, 6*(2), 157–167. doi:10.1177/1756283X12467564

Silani, V., Kasarskis, E. J., & Yanagisawa, N. (1998). Nutritional management in amyotrophic lateral sclerosis: A worldwide perspective. *J Neurol*, *245*(Suppl. 2), S13–S19; discussion S29.

Singer, P. A., Thiel, E. C., Naylor, C. D., Richardson, R. M., Llewellyn-Thomas, H., Goldstein, M., . . . Mendelssohn, D. C. (1995). Life-sustaining treatment preferences of hemodialysis patients: Implications for advance directives. *J Am Soc Nephrol*, *6*(5), 1410–1417.

Smedira, N. G., et al. (1990). Withholding and withdrawal of life support from the critically ill. *N. Engl. J. Med*,*322*(5): 309–315. doi:10.1056/NEJM199002013220506.

Sottile, F. D. (1995). Managing dying patients and paralytic agents. *Chest*, *108*(3), 887.

Stewart, T. E., Meade, M. O., Cook, D. J., Granton, J. T., Hodder, R. V., Lapinsky, S. E., . . . Slutsky, A. S. (1998). Evaluation of a ventilation strategy to prevent barotrauma in patients at high risk for acute respiratory distress syndrome. Pressure- and Volume-Limited Ventilation Strategy Group. *N Engl J Med*, *338*(6), 355–361. doi:10.1056/NEJM199802053380603

Sulmasy, D. P. (2008). Within you/without you: Biotechnology, ontology, and ethics. *J Gen Intern Med*, *23*(Suppl. 1), 69–72. doi:10.1007/s11606-007-0326-x

Taboada, P., Palma, A., & Shand, B. (2010). Ethics and medically assisted nutrition and hydration. In E. Del Fabbro (Ed.), *Nutrition and the cancer patient* (pp. xiv, 295–318). Oxford; New York: Oxford University Press.

Tangri, N., Grams, M. E., Levey, A. S., Coresh, J., Appel, L. J., Astor, B. C., . . . CKD Prognosis Consortium. (2016). Multinational assessment of accuracy of equations for predicting risk of kidney failure: A meta-analysis. *JAMA*, *315*(2), 164–174. doi:10.1001/jama.2015.18202

Truog, R. D., Arnold, J. H., & Rockoff, M. A. (1991). Sedation before ventilator withdrawal: Medical and ethical considerations. *J Clin Eth*, *2*(2), 127–129.

Truog, R. D., Burns, J. P., Mitchell, C., Johnson, J., & Robinson, W. (2000). Pharmacologic paralysis and withdrawal of mechanical ventilation at the end of life. *N Engl J Med*, *342*(7), 508–511. doi:10.1056/NEJM200002173420712

Truog, R. D., Cist, A. F., Brackett, S. E., Burns, J. P., Curley, M. A., Danis, M., . . . Hurford, W. E. (2001). Recommendations for end-of-life care in the intensive care unit: The Ethics Committee of the Society of Critical Care Medicine. *Crit Care Med*, *29*(12), 2332–2348.

United States Conference of Catholic Bishops. (2009). *Ethical and religious directives for Catholic health care services* (5th ed.). Washington, DC: USCCB Publications.

Verberne, W. R., Geers, A. B., Jellema, W. T., Vincent, H. H., van Delden, J. J., & Bos, W. J. (2016). Comparative survival among older adults with advanced kidney disease managed conservatively versus with dialysis. *Clin J Am Soc Nephrol*, *11*(4), 633–640. doi:10.2215/CJN.07510715

Vermont Ethics Network. (2016). Advance directive, short form. Retrieved from http://www.vtethicsnetwork.org/forms/advance_directive_short_form.pdf

Wachterman, M. W., Marcantonio, E. R., Davis, R. B., Cohen, R. A., Waikar, S. S., Phillips, R. S., & McCarthy, E. P. (2013). Relationship between the prognostic expectations of seriously ill patients undergoing hemodialysis and their nephrologists. *JAMA Intern Med*, *173*(13), 1206–1214. doi:10.1001/jamainternmed.2013.6036

Warr, J., Thiboutot, Z., Rose, L., Mehta, S., & Burry, L. D. (2011). Current therapeutic uses, pharmacology, and clinical considerations of neuromuscular blocking agents for critically ill adults. *Ann Pharmacother*, *45*(9), 1116–1126. doi:10.1345/aph.1Q004

Wee, B. L., Coleman, P. G., Hillier, R., & Holgate, S. H. (2006). The sound of death rattle I: Are relatives distressed by hearing this sound? *Palliat Med*, *20*(3), 171–175. doi:10.1191/0269216306pm1137oa

Weissman, D. (2013). Swallow studies, tube feeding and the death spiral. Retrieved from http://www.mcw.edu/FileLibrary/User/jrehm/fastfactpdfs/Concept084.pdf

Zellner, R. A., Aulisio, M. P., & Lewis, W. R. (2009). Should implantable cardioverter-defibrillators and permanent pacemakers in patients with terminal illness be deactivated? Deactivating permanent pacemaker in patients with terminal illness: Patient autonomy is paramount. *Circ Arrhythm Electrophysiol*, *2*(3), 340–344; discussion 340. doi:10.1161/CIRCEP.109.848523

7

Pain and Symptom Management at the End of Life

Death is an inevitable aspect of the human condition. Dying badly is not.
(JENNINGS, RYNDSE, D'ONOFRIO, & BAILY, 2003)

Case Study

A seventy-year-old woman has advanced cancer including bone metastases. Despite intensive treatment with opioids at home—including a fentanyl patch and appropriate breakthrough dosing of oxycodone—her pain becomes intolerable, and she is admitted to the hospital for pain management and end-of-life care. Her opioids are titrated upward and adjuvant analgesics added, achieving slightly improved pain control. However, her respiratory status worsens. Her physicians are concerned that if they increase her opioid dosing further, she may experience respiratory failure. But if they do not increase her opioid dose, her suffering will continue. They request an ethics consultation to provide additional guidance.

Historicolegal Background

For most of the history of Western medicine, there was little attention paid to the treatment of symptoms at the end of life. There were very few ways of keeping patients alive, and thus death tended to be more precipitous, especially compared to the often drawn-out dying processes of today (p. 13). While attention to the spiritual aspects of death was quite sophisticated—and, in many cases, strictly prescribed—management of physical symptoms lagged far behind.

This is not because no treatments were available, as the pharmacologic effects of the poppy plant have been known since Neolithic times (Booth, 1998). It is unclear, however, whether Hippocrates appreciated its analgesic—as opposed to the sedative and hypnotic—effects (Prioreschi, Heaney, & Brehm, 1998). These certainly came to be recognized by the time of the Roman Empire (Tallmadge, 1946) but subsequently fell out of practice after the Empire's fall. While Muslim physicians explored the analgesic use of opioids from the ninth century onward (Al-Mazroa & Abdel Halim, 1989), in the West they were only rediscovered at the beginning of the sixteenth century by Paracelsus, who stated that "among medicines offered by Almighty God to relieve human suffering none is so universal and effective as opium" (Baraka, 2000).

Sydenham's laudanum was among the most common opium-containing compounds in Great Britain and the Americas in the ensuing centuries (Hamilton & Baskett, 2000), with the nineteenth century seeing deeper understanding of the mechanism of its analgesic effects (Haller, 1989) as well as the first formulation of morphine by Sertürner (Macht, Herman, & Levy, 1915). Parenteral administration followed soon thereafter (Howard-Jones, 1947), and morphine was used to treat battlefield injuries both in the American Civil War as well as other conflicts (Howard-Jones, 1947).

The risks of opioid abuse soon became apparent, however, with opium overdose representing a frequent cause of death in the West (Booth, 1998), and the Chinese opium wars occurring in the East. For this reason, many felt that opioids were too addictive to be of widespread utility, especially in end-of-life (EOL) care.

This view remained prevalent in the West through the end of World War II when a new approach formed, led by John Bonica (1953) based on his experience treating soldiers in pain and his own personal experience with chronic pain as a professional wrestler. The profound impact of pain on one's quality of life was increasingly recognized, as Albert Schweitzer (1948) famously put it: "Pain is a more terrible lord of mankind than even death himself."

Recognizing the obligation to help patients who "scream in pain and suffer in silence" (Reich 1989), the role of opioids came to be reconsidered, especially in EOL care. Cicely Saunders (1963) took the lead in this area, and when her groundbreaking paper on the subject was published, everything changed. There was now empiric evidence that intense pain and dyspnea at the end of life could be treated effectively and safely, and upward titration proved beneficial in managing refractory pain.

However, there remained a concern that opioids might not only provide comfort as death approached but could also hasten the timing of death. In cases of extreme pain requiring administration of high doses of opioids, the well-known side effect of respiratory depression could cause a patient to stop breathing. This is especially true when benzodiazepines—another staple of EOL care, used to treat anxiety—are simultaneously administered, given their synergistic depressive effect on respiratory drive. As the AMA's

Council on Ethical and Judicial Affairs (1992) notes, "the level of analgesia necessary to relieve the patient's pain . . . may also have the effect of shortening the patient's life."

In order to avoid any possibility of hastening death, some physicians were extremely cautious in treating patients with opioids, either choosing a very low dose, giving it at unnecessarily long intervals, or titrating up too slowly. Such *opiophobia*—referring to an irrational fear of treating with opioids (Bennett & Carr, 2002)—can be prompted not only by clinical concerns for respiratory depression but also by medicolegal concerns if the treatment were felt to represent euthanasia. Some commentators took these concerns so far as to recommend *against* intensive pain treatment: "Just as a physician must learn that lack of a cure does not equate with failure, a nurse must learn that the presence of pain [in the dying patient] does not mean failure" (Pohlman, 1990).

The impact of opiophobia on patient care can hardly be overstated. The SUPPORT study—in addition to noting the degree to which patients' wishes were either unrecognized or, if recognized, were not heeded—clearly documented the amount of needless suffering that was occurring for lack of adequate analgesia (p. 10). Half of the conscious patients in the study experienced moderate to severe pain in the last three days of their lives (Desbiens & Wu, 2000), largely for wont of effective opioid management.

This led to increased attention to pain, including the classification of pain as the "fifth vital sign" (Davis & Walsh, 2004). Physicians and nurses were expected to inquire about the patient's pain level, document the answer, and respond appropriately. The World Health Organization (2017) devised an analgesic ladder, with the second and third steps composed primarily of opioid medications. The American Board of Anesthesiology recognized "pain medicine" as a certificate of added qualifications in 1991, followed a decade later by subspecialty certification by the American Boards of Psychiatry and Neurology and of Physical Medicine and Rehabilitation (Cope, 2010). During this period a wide variety of new opioids—administered through different routes and with varying durations of action—were developed.

Recently, however, the pendulum has begun to swing back in the other direction, but not because of the use of opioids in EOL care. Rather, the concern relates to the opioid "epidemic" in the United States. Despite representing only 5% of the world's population, the United States consumes 80% of the world's opioids (Express Scripts, 2014). To some degree, this has been attributed to the emphasis on lowering the patient's self-reported pain rating, rather than focusing on functional measures and admitting that not all pain can be reduced to "zero," at least by opioids alone (Younger, McCue, & Mackey, 2009).

A variety of steps have been taken to address the opioid epidemic. Drug manufacturers can be required to implement a risk evaluation and mitigation strategy to ensure that the benefits of a medication outweigh its risks (Food and Drug Administration [FDA], 2017). Prescription drug monitoring programs help ensure that prescriptions are not falsified and also identify patients who may be receiving opioids from multiple providers or pharmacies (Islam & McRae, 2014). "Daily milligram limits" on opioid use—generally approximately 90 milligrams of oral morphine equivalents—have been established, with greater scrutiny of higher dosing (Dowell, Haegerich, & Chou, 2016).

These are all prudent steps in response to a serious health crisis, but they can also have unintended negative consequences on the practice of palliative care. A blanket indictment of opioid prescribing falsely equates the use of opioids for chronic pain—where they may not be indicated and for which they carry significant long-term side effects (Dowell et al., 2016)—and for EOL care. To a large degree, the opioid epidemic was fueled by the failure to make this very distinction, extrapolating from the well-documented benefits of opioids in EOL care to their widespread and injudicious use in other contexts. The response to the epidemic threatens to make the same error only in the reverse direction, projecting the well-documented risks of long-term opioid use and frequent prescribing in chronic, nonmalignant contexts onto EOL care. For instance, a daily milligram limit on opioid use might make sense for chronic pain—and helpfully redirect the attention to non-opioid (and especially nonpharmacologic) pain management—but such a limit can represent a barrier to appropriate upward titration of opioids at the end of life.

The stakes in this debate could not be higher, ranging from addiction and even death in the context of opioid overuse, to unnecessary and extreme suffering at the end of life for underuse. It is crucial, therefore, to develop strategies which effectively address the former while not unintentionally turning back the clock to the days when pain at the end of life was inadequately treated.

Clinical

Palliative care is often associated with pain management, and this is certainly a common reason for palliative care consultation. However, there are many physical symptoms beyond pain that require treatment in patients receiving palliative care, including fatigue, weakness, loss of appetite, and loss of energy (Teunissen et al. 2007). Sometimes treatments for either the underlying disease (e.g., chemotherapy) or for the physical symptoms related to the disease (e.g., opioids for pain) can cause additional or worsened symptoms, such as nausea or pruritis. The reason for focusing on management of pain here is the potentially lethal side effect of respiratory depression due to opioids.

Pain is multifaceted, not limited to physical suffering. Patients may also experience other types of pain, including social (isolation), spiritual (wondering why this has befallen them), and psychological (demoralization and depression). These phenomena are not mutually exclusive (Cherny, Coyle, & Foley, 1994): intense physical pain can lead to isolation and metaphysical questioning, and by the same token depressed mood can heighten the perception of physical pain (Saunders, 1984). Saunders (1964) thus coined the term "total pain," which is an accurate description of what many patients with life-threatening illness may endure.

This underscores the significance of recognizing the type of pain(s) that one is treating, because opioid analgesics are effective in some cases but not others. Spiritual pain calls for spiritual care and emotional pain for psychological support (and perhaps antidepressant or anti-anxiety treatment). Some have gone so far as to argue that certain aspects of suffering fall outside the physician's purview altogether. For instance, Ahmedzai (1997) writes, "Ultimately, suffering from losses, lack of love, existential doubts as well as from poverty and cruelty are not medical issues, and the response to them is not necessarily the responsibility of any healthcare discipline." A similar point is made by critics of using palliative sedation to treat existential distress (p. 265).

This seems, though, to overlook the transdisciplinary and comprehensive nature of palliative care in addressing suffering in all its forms. To be sure, opioids (or any pharmacologic modality) are not the "cure" for pain of every stripe, but the palliative care team's role extends far beyond the prescription pad. To say that certain forms of individual suffering—acknowledging that societal ills such as poverty are broader questions—are not the "responsibility of any health care discipline" overlooks the uniqueness of palliative care, which intentionally takes up that broader mantle. To be sure, not all suffering can be "solved," and those forms that can be may well lie outside the sphere of the palliative care team. In its most fundamental form, "Suffering is not a question that demands an answer; it is not a problem that demands a solution; it is a mystery which demands a presence" (Wyatt, 2009). But that does not mean that suffering of every form should not be taken seriously and attempts made to address (if not eradicate) it.

In terms of physical suffering, opioids are commonly used not only for pain but also for dyspnea, and initially in small doses. These are usually increased over time, both in response to disease progression but also because of the development of *tolerance*. This refers to the physiologic need for higher doses to achieve the same effect, as the body adapts to the current dose of opioid medication. The need for increasing doses, therefore, does not necessarily reflect either disease progression or "addiction" but may simply be the body becoming accustomed to the current dose and requiring an increase to achieve the same effect.

Ongoing use of opioids also leads to *physiologic dependence*, defined as having a negative reaction if the medication were to be discontinued (i.e., *withdrawal*). This is distinct from *addiction*—what some have described as "psychological dependence"—which "is characterized by inability to consistently abstain, impairment in behavioral control, craving, diminished recognition of significant problems with one's behaviors and interpersonal relationships, and a dysfunctional emotional response" (American Society of Addiction Medicine, 2011).

The distinction between physical and psychological dependence is crucial, because sometimes undertreated pain can prompt behavior which resembles that caused by addiction. Such *pseudoaddiction* is characterized by reports of continued pain despite currently receiving treatment, emphatic demands for higher doses of opioids, and querying multiple physicians (so-called "doctor shopping") when initial responses are insufficient to control the pain (Weissman & Haddox, 1989). In such cases, a physician must determine whether the patient's pain is, indeed, being undertreated, for the proper response to pseudoaddiction is an optimized analgesic regimen. The proper response to true addiction is, of course, extremely different.

Another unique aspect of opioids is that there is no "correct dose." For most medications, there is a standard dose, often determined by the patient's weight or body surface area, with modifications made for impaired organ function. Sometimes there are multiple tiers of dosing, as in the case of high-dose steroids. But for the most part, if a medication does not have the desired effect at the recommended dose, it is considered a treatment failure, and another medication (or form of treatment) is tried.

Opioids for pain or dyspnea are an exception to this rule, for the "correct dose" is the one that controls the patient's symptoms. While the basic rule is to "start slow and go slow" in titrating upward—given side effects such as sedation and respiratory depression—rapid titration is often necessary to relieve severe symptoms. The doses that are reached can be stunningly high, especially if the patient has developed tolerance over time. Standard teaching is to increase the dose by as much as 50% for moderate unrelieved pain and 75% or more for severe unrelieved pain (Schneider, Yale, & Larson, 2003). This highlights the problem with a daily milligram limit, because judicious upward titration over time—especially in the face of advancing disease—can exceed that by an order of magnitude or more.

While most of this chapter focuses on pain, other symptoms present similar clinical and ethical challenges. In particular, management of dyspnea can be quite challenging. Many of the principles identified in relation to pain management also apply to dyspnea, for opioids are a mainstay of the treatment for both. Appropriate upward dose titration to manage symptoms—in light of the risk of respiratory depression—as well as the challenge of distinguishing suffering from either pure dyspnea or pain require clinical expertise as well as ethical nuance and insight.

Ethical

While simultaneously acknowledging the physiologic efficacy of opioids in treating pain and dyspnea, significant concerns have been expressed regarding potentially hastened death from the side effect of respiratory depression. Some have gone so far as to refer to high-dose opioid administration at the end of life as "indirect euthanasia" (Huang & Emanuel, 1995; Smith, Orlowski, Radey, & Scofield, 1992) or "accidental euthanasia" (Lundberg, 1988).

So what is the medical team to do, when clinical guidelines recommend upward titration of opioids which could compromise the patient's respiratory drive and hasten her death? One potential response, of course, is to risk undertreating pain, as the SUPPORT study revealed (p. 10) (SUPPORT Principal Investigators, 1995). Opiophobia is common: nearly half of physicians and nurses in another study acknowledged the prevalence of opiophobia by agreeing that "clinicians give inadequate pain medication most often out of fear of hastening a patient's death" (Solomon et al., 1993). The end result is unnecessary—and often extreme—patient suffering, leading Grond, Zech, Schug, Lynch, and Lehmann (1991) to conclude that "most doctors are much more aware of the side effects of opioids . . . than of the side effects of pain." Such physicians are not unsympathetic to the plight of patients, but likely are concerned about violating professional (not to mention legal) obligations to the degree that it influences their clinical practice.

To ensure optimal pain management of patients, then, physicians need to be reassured that it is not unethical to treat pain at the end of life aggressively with opioids that may risk hastening death. Quite the contrary, it is an ethical obligation to do so, and here the Rule of Double Effect (RDE) can provide valuable guidance.

Rule of Double Effect

First formulated by Thomas Aquinas (2012) in relationship to killing in self-defense, the RDE is used to determine whether an action that has two effects—one good and one bad—is morally permissible. The RDE has four basic components:

1. The act itself must be, at worst, morally neutral.
2. The bad effect cannot be the means to the good effect.
3. The good effect must outweigh the bad effect (principle of proportionality).
4. The agent must only intend the good effect, although the bad effect may be foreseen (Garcia, 1994).

In a medical context, the RDE has been applied to several situations. Since it grew out of Roman Catholic theology, historically one application has been to delineate contexts where ending a pregnancy is morally acceptable. The standard "termination to save the life of the mother" would not fulfill all four requirements, since the "bad effect" (in this case, terminating the fetus) is the means to the good effect (in this case, improved health of the formerly pregnant woman). Performing a hysterectomy on a pregnant woman with uterine cancer, however, would fulfill the requirements, since the intention is to treat cancer and the end of the pregnancy is an anticipated—but not intended—side effect of hysterectomy (Shaw, 2002).

The most common modern medical application of the RDE pertains to the use of opioids at the end of life, given the potential side effect of depressing respiratory drive (AMA Council on Ethical and Judicial Affairs, 1992; Foley, 1997; Pellegrino, 1992; President's Commission for the Study of Ethical Problems in Medicine and Biomedical and Behavioral Research, 1983; The Hastings Center, 1987). If analgesia is the good effect and hastened death is the bad effect, the RDE is applied to opioid administration in the following way:

1. The act of administering an FDA-approved medication for a condition it is indicated for is not morally bad.
2. Pain is not relieved through the patient's death but rather through direct action of the medication.

3. In cases where the pain is severe and the patient's prognosis is poor, the benefit of analgesia can outweigh the harm of hastened death.
4. In appropriately titrating the opioids, the physician's intention is to treat pain, with the foreknowledge—though not the intention—that death might be hastened.

The first component recognizes the obvious, but the latter three provide important clarifications.

The second component draws a sharp distinction between intensive analgesia and euthanasia. Whereas the latter "puts the patient out of her misery" (i.e., ends her life in order to end her pain), opioids directly treat pain or dyspnea. Relief of symptoms may well occur absent the death of the patient—indeed, that is the overriding objective—and thus the bad effect is not the means to the good effect.

The third component underscores that the discussion is only about extreme symptoms at the end of life. A patient whose symptoms are more moderate—or who could survive for a long period if she gets through an intense period of her disease—would not meet the proportionality requirement of the RDE.

The final component emphasizes the physician's intention, which—again in contrast to euthanasia—is not to end the patient's life. Rather, it is to effectively treat pain, with the recognition that this could possibly hasten the patient's death.

The second and fourth conditions of the RDE, in particular, distinguish intensive symptom management from euthanasia. This is based on the presumption that euthanasia is not ethically permissible (p. 143), and thus intensive symptom management must somehow be intrinsically different for it to be acceptable. If euthanasia were permissible, there would be no need to appeal to the RDE because there would be no "bad effect" that requires justification (Sulmasy & Pellegrino, 1999).

Criticisms of the RDE

The RDE is not without controversy, however, with critics leveling several criticisms against it (Quill, Dresser, & Brock, 1997). The first pertains to its origin in a particular religious tradition, whose beliefs many people in a multicultural society do not share. Why should a Thomistic theory—applied to a modern problem—be persuasive for persons who do not share its theological presuppositions?

This, however, seems a weak accusation, since the RDE makes no explicit appeal to any religious text or set of beliefs. The fact that its historical origin lies in a religious context is irrelevant if its basic claims are reasonable and argumentation valid. The US Supreme Court seems to believe this to be the case, implicitly referencing the RDE in drawing a distinction between intensive symptom management and physician-assisted dying: "It is widely recognized that the provision of pain medication is ethically and professionally acceptable even when the treatment may hasten the patient's death if the medication is *intended to alleviate pain* and severe discomfort, not to cause death" (*Vacco v. Quill*, 1997, emphasis added).

Even if the RDE were confined in its applicability to people who share the religious beliefs out of which it arose—thus limiting its scope—this would not negate its validity to that specific group. Physicians who have no moral qualm about potentially hastening death—viewing symptom management as an overriding obligation or perhaps even approving of euthanasia—have no need for the RDE to counteract an opiophobia from which they do not suffer. Rather, it is precisely those physicians who *are* concerned about hastening death—and who might well share the same spiritual heritage as the formulators of the RDE—who rely on the rule for reassurance. As Sulmasy and Pellegrino (1999) observe, for clinicians who are "fearful of unwittingly participating in euthanasia if a patient's death is hastened, . . . the rule of double effect provides moral reassurance and thus encourages optimal care of the dying."

A second criticism has to do with the physician's intention, which is not always monolithic (Brody, 1993; Quill, 1993). When a patient is suffering and has expressed a wish for hastened death, can a physician honestly say that his *only* intention in treating pain aggressively is analgesia? If he would not be saddened to see a patient—whose quality of life may be so poor that she longs for death—die sooner, does that amount to "intending" the patient's death and thus violate the last condition of the RDE?

Critics are surely right in questioning the purity of intention because it is possible to intend multiple things to various degrees. But this does not invalidate the RDE. Just because a physician would not be saddened to see a patient die sooner does not mean that he is acting purposefully to achieve that goal. The key here is not the purity of intention but rather the *primacy* of intention, which should be on relief of suffering. As Foley (1997) writes, "Saying that physicians struggle with doubts about their intentions is not the same as saying that their intention is to kill."

Another criticism has to do with responsibility, noting that people are generally held to account not only for what they intended to do but also what could have reasonably been foreseen as a result of their actions. As the President's Commission for the Study of Ethical Problems in Medicine and Biomedical and Behavioral Research (1983) put it, "People are equally responsible for all of the foreseeable effects of their actions, thereby having no need for a policy that separates 'means' from 'merely foreseen consequences.'" The most important component, critics argue, is not the physician's intended outcome but the proportionality of the sought-after good with the risked "bad effect" (Quill et al., 1997). The moral value of an action would not, therefore, depend on the motivation that prompts it, but rather on the consequences it predictably results in.

The RDE certainly recognizes the limits of intention, with the requirement of proportionality providing a substantial safeguard. Intending to eradicate pain is insufficient justification for placing *any* patient at risk of hastened death, especially when that patient could have lived for a long period after the pain eventually subsided. Only patients whose symptoms and prognosis meet the proportionality requirement are "covered" by the RDE, and the emphasis on intention ensures judicious upward titration, thus minimizing the risk of serious side effects.

Even admitting that good intentions—which, as the old saying goes, pave the road to hell (Boswell, 1791)—are no defense for an act that leads to excessive harm, this does not mean that intention does not matter. Imagine, for example, two physicians working in the intensive care unit, both caring for patients in extreme pain at the end of life. Physician A judiciously titrates opioid dosing in an attempt to control the patient's pain, starting at 5 mg per hour and eventually reaching 50 mg per hour. At that point the patient is comfortable but breathing quite slowly and soon thereafter dies peacefully. Physician B, on the other hand, has many other responsibilities, acknowledges that the patient is going to die anyway and thus gives a 50 mg bolus of morphine to "get this over with." Although the end result is the same, there exists a moral difference between these two physicians' actions, especially as viewed through the lens of virtue ethics (p. 40).

The next criticism of the RDE is directly related to this focus on physician intention, arguing that the rule implicitly prioritizes the physician's own professional responsibility over the patient's autonomy, which should be the primary emphasis (Meisel & Cerminara, 2004). What if the patient in the aforementioned example preferred to be "put out of her misery," rather than waiting for Physician A to gradually titrate the opioid dose?

This criticism takes a rather simplistic view of autonomy, however, essentially equating it to "what the patient wants, the patient gets." As noted in chapter 2, professional codes and obligations also play an important role in the discussion, if only to assure other patients that the treatments being offered are clinically indicated and ethically defensible. The RDE is not merely a salve for the physician's conscience; it is also a valuable guide—in applicable situations—for navigating complex situations.

A final criticism focuses on the unintended consequences of the RDE itself, which could actually impede—rather than make possible—optimal pain management. For instance, a physician might recognize that he would be relieved if a long-suffering patient died and thus be concerned that administering high doses of opioids could reflect an intention to hasten death. Rather than reassuring the physician, the RDE's focus on intention could discourage him from effectively treating the patient's pain, out of concern for violating the fourth requirement.

Here it is important to acknowledge the multifaceted nature of intention and focus on the primacy rather than purity of it. If a patient truly wished to have her life end, the physician's sharing in that hope is a sign of empathy, not unethicality. As long as this is not the primary reason for upward titration of opioids—and effective symptom management is—this should not represent a barrier to optimal care at the end of life.

This reveals another unintended consequence of relying on the RDE: the perpetuation of the misperception that intensive symptomatic treatment is likely to hasten death. The purpose of the RDE (related to palliative care) is to empower physicians to optimally treat suffering at the end of life, unencumbered by ethical concerns that unintentionally hastening death constitutes euthanasia. But while this may be extremely important reassurance to those who would otherwise be burdened by this concern, routinely appealing to the RDE as justification for intensive symptom management could perpetuate the belief that high-dose opioids are *likely* to hasten death. Indeed, some have gone so far as to call describe intensive pain treatment as "double effect euthanasia" (Vaux, 1989).

Yet while the physiologic mechanism by which opioids depress respiratory drive—especially upon their initiation (Hill 1993)—is well-established, the probability that they will hasten death by this mechanism is actually quite low (Whittaker, 2013). Pain itself is a significant respiratory stimulant, which explains why a person hyperventilates when he strikes his thumb with a hammer. It also explains why a patient in severe pain will continue to breathe—comfortably—after receiving an opioid dose that would have led to frank apnea in a healthy patient who is free of pain.

In point of fact, rather than being likely to hasten death, intensive symptom management may actually prolong life. Opioids have been shown to prolong survival after ventilator withdrawal (Edwards, 2005), likely by decreasing oxygen demand (Bakker, Jansen, Lima, & Kompanje, 2008). Indeed, a large study of hospice patients found that opioid use was directly—rather than inversely—correlated with duration of life for terminally ill patients (Portenoy et al., 2006). Editorials in leading medical journals have put it even more succinctly: "Morphine kills the pain, not the patient" (Sykes, 2007). Thus Fohr (1998) concludes: "In the case of medication to relieve pain in the dying patient, the RDE should be rejected not on ethical grounds, but for a lack of medical reality."

This empirical data suggests that overreliance on the RDE to justify pain management at the end of life may be counterproductive. In attempting to reassure a select few who fear stepping over the line into euthanasia that they are not doing anything wrong, a great many others may be led to believe that hastened death is inevitable, rather than rare. Ethicists may bear some responsibility for this perception. A recent study of medical school ethics educators found that one-third believed that opioids were "likely to cause significant respiratory depression that could hasten death" (Macauley, 2012). Understandably—based on this misperception—the RDE was routinely appealed to as justification for such intensive pain management.

In light of the uncertain correlation between opioids and hastened death, some have argued that appealing to the RDE to justify optimal EOL care may not only be counterproductive but also *unnecessary*. After all, the RDE is designed to justify actions which inevitably lead to both good and bad effects (Von Gunten, 2015), such as hysterectomy for uterine cancer in a pregnant woman. But in the case of symptomatic treatment at the end of life, the worst that can be said about opioids is that they could *possibly* hasten death. Where a bad effect is merely possible, it should be evaluated as a risk of treatment. In this respect, symptomatic treatment at the end of life is no different than any nearly every other medical treatment, which involves a balancing of the hoped-for benefit with the possible complications or side effects (Emanuel, Ferris, & von Gunten, 2002). And while the bad effect (i.e., death) is indeed serious, this is also a risk of many other medical procedures. As Bleich observes (1994), "[The] assumption of prudent risk is synonymous with life. It is only when the bad or immoral effect of an action is foreseeable as a matter of certainty, near certainty or strong likelihood that a moral dilemma arises."

Given the uncertain—or even *unlikely*—correlation between opioid treatment at EOL and hastened death, the RDE should not provide the sole justification of the former. Of course, some of the elements of the RDE would naturally factor into one's analysis, such as whether the benefits of the treatment outweigh the risks. And to those with heightened concern about the ethicality of potentially hastened death, the RDE could provide valuable reassurance, especially given its roots in a religious tradition that might have prompted that very concern.

But for most physicians, all four components of the RDE need not necessarily be satisfied to justify a treatment with only *potential* complications. Otherwise, overreliance on the RDE could actually perpetuate the very injustice it is designed to prevent. As Angell (1982) notes, "I can't think of any other area in medicine in which such an extravagant concern for side effects so drastically limits treatment."

Patient or Surrogate Refusal of Symptom Management

Regulatory barriers and physicians' opiophobia are not the only impediments to optimal pain management at the end of life. Patients and their surrogates might also refuse symptomatic treatment that is offered. The proper response to such a refusal depends on correctly identifying the basis for it, which can be classified into three general categories with some degree of overlap (Figure 7.1).

One medical reason for refusal of opioids is the stigma associated with them. The opioid epidemic frequently makes headlines, and some medications (such as Oxycontin) have been mentioned by name (Ryan, Girion, & Glover, 2016). While hospice clinicians recognize methadone as an inexpensive, broadly effective, and exceedingly well-absorbed pain reliever (Chhabra & Bull, 2008), many patients only know it only as treatment for patients suffering from opioid addiction. If a patient is reluctant to receive opioids based on fear of stigma, the team can reiterate that the treatment is medically indicated and review the benefits of it. It may also be helpful to rotate to another medication that achieves the same goal of pain relief but might be less commonly known or carry less negative connotations (e.g., hydromorphone).

Beyond the stigma of opioids, some patients may be concerned about becoming addicted themselves, in spite of their limited life expectancy. They might also have

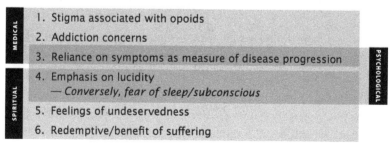

FIGURE 7.1 Reasons for refusing symptomatic treatment

misinterpreted a discussion of tolerance and physiologic dependence as equivalent to addiction, or view any dependence on medication as a sign of weakness. This concern might also betray an unspoken hope of exceeding the prognostic models, thus making addiction more of a relevant concern over a longer period of time.

Here it is important to distinguish between addiction, physiological dependence, and tolerance, stressing that the latter two are normal physiological mechanisms. With regard to physiologic dependence in particular, it may also be helpful to note that this phenomenon is not unique to opioids, as patients may become accustomed to—a more pleasant term than "dependent on"—other medications and thereby suffer negative effects from their discontinuation. For instance, a patient receiving long-term steroids will experience an adrenal crisis if they are withdrawn precipitously, but there is (properly) no stigma attached to this. Reasoning by analogy, just as one would never say that a patient with diabetes is "addicted" to insulin—even though the patient is dependent on that medication for health and to avoid negative symptoms—so also we should not say that a patient physiologically dependent on opioids is "addicted" to them.

Another reason that a patient might refuse optimal symptomatic treatment—which blurs the line between the medical and psychological—is her reliance on pain as a "marker of disease." If at least some of the symptom remains, then resolution of it signifies the improvement of the underlying disease, while a worsening may reflect disease progression. If analgesics completely eradicate pain—so the argument goes—then improvement in the underlying condition would not be noticeable. By the same token, if the patient were receiving too much analgesia, then incremental worsening of the condition would not be identified.

In such cases, patients can be reassured that there are other ways to mark the course of the disease beyond symptomatology. This might include blood counts or radiological scans. Focusing more on the psychological impetus for treatment refusal, it is reasonable to offer psychotherapy and empathic listening to directly address the patient's anxiety, while reassuring her that she will be fully informed of any developments in her condition.

In some cases, though, patients may still prefer to have some minor level of discomfort for the resulting "peace of mind." In cases such, it may not be appropriate to say that the patient is "suffering" from the symptom, since she has decided that she is on the whole more content with a small level of discomfort than being entirely symptom-free. Ideally ongoing conversations can identify the optimal balance of analgesia and reassurance for the patient, addressing whatever psychological or spiritual concerns make monitoring disease progression so important.

This highlights the distinction between pain or dyspnea on the one hand and suffering on the other. Certainly these terms are related, as both pain and dyspnea can cause suffering. But neither is synonymous with suffering, as some patients who might be experiencing high levels of pain or dyspnea would not report extreme suffering, while others would report it in the context of lesser measured levels of pain or dyspnea.

Ultimately, suffering is a broader concept than pain, taking into account nonphysical considerations that surpass the ability of quantitative scales to measure. It is just as subjective as either pain or dyspnea, and even more individual. If, indeed, "pain is whatever the experiencing person says it is, existing whenever the experiencing person says it does" (McCaffery & Beebe, 1989), suffering is at least equally so, encompassing both the physical and non-physical realms. It is ultimately up to the patient to determine what will increase or ameliorate her suffering, and the analgesic regimen should be tailored to optimally achieve the latter.

A classic example of this involves the patient who values lucidity over comfort. Sedation is a well-known—and, unlike respiratory depression, inevitable—side effect of opioids. In certain cases there needs to be a "trade-off" between lucidity and analgesia, with the severity of the patient's symptoms sometimes making it impossible to achieve both. Studies have shown that when faced with that choice, physicians generally prioritize comfort over lucidity, while patients are more likely to value lucidity even at the price of some degree of pain (Steinhauser et al., 2000).

Here it is important to clearly delineate what the primary goal of treatment is through direct discussion of this potentially tenuous balance. Palliative care should strive to minimize suffering, not merely physical pain. A patient who is pain-free could suffer greatly for wont of the opportunity to meaningfully engage with her loved ones at the end of her life. In an attempt to find the optimal balance, it may be possible to reduce the opioid dose without incurring extreme pain or to treat the sedation directly with a psychostimulant (Reissig & Rybarczyk, 2005).

Moving into the explicitly spiritual realm, another reason for refusing symptomatic treatment is a feeling of undeservedness. Some patients may have such a deep sense of past transgressions that they feel that the suffering they are experiencing is justified (Periyakoil, 2015). This is an explicitly spiritual issue which demands a spiritual response that addresses the underlying basis for this belief and identifies a way forward whereby the patient can make peace with her past while also (hopefully) receiving present-day relief of pain.

Lastly, a patient might believe that suffering is required by her religious tradition. This is not so much a question of deservedness as much as devoutness and thus merits a response rooted in that patient's religious tradition. The response to so-called "redemptive suffering" is addressed in detail later (p. 496).

All of the reasons cited so far can be voiced by patients themselves, and hopefully with attentive listening, accurate identification of the underlying issue, and focused discussion the patient's concerns can be addressed and allayed. If not, the clinician may be forced to accept the patient's request for suboptimal analgesia, at least temporarily. Admittedly, it can be very difficult to watch a patient endure pain "needlessly" when effective treatments are available. But if palliative care takes seriously the notion of "total pain," then it must recognize that increased physical discomfort may be the price that some patients are willing to pay for peace of mind or spirit. While one might wish it were not so, some patients find their balance in that place, and the job of palliative care clinicians is to simultaneously respect the patient's choice while also thoughtfully working with the patient to identify one that might better meet her physical as well as nonphysical needs (Macauley, 2011).

Clinicians should also take the time to reflect on the obligation they feel to eradicate suffering, specifically whose suffering it is that they are trying to address: the patient's, or their own? It is indeed a noble calling to ameliorate the suffering of another person, but when the drive to do so stems from the clinician's own need to discharge his moral duty, it runs the risk of prioritizing the clinician's values over those of the patient.

Up to this point, the discussion has assumed that the patient herself was refusing symptomatic treatment. But in some situations the patient might lack decision-making capacity and the refusal of symptom management is made by a surrogate decision-maker. As was the case with a patient's direct refusal of symptomatic treatment, a surrogate's refusal could stem from many reasons. The first step, once again, is to identify the precise reason why the surrogate believes the patient would refuse the treatment in question. Here the precise question is critical: *What do you think the patient would choose?* appropriately invokes substituted judgment, whereas *What do you think we should do?* opens the door for the surrogate to insert his own values (p. 63). Relevant factors include written advance directives, previous comments about the patient's own health status, and overall personal, spiritual, or religious values. The way in which the patient responded to previous episodes of discomfort or pain—including prior willingness to accept analgesia—are all relevant.

But none of these may be determinative. As noted earlier (p. 72), it is often not clear what the patient would have wanted. Most patients have not completed a written advance directive, and even those who did may have expressed rather general sentiments, or perhaps only named a health care agent. The majority of patients have done neither, leaving a surrogate—either identified through a state hierarchy or informally identified by the medical team (p. 62)—to make the decision. That surrogate necessarily has to rely on inferences from what the patient has said in the past and how that patient has lived her life.

The fact that the patient named that person as her decision-maker—or that that person is deemed by statute or practice as the appropriate surrogate—reflects not only the closeness of the relationship with the patient but also likely the overlap in their values. Thus, if the surrogate declines symptomatic treatment based on a notion of redemptive suffering, this could reflect a shared spiritual belief. He might also be deciding on the basis of a patient's longstanding aversion to taking medication or prioritizing of lucidity over pain relief.

The patient's context may have changed, though, since she espoused those beliefs. For instance, a patient who was generally averse to medication—during a period of good health and minimal symptomatology—might well be willing to accept medications when faced with severe symptoms. Similarly, concerns for addiction may fade in the face of a limited life expectancy.

218 | ETHICS IN PALLIATIVE CARE

The team, therefore, must also consider whether the surrogate could be acting based on his own values, which the patient may not share. A classic example is the stigma associated with opioids, especially if the surrogate has had personal experience with addiction. Similarly, when a surrogate prioritizes lucidity over analgesia, it can be challenging to determine whether he is doing so because that is what the patient would have done or because he himself is seeking something from the patient—such as forgiveness or simply additional moments of meaning—even at the price of the patient's increased suffering.

If this is the case, the general methods noted above for helping surrogate decision-makers navigate complexity and avoid excessive burden (p. 77) can be helpful. The surrogate may feel torn about advocating a course of action that violates his own personal beliefs, so reassurance that he is not really making the decision—rather, he is simply communicating what the patient would have chosen—can be helpful. Sometimes a surrogate may need to recuse himself if the sense of "moral complicity" is too great. In other situations, though, the surrogate may hold his ground and effectively demand that his instructions be followed, even though this would cause increased suffering to the patient.

Seeking additional input from others who know the patient may be helpful in such cases, not only from an informational point of view but also in terms of advocacy, as these additional stakeholders may have more sway with the primary surrogate than the clinical team does. If the impasse remains, however—and there is no clear evidence the surrogate is using appropriate substituted judgment—the medical team may have to prioritize beneficence by ensuring adequate symptomatic treatment. For while patients have the right to make "bad choices" for themselves, surrogates do not have the right to inflict suffering on patients based on their own value system.

There are several ways to accomplish this. The team could request an ethics consultation, in order to better delineate the surrogate's rights and the team's obligation. There may be other avenues to engage an impartial person to mediate the dispute. In extreme cases, an alternate surrogate may need to be identified. If the original surrogate is not specifically named in an advance directive as the primary agent, most states have a hierarchy of surrogates whereby others with some standing can challenge the decisions of the person at the top of the hierarchy (p. 62). In the few states without a hierarchy, there is nothing to prevent the clinical team from turning to someone else for medical decisions, unless the original surrogate opts to pursue guardianship in court. In that case, hopefully the court would take into account clinical concerns about undertreatment of suffering and appoint as guardian someone who is able to best advocate for the patient's comfort, as well as her values. This would also be the requisite course of action if the original surrogate decision-maker were the health care agent, thus requiring judicial appeal to displace him from that role.

Justice Concerns

True "opiophobia" inappropriately influences how a physician treats all his patients, and an individual patient's refusal of analgesia is her own choice. (Granted, one that might stem from misperceptions and certainly merits further exploration.) However, there are situations where inadequate analgesia may reflect personal or systemic discrimination against a certain subgroup of patients who are seeking relief of suffering. If all patients in pain are not treated the same, this raises profound justice concerns.

That this occurs in medical practice is irrefutable. Studies have shown that racial minorities, the poor, the elderly, women, and patients with HIV/AIDS are all less likely than white males to receive adequate chronic pain management (Nguyen, Ugarte, Fuller, Haas, & Portenoy, 2005). This could be due to a variety of factors, including an assumption that certain groups are more likely to be addicted to opioids and thus to seek them for secondary gain. Some groups are thought to have different "pain thresholds," suggesting that requests for opioid medications may be unwarranted by the level of pain experienced. Some physicians have even posited significant biological differences between groups. For instance, the majority of medical students and residents in one recent study believed there was a biological difference—such as altered sensitivity of nerve endings or skin thickness—between white and African American patients which influenced how they would treat pain in the latter (Hoffman, Trawalter, Axt, & Oliver, 2016).

Many of the ethical issues addressed in this textbook are complex and multilayered, requiring a balancing of competing obligations and identification of what in many cases is the "least bad option." This is not such an issue, for the ethics are clear: it is unjust to treat similar patients differently, based on nonclinical indicators such as the ones noted here.

It may be tempting to write off such discrimination as evidence of frank prejudice, but it is not as simple as that. There may exist genuine clinical misunderstanding which leads a physician to undertreat pain in a certain instance (such as by misdiagnosing undertreated pain as "addiction," thus leading to pseudoaddictive behavior). Or perhaps this a reflection of cognitive bias—especially attributive bias—whereby certain traits are attributed to specific groups (Saposnik, Redelmeier, Ruff, & Tobler, 2016).

The solution seems obvious, namely, to avoid such discrimination. But this is easier said than done, given the multifaceted nature of pain, the shifting focus from pain as "the fifth vital sign" to daily milligram limits meant to combat the opioid epidemic, and the lingering effects of opiophobia. Implicit bias, as the name suggests, is unrecognized by the physician, who may believe that he is not prejudiced in any way. Studies have shown, however, that implicit bias frequently impacts the clinical decisions physicians make (Blair, Steiner, & Havranek, 2011). Hopefully, raising the implications of this bias to consciousness can help prevent it from impacting patient care (Devine, Forscher, Austin, & Cox, 2012), as can establishing best practice standards for treating pain. Absent such recognition and direct engagement, however, there is no reason to believe that unjust disparities in pain treatment will not continue.

Return to the Case

The first thing the ethics consultant does is clarify that optimal pain relief is the primary goal in this case, given that some patients would prioritize lucidity and the meaningful interaction that permits. The patient's disease, however, is so far advanced at this point that meaningful interaction with her loved ones is essentially impossible: lucidity brings excruciating pain, and even inadequate pain control causes significant mental clouding and sedation.

While opioids are far from certain to hasten death in treating patients at the end of life, the doses necessary to relieve the extreme pain of the seventy-year-old woman with bone metastases could well cause respiratory depression. The clinicians have expressed significant moral qualms, concerned about violating their oath to "do no harm."

Responding to their concerns, the ethics consultant reviews the four components of the RDE. Administration of opioids is not morally bad, and the extreme nature of the patient's pain—in light of her short life expectancy—meets the proportionality requirement. The clinicians are clear that their intention is to appropriately titrate the opioids to treat the pain, rather than hasten death. Death would therefore not be the means to the good effect of analgesia but rather a separate and potential outcome.

The consultant confirms that the criteria of the RDE are met in this case and cites professional, ethical, and legal sources that endorse its application in situations such as this. He also notes the uncertainty about whether opioids would, in fact, hasten death, observing that they quite likely could actually prolong life.

The clinicians are relieved, and the patient receives effective analgesia and dies peacefully the following day.

Summary Points

- For most of the history of Western medicine, relatively little attention was paid to the treatment of symptoms at the end of life. This changed following World War II, and especially after the mid-century pioneering work of Cicely Saunders.
- Pain is multifaceted, going beyond physical discomfort to include emotional, psychological, and spiritual domains.
- Suffering is a deeper concept which recognizes varying pain tolerances as well as patient goals. In some cases, eradicating pain could cause greater suffering, if the patient's other goals are not respected.

- The primary justification for intensive treatment of pain and dyspnea at the end of life is the Rule of Double Effect.
  - Some have criticized the rule because of its theological roots, emphasis on physician intention and supposed deprioritizing of patient autonomy.
  - None of these criticisms is compelling. The rule can be used to justify intensive symptomatic treatment but it is largely unnecessary. Instead of hastening death, opioids frequently prolong life when used appropriately.
- Patients may refuse symptomatic treatment for a variety of medical, psychological, and spiritual reasons. Unless the true reason is identified, it is impossible to effectively address the patient's concerns.
- Surrogate refusal of symptomatic treatment is more concerning, as it may not reflect accurate substituted judgment. In such cases, it may be ethically requisite to override the refusal in order to minimize patient suffering.
- There exist profound justice-based concerns about inequitable treatment of pain across disease, racial, and ethnic groups. These can be caused either by overt or implicit bias or clinical misunderstandings.

References

Ahmedzai, S. (1997). Five years, five threads. *Prog Pall Care, 5*(6), 235–237.

Al-Mazroa, A. A., & Abdel Halim, R. E. (1989). Anesthesia 1000 years ago. *Royal Soc Med Intl Congress Symp Series, 134,* 46–47.

AMA Council on Ethical and Judicial Affairs. (1992). Decisions near the end of life. *JAMA, 267*(16), 2229–2233.

American Society of Addiction Medicine. (2011). Definition of addiction. Retrieved from http://www.asam.org/for-the-public/definition-of-addiction

Angell, M. (1982). The quality of mercy. *N Engl J Med, 306*(2), 98–99. doi:10.1056/NEJM198201143060210.

Aquinas, T. (2012). *Summa theologiae secunda secundae, 1-91: The complete works of Saint Aquinas.* Lander, WY: Aquinas Institute for the Study of Sacred Doctrine.

Bakker, J., Jansen, T. C., Lima, A., & Kompanje, E. J. (2008). Why opioids and sedatives may prolong life rather than hasten death after ventilator withdrawal in critically ill patients. *Am J Hosp Palliat Care, 25*(2), 152–154. doi:10.1177/1049909108315511

Baraka, A. (2000). Historical aspects of opium. 1982. *Middle East J Anaesthesiol, 15*(4), 423–436.

Bennett, D. S., & Carr, D. B. (2002). Opiophobia as a barrier to the treatment of pain. *J Pain Palliat Care Pharamcother, 16*(1), 105–109.

Blair, I. V., Steiner, J. F., & Havranek, E. P. (2011). Unconscious (implicit) bias and health disparities: Where do we go from here? *Perm J, 15*(2), 71–78.

Bleich, J. D. 1994. On the ethics of pain management. *Cancer Invest, 12*(3), 362–363.

Bonica, John J. (1953). *The management of pain; with special emphasis on the use of analgesic block in diagnosis, prognosis, and therapy.* Philadelphia: Lea & Febiger.

Booth, M. (1998). *Opium: A history* (1st US ed.). New York: St. Martin's Press.

Boswell, J. (1791). *The life of Samuel Johnson, LL.D., comprehending an account of his studies and numerous works in chronological order . . . the whole exhibiting a view of literature and literary men in Great-Britain for near half a century during which he flourished.* London: H. Baldwin.

Brody, H. (1993). Causing, intending, and assisting death. *J Clin Ethics, 4*(2), 112–117.

Chhabra, S., & Bull, J. (2008). Methadone. *Am J Hosp Palliat Care, 25*(2), 146–150. doi:10.1177/1049909107312597

Cherny, N. I., Coyle, N., & Foley, K. M. (1994). Suffering in the advanced cancer patient: a definition and taxonomy. *J Palliat Care, 10*(2), 57–70.

Cope, D. K. (2010). Intellectual milestones in our understanding and treatment of pain. In S. Fishman, J. Ballantyne, J. P. Rathmell, & J. J. Bonica (Eds.), *Bonica's management of pain* (4th ed., pp. 1–12). Baltimore, MD: Lippincott, Williams & Wilkins.

Council on Ethical and Judicial Affairs, American Medical Association. (1992). Decisions near the end of life. *JAMA, 267*(16), 2229–2233.

Davis, M. P., & Walsh, D. (2004). Cancer pain: How to measure the fifth vital sign. *Cleve Clin J Med, 71*(8), 625–632.

Desbiens, N. A., & Wu, A. W. (2000). Pain and suffering in seriously ill hospitalized patients. *J Amer Geratr Soc, 48*(5 Suppl.), S183–S186.

Devine, P. G., Forscher, P. S., Austin, A. J., & Cox, W. T. (2012). Long-term reduction in implicit race bias: A prejudice habit-breaking intervention. *J Exp Soc Psychol, 48*(6), 1267–1278. doi:10.1016/j.jesp.2012.06.003

Dowell, D., Haegerich, T. M., & Chou, R. (2016). CDC guideline for prescribing opioids for chronic pain—United States, 2016. *JAMA, 315*(15), 1624–1645. doi:10.1001/jama.2016.1464

Edwards, M. J. (2005). Opioids and benzodiazepines appear paradoxically to delay inevitable death after ventilator withdrawal. *J Palliat Care, 21*(4), 299–302.

Emanuel, L. L., Ferris, F. D., & von Gunten, C. F. (2002). EPEC. Education for physicians on end-of-life care. *Am J Hosp Palliat Care, 19*(1), 17; author reply 17–18.

Express Scripts. (2014). A nation in pain. Retrieved from http://lab.express-scripts.com/lab/publications/a-nation-in-pain

Fohr, S. A. (1998). The double effect of pain medication: Separating myth from reality. *J Palliat Med, 1*(4), 315–328. doi:10.1089/jpm.1998.1.315

Foley, K. M. (1997). Competent care for the dying instead of physician-assisted suicide. *N Engl J Med, 336*(1), 54–58. doi:10.1056/NEJM199701023360109

Food and Drug Administration. (2017). A brief overview of risk evaluation and mitigation strategies. Retrieved from https://www.fda.gov/aboutfda/transparency/basics/ucm325201.htm

Garcia, J. L. (1994). Double effect. In W. T. Reich (Ed.), *Encyclopedia of bioethics* (pp. 636–641). New York: Simon & Schuster.

Grond, S., Zech, D., Schug, S. A., Lynch, J., & Lehmann, K. A. (1991). Validation of World Health Organization guidelines for cancer pain relief during the last days and hours of life. *J Pain Symptom Manage, 6*(7), 411–422.

Haller, J. S. Jr. (1989). Opium usage in nineteenth century therapeutics. *Bull N Y Acad Med, 65*(5), 591–607.

Hamilton, G. R., & Baskett, T. F. (2000). In the arms of Morpheus: The development of morphine for post-operative pain relief. *Can J Anaesth, 47*(4), 367–374. doi:10.1007/BF03020955

Hill, C. S. Jr. (1993). The barriers to adequate pain management with opioid analgesics. *Semin Oncol, 20*(2 Suppl. 1), 1–5.

Hoffman, K. M., Trawalter, S., Axt, J. R., & Oliver, M. N. (2016). Racial bias in pain assessment and treatment recommendations, and false beliefs about biological differences between blacks and whites. *Proc Natl Acad Sci U S A, 113*(16), 4296–4301. doi:10.1073/pnas.1516047113

Howard-Jones, N. (1947). A critical study of the origins and early development of hypodermic medication. *J Hist Med Allied Sci, 2*(2), 201–249.

Huang, F. Y., & Emanuel, L. L. (1995). Physician aid in dying and the relief of patients' suffering: Physicians' attitudes regarding patients' suffering and end-of-life decisions. *J Clin Ethics, 6*(1), 62–67.

Islam, M. M., & McRae, I. S. (2014). An inevitable wave of prescription drug monitoring programs in the context of prescription opioids: Pros, cons and tensions. *BMC Pharmacol Toxicol, 15*, 46. doi:10.1186/2050-6511-15-46

Jennings, B., Ryndse, T., D'Onofrio, C., & Baily, M. A. (2003). Access to hospice care: Expanding boundaries, overcoming barriers. *Hastings Cent Rep*, Suppl., S3–S7, S9–S13, S15–S21 passim.

Lundberg, G. D. (1988). "It's over, Debbie" and the euthanasia debate. *JAMA, 259*(14), 2142–2143.

Macauley, R. (2011). Patients who make "wrong" choices. *J Palliat Med*, *14*(1), 13–16. doi:10.1089/jpm.2010.0318

Macauley, R. (2012). The role of the principle of double effect in ethics education at US medical schools and its potential impact on pain management at the end of life. *J Med Ethics*, *38*(3), 174–178. doi:10.1136/medethics-2011-100105

Macht, D. I., Herman, N. B., & Levy, C. S. (1915). A quantitative study of cutaneous analgesia produced by various opium alkaloids. *Proc Natl Acad Sci U S A*, *1*(12), 582–585.

McCaffery, M., & Beebe, A. (1989). *Pain: Clinical manual for nursing practice*. St. Louis, MO: Mosby.

Meisel, A., & Cerminara, K. L. (2004). *The right to die: The law of end-of-life decisionmaking* (3rd ed.). New York: Aspen.

Nguyen, M., Ugarte, C., Fuller, I., Haas, G., & Portenoy, R. K. (2005). Access to care for chronic pain: Racial and ethnic differences. *J Pain*, *6*(5), 301–14. doi:10.1016/j.jpain.2004.12.008

Pellegrino, E. D. (1992). Doctors must not kill. *J Clin Ethics*, *3*, 95–102.

Periyakoil, V. S. (2015). A never-ending battle. *N Engl J Med*, *373*(25), 2399–2401. doi:10.1056/NEJMp1505976

Pohlman, K. J. (1990). Pain control: Euthanasia or criminal act? *Focus Crit Care*, *17* (3), 260–261.

Portenoy, R. K., Sibirceva, U., Smout, R., Horn, S., Connor, S., Blum, R. H., . . . Fine, P. G. (2006). Opioid use and survival at the end of life: A survey of a hospice population. *J Pain Symptom Manage*, *32*(6), 532–540. doi:10.1016/j.jpainsymman.2006.08.003

President's Commission for the Study of Ethical Problems in Medicine and Biomedical and Behavioral Research. (1983). *Deciding to forego life-sustaining treatment: A report on the ethical, medical, and legal issues in treatment decisions*. Washington, DC: U.S. Government Printing Office.

Prioreschi, P., Heaney, R. P., & Brehm, E. (1998). A quantitative assessment of ancient therapeutics: Poppy and pain in the Hippocratic Corpus. *Med Hypotheses*, *51*(4), 325–331.

Quill, T. E. (1993). The ambiguity of clinical intentions. *N Engl J Med*, *329*(14), 1039–1040. doi:10.1056/NEJM199309303291414

Quill, T. E., Dresser, R., & Brock, D. W. (1997). The Rule of Double Effect—a critique of its role in end-of-life decision making. *N Engl J Med*, *337*(24), 1768–1771. doi:10.1056/NEJM199712113372413

Reich, W. T. (1989). Speaking of suffering: A moral account of compassion. *Soundings*, *72*(1), 83–108.

Reissig, J. E., & Rybarczyk, A. M. (2005). Pharmacologic treatment of opioid-induced sedation in chronic pain. *Ann Pharmacother*, *39*(4), 727–731. doi:10.1345/aph.1E309

Ryan, H., Girion, L., & Glover, S. (2016, May 5). "You want a description of hell?" OxyContin's 12-hour problem. *Los Angeles Times*. Retrieved from http://www.latimes.com/projects/oxycontin-part1/

Saposnik, G., Redelmeier, D., Ruff, C. C., & Tobler, P. N. (2016). Cognitive biases associated with medical decisions: A systematic review. *BMC Med Inform Decis Mak*, *16*(1), 138. doi:10.1186/s12911-016-0377-1

Saunders, C. (1963). The treatment of intractable pain in terminal cancer. *Proceed Royal Soc Med*, *56*, 195–197.

Saunders, C. (1964). The symptomatic treatment of incurable malignant disease. *Prescribers J*, *4*(4), 68–73.

Saunders C. M. (Ed.). (1984). *The management of terminal malignant disease*. London: Hodder Arnold.

Schneider, C., Yale, S. H., & Larson, M. (2003). Principles of pain management. *Clin Med Res*, *1*(4), 337–340.

Schweitzer, A. (1948). *On the edge of the primeval forest & More from the primeval forest. Experiences and observations of a doctor in equatorial Africa*. New York: Macmillan.

Shaw, A. B. (2002). Two challenges to the double effect doctrine: Euthanasia and abortion. *J Med Ethics*, *28*(2), 102–104.

Smith, M. L., Orlowski, J., Radey, C., & Scofield, G. (1992). A good death: Is euthanasia the answer? *Cleveland Clin J Med*, *59*(1), 99–109.

Solomon, M. Z., O'Donnell, L., Jennings, B., Guilfoy, V., Wolf, S. M., Nolan, K., . . . Donnelley, S. (1993). Decisions near the end of life: Professional views on life-sustaining treatments. *Am J Public Health*, *83*(1), 14–23.

Steinhauser, K. E., Voils, C. I., Clipp, E. C., Bosworth, H. B., Christakis, N. A., Tulsky, J. A. (2000). Factors considered important at the end of life by patients, family, physicians, and other care providers. *JAMA*, *284*(19), 2476–2482. doi:10.1001/jama.284.19.2476

Sulmasy, D. P., & E. D. Pellegrino. (1999). The Rule of Double Effect: Clearing up the double talk. *Arch Intern Med, 159*(6), 545–550.

SUPPORT Principal Investigators. (1995). A controlled trial to improve care for seriously ill hospitalized patients: The study to understand prognoses and preferences for outcomes and risks of treatments (SUPPORT). *JAMA, 274*(20), 1591–1598.

Sykes, N. P. (2007). Morphine kills the pain, not the patient. *Lancet, 369*(9570), 1325–1326. doi:10.1016/S0140-6736(07)60611-4

Tallmadge, G. K. (1946). Some anesthetics of antiquity. *J Hist Med Allied Sci, 1*(4), 515–520.

Teunissen, S. C., Wesker, W., Kruitwagen, C., de Haes, H. C., Voest, E. E., & de Graeff, A. (2007). Symptom prevalence in patients with incurable cancer: A systematic review. *J Pain Symptom Manage, 34*(1), 94–104. doi:10.1016/j.jpainsymman.2006.10.015

The Hastings Center. (1987). *Guidelines on the termination of life sustaining treatment and the care of the dying.* Bloomington: Indiana University Press.

Vacco v. Quill. (1997). U.S. 521 793.

Vaux, K. L. (1989). Mercy, murder, & morality: Perspectives on euthanasia. The theological ethics of euthanasia. *Hastings Cent Rep, 19*(1 Suppl.), 19–22.

Von Gunten, C. F. (2015). Morphine and hastened death. Retrieved from http://www.eperc.mcw.edu/EPERC/FastFactsIndex/ff_008.htm

Weissman, D. E., & Haddox, J. D. (1989). Opioid pseudoaddiction—an iatrogenic syndrome. *Pain, 36*(3), 363–366.

Whittaker, M. R. (2013). Opioid use and the risk of respiratory depression and death in the pediatric population. *J Pediatr Pharmacol Ther, 18*(4), 269–276. doi:10.5863/1551-6776-18.4.269

World Health Organization. (2017). WHO's cancer pain ladder for adults. Retrieved from http://www.who.int/cancer/palliative/painladder/en/

Wyatt, J. (2009). *Matters of life & death: Human dilemmas in light of the Christian faith.* Nottingham, England: Inter-Varsity Press.

Younger, J., McCue, R., & Mackey, S. (2009). Pain outcomes: A brief review of instruments and techniques. *Curr Pain Headache Rep, 13*(1), 39–43.

8

Physician-Assisted Dying

Case Study

A seventy-seven-year-old Vermont resident was diagnosed with thryoid cancer approximately two years ago. First-line chemotherapy was initially effective, but then his disease progressed. Other disease-directed therapies are highly unlikely to help, and his life expectancy is measured in months. He enrolls in hospice and his moderate pain and nausea are well-controlled. Knowing what lies ahead of him, he does not want to "wither away" and asks his physician, "Will you help me die?"

Terminology

The terminology of a practice often evolves over time. This may be to avoid any inaccurate associations, as in the case of the transition from "terminal sedation" to "palliative sedation" (p. 252). Alternatively, it may strive to distinguish a specific practice from something that is more ethically contentious, as in the transition from "passive euthanasia" to "letting die" (p. 140).

In probably no other case is the terminology so charged as in the case of the practice of a physician prescribing a lethal dose of a drug[1] to a competent, terminally ill patient at the patient's request, which the patient then has the option of self-administering for

---

1. Many commentators use the term "medicine" to refer to what is prescribed. That word has a very positive connotation, however, suggesting it is safe to use and treats a disease (neither of which are true in this case). This handbook uses neutral—and more accurate—terms related to physician-assisted dying, in this case "prescription" and "drug."

the purpose of hastening his death. The term that one uses to describe this practice likely reflects that person's ethical view of the practice.

For many years this practice was referred to as physician-assisted suicide (PAS), which is etymologically correct since suicide is derived from the Latin *-cidius* (killing) and *sui* (of oneself). Despite the fact that there are courageous instances of self-killing—such as a soldier throwing himself on a grenade to save his comrades—the use of the word "suicide" carries with it strongly negative connotations, often suggesting the presence of mental illness or instability. Advocates of the practice are generally averse to using the "S-word" because they claim the true cause of death is the terminal (qualifying) diagnosis. Further, they believe that the term casts judgment on a terminally ill patient making an informed choice that reflects his values. This is one of the reasons why laws passed in Oregon, Washington, Vermont, California, Colorado, and the District of Columbia assiduously avoid any reference to "suicide," other than to specify that the legal cause of death after ingestion of the prescribed drug is *not* to be considered suicide.[2]

Whereas a person who uses the term "physician-assisted suicide" is likely opposed to the practice, those in favor of it choose alternate terms that are at least neutral, if not positive. These include "physician aid in dying." "physician-assisted death," and "death with dignity." The last of these is a classic example of choosing a term that, when taken at face value, no one could disagree with. (This is reminiscent of the abortion debate, with one side claiming the "pro-choice" mantle and the other that of being "pro-life.") Who, after all, would *not* wish to die with dignity? As a term, though, it is calculated and imprecise. It does not specify the practice to which it has come to commonly refer and could even be taken to imply that patients who do not seek hastened death do *not* die with dignity.

Because of the overwhelmingly negative connotation of PAS and the similarly positive connotations associated with death with dignity, this textbook will seek a terminologically neutral middle ground by referring to the practice as physician-assisted dying (PAD), in keeping with the practice of several professional bodies (e.g., American Academy of Hospice and Palliative Medicine, 2016). It should be noted, however, that some professional bodies consciously continue to use the term PAS, reflecting their opposition to its legalization and implementation (American Medical Association, 2010–2011).

Historicolegal Background

The ethicality of suicide has been hotly debated for millennia. In the pre-Christian era it was generally felt to be an ethically acceptable option. Indeed, Socrates, the "father" of Western philosophy, took his own life on principle. While Plato (1984) generally condemned suicide,

---

2. This is significant from a medicolegal perspective, as some life insurance policies are rendered void if the patient is deemed to have committed suicide.

he allowed for several exceptions, including in cases of extreme and unavoidable personal misfortune. Aristotle (1953) condoned suicide as long as it was voluntary. Some philosophical schools—notably the Stoics—went so far as to view suicide as a potentially courageous decision. As Cicero (1968) said: "When [a man] possesses or sees in prospect a majority of [things contrary to nature], it is appropriate for him to depart from life."

With the rise of Christianity, however, the prevailing sentiment began to shift. Augustine (2006) was the first Christian theologian to formatively address suicide, deeming it a violation of the commandment not to kill. Thomas Aquinas (2012) concurred, arguing that suicide was contrary to self-love, injures the community, and violates our duty to value God's gift of life. The Roman Catholic Church (1994) continues to follow this line of thought, deeming active steps to end one's life a mortal sin. While broad eternal judgments and injunctions against church burials for victims of suicide have been revised (Catholic Church, 1994), the religious stigma clearly remains.

Some philosophers (Kant, 1964) concur with this view, but many do not. Michel de Montaigne (1958), for example, made frequent reference to Roman writers praising suicide. David Hume (1934)—foreshadowing the compassion-based defense of PAD— believed that sympathy was a more reliable virtue than reason, which he felt should be "sympathy's slave." Even John Donne (1977)—an ordained minister—defended suicide by claiming it was not, in fact, contrary to God's law. Idealist (Schopenhauer, Norman, Welchman, & Janaway, 2010) and liberal (Szasz, 2002) philosophers have gone so far as to proclaim suicide an inalienable human right and one that can reasonably be exercised when a person is unable to live according to his own values and beliefs.

Society's views of suicide over time may be interesting from a broad-ranging academic standpoint, but they are not directly relevant to the question of PAD. In the first place, in the aforementioned analyses there was little consideration of a person being seriously ill, let alone with a life expectancy of six months or less. The philosophical debate thus includes somatically healthy people, as well as people in unique situations—such as being surrounded by enemies in time of war—that are not applicable to this discussion.

The second reason is that for all the thoughtful analysis of suicide as a concept and practice, up until the nineteenth century—when use of analgesics and anesthetics became more widespread—there was no serious consideration of *physician assistance* in suicide. Suicide up until that point was a private act, accomplished by any number of means without the involvement—let alone assistance—of a medical professional. Indeed, the Hippocratic Oath expressly forbids the practice: "I will give no deadly medicine to anyone if asked, nor suggest any such counsel" (Hippocrates, 1923). Most medical schools no longer administer the Hippocratic Oath (Kao and Parsi, 2004), however, as some of its methodologies are now outdated (such as its recommended treatment for kidney stones). So, too, some would argue, are its moral injunctions (such as against performing abortions). Just as society has come to accept physicians' role in termination of pregnancy—once forbidden—so also hastened death could become acceptable for physicians to participate in.

From a legal perspective, suicide is not illegal in any of the United States, if for no other reason than it is impossible to punish the person who committed the crime. *Assisted* suicide generally is illegal, however, either based on state statute or common law. Even where it is not specifically criminalized, concern for legal or professional sanction often leads physicians to refrain from participating in PAD, or at the very least do so in a covert fashion.

In 1967, at around the same time that suffering at the end of life began to be increasingly recognized—and before the right to refuse treatment had been codified in US law—the first bill to legalize PAS (as it was called then) was introduced in Florida. Even though it failed to pass, the conversation continued. The years that followed saw many of the famous "right to die cases" (*Cruzan v. Director, Missouri Department of Health*, 1990; *In re Quinlan*, 1976).[3] Advocacy groups were formed, beginning with the Hemlock Society in 1980, which later changed its name to End of Life Choices and subsequently merged with Compassion in Dying in 2005 to become Compassion and Choices (Humphry, 2005).

During this period several events garnered significant public attention. Jack Kevorkian (known to some as "Dr. Death") was a retired pathologist who believed patients should be able to end their own lives. He created a euthanasia machine which was used by a terminally ill patient named Janet Adkins in 1990, thus providing a "face" for the movement to legalize PAD. Kevorkian subsequently went on to assist approximately 150 patients in hastening their deaths and was charged with and acquitted of assisting in suicide on several occasions. He was ultimately found guilty of second-degree murder when he crossed the line from PAD to active euthanasia by administering a lethal injection to Thomas Youk, a fifty-two-year-old patient with amyotrophic lateral sclerosis (Lou Gehrig's disease), an act that was broadcast in 1998 on *60 Minutes*.

Another important personal story was that of "Diane," the patient described by the noted palliative care clinician and ethicist Timothy Quill, in a 1991 article in the *New England Journal of Medicine*. Quill was Diane's long-time physician and ultimately provided her with a lethal prescription to hasten her death. His decision to write about the case stemmed from his belief that PAD deserved more serious discussion (beyond Kevorkian's sensationalism). Charges were brought against Dr. Quill but the grand jury declined to indict, and the state medical board not only permitted him to keep his license but also recommended that the subject be studied by a state ethics panel.

That same year Derek Humphry (1991) published *Final Exit*, essentially a how-to manual for patients wishing to end their lives. Other similar books have since followed, including Philip Nitschke and Fiona Stewart's (2010) *The Peaceful Pill Handbook*. Meanwhile, ballot measures were introduced in several states (including Washington, California, Michigan, and Maine), only to be rejected (at least initially).

---

3. These cases involve the *negative* right to die (i.e., the right to refuse life-sustaining medical treatment) while the PAD debate involves a positive right to die (i.e., the right to active assistance in hastening death).

In 1994 Oregon became the first state to legalize PAD, by way of a voter referendum that approved the Oregon Death with Dignity Act with 51% of the vote. This act legalized PAD for patients who met several criteria:

- Life expectancy of six months or less, confirmed by a second physician
- Resident of the state
- Age eighteen or older
- One written request
- Two oral requests for a lethal prescription, separated by at least fifteen days
- Explicit opportunity to rescind request after completing above steps, with a forty-eight-hour waiting period
- Sufficient decision-making capacity (DMC) to choose PAD. If this is in question, referral to a mental health professional is indicated, but this is not a requirement for all patients.

The law specifically states that no physician is obligated to write a lethal prescription if asked to do so. Hospice and palliative care services should be offered, but the patient need not accept them. Similarly, the physician may encourage the patient to involve—or, at least, inform—his family, but the patient is not required to do so. The cause of death on the death certificate is the patient's underlying disease, rather than "suicide."

An injunction delayed implementation of the law pending a subsequent ballot initiative to repeal the law, which was considered in 1997 in the aftermath of two pivotal Supreme Court decisions. The first was *Washington v. Glucksberg*, where four physicians (including Dr. Glucksberg) and three terminally ill patients challenged Washington state's ban on assisted suicide in the state's Natural Death Act (State of Washington, 1979), appealing to the Due Process Clause of the Fourteenth Amendment. They argued that the right to suicide was a fundamental liberty interest which could not be infringed upon without due process of law.

Both the District Court and the Ninth Circuit Court of Appeals (upon hearing it *en banc*) ruled with the plaintiffs. As the Appeals court concluded, "A competent, terminally ill adult, having lived nearly the full measure of his life, has a strong liberty interest in choosing a dignified and humane death rather than being reduced to a state of helplessness, diapered, sedated, incompetent."

Simultaneously in *Vacco v. Quill*, Dr. Quill—who had written the seminal article several years earlier in the *New England Journal of Medicine*—joined several other physicians in challenging New York's ban on assisted suicide by appealing to a different aspect of the Fourteenth Amendment: the Equal Protection Clause. The District Court rejected their argument that since terminally ill patients who were dependent on life-sustaining medical treatment (LSMT) could end their lives by refusing treatment—based on the negative right to die which had already been established—patients who were *not* dependent on

LSMT should have the same right. The Second Circuit of Appeals, however, reversed the decision, siding with the plaintiffs.

Both cases were appealed to the Supreme Court, which unanimously rejected both claims to a constitutional right to assistance in dying. With regard to the Equal Protection Clause, the Supreme Court found that there is a substantive difference between allowing a patient to die and causing him to die. The Court noted that the distinction between assisting suicide and withdrawing LSMT is "widely recognized and endorsed in the medical profession and in our legal traditions [and] is both important and logical" (*Vacco v. Quill*, 1997).

With regard to the due process argument, the Court cited compelling state interests which could justify a prohibition of PAD. These included the preservation of human life, the sanctity of the doctor-patient relationship, and concern for coercion of the vulnerable. The Court also expressed concern about a slippery slope beginning at PAD and ultimately extending to euthanasia, even involuntary euthanasia.

Three important points need to be made regarding these Supreme Court decisions. The first is that the Court found that there was no *constitutional* right to aid in dying, but this in no way prevents individual states from establishing such a right through statute. Chief Justice Rehnquist concluded the *Glucksberg* decision by observing that "throughout the Nation, Americans are engaged in an earnest and profound debate about the morality, legality, and practicality of physician-assisted suicide. Our holding permits this debate to continue, as it should in a democratic society" (*Washington v. Glucksberg*, 1997). Indeed, that is precisely what Oregon did in 1997, when voters upheld the Death with Dignity Act with 60% of the vote.

Second, the Court opened the door to its own subsequent reconsideration of the issue. In his concurring opinion, Justice Stevens acknowledged the

> possibility that an individual plaintiff seeking to hasten her death, or a doctor whose assistance was sought, could prevail in a more particularized challenge. However, . . . such a claim would have to be quite different from the ones advanced . . . here. (*Washington v. Glucksberg*, 1997)

Finally, while the Court did not find a constitutional right to aid in dying, it did appear to establish a constitutional right to palliative sedation (p. 253). Justice O'Connor wrote: "A patient who is suffering from a terminal illness and who is experiencing great pain has no legal barriers to obtaining medication, from qualified physicians, to alleviate that suffering, even to the point of causing unconsciousness and hastening death" (*Washington v. Glucksberg*, 1997). One might say that in rejecting a constitutional right on the question they were asked, the justices affirmed such a right on a question they weren't (Orentlicher, 1997).

Four states subsequently adopted laws modeled on Oregon's: Washington and Colorado by voter referendum in 2008 and 2016, respectively, and Vermont and California by legislative passage in 2013 and 2015, respectively. The District of Columbia also passed a law permitting it in 2016.

One other state has taken steps to legalize PAD,[4] this time through a court decision. In 2009 Montana's First Judicial District Court rejected the claim of a terminally ill patient and four physicians that the state constitution established a right to aid in dying. The court did assert, though, that PAD was not against public policy, concluding that the "constitutional rights of individual privacy and human dignity, taken together, encompass the right of a competent terminally-ill patient to die with dignity" (*Baxter v. Montana,* 2009).

Among professional groups, some are opposed to legalization of PAD (American College of Physicians, 2017; American Medical Association, 2010–2011; National Hospice and Palliative Care Organization, 2005), while others favor it (American Medical Student Association, 2008; American Medical Women's Association, 2007; American Public Health Association, 2008). Still others have taken a position of "studied neutrality," which neither supports nor opposes legalization (American Academy of Hospice and Palliative Medicine, 2016).

Global Perspective

While the Netherlands is the country most associated with PAD—as well as euthanasia— Switzerland was actually the first country to legalize "assisted suicide." Its penal code has long held that "every person who, *for selfish reasons,* incites or assists someone to commit suicide, shall be sentenced to imprisonment of up to five years or a fine" (Swiss Federal Criminal Code, 1937, emphasis added). This has generally been thought to exclude people who have assisted a person for altruistic—or, at least, nonselfish—reasons in ending his life.

Swiss law is unique in two respects (Andorno, 2013). One is that while "assisted suicide" is legal (at least in certain cases), it is generally implemented by non-physicians. A physician is required to write the lethal prescription—and thus must examine the patient, according to the Swiss Law on Pharmaceutical Products—but organization and implementation of assisted death are accomplished by non-physicians. The second unique aspect is that the only requirement for the patient is that he possess sufficient DMC to choose assisted death (i.e., he need not be terminally ill).

Two organizations in Switzerland facilitate most of the assisted deaths there, either in their own accommodations, in apartments rented for that specific purpose, or in hospitals in Geneva and Lausanne where this is permitted. The organization Exit (created in 1982) caters exclusively to residents of Switzerland, and in addition to sufficient DMC— as mandated by law—also requires people to be consistent in their expressed wish for suicide and also be experiencing "unbearable suffering, or be disabled in a serious manner."

---

4. A district judge in New Mexico concluded in 2014 that PAD was a right under the state constitution, but this decision was overturned on appeal (*Morris v. Brandenburg,* 2016).

Dignitas (created in 1998), on the other hand, works with nonresidents who for a fee can obtain assistance in ending their lives. This organization has generated significant controversy for its methods as well as the apparent "health" of some people it has assisted (Konnolly, 2008; Ledig & Samuel, 2007). Indeed, in a recent study nearly one out of four people who died in Switzerland through aid in dying had no significant medical illness but were simply old or "tired of life" (Fischer et al., 2008).

As noted (p. 146), euthanasia—and, by logical extension, PAD—has been unofficially permitted in the Netherlands since the 1970s. The situation was clarified in 2001 by the passage of the Termination of Life on Request and Assisted Suicide Act (2001) which established requirements for both euthanasia and PAD. These include unbearable suffering, voluntariness, sufficient decisional capacity, and a minimum age of twelve.

The following year Belgium approved both euthanasia and PAD for adult patients (as well as emancipated minors) with a "futile medical condition of constant and unbearable physical or mental suffering that cannot be alleviated" (Aviv, 2015). Luxembourg followed suit in 2009, and Belgium expanded this option to include children (with their parents' permission) in 2014.

Canada is the most recent country to legalize PAD and euthanasia. In 2014, the Quebec legislature passed the "medical aid in dying law" which made the practice legal in that province only. The following year the Supreme Court of Canada unanimously struck down the prohibition on PAD as unjustifiably infringing on the Canadian Charter of Rights and Freedoms (*Carter v. Canada*, 2015). Implementation of this decision was deferred, however, to permit time for legislation to be passed in order to appropriately regulate and monitor the practice.

That legislation subsequently established requirements for PAD which are very similar to those in the United States, with three notable exceptions. One is that the patient need not have a prognosis of six months or less to live; rather, he must have a "grievous and incurable medical condition," which is further defined as serious and incurable, in an advanced rate of incurable decline, and causing "intolerable" physical or psychological suffering "that cannot be relieved under conditions that [he considers] acceptable." The second difference is that the waiting period is ten days rather than fifteen and can be shortened if "the person's death, or the loss of [his] capacity to provide informed consent, is imminent." And, finally, the law allows for both PAD as well as active euthanasia (Bill C-14, 2016).

Clinical

From a clinical standpoint, ending one's own life is not simple. First, despite the extensive debate about PAD, the specific clinical regimen used to effect it is not well-known among physicians, even in states where the practice is legal. Generally, a lethal dose of a barbiturate (e.g., nine grams of secobarbital) is used to induce unconsciousness and ultimately respiratory arrest. The drug needs to be consumed relatively rapidly, however, so that the patient does not lose consciousness before consuming a lethal amount. But if a patient ingests too quickly, there is a risk of vomiting. (Approximately 3% of Oregonians who ingest a lethal prescription have experienced a complication, such as regurgitation.) For this reason, most protocols include taking an anti-emetic up to an hour before the lethal ingestion. The regimen is quite effective, with only 0.6% of Oregonians who ingest the lethal prescription ultimately regaining consciousness (State of Oregon, 2016).

Access is also an issue. The lethal dose is so large that it can become quite expensive, even more so now that one of the standard medications (secobarbital) is only produced by a for-profit company renowned for jacking up drug prices (Dembosky, 2016). A lethal dose has been estimated to cost up to $5,000, and taking pentobarbital is even more expensive (as much as $25,000, up from only $500 as recently as 2012).[5] Further, federal programs such as Medicare do not pay for the lethal prescription. Given the relatively small number of patients availing themselves of the law, some pharmacies have been known to provide the drug free of charge or at a significant discount.

Most states that have legalized PAD keep very detailed records of who obtains lethal prescriptions. The data from Oregon is particularly enlightening, since it has the longest history with PAD. Between 1997 and 2016, a total of 1,749 people had Death with Dignity Act (DWDA) prescriptions written and 1,127 patients died from ingesting drugs prescribed under the DWDA. The rate of growth in the number of prescriptions was relatively steady for the first sixteen years (at approximately 12% per year), but in 2014 and 2015 it grew at more than twice that rate before leveling out in 2016 (State of Oregon, 2016). Despite this increase, deaths via PAD still represent only 1 in 300 deaths in the state.

Hospice enrollment and PAD are not mutually exclusive. Over three-quarters of patients who died through DWDA had cancer, and the vast majority were enrolled in hospice (90%) and ultimately died at home (94%). As Constance Putnam (2002) notes, the question is not a false choice between "hospice or hemlock."

While many people assume that unrelieved pain is the primary reason cited for engaging in PAD, the data from Oregon do not bear this out. In fact, only one-quarter of patients cited "inadequate pain control or concern about it" as a reason for PAD. Instead, approximately 90% patients cited loss of autonomy and decreasing ability to engage in enjoyable activities, with nearly 80% also citing loss of dignity.

There is a very wide range in the length of the preexisting physician-patient relationship, from zero to almost two thousand weeks. In other words, some patients requested the lethal prescription the first time they met the prescribing physician, and others had known that physician for close to forty years.

There is also significant range in the time from the first request for the lethal dose until the patient ingested it (15–1,009 days). In other words, some patients ingested it on the first possible day—recalling the fifteen-day minimum period between first and second oral requests—while some waited nearly three years. This is particularly notable since in order to qualify under the DWDA, patients cannot have a life expectancy greater than six months. This does not mean that someone "gamed the system," only that prognostication

---

5. Some newer drug combinations recently introduced in Oregon cost much less, on the order of $500 (Death with Dignity, 2016).

is an inexact science (Christakis, 1999). While physicians generally tend to overestimate prognosis (p. 86), clearly there are times when they also underestimate it.

Ethical

From an ethical perspective, PAD can be distinguished from both potential respiratory depression from intensive pain medication (chapter 7) as well as continuous sedation to unconsciousness (chapter 9) because the intent of both of these is to relieve symptoms. In terms of intention, PAD is more similar to euthanasia, since the goal is to end the patient's life. As such, it does not fall under the well-accepted definition of palliative care, which does not seek to hasten death (World Health Organization, 2013). PAD is distinct from euthanasia, however, because the lethal dose is administered by the patient himself (rather than by the physician).

Arguments in Favor of PAD
Autonomy and Compassion

The primary argument in favor of PAD is based on two considerations: autonomy and compassion. If suffering is (as palliative care claims) truly a subjective phenomenon which only the patient himself can assess, and a competent, terminally ill patient determines that life is no longer worth living, why should a physician withhold a requested intervention—in this case, a lethal prescription—which she has the knowledge and ability to provide?

The personal narratives offered by advocates of PAD are incredibly moving. They describe patients in their last days or weeks or months of life, who simply wish to be delivered from their suffering and end life on their own terms. They are not dependent on LSMT, the withdrawal of which could have hastened their death. They do not have intolerable, refractory symptoms that would justify palliative sedation (p. 251). They do not wish to "linger" and ultimately die of dehydration through voluntarily stopping eating and drinking (VSED, p. 152). Rather, they wish to die on their own terms, at their chosen time, ideally at home surrounded by loved ones. Without the option of PAD, proponents argue that such patients would be left with only two choices: live out the remainder of a life they deem to be without quality, or end their lives by a much more violent—and emotionally traumatic—means.

A well known example of such a patient is Brittany Maynard. In early 2014, at the age of twenty-nine, she was diagnosed with brain cancer, which recurred several months later despite treatment. Given less than six months to live, she moved from her home state of California—which would not legalize PAD until the following year—to Oregon, so that she might utilize the PAD law there. In the meantime she became an outspoken and articulate advocate for Compassion and Choices, establishing a fund to raise money to support legalization and penning an eloquent reflection on what led to her decision to utilize the law later that same year (Maynard, 2014). In the process she became the "new face" of PAD (Angell, 2014) and "changed the optics of the debate" (Caplan, 2014).

Taken to an extreme, the argument from autonomy and compassion could lead physicians to feel *compelled* to participate in PAD, out of respect for the patient's autonomy (Kass, 2002). This, however, makes patient autonomy not only a positive right (p. 36) but an absolute one, whereby the patient must receive whatever he requests. That view has been rejected throughout this textbook, as there are many things which a patient might want that a physician is not obligated to provide (such as antibiotics for a viral infection). And even proponents of PAD are very clear that no physician is obligated to participate in the practice.

Proponents of PAD also claim that legalization not only benefits terminally ill patients who choose to hasten their death through PAD but also those patients who do not so choose yet still derive comfort and reassurance from knowing this is an option for them. Indeed, data from Oregon—where PAD has been legal for the longest period of time in the United States—reveals that only 56% of patients who received a lethal prescription in 2016 were known to have self-administered it. Not only would the other 44% purportedly gain assurance in having the prescription in hand, proponents also cite the untold—and unmeasured—others who might derive comfort from this "insurance policy" (i.e., the belief that they *could* get a prescription, if it became necessary).

Whether or not those other patients could, in fact, obtain a prescription is an important question. Studies have shown that less than 20% of patients who request a prescription actually receive one, with the remainder either not qualifying for the law, changing their minds, dying during the waiting period, or having their doctor decline the request on personal moral grounds (Ganzini et al., 2000). Yet the reason insurance (of any sort) offers piece of mind is the confidence that it will "pay off" when the time comes. One might reasonably wonder what comfort exists in an insurance policy that only pays off 20% of the time.

Viewed in this light, the very safeguards built into every state law legalizing PAD—which were necessary to achieve passage of the bills—effectively undercut the "insurance policy" argument. Patients who have a lethal prescription in hand might reasonably be reassured by possessing it, but those who have not yet received one might well be taking comfort in a false belief (i.e., that they could get such a prescription if they requested it).

Justice

The US Supreme Court may have concluded (*Vacco v. Quill*, 1997) that laws against PAD do not violate the Equal Protection Clause of the Fourteenth Amendment, but that has not stopped people from making an ethical argument to that effect. Why should a suffering, terminally ill patient be "condemned" to live out the rest of his days simply by virtue of the fact that he is not dependent on LSMT, which would have provided an "exit ramp"?

This argument essentially holds that there is no morally significant difference between doing something that might hasten a patient's death and *not* doing something that could keep the patient alive. In support of this argument, advocates of PAD note that there is nothing "passive," for instance, about removing someone from a ventilator (Edwards & Tolle, 1992). They also claim that VSED—which is acknowledged as ethically acceptable—does not passively let nature take its course because it is dehydration that kills (not the disease) and it would kill anyone, even someone who was not sick.

This is essentially the same argument classically put forth by Rachels (1975), who called into question the permissibility of limitation of LSMT. He likened it to active euthanasia—which at that time was acknowledged as clearly wrong—forcing defenders of palliative care to distinguish what was then known as "passive euthanasia" (and now is called "letting die") from actively hastening death (p. 140). But now that letting die is so widely accepted, proponents of PAD claim that it is not so different from actively hastening death after all. What began as an attempt to not let the negative connotation of hastened death taint letting die has transformed into trying to extend the positive connotation of letting die to encompass hastened death through PAD (p. 142).

One problem with this argument is that it is nearly impossible to "hold the line" between active forms of hastened death. If PAD is acceptable because active means are appropriate in some situations, why not also active euthanasia? To be sure, PAD—and the laws pertaining to its use—provide additional safeguards over active euthanasia, including assuring voluntariness. But there would still be no moral distinction between PAD and truly voluntary active euthanasia. Some advocates of PAD admit this and appear to view PAD as a "stepping stone" to euthanasia (Brock, 1992), but the latter is still rejected by the vast majority of countries and cultures (p. 144).

Another problem is the risk this argument poses to the progress of the past four decades. By linking actively hastened death—whether in the form of active euthanasia or PAD—to currently accepted practices (such as forgoing LSMT), instead of all of these practices being embraced, they may instead all be rejected, setting the whole end-of-life debate back decades (Kamisar, 1995; Teno & Lynn, 1991). In some ways, it is a gamble that society is more committed to "letting die" than opposed to actively hastening death, which is far from clear.

Non-abandonment

Another argument made in favor of legalized PAD is non-abandonment. A physician's sacred role is to care for a patient through times of illness as well as health, and the request for aid in dying is a sign of both the patient's need as well as his trust in the physician. Data from Oregon make clear that some physician-patient relationships have been in place for nearly forty years when that request is made. To deny such a heartfelt plea could amount to abandoning the patient at the moment of his greatest need. As Quill (2014) writes in describing just such a situation: "Because I had made a commitment not to abandon Cynthia at this critical moment, my obligation as her physician was to help her meet death on her own terms as much as possible."

Some physician-patient relationships are not as longstanding, however, including some which were initiated by the request for a lethal prescription. It is hard to imagine "abandoning" a patient when no prior relationship exists. Further, "abandonment" suggests that the physician ignores the patient's plight and does not attempt to assist in any way. In states where PAD is not legal, one would hope that physicians would meet requests for hastened death with compassion and concern, doing what is in their power to alleviate the patient's suffering and stand by that patient until the end—in other words, provide palliative care (of which PAD is not an element).

Even if PAD is legal, physicians still have the right not to participate. In arguing that PAD should be legal everywhere based on non-abandonment, advocates risk condemning nonparticipating physicians as "abandoners." They also risk reducing the physician-patient relationship to a willingness to write a lethal prescription, when in fact it is much more than that.

Transparency

The final primary argument in favor of legalization is based on transparency. Even though PAD is explicitly legal in only five states—and as recently as 1994 was legal in none—it continues to occur in states where it is not. Even before PAD was first legalized in Oregon in the 1990s, some physicians worked under the rubric of "don't ask, don't tell," surreptitiously advising terminally ill patients experiencing great suffering not to take more than a certain number of pills to "avoid the risk" of hastened death (Quill & Greenlaw, 2008). According to one study, 3% of physicians in the United States had been party to PAD at least once (Meier et al., 1998).

This proves that PAD is going to happen, whether it is legal or not. Acknowledging this, some argue that it is better to bring the practice out into the open, establish safeguards, and measure it. This would highlight at-risk populations or abuses of the system, for in the absence of specific regulations—which must be followed in order to spare the physician risk of criminal or civil prosecution in states where it is now legal—such acts might involve impetuous decisions by patients whose DMC is compromised. Analogous to Prohibition or pre-*Roe v. Wade* abortion bans, criminalizing a morally contentious practice will not eradicate it from society; rather, it will drive it underground and make it more dangerous for all involved.

What this argument fails to recognize is that legalization will make PAD more common, since there would be no legal injunction against it. For even if criminalization does not completely eradicate the practice, it surely provides a disincentive for physicians to participate in it. Legalization thus increases the risk that some patients who "shouldn't" have access to PAD will, while at the same time assuming that in the absence of legalization patients who "should" have access to it might not. Both of these assumptions are addressed later (p. 242).

Arguments Against PAD
Wrongness of Killing

The most fundamental argument against PAD is that it involves the killing of a patient.[6] For while the physician does not administer the lethal dose—as in the case of euthanasia—she does intentionally provide the means by which the patient can end his life. Even though physicians generally do not take the Hippocratic Oath anymore, most physicians' oaths—and current codes of ethics—still contain a primary injunction against causing harm to the patient (*primum non nocere*) (Gaylin, Kass, Pellegrino, & Siegler, 1988).

Some advocates would dispute the equivalence of PAD and killing. Battin and Quill (2004) contend that "PAD is certainly not 'killing' in the pejorative sense of robbing someone of a life he or she values and that could otherwise continue." Yet unlike murder—which has been defined as the killing of an innocent person—"killing" is a broad term that encompasses both acceptable and unacceptable versions. Some forms of killing may be laudable (e.g., to rescue another person threatened by someone else's immoral acts), while others are at the very least excusable (e.g., in self-defense). It would seem more honest to admit that PAD—like euthanasia—represents killing, and then attempt to defend it as one of the exceptions to the general rule. The fact that proponents go to such lengths to claim—contrary to what appears obvious—that PAD does not represent self-killing underscores the difficulty in defending it for what it really is.

Physician-Patient Relationship

In contrast to the non-abandonment argument in favor of legalizing PAD, some have argued that consideration of PAD taints the physician-patient relationship by introducing a layer of complexity that is often unspoken yet nevertheless significant. Consider the following example: A patient has just been diagnosed with a terminal illness and goes to see his long-time primary doctor. Upon hearing of the diagnosis, the physician asks, "How can I help?" If PAD were not a legitimate consideration, this question would be interpreted in light of the basic goals of medicine: to help patients live longer and/or live better (in terms of function and quality of life). The physician might be asking if the patient wants to try disease-modifying therapy in the hopes of prolonging life, or if he wishes to focus on comfort in the time he has left. The physician is also offering emotional support at an extremely difficult time.

But if PAD *is* a consideration, perhaps the physician is inquiring about something else: "Do you want me to help you die sooner?" Even if the physician is not actually asking

---

6. Some might use the term "sanctity of life" to describe this argument, but often that term is taken too far. It has been used as justification for maximal treatment in every situation when life can possibly be prolonged, which overlooks a competent patient's right to refuse LSMT when the burdens of treatment outweigh the benefits. To some, it suggests that life itself is the ultimate consideration, without regard for the quality of that life. Of all medical specialties, palliative care in particular recognizes that a patient's goals and values matter just as much as his physiologic existence, and thus the more measured term "wrongness of killing" is used (Quill & Greenlaw, 2008).

that, the patient may *think* she is. For a patient who is not interested in PAD, this may be off-putting or even threatening. And in contrast to the "insurance policy" argument noted earlier—which inaccurately asserts that legalization of PAD would provide comfort to all patients, even those who might never access it—the *possibility* of PAD does affect every patient, with regard to the unspoken assumptions and subtext which pervade important conversations with their physicians.

The key point here is not that the physician-patient relationship becomes more "complex"—which is not necessarily a bad thing—but rather it becomes something different than it once was. Universally accepted norms (e.g., that physicians must not intentionally hasten death) would no longer hold. At a point where the patient is most vulnerable, the relationship that should sustain him may, instead, introduce doubt and mistrust. As Kass (2002) writes, "Anyone who understands even a little of the subtle psychodynamics of the doctor-patient relationship can see immediately the corrosive effects of doubt and suspicion that will be caused by explicit (or avoided) speech about physician-assisted death." For this reason, the American Medical Association (2010–2011) concludes, "Physician-assisted suicide is fundamentally incompatible with the physician's role as healer."

Exploitation of the Vulnerable

The "poster child" for the legalization of PAD is a terminally patient in unrelenting pain who is receiving hospice care, has thoughtfully considered all of his options, and has—with fully intact DMC—elected to hasten death through PAD. As noted, some of these characteristics are true of most patients who end their life through PAD (such as hospice enrollment), while others are not (such as unrelenting pain). But the one that should, given legal requirements, be common to all patients is having sufficient DMC to voluntarily choose PAD.

Some opponents of PAD have cited specific cases where they claim patients have been coerced into PAD or been inappropriately assisted in ingesting the lethal dose (Foley & Hendin, 2002). Advocates, understandably, have questioned these accusations, and it is beyond the scope of this textbook to investigate their veracity. From personal experience, though, clinicians who are advocates of legalization of PAD—and are willing to write a lethal prescription—generally are extremely prudent in their application of the law. A far cry from Jack Kevorkian's "Dr. Death," pro-PAD clinicians are methodical in attempting to address the patient's suffering without ultimately resorting to PAD. It is not uncommon for them to decline requests to prescribe the lethal dose even for a patient who legally qualifies when they believe that the patient might benefit from a different type of treatment.

Rather than relying on anecdotal cases of purported abuse, it is more appropriate to look at aggregate data to evaluate concerns for exploitation of the vulnerable. And that data from Oregon is concerning, especially with regard to screening for depression. Studies have shown that more than half of patients with a genuine desire for death are depressed, a more direct connection than either pain or low family support (Chochinov et al., 1995). Indeed, in one Oregon study, one in five patients who requested PAD were found to be depressed (Ganzini et al., 2000).

Legally, there is no requirement to seek mental health evaluation for all patients requesting PAD but only those in whom the physician is concerned for depression or impaired DMC. Over time, however, the percentage of patients who received psychiatric evaluation before they received their PAD prescription and took the lethal dose has markedly declined. Over 30% underwent psychiatric evaluation in the first two years that PAD was legal in Oregon, but less than 4% did so in 2016. (The average over the entire span was approximately 5%; State of Oregon, 2016.)

There is no reason to believe that patients requesting PAD have greater DMC now than twenty years ago. A more reasonable conclusion is that clinicians are becoming more comfortable—some might even say "complacent"—as PAD becomes more accepted in that environment. Even if clinicians are vigilant, studies have shown that less than one in seven are able to identify depression in cancer patients with moderate to severe depression (Passik et al., 1998). Even psychiatrists are hard-pressed to diagnose the condition in a single visit (Ganzini & Fenn, 1996). Depression is notoriously underassessed and undertreated in elderly patients in particular (Conwell & Caine, 1991). When treated, however, depressed patients who had requested PAD often change their minds (Emanuel, Fairclough, & Emanuel, 2000).

In addition to potentially missing cases of incapacitating depression, another concern involves populations who historically have been undertreated by the medical profession: disabled persons, women, and minorities. The first group, in particular, has been extremely vocal in their opposition to legalization of PAD. Disability rights groups such as "Not Dead Yet" have expressed concern about external judgments about quality of life, which could lead disabled persons to feel pressured—or even expected—to hasten their own deaths. As Coleman (2002) writes, "As human beings, by now we should know ourselves and each other well enough to recognize that people, whether individuals or corporations, cannot be trusted with the right to kill other people, especially people who are socially devalued."

In addition to disabled persons, women and minorities are other groups that may suffer discrimination in the face of legalized PAD. Studies have shown that African Americans are less likely to favor PAD (Lichtenstein, Alcser, Corning, Bachman, & Doukas, 1997), and some feminist commentators have observed that women are at greater risk because they live longer, are more likely to be poor or uninsured, and are less likely to have pain treated than men (Wolf, 1996). This is precisely the point made by the Supreme Court in *Washington v. Glucksberg*:

> The State's assisted suicide ban reflects and reinforces its policy that the lives of terminally ill, disabled, and elderly people must be no less valued than the young and the healthy, and that a seriously disabled person's suicidal impulses should be interpreted and treated the same way as anyone else's.

For all the concerns about exploitation of the vulnerable, however, there is no empirical evidence that disabled persons, women, or minorities have, in fact, been exploited. Data from Oregon show that the vast majority of patients who have hastened their death through PAD are financially stable, well-educated, and enrolled in hospice.

Notably, some advocates of PAD also express concern about discrimination in its implementation, but not because certain groups might be coerced into engaging in it; rather, advocates are concerned that these groups might be deprived of *their right* to PAD. For instance, the requirement that the patient self-administer the lethal dose was intended as a safeguard against abuse, but some have argued that it is actually discriminatory because it precludes patients with certain disabilities—such as quadriplegia—from exercising their right to assistance in dying (Batavia, 2004). While some disability rights groups (such as Not Dead Yet) are opposed to legalization of PAD, others (such as AUTONOMY, Inc.) are in favor of it, concerned that disabled persons will be deprived of yet another fundamental human right (in this case, the right to assistance in hastening death).

This reversal of the discrimination argument logically raises the final—and perhaps most compelling—argument against PAD: the slippery slope.

Slippery Slope

The statutory requirements for PAD in the states where it has been legalized are quite standardized and rather rigorous. Over time, though, it is very possible that monitoring and requirements restrictions will begin to ease. Indeed, this is precisely what appears to have occurred in Oregon with regard to screening for potential depression. Even as there are few—if any—clear examples of abuse of current regulations, some advocates are lobbying for a broadening of the "right" to PAD, softening the requirements for self-administration, life expectancy of less than six months, and intact DMC.

After all, if the primary arguments in favor of PAD are autonomy and compassion, why restrict such noble sentiments to patients at the end of their lives? Shouldn't someone facing *years* of diminished autonomy and dignity be even more deserving of PAD, should he request it (Kamisar 1995)? Given physicians' well-documented deficiencies in the area of prognostication (p. 85), under current law many patients who will die within six months would be prevented from utilizing PAD because of overestimates of their life expectancy.

And why should patients with dementia who previously expressed a wish for PAD be prevented from obtaining it, simply because they currently lack DMC? Or patients with serious mental illness that is clearly causing great suffering? Indeed, some proponents of legalization of PAD in its current form specifically envision the possibility of expansion of the law to include groups currently excluded. Brock (2004) writes, "*Initially* restricting assisted suicide to the terminally ill would allow assessment of how realistic the risks and abuses feared by opponents are before extending the practice to patients who are not terminally ill" (emphasis added).

This highlights a logical inconsistency in the argument for legalization of PAD: if compassion and respect for autonomy are the prevailing concerns—essentially reducing the entire question to one of *voluntariness*—why limit who is able to utilize PAD? If PAD is okay for anyone, it should be okay for *everyone* regardless of their life expectancy or current level of DMC (Ackerman, 1998). And if surrogate decision-making is sufficient to forgo LSMT—which also leads to a patient's death—shouldn't it also be sufficient to authorize PAD (Cohn & Lynn, 2002), especially if the two are ethically equivalent as PAD advocates argue?

The slippery slope seems an apt description of PAD in both the Netherlands and Belgium. PAD (and euthanasia) began as a commonly accepted though extralegal prac- tice in the Netherlands and subsequently has been legalized and expanded in use to even include euthanasia of impaired newborns (p. 326). Similarly in Belgium, a practice that had once been reserved for competent adults now permits children with severe depres- sion to hasten their deaths, even as supporters of PAD advocate for expanding access to severely demented patients who previously requested it (p. 151).

Defenders of PAD will point to the cultural differences between the Benelux coun- tries on the one hand and the United States on the other. They also claim that data from Oregon should dispel concerns about the slippery slope. Yet while nineteen years (as of this writing) may seem like a long time, in the course of cultural change it is not, as the expansion of laws in those countries over time attests. To assert that the current form of PAD in the United States will never expand seems short-sighted at best and disingenuous at worst (especially in light of advocates' expressed intentions to do precisely that).

Conclusions

There would seem to be four possible positions on the issue of PAD:

1. PAD and active euthanasia should both be legal.
2. PAD should be legal, although active euthanasia should not be.
3. PAD should be illegal but in some cases may be ethical.
4. PAD should be illegal and is always unethical. (Fins, 2006)

The first option is not acceptable, for the reasons cited previously (p. 150). And while some have advocated for the fourth option (Yang & Curlin, 2016), this seems too ex- treme. There is a good reason that Brittany Maynard became "the new face" of PAD: she was articulate, intelligent, and thoughtful, and was facing a certain and debilitating death. She should not be judged, nor should anyone else who has availed themselves of PAD. The question—at least from a public policy perspective—is not whether PAD is ever eth- ically justified but rather whether it should be *legalized*.

In determining that, it is worth noting the stark contrast between pro-PAD and anti-PAD arguments. The latter tend to be philosophical (the physician's moral duty), theoretical (the slippery slope), and difficult to quantify (the effect on the physician-patient relationship). By contrast, arguments in favor are often heart-wrenching and personal, like the story of Brittany Maynard. For some people, one compelling example determines the conclusion. If even a single patient suffers unnecessarily by virtue of being deprived of PAD, then it should be legalized. To oppose legalization seems to overlook the suffering of people like Ms. Maynard and to condemn them for doing what they believed in their hearts was right.

Yet, as Pellegrino (2002) observes, "even an emotion so powerful, necessary, and ubiquitous [as compassion] needs the restraint of reason." Sometimes the step necessary to give one person what they need ends up harming a great many others. For example, imagine a patient with metastatic cancer and extreme pain that is managed with high doses of oral morphine. Further imagine that the patient has run out of medication and discovers at the pharmacy that no refills remain on his prescription. The patient's physician is unavailable and the nearest emergency department is far away.

This is a terrible situation, but the appropriate response is not to alter the law to allow patients to write their own morphine prescriptions. That would certainly have saved this patient from suffering needlessly, but it would cause incalculable harm to other patients. As the old saying goes, "Hard cases do not make good laws" (Holdsworth, 1926).

Applied to PAD, this means that legalization does not just enable patients who "should" have access to PAD to get it; it also allows other patients to hasten their deaths who "should not" (not to mention the impact on patients who would never want PAD but whose relationship with their physician is altered by it being a legal consideration). Whereas the poster child for PAD is a hospice patient who continues to suffer from extreme pain and—with full capacity—chooses PAD and informs his family of this, the poster child for the other side is a terminally ill patient who is in no pain at all, has refused hospice care, is grappling with the future loss of independence, and has not told any of his loved ones of his intention to hasten his death. Both patients legally qualify for PAD, but the second might even give ardent advocates pause.

Some have argued that this objection is out of proportion to reality. They claim that those who would be improperly deprived of PAD by a blanket prohibition "would undoubtedly be . . . vastly greater" than the number of people who would "mistakenly" receive assistance (Dworkin et al., 1997). Even if this is true—and it is far from clear that it is—the objection is not a simple calculation of which "side" is numerically greater. Certain errors are so egregious that extensive steps must be taken to prevent them from occurring, even at the risk of limiting the options of others. To take a legal example, the American criminal justice system is predicated on the belief that no innocent person should ever be punished, even at the cost of allowing guilty people to go free on technicalities. Analogously, shouldn't the legal system do everything in its power to eliminate the possibility that even one person's death be hastened improperly?

There are other options available to people who seek PAD, after all. The argument that without PAD a patient would be condemned to live out a burdensome existence overlooks other so-called "exit ramps." Even if a terminally ill patient does not currently require LSMT, complications—such as pneumonia—invariably arise as a condition progresses. When this occurs, the patient has an undeniable right to refuse LSMT and even transfer to the hospital. As Diane Meier was quoted as saying, "The notion that if people don't kill themselves they're going to die on a ventilator in the hospital would be humorous if it weren't so serious" (Aviv, 2015).

Prior to that—or in the absence of a terminal diagnosis—VSED is an ethically acceptable option (p. 154). Granted, it requires more time, but it also confirms voluntariness in ways that a one-moment-in-time ingestion cannot. VSED also will lead to death more quickly than PAD, given the legally mandated waiting periods of the latter. Advocates of PAD cannot, therefore, claim that patients requesting it have no other option to hasten their deaths. There is at least one other option, although it may not be their preferred one.

Just because PAD is not legal does not mean it never happens, or even that it should not happen. To some, ethics and the law are so closely entwined that it would be unthinkable to break the law. But there are clear examples where it is highly ethical to break the law, such as in the case of nonviolent civil disobedience (Macauley, 2005). And given the stakes involved in PAD—especially the risk that a patient may end his life in a violent manner if denied it—there could be instances where a physician feels ethically compelled to defy the law and write a lethal prescription (Fins, 2006).

It may appear inconsistent to argue that PAD should be illegal yet nevertheless endorse it in some cases. But from a public policy perspective, this may be the only way to ensure that the bar for providing PAD is so high as to prevent those who should not have access to it from hastening their deaths. There are some medical practices which are right so rarely that it makes sense to keep them illegal, thereby ensuring that physicians only engage in them when the stakes are sufficiently high that it is worth risking the legal consequences (Ramsey, 1970). This is precisely the position of certain Belgian physicians who—despite many having practiced euthanasia when it was illegal—nevertheless generally opposed legalization because they did not want to make "the exception the rule" (Aviv, 2015).

Up to now, the discussion has focused on whether PAD should be legalized and how physicians who might wish to prescribe a lethal dose should respond if it is not. But what of the physician who is morally opposed to the practice, yet works in a state where it *is* legal? Clearly, there is no legal requirement that she participate in PAD, although she may choose to set aside her moral reservations so as not to feel like she is "abandoning" her patient. She may also choose to refer the patient to another physician who is willing to prescribe.

But what if the physician's moral opposition is so deep that she would feel complicit by referring? This is analogous to physicians who are opposed to abortion and feel conflicted about referring pregnant women seeking termination to a provider who is willing to provide it. Some physicians even go so far as to withhold information about the practice itself, whether it be abortion or PAD (Curlin, Lawrence, Chin, & Lantos, 2007). What is the best way to balance the patient's right to receive a legal procedure with the physician's right of conscience, especially with regard to PAD which—unlike abortion for the pregnant patient—a terminally ill patient may not know is even an option?

Fortunately, in the case of PAD, advocacy organizations exist whose mission is to make sure that patients are informed about what PAD is, who qualifies for it, and which physicians participate in it. The last of these is often not commonly known, for fear that opponents of the practice might target those clinicians just as abortion providers have been. So when a physician who is not willing to participate in PAD refers the patient to such an organization, it is not abdication of her professional responsibility, and (hopefully) also not a violation of his personal beliefs. It is an honest response to the patient's inquiry, through which the patient will be able to receive information and services that the physician herself cannot provide.

This raises the final point: Why should be physicians be involved at all? After all, for most of Western history discussions of suicide and assisted suicide never envisioned the involvement of physicians. And lest anyone question whether non-physicians have sufficient knowledge to assist patients in hastening their own deaths, one need only look to Switzerland's practice, or the fact that most physicians in states where PAD has recently been legalized need to call advocacy organizations to learn what drugs to prescribe.

The only parts of PAD that truly require physician participation are establishing prognosis and confirming capacity. From that point on, no other legal requirements (such as verifying age and state residency) require medical training. One could envision a system where the physician provides the patient with a signed form attesting that the patient has six months or less to live—analogous to confirming hospice eligibility—and has sufficient DMC to make his own end-of-life decisions. The patient could then take the form to a regulated entity—one might call it a "Thanatology Center"—where other legal requirements would be verified and the patient's oral and written requests for assisted death could be tracked. Once the patient completes all the requirements, the Thanatology Center would dispense the lethal packet, containing standard doses of barbiturate and anti-emetic as well as instructions on how to use them.

Some might recoil at this concept. Doesn't something as important and irrevocable as assisted death require the integral involvement of a trusted physician? This assumes, of course, that there is a relationship between the patient and the physician that goes beyond the request for assisted dying which is not always the case. But even if there is, on the proposed model the physician can still provide guidance, perspective, and recommendations. The physician would not be unaware of the patient's intention; she would just not be intimately involved in accomplishing it. As a result, some of the objections to PAD—like its impact on the physician-patient relationship—would no longer be relevant.

But, more importantly, the implicit approval of the medical profession would vanish. And despite all the emphasis on PAD being the patient's decision and physicians having the right not to participate, the imprimatur of the physician is critical to societal acceptance.[7] This keeps PAD in the clinical realm, under the broader auspices of a healing profession and perhaps (inaccurately) even palliative care itself. Removed from that context and clarified as a service provided by an entity whose sole purpose is the hastening of death, assisted dying—AD with the "P" no longer attached—might well be viewed in a much less positive light.

Return to the Case

"Will you help me die?" is never a yes or no question. It can mean a great many things, including whether the patient has the right to refuse life-sustaining treatment, whether the patient will suffer at the end of life, or whether the physician will stand by him until the very end. In some cases it represents an explicit request for either PAD (which is legal in the state where this patient resides) or euthanasia (which is not legal in any state). The physician's appropriate response is to ask what the patient means by that question and what prompted him to ask it.

The patient explains that he has read about Vermont's PAD law and wants to use it. He qualifies for it based on his prognosis, and the physician believes his DMC is intact. The physician reviews other options and explores his reasons for requesting PAD, which seem extremely well thought out. She explains the mandated process and refers him to another physician for a second opinion, who confirms her impressions. The patient makes his first oral request for lethal medication and follows up with a written request and then a second oral request approximately three weeks later.

The physician sends the lethal prescription to the pharmacy, which the patient picks up later in the week. His condition continues to deteriorate, but his symptoms are well controlled. He considers taking the lethal dose many times but ultimately decides not to. He dies approximately two months later, and his family reports that he gained significant consolation from knowing that the lethal dose was "there if he needed it."

Summary Points

- The terminology used for the practice discussed in this chapter likely reflects one's position: those who refer to "physician-assisted suicide" are generally opposed and those who refer to "death with dignity" are in favor. "Physician-assisted dying" is a more neutral—as well as accurate—term.

7. This is the same reason why advocates refer to the lethal dose of a drug as "medicine."

- The US Supreme Court unanimously rejected arguments that there was a constitutional right to PAD based either on the Due Process Clause or the Equal Protection Clause of the Fourteenth Amendment. States are free to legalize the practice, however.
- PAD was first legalized in the United States in 1994 in Oregon, and as of 2017 is also legal in Washington, Vermont, California, Colorado, and the District of Columbia.
- Arguments in favor of legalizing PAD include autonomy, compassion, justice, non-abandonment, and transparency.
- Arguments against legalizing PAD include the wrongness of killing, the impact on the physician-patient relationship, exploitation of the vulnerable, and the slippery slope.
- It is inaccurate to claim that PAD represents the only recourse for patients who are not dependent on life-sustaining medical treatment, as voluntarily stopping eating and drinking is an option, as is palliative sedation for refractory symptoms.
- It is possible to oppose legalization of PAD without believing that it is ethically wrong in every case. This serves to "raise the bar" for PAD such that only the most exceptional of situations merit it, thereby protecting others who might avail themselves of it inappropriately.

References

Ackerman, F. (1998). Assisted suicide, terminal illness, severe disability, and the double standard. In M. P. Battin, R. Rhodes, & A. Silvers (Eds.), *Physician assisted suicide: Expanding the debate* (pp. 149–162). New York: Routledge.

American Academy of Hospice and Palliative Medicine. (2016). Physician-assisted dying position statement. Retrieved from http://aahpm.org/positions/pad

American College of Physicans. (2017). Ethics and the legalization of physician-assisted suicide. *Ann Intern Med, 167*(8), 576–578. doi:10.7326/M17-0938

American Medical Association. (2010–2011). Code of medical ethics, annotated current opinions. Chicago: American Medical Association.

American Medical Student Association. (2008). Preambles, purposes, principles: Principles regarding physicain aid in dying. Retrieved from http://www.amsa.org/wp-content/uploads/2015/03/PPP-2015.pdf

American Medical Women's Association. (2007). Position paper on aid in dying. Retrieved from https://www.amwa-doc.org/wp-content/uploads/2013/12/Aid_in_Dying1.pdf

American Public Health Association. (2008). Patients' rights to self-determination at the end of life. Retrieved from https://www.apha.org/policies-and-advocacy/public-health-policy-statements/policy-database/2014/07/29/13/28/patients-rights-to-self-determination-at-the-end-of-life

Andorno, R. (2013). Nonphysician-assisted suicide in Switzerland. *CQ, 22*(3), 246–253. doi:10.1017/S0963180113000054

Angell, M. (2014, October 31). The Brittany Maynard effect: How she is changing the debate on assisted dying. *The Washington Post.*

Aquinas, T. (2012). *Summa theologiae secunda secundae, 1-91: The complete works of saint aquinas.* Lander, WY: Aquinas Institute for the Study of Sacred Doctrine.

Aristotle. (1953). *The Nicomachean ethics.* London: Allen & Unwin.

Augustine. (2006). *The city of God* (The Barnes & Noble Library of Essential Reading). New York: Barnes & Noble.

Aviv, R. (2015, June 22). The Death Treatment. *The New Yorker.*

Batavia, A. I. (2004). Disability and physician-assisted dying. In T. E. Quill & M. P. Battin (Eds.), *Physician-assisted dying: The case for palliative care and patient choice* (pp. 55–74). Baltimore: Johns Hopkins University Press.

Baxter v. Montana. (2009). In *Mont. Sup. Ct.*: MT 449, 354 Mont. 234, 224 P.3d 1211.

Brock, D. W. (1992). Voluntary active euthanasia. *Hastings Cent Rep, 22*(2), 10–22.

Caplan, A. L. (2014). Terminally ill woman chooses suicide, may influence a new generation. Retrieved from http://www.medscape.com/viewarticle/833603

Carter v. Canada. (2015). 2015 SCC 5, 1 S.C.R. 331.

Catholic Church. (1994). *Catechism of the Catholic Church.* Chicago: Loyola University Press.

Chochinov, H. M., Wilson, K. G., Enns, M., Mowchun, N., Lander, S., Levitt, M., & Clinch, J. J. (1995). Desire for death in the terminally ill. *Am J Psychiatr, 152*(8), 1185–1191.

Christakis, N. A. (1999). *Death foretold: Prophecy and prognosis in medical care.* Chicago: University of Chicago.

Cicero, M. T. (1968). *De finibus bonorum et malorum.* (James S. Reid, Trans.). Hildesheim: G. Olms.

Cohn, F., & Lynn, J. (2002). Vulnerable people. In K. M. Foley & H. Hendin (Eds.), *The case against assisted suicide: For the right to end-of-life care* (pp. 238–260). Baltimore: Johns Hopkins University Press.

Coleman, D. (2002). Not dead yet. In K. M. Foley & H. Hendin (Eds.), *The case against assisted suicide: For the right to end-of-life care* (pp. 213–237). Baltimore: Johns Hopkins University Press.

Conwell, Y., & Caine, E. D. (1991). Rational suicide and the right to die: Reality and myth. *N Engl J Med, 325*(15), 1100–1103. doi:10.1056/NEJM199110103251511

Cruzan v. Director, Missouri Department of Health, 497 261 (S.Ct. 1990).

Curlin, F. A., Lawrence, R. E., Chin, M. H., & Lantos, J. D. (2007). Religion, conscience, and controversial clinical practices. *N Engl J Med, 356*(6), 593–600. doi:10.1056/NEJMsa065316

Death with Dignity. (2016). For healthcare providers. Retrieved from https://www.deathwithdignity.org/learn/healthcare-providers/.

Dembosky, A. (2016). Drug company jacks up cost of aid-in-dying medication. Retrieved from https://www.npr.org/sections/health-shots/2016/03/23/471595323/drug-company-jacks-up-cost-of-aid-in-dying-medication

Donne, J. (1977). *Biathanatos: The Literature of death and dying.* New York: Arno Press.

Dworkin, R., Nagel, T., Nozick, R., Rawls, J., Scanlon, T., & Thomson, J. J. (1997). Assisted suicide: The philosophers' brief. *The New York Review of Books,* 41–47.

Edwards, M. J., & Tolle, S. W. (1992). Disconnecting a ventilator at the request of a patient who knows he will then die: The doctor's anguish. *Ann Intern Med, 117*(3), 254–256.

Emanuel, E. J., Fairclough, D. L., & Emanuel L. L. Attitudes and desires related to euthanasia and physician-assisted suicide among terminally ill patients and their caregivers. (2000). *JAMA, 284*(19), 2460–2468.

Fins, J. (2006). *A palliative ethic of care: Clinical wisdom at life's end.* Sudbury, MA: Jones and Bartlett.

Fischer, S., Huber, C. A., Imhof, L., Mahrer Imhof R., Furter, M., Ziegler, S. J., Bosshard, G. (2008). Suicide assisted by two Swiss right-to-die organisations. *J Med Ethics, 34*(11), 810–814. doi:10.1136/jme.2007.023887

Foley, K. M., Hendin, H. (2002). The Oregon experiment. In K. M. Foley & H. Hendin (Eds.), *The case against assisted suicide: For the right to end-of-life care* (pp. 144–174). Baltimore: Johns Hopkins University Press.

Ganzini, L., & Fenn, D. S. (1996). Attitudes of Oregon psychiatrists toward physician-assisted suicide. *Am J Psychiatr, 153*(11), 1469–1475.

Ganzini, L., Nelson, H. D., Schmidt, T. A., Kraemer, D. F., Delorit, M. A., & Lee, M. A. (2000). Physicians' experiences with the Oregon Death with Dignity Act. *N Engl J Med, 342*(8), 557–563. doi:10.1056/NEJM200002243420806

Gaylin, W., Kass, L. R., Pellegrino, E. D., & Siegler, M., (1988). "Doctors must not kill." *JAMA, 259*(14), 2139–2140.

Hippocrates. (1923). *Hippocrates.* London, New York,: W. Heinemann; G.P. Putnam's Sons.

Holdsworth, W. S. (1926). *History of English law.* Vol. IX. Boston: Little, Brown.

Hume, D. (1934). *A treatise of human nature* (Ernest Rhys, Ed.). 2 vols. (Everyman's Library). New York: E.P. Dutton.

Humphry, D. (1991). *Final exit* [Sound recording]. Beverly Hills, CA: Dove Audio.

Humphry, D. (2005). Farewell to hemlock: Killed by its name. Retrieved from http://www.assistedsuicide.org/farewell-to-hemlock.html

In re Quinlan, 70 10 (N.J. 1976).

Kamisar, Y. (1995). Against assisted suicide—even a very limited form. *Univ Detroit Mercy Law Rev, 72*(4), 735–769.

Kant, I. (1964). *The doctrine of virtue. Part II of the Metaphysic of morals* (Harper Torchbooks, The Cloister Library). New York: Harper & Row.

Kao, A. C., & Parsi, K. P. (2004). Content analyses of oaths administered at U.S. medical schools in 2000. *Acad Med, 79*(9), 882–887.

Kass, L. (2002). I will give no deadly drug: Why doctors must not kill. In K. M. Foley & H. Hendin (Eds.), *The case against assisted suicide: For the right to end-of-life care* (pp. 17–40). Baltimore: Johns Hopkins University Press.

Konnolly, K. (2008, March 21). Dignitas attacked for new assisted suicide method. *The Guardian.*

Ledig, M., & Samuel, H. (2007, November 9). Swiss suicide group operates in car parks. *The Telegraph.*

Lichtenstein, R. L., Alcser, K. H., Corning, A. D., Bachman, J. G., & Doukas, D. J. (1997). Black/white differences in attitudes toward physician-assisted suicide. *J Natl Med Assoc, 89*(2), 125–133.

Macauley, R. (2005). The Hippocratic underground: Civil disobedience and health care reform. *Hastings Cent Rep, 35*(1), 38–45.

Maynard, B. (2014, October 27). My decision to die. *People.*

Meier, D. E., Emmons, C. A., Wallenstein, S., Quill, T., Morrison, R. S., & Cassel, C. K. (1998). A national survey of physician-assisted suicide and euthanasia in the United States. *N Engl J Med, 338*(17), 1193–1201. doi:10.1056/NEJM199804233381706

Montaigne, M. de. (1958). *Complete essays.* Stanford, CA: Stanford University Press.

Morris v. Brandenburg. (2016). 376 N.M. P.3d 836.

National Hospice and Palliative Care Organization. (2005). Commentary and resolution on physician assisted suicide. Retrieved from http://www.nhpco.org/sites/default/files/public/PAS_Resolution_Commentary.pdf

Nitschke, P., & Stewart, F. (2010). *The peaceful pill handbook.* Bellingham, WA: Exit International US.

Orentlicher, D. (1997). The Supreme Court and physician-assisted suicide—rejecting assisted suicide but embracing euthanasia. *N Engl J Med, 337*(17), 1236–1239. doi:10.1056/NEJM199710233371713

Passik, S. D., Dugan, W., McDonald, M. V., Rosenfeld, B., Theobald, D. E., & Edgerton, S. (1998). Oncologists' recognition of depression in their patients with cancer. *J Clin Oncol, 16*(4), 1594–1600.

Pellegrino, E D. (2002). Compassion is not enough. In K. M. Foley & H. Hendin (Eds.), *The case against assisted suicide: for the right to end-of-life care* (pp. 41–51). Baltimore: Johns Hopkins University Press.

Plato. (1984). *Four texts on Socrates: Plato's Euthyphro, Apology, and Crito, and Aristophanes' Clouds.* Ithaca, NY: Cornell University Press.

Putnam, C. E. (2002). *Hospice or hemlock? Searching for heroic compassion.* Westport, CT: Praeger.

Quill, T., & Greenlaw, J. (2008). Physician-assisted death. In M. Crowley (Ed.), *From birth to death and bench to clinic: The Hastings Center bioethics briefing book for journalists, policymakers, and campaigns* (pp. 137–142). Garrison, NY: The Hastings Center.

Quill, T. E. (2014). Physician-assisted death. In T. E. Quill & F. G. Miller (Eds.), *Palliative care and ethics* (pp. 247–265). New York: Oxford University Press.

Quill, T. E., & Battin, M. P. (2004). False dichotomy versus genuine choice: The argument over physician-assisted dying. In T. E. Quill & M. P. Battin (Eds.), *Physician-assisted dying: The case for palliative care and patient choice* (pp. 1–14). Baltimore: Johns Hopkins University Press.

Rachels, J. (1975). Active and passive euthanasia. *N Engl J Med, 292*(2), 78–80. doi:10.1056/NEJM197501092920206

Ramsey, P. (1970). *The patient as person; Explorations in medical ethics* (The Lyman Beecher Lectures at Yale University). New Haven, CT: Yale University Press.

Schopenhauer, A., Norman, J., Welchman, A., & Janaway, C. (2010). *The world as will and representation* (The Cambridge Edition of the Works of Schopenhauer). Cambridge, UK; New York: Cambridge University Press.

State of Oregon. (2016). *Death with Dignity Act.* Retrieved from http://public.health.oregon.gov/ProviderPartnerResources/EvaluationResearch/DeathwithDignityAct/Pages/index.aspx

State of Washington. (1979). Natural Death Act. Chapter 70.122 RCW.

Swiss Federal Criminal Code. (1937). Article 115.

Szasz, T. (2002). *Fatal freedom: The ethics and politics of suicide.* Syracuse, NY: Syracuse University Press.

Teno, J., & Lynn, J. (1991). Voluntary active euthanasia: The individual case and public policy. *J Amer Geriatr Soc, 39*(8), 827–830.

Termination of Life on Request and Assisted Suicide (Review Procedures) Act. (2001). *Ethic Perspect, 9*(2–3), 176–181.

Vacco v. Quill. (1997). 521 U.S. 793.

Washington v. Glucksberg. (1997). 521 U.S. 702.

Wolf, S. M. (1996). Gender, feminism, and death: Physician-assisted suicide and euthanasia. In S. M. Wolf (Ed.), *Feminism & bioethics: Beyond reproduction* (pp. 282–317). New York: Oxford University Press.

World Health Organization. (2002). WHO definition of palliative care. Retrieved from www.who.int/cancer/palliative/definition/en/

Yang, Y. T., & Curlin, F. A. (2016). Why physicians should oppose assisted suicide. *JAMA, 315*(3), 247–248. doi:10.1001/jama.2015.16194

9

Palliative Sedation

Case Study

A sixty-three-year-old woman with metastatic stomach cancer is admitted to the hospital because her abdominal pain and nausea could not be managed adequately at home. She is receiving escalating doses of opioids, but she still rates her pain as 10 out of 10. There are concerns for opioid-induced hyperalgesia, which has not improved with opioid rotation. Even maximal treatment with anti-emetics is not helping her nausea, which is worsened by the opioids.

The patient is unable—and has shown no desire—to eat or drink, and the only IV fluids she is receiving are those necessary to deliver her medications. She is not dependent on any life-sustaining treatment that can be withdrawn. A do not attempt resuscitation/do not intubate (DNAR/DNI) order is in place.

Her doctors believe she has only a matter of days to live, and her loved ones are distraught over her suffering. Her son asks the attending physician, "Isn't there something else you can do to help her?"

Historical Background

Two developments in the 1960s and 1970s substantially reduced suffering at the end of life. The first was increased appreciation and utilization of opioids for pain (Saunders, 1963). The other was codification in the United States of the legal right of competent patients to refuse treatment, even if the treatment was life-sustaining (*In re Quinlan*, 1976; Natural Death Act, 1976). These seminal developments led many to conclude that all suffering at the end of life was "treatable." Even severe pain was responsive to opioids, and in exceptional cases extremely high doses which (in rare cases) could depress respiratory drive were deemed ethically acceptable (p. 209). When suffering became intolerable, life-sustaining medical treatment (LSMT)—such as ventilators, pressors, or dialysis, which many critically ill patients were dependent on—could be discontinued.

Several barriers to optimal symptom management remained, however. Some were educational, such as a lack of expertise in pain management among many physicians. This can manifest itself in "opiophobia," or a fear of using opioids out of undue concern that they might cause the patient to stop breathing and thus amounted to euthanasia (Zylicz, 1993). But even in situations where opioids—as well as other pain treatments, both pharmacologic and interventional—were used appropriately, there remained cases where patients continued to suffer, despite maximal intervention. This could be because the treatment was ineffective at relieving pain, or perhaps the treatment itself caused intolerable side effects (such as opioid-induced hyperalgesia). For patients with no LSMT to withdraw, this seemed to condemn them to intolerable suffering for however long they continued to live.

Another barrier to optimal symptom management is that pain is only one of many causes of suffering at the end of life. Other symptoms can be even more difficult to treat, such as nausea, anxiety, depression, pruritis, and others. When such symptoms are "refractory" or "intractable"[1] —and the patient is not receiving LSMT that may be forgone— the only way to prevent the patient from suffering from a symptom may be to depress the patient's consciousness to the point where she is no longer suffering from it.

Compared to active euthanasia (p. 143), the Rule of Double Effect (p. 209), or physician-assisted dying (PAD, p. 225), intentionally depressing the level of a patient's consciousness for symptom control is a relatively new concept. The fact that it is a consideration at all is due in no small part to the evolving recognition of the moral imperative to treat suffering that came out of the work Cicely Saunders and others. Advances in pharmacology and medication delivery—since this level of sedation is usually accomplished intravenously—served to make it possible. The fact that actions which intentionally hasten the patient's death (such as PAD) are hotly debated made an action that does *not* do so—yet still addresses significant suffering—more palatable.

This concept was first described in the medical literature in 1991 under the name "terminal sedation," referring to "the intention of deliberately inducing and maintaining deep sleep, but not deliberately causing death in very specific circumstances" (Enck, 1991). The choice of the modifier "terminal" reflected its relationship to end-of-life care, but some were concerned that this might suggest that the sedation—rather than the underlying disease—was the cause of death (Broeckaert & Nunez-Olarte, 2002). It also does not clearly indicate that the purpose of the sedation is symptom control.

---

1.   In common use some might use "refractory" to refer to symptoms that have not responded to initial treatment, with "intractable" referring to symptoms that have continued despite all available treatments. In this text, these terms are used interchangeably to refer to symptoms that have not responded to appropriate treatment.

Over time the concept has come to be referred to in many other ways, such as "controlled sedation" (Mercadante et al., 2009) and "continuous sedation" (Papavasiliou, Payne, Brearley, Brown, & Seymour, 2012). At present there seems to be an evolving consensus to refer to the practice as "palliative sedation therapy" (Morita, Tsuneto, & Shima, 2001) or simply "palliative sedation" (Materstvedt & Kaasa, 2011). The latter term is used here to refer to "the use of sedative medications to relieve intolerable suffering from refractory symptoms by a reduction in patient consciousness" (de Graeff & Dean, 2007).

Legal and Professional

The definitive legal determination related to palliative sedation came in the context of the pivotal Supreme Court decisions in 1997 dealing with PAD. In *Vacco v. Quill*, the Court found that there was a difference between allowing a patient to die and causing that patient to die. As a result, the Court concluded that there was no constitutional right to aid in dying because state laws prohibiting PAD did not violate the Equal Protection Clause of the Fourteenth Amendment.

Although this case—as well as *Washington v. Glucksberg*, decided in the same fashion in the same year—was primarily concerned with PAD, the Court also weighed in on the practice of palliative sedation, without using that specific term.

> The pain of most terminally ill patients can be controlled throughout the dying process without heavy sedation or anesthesia. . . . For a very few patients, however, sedation to a sleep-like state may be necessary in the last days or weeks of life to prevent the patient from experiencing severe pain. (*Vacco v. Quill*, 1997)

One might say, then, that in rejecting a constitutional right on the question they were asked, the Court affirmed such a right on a question they were not, namely, the legality of palliative sedation (Orentlicher, 1997).

To be sure, the Court's observation does not represent an in-depth exploration of the concept of palliative sedation. It makes specific reference to "severe pain" without elaborating on the use of less significant steps to control that pain before palliative sedation is considered, and it does not mention other symptoms (such as delirium) that might justify the use of palliative sedation. It also does not specify the precise life expectancy that would justify palliative sedation, instead using the phrase "last days or weeks of life."

As a position statement the Court's position leaves much to be desired. But in terms of establishing a precedent that palliative sedation is legal in certain circumstances, the Court's decision is of indisputable significance. No longer can one claim that palliative sedation is illegal. One can, however, debate whether *specific instances* of palliative sedation comport with the brief description the court offered.

From a professional perspective, a wide range of bodies have asserted the ethical permissibility of palliative sedation, including the American Medical Association

(2010–2011), the American College of Physicians (Quill & Byock, 2000a), the American Academy of Hospice and Palliative Medicine (2014), the National Hospice and Palliative Care Organization (2010), the Veterans Administration (Veterans Health Administration National Ethics Committee, 2006), and the American Academy of Pain Medicine (2003), as well as various consensus panels (de Graeff & Dean, 2007). Some requirements are common to all of these position statements, such as that the symptom be refractory and intolerable, that the sedation be proportionate and a last resort, and that proper informed consent be obtained. There is significant variation in other relevant factors, however, such as the patient's prognosis and whether the suffering is physical, emotional, or existential.

Clinical

Defining what precisely the term "palliative sedation" means remains a challenge. For instance, sedation is a well-known side effect of many medications that are used frequently in palliative care (such as opioids for pain and benzodiazepines for anxiety, which have additive effects when used in combination). All medications have side effects, though, and just as it would not be reasonable to refer to the pleasure some patients experience from opioids as "palliative euphoria," similarly it makes little sense to refer to the expected and usually mild side effect of sedation as "palliative sedation." A better term for this is "ordinary sedation" (Quill, Lo, & Brock, 1997).

The concept that Enck (1991) originally defined as "inducing and maintaining deep sleep" has, over time, been refined to refer to the intentional depression of consciousness to treat suffering, either as a primary or side effect of a medication. It can be further classified based on the depth and duration of the sedation. With regard to *depth*, "mild" sedation refers to a state where a patient's level of consciousness is only slightly depressed (while still sufficient to control symptoms). The patient may appear sleepy but is able to recognize and communicate with others, and may even be able to eat and drink small amounts. Under "moderate" sedation patients have decreased extent and duration of interactivity. Only "deep" sedation entails rendering the patient entirely unconscious, as Enck originally described. Thus not all palliative sedation deprives the patient of the ability to interact, eat and drink, and participate in decision-making, which as noted later are the ethically relevant components of the practice.

With regard to *duration*, palliative sedation can be either intermittent or continuous. One form of intermittent sedation ("emergency sedation") temporarily reduces consciousness in the face of overwhelming symptoms, essentially buying time for targeted symptomatic treatment to achieve sufficient effect (Shlamovitz, Elsayem, & Todd, 2013). "Respite sedation" is another form of intermittent sedation, where a patient who is exhausted or demoralized by an unremitting symptom is sedated to provide temporary relief from suffering. Sedation is then lightened after a previously established period of time (such as forty-eight hours), at which point the patient's mental outlook and symptomatology may have improved (Mazzotta, 2012). By contrast, "continuous sedation" is maintained until the patient dies, unless another symptomatic treatment becomes available.

Given the various delineations of palliative sedation, a broad and generally acceptable definition would be "the use of sedative medications to relieve intolerable suffering from refractory symptoms by a reduction in patient consciousness" (de Graeff & Dean, 2007). The definition is broad enough to encompass sedation of various durations and depths, while also including one of the generally accepted requirements for palliative sedation (i.e., that the symptom be refractory and intolerable). As noted later, only continuous sedation to unconsciousness (CSU) is ethically contentious, by virtue of its impact on decision-making capacity, lucidity, and (potentially) life expectancy.

Precisely because of what is lost due to CSU, it is never the first response to suffering. Symptom management should always begin with targeted treatment (e.g., analgesics for pain, antiemetics for nausea). Depending on the symptom, medication dosages may be titrated upward and other medications used in addition to—or in lieu of—those that have not achieved sufficient relief. It is important to note that pain is not the only symptom that may become intolerable and refractory. In fact, delirium was the justification for the majority of cases of palliative sedation in a recent meta-analysis, with dyspnea and psychological distress also being more common reasons than pain (Maltoni et al., 2012).

This raises the question of what medication to use to effect CSU, if it is deemed necessary. By the time CSU is being considered, the patient is likely on several medications targeted at the intolerable symptom. Many medications used in palliative medicine have the side effect of sedation. Thus an elegant and efficient way of achieving CSU is to continue upward titration of sedating medications already in use, no longer with the intent of controlling symptoms—which has proven impossible—but rather to achieve unconsciousness. This is referred to as *secondary palliative sedation* and is reflected by the fact that benzodiazepines—a staple of end-of-life care and first-line treatment for anxiety—are the most common medications used to achieve CSU (de Graeff & Dean, 2007). One specific benzodiazepine, midazolam, is specifically recommended in the majority of published guidelines (Schildmann, Schildmann, & Kiesewetter, 2015).

In other cases, medications in use for the intolerable symptom may not be sufficiently sedating—or the side effects of upward titration are too great—so another class of medications is required to achieve CSU. Generally these medications are "pure sedatives" (such as barbiturates) which are added to the original treatment regimen for the express purpose of achieving CSU. Other options include atypical antipsychotics such as levomepromazine (Alonso-Babarro, Varela-Cerdeira, Torres-Vigil, Rodriguez-Barrientos, & Bruera, 2010) or anesthetics such as propofol (Anghelescu, Hamilton, Faughnan, Johnson, & Baker, 2012). This is referred to as *primary palliative sedation*.

Once CSU is achieved, it can be maintained either by a steady infusion or regularly scheduled bolus doses of medication, either intravenously or subcutaneously. This can certainly be achieved in the hospital or inpatient hospice setting and, depending on the supports available, potentially also in the home.

Ethical

As noted, essentially all professional position statements include several core requirements for CSU.

1. The symptom must be refractory and intolerable.
2. Sedation must be proportionate to the symptom.
3. Complete sedation to unconsciousness should be a last resort.
4. Informed consent must be obtained.

Before exploring the more contentious aspects of the practice, these minimum requirements warrant additional exploration.

Minimum Requirements

The two primary clinical characteristics of a symptom warranting CSU are that it be *refractory* and *intolerable*.[2] Refractoriness requires that all other reasonable treatments for that symptom be tried and have failed to relieve the symptom in question. By logical inference, then, CSU can only be implemented by—or in consultation with—expert palliative care clinicians. Less experienced clinicians may not be familiar with the complete array of therapeutic modalities and thus will not be able to determine whether all reasonable measures have been used in an attempt to control a symptom prior to initiation of CSU.

The requirement of refractoriness should not be taken as a requirement that *every* possible treatment for that symptom be tried before pursuing palliative sedation. Some potential treatments may have such a low probability of working, significant side effects, or lag time before taking effect that they are not reasonable considerations for a patient who is approaching the end of her life. Cherny and Portenoy (1994) recognize this in their widely-accepted definition of a "refractory symptom" as one "for which all possible treatment has failed, or it is estimated that no methods are available for palliation within the time frame and the risk-benefit ratio that the patient can tolerate."

The other requirement is that the symptom be *intolerable*. This is obviously a very subjective concept, since some people have a higher tolerance for pain or other symptoms than others. But, unlike other medical specialties, palliative care relies heavily on subjective measurement (Stiel et al., 2011). Self-report is the gold standard for symptom assessment. As McCaffery (1986) famously wrote, "Pain is what the person says it is and exists whenever he or she says it does." Based on patient report, 5% to 35% of hospice patients suffer from "severe" pain in the last week of life, and 25% describe shortness

---

2. While there is general consensus among the requirement that CSU only be considered if a patient's symptoms are both refractory and intolerable, professional bodies use slightly different terminology, including "unrelieved" (Quill & Byock, 2000b), "unrelenting and unendurable" (Hospice and Palliative Nurses Association, 2008), "severe and intractable" (American Academy of Hospice and Palliative Medicine, 2014), and "intractable and intolerable" (National Hospice and Palliative Care Organization, 2010). This requirement has also been noted by consensus panels (de Graeff & Dean, 2007) and other commentators (Braun, Hagen, & Clark, 2003).

of breath as "unbearable," despite the extensive symptom-treatment resources available (Coyle, Adelhardt, Foley, & Portenoy, 1990). These are precisely the situations where CSU is an appropriate consideration. (The specific instance of "existential suffering" as an intolerable symptom is addressed later on p. 265.)

Once a symptom is deemed refractory and intolerable, palliative sedation can be considered. Recognizing that some important abilities (e.g., interactiveness) may have to be sacrificed for symptom control, all forms of palliative sedation must also be *proportionate*, only deep enough to eliminate—or substantially diminish—the symptom being treated (Claessens, Menten, Schotsmans, & Broeckaert, 2012). The appropriate duration and depth of sedation is the amount necessary to ensure the patient no longer suffers from that symptom. In many cases, this does not require CSU. Emergency or respite sedation may "buy time" for other treatments to work, or in the hopes that the patient's condition may improve as a result of much needed rest and relief. If continuous sedation is required, the depth should be titrated so as to maximize consciousness as far as possible while still providing relief from the symptom. In many cases, mild or moderate sedation is sufficient to accomplish this task. Only when the intolerable symptom is also refractory to sedation of lesser duration and depth is CSU justified. As such, it is considered an intervention of *last resort* (Veterans Health Administration National Ethics Committee, 2006).

The final consensus requirement is *informed consent*. If the patient has sufficient DMC, it is critical to engage in a thoughtful discussion given the fact that the patient will not be able to change her mind once CSU is instituted. Identification of a surrogate and clear instructions as to when—if ever—CSU should be reconsidered must be part of the discussion.

If the patient lacks sufficient DMC to give informed consent, standard procedure is followed by seeking input from a surrogate decision-maker (Quill & Byock, 2000b), Notably, only select guidelines specifically mandate the consent of the surrogate (Veterans Health Administration National Ethics Committee, 2006). Cultural norms also play a role, as guidelines in countries that have a less autonomy-centered model—or where there are expanded options for suffering at the end of life—may ultimately defer to the physician's decision (Royal Dutch Medical Association, 2009).

If the minimum requirements are met, one might reasonably ask why palliative sedation—given the conditions noted previously—is ethically debatable. If there is a moral imperative to treat suffering, then wouldn't it be ethically *obligatory* to provide proportionate sedation, if less extreme methods have been tried and failed to treat intolerable suffering, and sedation is requested by the patient or family?

Yet while the benefit of palliative sedation is clear, it also has several potential drawbacks that have ethical implications (Douglas, 2014):

- inability to participate in subsequent decision-making
- inability to interact with others
- (potentially) shortened life expectancy

DURATION	DEPTH		
	Mild	Moderate	Deep
Emergency	Permissible	Permissible	Permissible
Respite	Permissible	Permissible	Permissible
Continuous	Permissible	Generally permissible	Complex

FIGURE 9.1 Ethical permissibility of various forms of palliative sedation

As with any medical intervention, in determining whether to proceed, the benefits need to be weighed against the drawbacks.

It is important to note that these ethically relevant implications do not apply to all forms of palliative sedation. For instance, sedation that is administered either emergently—to gain time to get symptoms under control—or for the purpose of respite would not permanently impact any of these aspects. (Indeed, temporarily induced unconsciousness is a common occurrence in the medical world, in the form of general anesthesia for surgery.) Similarly, mild or even moderate sedation may offer the possibility of at least occasional meaningful interaction and the expression of one's goals. The patient would be better able to protect her airway than under deep sedation and perhaps even drink liquids. As classified in terms of duration and depth, only CSU invokes ethically relevant considerations (Figure 9.1). The ethical analysis in this chapter therefore focuses exclusively on this specific type of palliative sedation.

Inability to Participate in Decision-Making

One ethically relevant aspect of CSU is the inability to participate in subsequent medical decision-making. Autonomy is not a one-time event, whereby a patient makes a decision and subsequently loses authority to alter the course of her medical care. Ideally, a patient will be able to make subsequent decisions based on ensuing developments, which would include the right to change her mind if the intermediate outcomes are not what she was hoping for. As noted, there is no ethical or legal difference between withdrawing and withholding medical treatment (p. 156). Just as a patient has the option of refusing to initiate a certain treatment, she would also have the option of refusing to *continue* that treatment once it is initiated, if it is not achieving the patient's goals.

Often a patient's chosen treatment involves decreased consciousness and resulting incapacity, such as consenting to major surgery involving general anesthesia. But there are two important differences between this and CSU. The first is that decreased consciousness is not the primary goal of these other procedures but rather a necessary component of a broader treatment plan. Second, the resulting incapacity is intended to be temporary, although in serious situations it is recognized that if things do not go well the patient might never regain the ability to make her own decisions. In CSU, however, decreased consciousness is the primary goal of the therapy, and there is no expectation that the patient will ever regain her DMC. Indeed, the treatment is specifically intended to prevent this from happening.

Clearly, then, the stakes are much higher in opting for CSU than for a treatment which affords the possibility of reconsideration. This does not mean, though, that a patient should not be permitted to make such a decision. The stakes are already extremely high by virtue of refractory and intolerable symptoms, in the context of a very limited life expectancy. Since CSU is the last resort, it should not come as a surprise that some options being considered have implications on autonomy that are not frequently encountered in the rest of medical care.

If a patient has sufficient DMC to consent to CSU, the implication of such a choice on future decisions needs to be stressed. CSU, by definition, is irrevocable by the patient once instituted, but it is not unique in that respect among medical decisions (e.g., amputation). Full information needs to be provided and thoughtful discussion held, to the degree permitted by the burden of symptoms and with specific mention of irrevocability of the decision. As long as this is provided, it would seem illogical to use concern for autonomy as a justification for *limiting* a patient's autonomy, given the seriousness of the situation and the time-sensitive nature of the decision. If nothing else, respect for autonomy requires the clinical team to accept the patient's decision, while also clarifying with the patient who her appropriate surrogate decision-maker is and under what conditions (if any) the decision to institute CSU should be reevaluated.

Often, though, by the time a symptom is deemed refractory and intolerable, the patient's DMC is sufficiently compromised that she is unable to give informed consent for CSU. It is necessary in such situations for the appropriate surrogate decision-maker to offer substituted judgment. CSU is not a uniquely serious decision in this respect, as surrogates frequently are called upon to make decisions involving withdrawal of LSMT, such as in the case of compassionate extubation.

In many ways, a surrogate's decision to institute CSU is less emotionally fraught than a decision to withhold LSMT. In the first place, there is usually less temporal connection between the decision and the patient's death compared, for instance, to compassionate extubation. If CSU is reserved for situations of extremely limited life expectancy, it should not hasten the patient's death (p. 262). In addition, while compassionate extubation is often a response to a lack of clinical improvement, CSU promptly relieves suffering from a previously intolerable symptom.

The Quality of an Unconscious Life

The second ethically relevant consideration in implementing CSU is the loss of consciousness. When receiving CSU, the patient is no longer able to interact with others or express her goals and values. For some patients this is too steep a price. They place a great emphasis on lucidity, even if that precludes optimal symptom relief. Studies have shown that patients attribute greater importance to being "mentally aware" at the end of life, while physicians tend to stress comfort at the expense of lucidity (Steinhauser et al., 2000). Reasons for this include a desire to maintain relationship with those close to them, a spiritual priority on lucidity at the very end of life, and a belief in redemptive suffering (p. 496). As Battin (1983) writes, "Although it is always technically possible to achieve relief from pain, at least when the appropriate resources are available, the price may be functionally and practically equivalent, at least from the patient's view, to death."

Other patients, however, do not view loss of consciousness—especially in the context of a heavy symptom burden—as a huge sacrifice. For while patients generally value lucidity more than physicians, not all do. This is significant because loss of consciousness is one of the ethical considerations that justifies limiting CSU to exceptional cases. If loss of consciousness were not ethically relevant, then some of the minimum considerations for CSU would no longer be required. Berger (2010) rightly observes:

> Guidelines that include the criterion of symptom refractoriness impose a value judgment that may not be uniformly shared by patients. [CSU] guidelines put a priority on preserving consciousness. This compels patients to conform to the view that maintaining consciousness is valued over immediate relief from symptoms.

Following this line of argument, some commentators have shifted the question from whether refractory, intolerable suffering is sufficient to justify CSU to wondering if it is even necessary to justify the practice.

Here it is important to note that "intolerability" is inherently a subjective judgment. If "pain is what the patient says it is," then a patient's declaration that a symptom is intolerable should be sufficient. Generally this takes into consideration not only the severity of the symptom but also the countervailing benefits of consciousness, with regard to awareness and personal interactions. For a patient who puts great emphasis on being aware of her surroundings, a refractory symptom may be "tolerable" when the only alternative is unconsciousness; for a patient who does not so value lucidity, it may be deemed intolerable. So rather than dispensing with the core requirement of intolerability, it is more appropriate to respect a patient's individual values—including the degree to which lucidity is valued—which necessarily influence what she considers tolerable and should be part of the required informed consent process.

The same can be said for the requirement of refractoriness. As noted (p. 256), this does not mean that every possible treatment be tried, as some are overly burdensome, may not be locally available, or would take too long to work. As such, there is often some measure of value judgment in an assessment of refractoriness, based on the patient's expressed level of suffering, nature of other potential treatments, and the degree to which the patient values consciousness. Once again, rather than doing away with a minimum requirement, it is more appropriate to recognize the degree to which considerations of consciousness are already built into what is considered refractory.

Impact on Life Expectancy

The final—and most complex—ethically relevant aspect of palliative sedation is its potential impact on life expectancy. Someone who is under deep sedation has diminished ability to protect her airway, thus increasing the risk of aspiration. Such a patient is also unable to eat or drink, rendering her dependent on MANH to prevent dehydration. Patients receiving CSU generally refuse life-prolonging measures such as MANH, concluding that continued existence in an unconscious state provides insufficient quality of life. In contrast to voluntarily stopping eating and drinking (VSED), in CSU medication makes it impossible for the patient to eat or drink.

Studies have shown that an otherwise well-hydrated patient will usually die within two weeks if she does not drink and supplemental fluids are not provided (Ganzini et al., 2003). Logically, then, if a patient dies a few days after initiation of CSU, it is highly likely that she died of the underlying disease process (Chabot & Goedhart, 2009). If she dies ten to fourteen days later, however, the proximate cause of her death may well have been dehydration, which was made inevitable by CSU in the absence of MANH.

Is it possible, then, that palliative sedation not only minimizes suffering but might also shorten life, which would conflict with palliative care's stated goal of not hastening death (World Health Organization, 1990)? If so, CSU could be more properly termed "slow euthanasia," which Billings and Block (1996) define in this way:

> In slow euthanasia . . . regardless of how well the patient's pain or other physical distress is controlled, the dosage is maintained or adjusted upward gradually to assure at least somnolence, often to produce obtundation, coma and even apparent respiratory distress.

It is important to note, however, that this description does not comport with the modern concept of CSU. "Slow euthanasia" is not proportionate to the symptoms, as sedation is maintained or increased without regard for the patient's level of suffering. But the general accusation of CSU being akin to euthanasia—albeit over a longer time frame—remains relevant, both in terms of inevitability (of death) as well as appearance.

A critically important consideration, therefore, is the patient's life expectancy before CSU is initiated. The sooner the patient dies after CSU begins, the less likely it is that dehydration contributed to her death. In a patient who is actively dying, withholding MANH should not impact duration of life. For this reason, many professional bodies limit consideration of CSU to patients whose life expectancy is already extremely limited, such as "hours to days" (Hospice and Palliative Nurses Association, 2008) or "final stages of terminal illness" (American Medical Association, 2010-2011).

Where does that leave the terminally ill patient with intolerable and refractory symptoms who has weeks or longer to live? Assuming the patient is not dependent on LSMT which could be withdrawn, the other options for hastened death both take time: likely a week or longer for VSED, and at least fifteen days to obtain a lethal prescription in the case of PAD (if it is even available). In the meantime, neither ameliorate the patient's intolerable symptoms. Palliative sedation may be the patient's only way to avoid intolerable suffering.

Recognizing this, some have argued that the moral imperative for CSU is even *greater* in situations such as this—despite the potential impact on duration of life—because it could spare the patient weeks or months of suffering. For this reason, some commentators and professional bodies do not restrict CSU to patients who are imminently dying. Suggested time frames include up to two weeks (National Hospice and Palliative Care Organization, 2010; Royal Dutch Medical Association, 2009) and "days to weeks" (Quill & Byock, 2000b).

Three arguments have been offered in support easing life expectancy requirements for CSU:

1. Denying that CSU hastens death
2. The Rule of Double Effect
3. Distinguishing between CSU and forgoing MANH

Only the last of these, however, is compelling.

Denying that CSU Hastens Death

Is it really safe to assume that CSU hastens death? Certainly this assumption makes intuitive sense, since if a patient cannot drink and no supplementary hydration is provided, then dehydration, hypotension, uremia, and death will inevitably follow. However, the data may not bear this out. In a recent meta-analysis, Maltoni et al. (2012) reviewed relevant studies of palliative sedation and found that in only one did palliative sedation have a statistically significant effect on duration of life. And in that one study (Mercadante et al., 2009) patients undergoing palliative sedation actually lived *longer* than those who were not sedated (6.6 vs. 3.3 days).

There are three potential reasons for this finding. One is that suffering—whether from pain, dyspnea, delirium, or some other burdensome symptom—can itself hasten death, which is a phenomenon suggested by other studies (Sykes & Thorns, 2003; Walsh, 1984). The simple fact that the patient is no longer suffering could conceivably have a positive impact on life expectancy, which might compensate for any negative impact from CSU. Similarly, withholding MANH could help prevent some complications, since a patient who is not well-hydrated will have decreased secretions, thereby reducing the risk of aspiration pneumonia.

An alternative explanation for the findings is that Maltoni et al. (2012)—as a meta-analysis of several other studies—addresses palliative sedation in general, not CSU in particular. Since patients undergoing mild or moderate sedation are better able to protect their airway and can potentially drink some liquids, their risk of hastened death would be less than if they were undergoing CSU. By including these shallower forms of sedation in the overall analysis, average survival would logically be increased. Indeed, some patients in the studies examined survived for so long (up to six months) that some hydration—whether oral or medically administered—must have been provided.

The most logical explanation, though, is that CSU could well hasten death—simply because the patient is unable to eat or drink and is likely to refuse MANH—but only when the patient is likely to live long enough to potentially die of dehydration, rather than her underlying disease. If so, the patients in the meta-analysis who did undergo CSU might not have died sooner precisely because sufficiently strict criteria for CSU were used. In other words, their life expectancy was already so limited that there was not enough time for dehydration to impact survival.

If so, the results of the meta-analysis should be viewed with some caution, because if one were to assume that palliative sedation never hastens death—and on this basis ease the requirements to include patients with weeks or months to live—then palliative sedation might end up doing just that in subsequent cases. This is precisely the reason why it is crucial to limit CSU without MANH to patients with an extremely limited life expectancy.

Rule of Double Effect

Acknowledging that CSU could impact life expectancy when a patient might otherwise have weeks or longer to live, some have appealed to the Rule of Double Effect (RDE) to justify its use in such situations. As noted (p. 209), the RDE justifies an action which has both a good effect (in this case, relief of suffering) and a bad effect (in this case, potentially hastened death), as long as certain conditions apply. The argument goes this way:

1. Sedating a patient to unconsciousness is not morally bad, in and of itself.
2. The intention is to relieve suffering, not to hasten death.
3. In the context of terminal illness and refractory symptoms, the benefit (i.e., relief of suffering) is proportionate to the risk of hastened death.
4. Unlike euthanasia or PAD, suffering is relieved through unconsciousness, not through death. (In other words, the bad effect is not the means to the good effect.)

To be sure, the same criticisms that have been leveled against the RDE as justification for intensive opioid therapy at the end of life (p. 210) could be leveled against its application to CSU (e.g., the complexity of "intention"). The ultimate result is, after all, the same as for euthanasia: the death of the patient as a foreseeable consequence of the action of the physician. Viewed in this light, some would say that appealing to the RDE does not ethically justify the practice of CSU but merely serves to soothe the consciences of the clinicians administering it. As Billings and Block (1996) write,

> Insofar as our first duty in care at the end of life is to help patients and their families meet their personal goals, slow euthanasia can seem like a severe compromise, a diversion of attention toward professional caregivers' concerns, possibly at the expense of those who are facing intense personal loss.

Yet even if one grants the legitimacy of the RDE—which many do not (Quill, Dresser, & Brock, 1997)—it is not necessary to justify the use of CSU. For the mechanisms by which CSU may shorten life are impaired airway protection and the inability to eat and drink. Both of these are easily "treatable" by intubation and MANH, respectively. Viewed independently, CSU itself is highly unlikely to shorten life expectancy. It is rather the forgoing of other LSMT—admittedly, that CSU renders the patient dependent on (and will be discussed in the following section)—that could hasten death.

It is very difficult to argue that withholding LSMT from a patient sedated to unconsciousness can be justified according to the RDE. The patient is unable to experience the burdens of LSMT, and thus the intention cannot be to relieve suffering (as this was already relieved by the sedation). Fortunately, it is not necessary to appeal to the RDE to justify forgoing LSMT. That is a right granted to all patients and logically leads to the third (and most compelling) argument in favor of easing life expectancy requirements for CSU.

The Distinction between CSU and Forgoing MANH

While it is true that most patients undergoing CSU refuse MANH, this is not an absolute requirement. Certain religious groups, for instance, believe that any life—even an unconscious one—is better than no life, often based on religious beliefs related to the sacredness of the image of God which is inherent in every person, regardless of sentience (Fletcher, 1951). So-called "vitalists" could reasonably accept CSU to control intolerable symptoms while also continuing to receive MANH. Such patients could be maintained in that condition until the underlying disease takes their lives or some complication (other than dehydration) occurs.

In and of itself, therefore, CSU does not provoke concerns of hastened death. While inability to participate in decision-making and loss of consciousness remain relevant considerations, CSU need not substantially impact life expectancy, and thus remains an ethical option for patients with refractory, intolerable suffering, even if they are not in the last hours to days of their lives.

It is, more precisely, the *forgoing of MANH* in the context of CSU that legitimately raises concerns for hastened death in patients who otherwise might have lived for weeks or longer. Administering CSU in this context runs the very real risk of tainting the practice of palliative care in general. As the death panel controversy (p. 510) revealed, if an uncontentious practice like patient-centered advance care planning can precipitate outrage and backlash, then a nuanced practice such as CSU—if too broadly applied—would likely prompt much worse. Attempts to delineate the ethically subtle distinction between two practices that are often but not invariably associated (i.e., CSU and forgoing MANH) would surely be lost on the general public, drowned out by pundits with an agenda that negatively impact the mission of palliative care (Politifact, 2009).

This highlights the importance of requiring a very limited prognosis—on the order of hours to days—for CSU in its usual form (i.e., forgoing MANH). While it is impossible to say with absolute certainty whether dehydration will ultimately contribute to a patient's death in those situations—especially given the challenges of prognostication (p. 84)—death over the ensuing hours to days would almost surely be due to the underlying disease.

Patients with a longer prognosis who seek CSU are not condemned to endure refractory and intolerable suffering. Rather, they are simply required to accept the concomitant administration of MANH, to insulate palliative care against accusations of "slow euthanasia." This should not be taken as an indictment of patients' right to refuse MANH, which is well-established (p. 185). Rather, it is simply an example of an intervention—in this case, CSU—whose balance of burdens and benefits shifts upon a patient's refusal of LSMT, such that the intervention may no longer be appropriate if interventions to address its sequelae are refused.

In this respect, it is analogous to a patient's code status in the operating room. A patient certainly has the right to refuse CPR, but a surgeon also has the right to refuse to operate on such a patient if that decision sufficiently negatively impacts the likely outcomes of the surgery. So also a palliative care clinician has the right to refrain from administering CSU to a patient who refuses MANH, if by virtue of prognosis this combination is likely to hasten the patient's death.

A patient who is steadfast in her refusal of MANH should not be left to suffer. Respite sedation can provide crucial (if temporary) relief of symptoms. VSED is always an option, thus reducing the duration—if not the intensity—of suffering. PAD may also be, depending on where the resides. And when the patient's life expectancy eventually reaches "hours to days," CSU—in the continuing absence of MANH—becomes an ethically appropriate option.

Return to the Case

The patient's abdominal pain and nausea are intolerable to the patient and have proven refractory to every available treatment, under the direction of a palliative care specialist. With the informed consent of the patient, a midazolam drip is instituted to provide primary, proportionate palliative sedation. The rate of infusion is gradually titrated upward, and sedation to unconsciousness is necessary to achieve relief of symptoms. MANH is not provided as it is not consistent with her goals of care, and her prognosis makes it highly unlikely that dehydration will cause her death.

The patient dies peacefully two days later with her family at her side. Given the time course, it is quite clear that CSU and forgoing MANH did not hasten his death.

Special Considerations
Palliative Sedation for Existential Distress

Up to this point the discussion has focused on symptoms such as delirium and pain which are directly related to a terminal condition, can be quantitatively measured (at least by self-report), often have clinical signs that can be externally evaluated, and have clinically proven treatments that may provide relief in short order. This is not to say that the symptom itself is the only source of the patient's suffering—which encompasses emotional, social, and spiritual domains as well—but it is the component that is identifiable, intolerable, and refractory to known treatments, thereby justifying CSU.

In some cases, though, a patient may report suffering not from an identifiable physical symptom but rather from an overall sense of purposelessness, lack of meaning, and emptiness. It is not difficult to understand why, especially if the patient has a terminal illness. This has been termed "existential distress," which the American Medical Association defines as "the experience of agony and distress that results from living in an unbearable state of existence including . . . death anxiety, isolation, and loss of control" (Council on Ethical and Judicial Affairs, 2008).

Studies have shown that palliative care clinicians are less comfortable instituting CSU for existential distress than for physical symptoms. This is not isolated to the United States (Putman, Yoon, Rasinski, & Curlin, 2013) but also has been seen in Canada (Blondeau, Roy, Dumont, Godin, & Martineau, 2005) and Europe (Beauverd et al., 2014).

There are two potential reasons for this. The first is the claim that treatment of such distress falls outside the goals of medicine (Illich, 1982). Thus Randall and Downie (2006) make the distinction between the intrinsic aim of palliative care (which they define as "the medical good") and the extrinsic aim (which refers to the "psychological good"), arguing that treatment modalities should focus on the former. Following the same line of argument, Jansen and Sulmasy (2002) assert that

> a primary goal of medicine is not simply to relieve suffering, but also to restore the patient to a state of health. . . . Accordingly, the appropriate intervention for patients experiencing non-terminal [existential] suffering . . . will be one that restores them to a state of psychosocial well-being. And quite clearly providing them with sedating doses of opioids will not further this goal.

Other commentators disagree. They argue that the fact that palliative care aspires to address "total suffering" (not only physical symptoms) seems to underscore—not undermine—the obligation to use every available modality to treat existential suffering, as well. Cassell and Rich (2010) observe that "suffering . . . variously destroys the coherence, cohesiveness, and consistency of the whole. It is in this sense that the integrity of the person is threatened or destroyed." Someone suffering existentially would therefore be just as in need (and just as entitled to) relief of suffering—up to and including CSU—as someone experiencing purely physical pain.

Ideally, transdisciplinary care should be able to relieve existential distress without resorting to CSU. Yet just as there are exceptional cases where pain or other physical symptoms prove refractory to expert palliative care, so also there are cases where existential distress persists despite all available treatment. Indeed, this is a standard requirement for consideration of CSU (i.e., that the intolerable symptom be refractory). To reject outright the use of CSU for existential distress would seem to call into question the overarching goal of palliative care to treat total suffering by carving out one type of suffering where the "last resort" tool of palliative care is not appropriate to use.

A distinct concern has to do with the risk of hastening death based on the patient's underlying life expectancy. As noted, the use of CSU in situations where the patient might otherwise survive for weeks or longer may prompt concerns about hastening death and endanger public acceptance of palliative care. Because existential distress need not be associated with imminent death—or even with terminal illness at all—the probability of hastened death is much higher.[3] For these reasons, several professional bodies have rejected the use of CSU for existential distress (American College of Physicians, 2005; Veterans Health Administration National Ethics Committee, 2006).

It is crucial to identify which of the two reasons for rejecting CSU is operative, and here a hypothetical case may be illustrative. Imagine that the patient in this chapter's case—terminal stomach cancer, life expectancy of hours to days—achieves adequate control of her physical symptoms. Her pain and nausea are well managed, but she is overwhelmed by a sense of meaningless and despair. She cannot bear the thought of "withering away," and each moment is excruciating in its overwhelming sense of loss. Her suffering, therefore, is existential rather than physical.

Further suppose that this suffering is refractory to standard treatments such as counseling, spiritual care, and even psychostimulants for possible underlying depression. It is unlikely that other treatments will be effective in ameliorating her distress, based on the likelihood of efficacy and also the time required for medications to take effect. (Typical antidepressants, for instance, often take four to six weeks, which she does not have.) This leaves CSU as the "last resort," and she is requesting to be rendered unconscious for her last remaining hours to days. She even quotes Woody Allen (1986) in support of her request: "It's not that I'm afraid to die, I just don't want to be there when it happens."

This patient is clearly suffering with minimal prospect of relief, at least in the time that she has left. While one might hope she could find meaning in her final days through human connection and reflection on her life (what some refer to as "transcendence"), it seems unlikely to occur (ten Have & Welie, 2014). Although clinicians may be generally more reluctant to institute palliative sedation for existential rather than physical distress, in a recent meta-analysis "psychological distress" was the third-most common indication for palliative sedation (Maltoni et al., 2012). (This may reflect the fact that there are more focused and effective treatments available for physical symptoms than for

---

3. Here assuming that CSU is instituted in its most common form, without MANH. Were MANH to be administered concomitantly, concerns for hastened death would be much less relevant.

existential ones.) Ultimately many palliative care clinicians would be willing to consider palliative sedation for this patient.

But if her life expectancy were measured not in days but in months, the response would be significantly different. This time frame permits greater opportunity for potentially meaningful experiences to occur or medications to work. Particularly relevant from an ethical perspective, instituting CSU without MANH would almost certainly hasten her death, thus calling into question palliative care's fundamental assertion that it does not intend to do so (World Health Organization, 2002). It would also violate relevant professional position statements, including that of the American Academy of Hospice and Palliative Medicine (2014): "If palliative sedation is used for truly refractory existential suffering, as for its use for physical symptoms, it should not shorten survival."

Such an action thus risks tumbling down the slippery slope, for if CSU is deemed appropriate for refractory and intolerable existential distress in the context of terminal illness where death is not imminent, one might reasonably wonder why it should be limited to those patients who are deemed "terminal." The distress is no less intolerable and refractory for patients with *serious* physical illness, without a clear life expectancy. Indeed, the suffering could be even worse because it might seem unending.

Of course, CSU with concomitant MANH would be an ethically acceptable alternative, as this would obviate concerns about potentially hastened death. Admittedly, this is a less attractive option for many patients. While it effectively addresses the presenting symptom, it can create a host of other concerns, including vulnerability (in a sedated state for an indefinite period of time), feasibility (especially at home over a long period of time), family burden, and cost. For all these reasons, other options—such as VSED—would be more expeditious and thus potentially preferable to the patient.

Pediatric Implications

Relatively little has been written about CSU in the pediatric population (Anghelescu, Hamilton, Faughnan, Johnson, & Baker, 2012; Kenny & Frager, 1996; Kiman, Wuiloud, & Requena, 2011; Naipaul & Ullrich, 2011; Postovsky, Moaed, Krivoy, Ofir, & Ben Arush, 2007; Pousset, Bilsen, Cohen, Mortier, & Deliens, 2011). This may have to do with the fact that far fewer children die than do adults, as well as the fact that pediatrics carries with it the presumption of maximal treatment because "children aren't supposed to die." Given that palliative sedation is an ethically charged—and infrequently utilized—intervention even in the adult population, pediatric units may not have extensive experience or comfort with it. The patient's informed consent is also often impossible to obtain, as children are generally unable to make their own medical decisions. Finally, because so much of a child's life is based in activity—and *inter*activity—to a parent authorizing CSU may feel like what was distinctive and personal about their child is forever lost.

Despite these barriers, children are just as susceptible to refractory and intolerable suffering as adults. For adults who have lost DMC, surrogate decision-makers are permitted to consent to CSU, assuming all the other requirements are also met. It would be unfair to withhold the "last resort" therapy simply because of the complexity of issues involved. The American Academy of Pediatrics (2000) recognizes this fact, stating, "Rarely, the relief of progressive symptoms may require deep sedation."

While the American Academy of Pediatrics does not provide practical guidance about which "rare" cases require CSU, there is no reason to believe that ethical requirements for use of CSU in adults—refractory and intolerable symptoms, proportionate sedation, last resort, and informed consent—would be in any different in children. Some modification is necessary, of course, with parental permission taking the place of surrogate consent based on substituted judgment (p. 285).

This, however, raises the deeper issue of whether a surrogate's informed consent should be required for palliative sedation of an incapacitated patient who is experiencing refractory and intolerable symptoms (Berger, 2017). Because if informed consent is required, then informed refusal must be honored. Are clinicians willing to stand by and watch a patient endure such suffering for wont of the informed consent of a surrogate, especially when the patient is a child?

This debate largely rests on an artificial distinction between where requisite symptom management ends and CSU begins. In some ways, CSU is a formal determination that the goals have shifted and comfort (even at the price of unconsciousness) is paramount. But even if a surrogate—which in the case of a child would generally be the parent—refuses CSU, the moral obligation to treat pain and suffering remains. This could involve upward titration of symptomatic medications that in some cases renders the patient unconscious (i.e., secondary palliative sedation), even absent a formal decision to institute CSU.

When symptom control is not possible in this way, primary palliative sedation may be the only recourse. Parental refusal of this recommendation should prompt reevaluation on a number of levels. For instance, the treating team might reconsider their reasons for concluding that the patient's suffering is truly "intolerable," when the parents clearly do not. It may also lead to frank discussions about the parent's reason for refusing CSU, and whether it may stem from misunderstanding, bias, or personal beliefs that the patient should not suffer as a result of (Macauley & Fritzler, 2014). Ultimately, the moral obligation to relieve suffering remains paramount, whether or not this meets the formal definition of CSU.

Risk of Heightened Suffering

Up to this point, the discussion—like most every other analysis of CSU—has assumed that it relieves suffering. Its primary purpose, after all, is to treat refractory and intolerable symptoms. It is the last resort when all other attempts at treating suffering have failed. And, unlike other modalities, it is also thought to be effective in treating existential distress, because if a patient is unconscious, how much distress could she be experiencing?

Some have called this fundamental assumption into question, however (Deschepper et al., 2013; Kon, 2011). One reason is that the gold standard for pain measurement (i.e., self-report) is no longer available in an unconscious patient. Observational pain scales are therefore used, and these have shown increased scores even in the presence of complete sedation (Gelinas, Tousignant-Laflamme, Tanguay, & Bourgault, 2011).

This observation is supported by recent discoveries based on both clinical assessment and more nuanced radiological studies, such as functional magnetic resonance imaging. Contrary to what was previously believed, high-level brain processing is present even during propofol sedation (Koelsch, Heinke, Sammler, & Olthoff, 2006). In the context of documented variation in the degree—and the quality of measurement—of palliative sedation in relation to the intolerable and refractory symptom (Brinkkemper et al., 2013), this raises profound questions as to whether CSU is always effective in relieving suffering.

In many ways this is a logical corollary to the more optimistic suspicion that patients who are in a coma or undergoing general anesthesia might still be able to perceive the world around them, including the presence or words of loved ones (Schwender et al., 1998). Is it consistent, then, to encourage families to continue to speak to their unconscious loved ones because they might be able (on some level) to perceive what is said, while at the same reassuring them that the patient is incapable of suffering in that state?

At present, the jury is still out as to whether deep sedation eliminates pain or in some cases merely masks the expression of it (p. 170). Reports of suffering while deeply sedated remain the exception rather than the rule, and since CSU represents the last resort of pain management, its use reflects the fact that all other reasonable treatments have already been tried and have failed. Hopefully over time there will be additional clarity as to the ultimate effectiveness of CSU, but in the meantime it remains the last, best resort for patients at the end of life whose symptoms are both intolerable and refractory.

Summary Points

- Palliative sedation refers to "the use of sedative medications to relieve intolerable suffering from refractory symptoms by a reduction in patient consciousness" (de Graeff & Dean, 2007).
- Palliative sedation can be subclassified in terms of both duration and depth. Only continuous sedation to unconsciousness (CSU) is ethically contentious, as it prevents the patient from participating in subsequent decisions, eliminates the possibility of meaningful interaction, and prevents the patient from eating and drinking.
- Minimum requirements for CSU include:
  - The symptom must be intolerable and refractory.
  - The degree of sedation must be proportionate to the symptom.
  - CSU should be a last resort.
  - Informed consent should be obtained.

- There exists significant concern about whether palliative sedation hastens death and is thus incompatible with the mission of palliative care.
  - Recent studies have shown that palliative sedation does not hasten death, but this is largely due to the fact that not all patients underwent CSU, and those who did likely were already in the last hours to days of life.
  - Easing the criteria for CSU (without MANH) to include patients who are not in the last hours to days of life therefore risks actually hastening death.
- Palliative sedation for existential distress is hotly debated, with some professional bodies amenable and others opposed. Arguments that this is outside the scope of palliative care are not compelling, but concerns of hastened death in cases of prolonged life expectancies are justified.

Acknowledgments

I am grateful to Donna Zhukovsky, Jessica Moore, and Francine Rainone for raising the important issue addressed in the "Risk of Heightened Suffering" section in their outstanding presentation at the 2014 International Congress of Palliative Care and for their generosity in sharing their slides.

References

Allen, W. (1986). *Without feathers*. New York: Ballantine.

Alonso-Babarro, A., Varela-Cerdeira, M., Torres-Vigil, I., Rodriguez-Barrientos, R., & Bruera, E. (2010). At-home palliative sedation for end-of-life cancer patients. *Palliat Med*, 24(5), 486–492. doi:10.1177/0269216309359996

American Academy of Hospice and Palliative Medicine. (2014). Palliative sedation position statement. Retrieved from http://aahpm.org/positions/palliative-sedation

American Academy of Pain Medicine. (2003). Ethics charter. Retrieved from http://www.painmed.org/files/ethics-charter.pdf

American Academy of Pediatrics. (2000). Palliative care for children. *Pediatrics*, 106(2 Pt 1), 351–357.

American College of Physicians. (2005). *Ethics manual* (5th ed.). Philadelphia: American College of Physicians.

American Medical Association. (2010–2011). Sedation to unconsciousness in end-of-life care. In *Code of medical ethics, annotated current opinions* (p. 2.201). Chicago: American Medical Association.

Anghelescu, D. L., Hamilton, H., Faughnan, L. G., Johnson, L. M., & Baker, J. N. (2012). Pediatric palliative sedation therapy with propofol: Recommendations based on experience in children with terminal cancer. *J Palliat Med*, 15(10), 1082–1090. doi:10.1089/jpm.2011.0500

Battin, M. P. (1983). The least worst death. *Hastings Cent Rep*, 13(2), 13–16.

Beauverd, M., Bernard, M., Currat, T., Ducret, S., Foley, R. A., Borasio, G. D., . . . Dumont, S. (2014). French Swiss physicians' attitude toward palliative sedation: Influence of prognosis and type of suffering. *Palliat Support Care*, 12(5), 345–350. doi:10.1017/S1478951513000278

Berger, J. T. (2010). Rethinking guideliens for the use of palliative sedation. *Hastings Cent Rep*, 40(3), 32–38.

Berger, J. T. (2017). The limits of surrogates' moral authority and physician professionalism: Can the paradigm of palliative sedation be instructive? *Hastings Cent Rep*, 47(1), 20–23. doi:10.1002/hast.665

Billings, J. A., & Block, S. D. (1996). Slow euthanasia. *J Palliat Care*, *12*(4), 21–30.

Blondeau, D., Roy, L., Dumont, S., Godin, G., & Martineau, I. (2005). Physicians' and pharmacists' attitudes toward the use of sedation at the end of life: Influence of prognosis and type of suffering. *J Palliat Care*, *21*(4), 238–245.

Brinkkemper, T., van Norel, A. M., Szadek, K. M., Loer, S. A., Zuurmond, W. W., & Perez, R. S. (2013). The use of observational scales to monitor symptom control and depth of sedation in patients requiring palliative sedation: A systematic review. *Palliat Med*, *27*(1), 54–67. doi:10.1177/0269216311425421

Broeckaert, B., & Nunez-Olarte, J. M. (2002). Sedation in palliative care: Facts and concepts. In H. ten Have & D. Clark (Eds.), *The ethics of palliative care: European perspectives* (pp. 166–180). Buckingham, UK: Open University Press.

Cassell, E. J., & Rich, B. A. (2010). Intractable end-of-life suffering and the ethics of palliative sedation. *Pain Med*, *11*(3), 435–438. doi:10.1111/j.1526-4637.2009.00786.x

Chabot, B. E., & Goedhart, A. (2009). A survey of self-directed dying attended by proxies in the Dutch population. *Soc Sci Med*, *68*(10), 1745–1751. doi:10.1016/j.socscimed.2009.03.005

Cherny, N. I., & Portenoy, R. K. (1994). Sedation in the management of refractory symptoms: Guidelines for evaluation and treatment. *J Palliat Care*, *10*(2), 31–38.

Claessens, P., Menten, J., Schotsmans, P., & Broeckaert, B. (2012). Level of consciousness in dying patients. The role of palliative sedation: A longitudinal prospective study. *Am J Hosp Palliat Care*, *29*(3), 195–200. doi:10.1177/1049909111413890

Council on Ethical and Judicial Affairs. (2008). Sedation to unconsciousness in end-of-life care. Retrieved from https://www.ama-assn.org/sites/default/files/media-browser/public/about-ama/councils/Council%20Reports/council-on-ethics-and-judicial-affairs/a08-ceja-palliative-sedation.pdf

Coyle, N., Adelhardt, J., Foley, K. M., & Portenoy, R. K. (1990). Character of terminal illness in the advanced cancer patient: Pain and other symptoms during the last four weeks of life. *J Pain Symptom Manage*, *5*(2), 83–93.

de Graeff, A., & Dean, M. (2007). Palliative sedation therapy in the last weeks of life: A literature review and recommendations for standards. *J Palliat Med*, *10*(1), 67–85. doi:10.1089/jpm.2006.0139

Deschepper, R., Laureys, S., Hachimi-Idrissi, S., Poelaert, J., Distelmans, W., & Bilsen, J. (2013). Palliative sedation: Why we should be more concerned about the risks that patients experience an uncomfortable death. *Pain*, *154*(9), 1505–1508. doi:10.1016/j.pain.2013.04.038

Douglas, C. (2014). Moral concerns with sedation at the end of life. *J Med Ethics*, *40*(4), 241. doi:10.1136/medethics-2012-101024

Enck, R. E. (1991). Drug-induced terminal sedation for symptom control. *Am J Hosp Palliat Care*, *8*(5), 3–5.

Fletcher, J. (1951). Our right to die. *Theol Today*, *8*, 202–212.

Ganzini, L., Goy, E. R., Miller, L. L., Harvath, T. A., Jackson, A., & Delorit, M. A. (2003). Nurses' experiences with hospice patients who refuse food and fluids to hasten death. *N Engl J Med*, *349*(4), 359–365. doi:10.1056/NEJMsa035086

Gelinas, C., Tousignant-Laflamme, Y., Tanguay, A., & Bourgault, P. (2011). Exploring the validity of the bispectral index, the Critical-Care Pain Observation Tool and vital signs for the detection of pain in sedated and mechanically ventilated critically ill adults: A pilot study. *Intensive Crit Care Nurs*, *27*(1), 46–52. doi:10.1016/j.iccn.2010.11.002

Hospice and Palliative Nurses Association. (2008). Palliative sedation position statement. Retrieved from https://www.hpna.org/PicView.aspx?ID=707

Illich, I. (1982). *Medical nemesis: The expropriation of health*. New York: Pantheon Books.

In re Quinlan, 70 10 (N.J. 1976).

Jansen, L. A., & Sulmasy, D. P. (2002). Proportionality, terminal suffering and the restorative goals of medicine. *Theor Med Bioeth*, *23*(4–5), 321–337.

Kenny, N. P., & Frager, G. (1996). Refractory symptoms and terminal sedation of children: Ethical issues and practical management. *J Palliat Care*, *12*(3), 40–45.

Kiman, R., Wuiloud, A. C., & Requena, M. L. (2011). End of life care sedation for children. *Curr Opin Support Palliat Care*, *5*(3), 285–290. doi:10.1097/SPC.0b013e3283492aba

Koelsch, S., Heinke, W., Sammler, D., & Olthoff, D. (2006). Auditory processing during deep propofol sedation and recovery from unconsciousness. *Clin Neurophysiol*, *117*(8), 1746–1759. doi:10.1016/j.clinph.2006.05.009

Kon, A. A. (2011). Palliative sedation: It's not a panacea. *Am J Bioeth, 11*(6), 41–42. doi:10.1080/15265161.2011.577513

Macauley, R., & Fritzler, L. (2014). Parental refusal of pain management: A potentially unrecognized form of medical neglect. *Palliat Med Care, 1*(2), 5–11.

Maltoni, M., Scarpi, E., Rosati, M., Derni, S., Fabbri, L., Martini, F., . . . Nanni, O. (2012). Palliative sedation in end-of-life care and survival: A systematic review. *J Clin Oncol, 30*(12), 1378–1383. doi:10.1200/JCO.2011.37.3795

Materstvedt, L. J., & Kaasa. (2011). Palliative sedation. In G. W. C. Hanks (Ed.), *Oxford textbook of palliative medicine* (4th ed., pp 304–319). Oxford; New York: Oxford University Press.

Mazzotta, P. (2012). Symptom management using methotrimeprazine: Expanding the definition of respite sedation. *J Palliat Care, 28*(2), 122–123.

McCaffery, M. (1968). *Nursing practice theories related to cognition, bodily pain and main environment interactions.* Los Angeles: University of California.

Mercadante, S., Intravaia, G., Villari, P., Ferrera, P., David, F., & Casuccio, A. (2009). Controlled sedation for refractory symptoms in dying patients. *J Pain Symptom Manage, 37*(5), 771–779. doi:10.1016/j.jpainsymman.2008.04.020

Morita, T., Tsuneto, S., & Shima, Y. (2001). Proposed definitions for terminal sedation. *Lancet, 358*(9278), 335–336. doi:10.1016/S0140-6736(01)05515-5

Naipaul, A. D., & Ullrich, C. (2011). Palliative sedation. In J. Wolfe, P. S. Hinds, & B. M. Sourkes (Eds.), *Textbook of interdisciplinary pediatric palliative care* (pp. 204–214). Philadelphia: Elsevier/Saunders.

National Hospice and Palliative Care Organization. (2010). National Hospice and Palliative Care Organization (NHPCO) position statement and commentary on the use of palliative sedation in imminently dying terminally ill patients. *J Pain Symptom Manage, 39*(5), 914–923. doi:10.1016/j.jpainsymman.2010.01.009

Natural Death Act, 7, California Health and Safety Code § 7185-95, 1 Stat. (1976).

Orentlicher, D. (1997). The Supreme Court and physician-assisted suicide—rejecting assisted suicide but embracing euthanasia. *N Engl J Med, 337*(17), 1236–1239. doi:10.1056/NEJM199710233371713

Papavasiliou, E., Payne, S., Brearley, S., Brown, J., & Seymour, J. (2012). Continuous sedation (CS) until death: Mapping the literature by bibliometric analysis. *J Pain Symptom Manage, 45*(6), 1073–1082 e1010. doi:S0885-3924(12)00341-7 [pii]10.1016/j.jpainsymman.2012.05.012

Politifact. (2009). McCaughey claims end-of-life counseling will be required for Medicare patients. Retrieved from http://www.politifact.com/truth-o-meter/statements/2009/jul/23/betsy-mccaughey/mccaughey-claims-end-life-counseling-will-be-requi/

Postovsky, S., Moaed, B., Krivoy, E., Ofir, R., & Ben Arush, M. W. (2007). Practice of palliative sedation in children with brain tumors and sarcomas at the end of life. *Pediatr Hematol Oncol, 24*(6), 409–415. doi:10.1080/08880010701451079

Pousset, G., Bilsen, J., Cohen, J., Mortier, F., & Deliens, L. (2011). Continuous deep sedation at the end of life of children in Flanders, Belgium. *J Pain Symptom Manage, 41*(2), 449–455. doi:10.1016/j.jpainsymman.2010.04.025

Putman, M. S., Yoon, J. D., Rasinski, K. A., & Curlin, F. A. (2013). Intentional sedation to unconsciousness at the end of life: Findings from a national physician survey. *J Pain Symptom Manage, 46*(3), 326–334. doi:10.1016/j.jpainsymman.2012.09.007

Quill, T. E., & Byock, I. R. (2000a). Responding to intractable terminal suffering. *Ann Intern Med, 133*(7), 561–562.

Quill, T. E., & Byock, I. R. (2000b). Responding to intractable terminal suffering: The role of terminal sedation and voluntary refusal of food and fluids. ACP-ASIM End-of-Life Care Consensus Panel. American College of Physicians-American Society of Internal Medicine. *Ann Intern Med, 132*(5), 408–414.

Quill, T. E., Dresser, R., & Brock, D. W. (1997). The rule of double effect—a critique of its role in end-of-life decision making. *N Engl J Med, 337*(24), 1768–1771. doi:10.1056/NEJM199712113372413

Quill, T. E., Lo, B., & Brock, D. W. (1997). Palliative options of last resort: A comparison of voluntarily stopping eating and drinking, terminal sedation, physician-assisted suicide, and voluntary active euthanasia. *JAMA, 278*(23), 2099–2104.

Randall, F., & Downie, R. S. (2006). *The philosophy of palliative care: Critique and reconstruction*. Oxford; New York: Oxford University Press.

Royal Dutch Medical Association. (2009). Guideline for palliative sedation. Retrieved from http://knmg. artsennet.nl/web/file?uuid=d57c9dec-49d3-43a2-9c4d-1b15005c615c&owner=a8a9ce0e-f42b-47a5-960e-be08025b7b04&contentid=66977

Saunders, C. (1963). The treatment of intractable pain in terminal cancer. *Proc R Soc Med, 56*, 195–197.

Schildmann, E. K., Schildmann, J., & Kiesewetter, I. (2015). Medication and monitoring in palliative sedation therapy: A systematic review and quality assessment of published guidelines. *J Pain Symptom Manage, 49*(4), 734–746. doi:10.1016/j.jpainsymman.2014.08.013

Schwender, D., Kunze-Kronawitter, H., Dietrich, P., Klasing, S., Forst, H., & Madler, C. (1998). Conscious awareness during general anaesthesia: Patients' perceptions, emotions, cognition and reactions. *Br J Anaesth, 80*(2), 133–139.

Shlamovitz, G. Z., Elsayem, A., & Todd, K. H. (2013). Ketamine for palliative sedation in the emergency department. *J Emerg Med, 44*(2), 355–357. doi:10.1016/j.jemermed.2012.08.026

Steinhauser, K. E., Christakis, N. A., Clipp, E. C., McNeilly, M., McIntyre, L., & Tulsky, J. A. (2000). Factors considered important at the end of life by patients, family, physicians, and other care providers. *JAMA, 284*(19), 2476–2482.

Stiel, S., Psych, D., Kues, K., Krumm, N., Radbruch, L., & Elsner, F. (2011). Assessment of quality of life in patients receiving palliative care: Comparison of measurement tools and single item on subjective well-being. *J Palliat Med, 14*(5), 599–606. doi:10.1089/jpm.2010.0473

Sykes, N., & Thorns, A. (2003). The use of opioids and sedatives at the end of life. *Lancet Oncol, 4*(5), 312–318.

ten Have, H., & Welie, J. V. (2014). Palliative sedation versus euthanasia: An ethical assessment. *J Pain Symptom Manage, 47*(1), 123–136. doi:10.1016/j.jpainsymman.2013.03.008

Vacco v. Quill. (1997). U.S. 521 793.

Veterans Health Administration National Ethics Committee. (2006). The ethics of palliative sedation as a therapy of last resort. *Am J Hosp Palliat Care, 23*(6), 483–491. doi:10.1177/1049909106294883

Walsh, T. D. (1984). Opiates and respiratory function in advanced cancer. *Recent Results Cancer Res, 89*, 115–117.

Washington v. Glucksberg, 521 U.S. 702 (1997)

World Health Organization. (1990). Cancer pain relief and palliative care (Technical Report Series Vol. 804). Geneva; Author.

World Health Organization. (2002). WHO definition of palliative care. Retrieved from www.who.int/cancer/palliative/definition/en/

Zylicz, Z. (1993). Opiophobia and cancer pain. *Lancet, 341*(8858), 1473–1474.

Pediatric Ethics and Palliative Care

10

Overview of Pediatric Ethics and Palliative Care

In many medical and ethics textbooks, pediatric issues are an afterthought. One explanation for this is proportionality. On a population basis, there are many more adults than children, so it is understandable that the majority of a general text would be devoted to the most commonly encountered problems. Yet, while it is true that sixty times as many adults as children die in the United States (Osterman et al., 2015), this does not mean that the more than 40,000 children who *do* die each year—not to mention the 500,000 others who are living with complex chronic conditions—do not deserve specific and thoughtful attention.

Further, in contrast to adults, most children die in hospitals, and the majority of these deaths occur in the intensive care unit often after undergoing interventions with little hope of benefit and associated with a degree of suffering that many adults would have rejected for themselves. To compound the problem, parents are then asked if they "want" to stop these interventions (Burns et al., 2000, Feudtner et al., 2002, Garros, Rosychuk, & Cox, 2003, Carter et al., 2004, Copnell, 2005, Tan, Totapally, Torbati, & Wolfsdorf, 2006, Lee, Tieves, & Scanlon, 2010), thus adding further grief and guilt to an already fraught scenario. There is, therefore, a great need for thoughtful and nuanced attention to how health care professionals think about, discuss, and address the particular issues pediatric patients and their families face.

Another reason that children are often overlooked in the palliative care literature is a failure to appreciate the distinctiveness of the ethical, practical, emotional, and social needs of children, including differences based on their age and experiences. Many people tend to assume that the same basic principles apply to adults as to children, and thus it is sufficient to address these principles in general, possibly with subtle modifications for the unique needs of the pediatric population. As the old saying goes, though, "Children are not little adults." Neither is pediatric palliative care (PPC) a diminutive version of adult palliative care; it is a distinct specialty with unique aspects that demand particular attention.

Differences between Pediatric and Adult Palliative Care

Distinct Diagnoses

The conditions and illnesses encountered in adult palliative care and PPC are often distinct. For instance, the majority of adults referred for palliative care have cancer, and thus many adult or general palliative care programs are situated within cancer centers. By contrast, genetic/congenital and neuromuscular conditions are the most common diagnoses in PPC (Figure 10.1). This difference from adult palliative care impacts both the focus of PPC clinical programs as well as the knowledge base required to provide optimal PPC.

It is not simply a question of certain diagnoses being more or less frequent in pediatrics. Some pediatric diagnoses (such as hydrops fetalis or spinal muscular atrophy type I) *never* occur in adults. Many others (like cystic fibrosis and severe forms of congenital heart disease) were once only seen in childhood, but thanks to advances in medical technology, patients are increasingly living into adulthood. This has left the health care system with two options: either have pediatricians care for young adults or expect adult physicians to become familiar with these conditions (ideally in collaboration with pediatric colleagues). Whichever route is chosen, expert knowledge of the issues facing children—not only physiological but also psychological, social, and spiritual—is crucial.

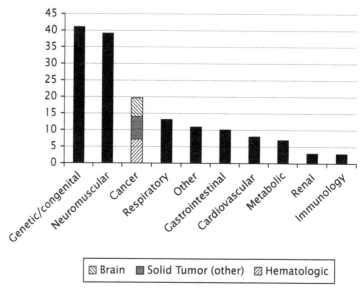

FIGURE 10.1 Percentage of patients referred for pediatric palliative care consultation, based on diagnoses (adapted from Feudtner et al., 2011)

Trajectory and Nature of Illness

Most adults die relatively soon after initial palliative care consultation—in some studies, on the order of weeks (Kamal et al., 2011)—primarily due to comorbidities and a frequent delay in palliative care referral. Therapeutic relationships must be formed quickly and last a relatively short period of time. End-of-life (EOL) conversations therefore play a very large role in adult palliative care, and there is appropriate emphasis on bereavement support.

By contrast, two-thirds of children survive for at least a year after PPC consultation (Feudtner et al., 2011). This is not a sign of earlier referral to palliative care; on the contrary, pediatric referrals often come even later than in adult palliative care because of the presumption toward aggressive treatment. Instead, this reflects the significant diversity in pediatric conditions that are appropriate for palliative care, which can be divided into four categories (Himelstein, Hilden, Morstad Boldt, & Weissman, 2004).

1. Conditions which *may* lead to a child's premature death, such as cancer. The illness trajectory of this group can mirror that of adult palliative care in general, although some childhood cancers which were once uniformly fatal—such as acute lymphoblastic leukemia—are now eminently treatable (Hunger et al. 2012).
2. Conditions that *will* lead to premature death, but life can be prolonged (often significantly) through medical treatment, such as cystic fibrosis.
3. Terminal conditions that are amenable only to palliative treatments, such as glycogen storage diseases.
4. Conditions that may not lead to premature death but do have significant impact on quality of life (QOL), such as profound static brain injuries.

The greater variability—and flatter trajectory in many cases—in disease progression creates both opportunities and challenges. On the one hand, there is greater potential for longitudinal relationship, built over a longer period of time. On the other hand, it can be difficult to pinpoint precisely when the patient is truly approaching the end of life. Prognostication—which is quite challenging even in adult palliative care (p. 84)—is even more complex in PPC. Some commonly used measures of prognostication (such as the surprise question, p. 87) have only recently begun to be studied in the pediatric population (Burke, Coombs, Menezes, & Anderson, 2017). The longer duration of the physician-patient relationship may further complicate matters, as this has been shown to impair the ability to accurately prognosticate the patient's expected survival, at least for adult patients (Christakis, 1999).

Unique Aspects of Treatment of Children

Formulating and implementing a treatment plan in pediatrics can be very complex. Unlike most adults, children—especially very young children—may not appreciate the need for treatment that requires suffering today for survival tomorrow and thus may require additional supports in order to accept it. This requires the involvement of a multidisciplinary team including child life specialists, child psychologists, and expressive therapists (such as art, music, or play).

Even if a child is willing to undergo treatment, determining what that treatment should be can be challenging. Since many conditions that affect children rarely affect adults, there may be little commercial incentive to develop treatments for such conditions. Treatments that do exist may not have been tested on children, forcing clinicians into off-label use with inherent uncertainty as to dosing and side effects (Pandolfini & Bonati, 2005). Some medications used frequently in adult palliative care have an increased risk of side effects in children (Stephenson, 2005). For instance, antidopaminergic medications for nausea and vomiting are less likely to cause dystonic reactions in adults than children, especially the youngest.[1] The difficulty in translating adult treatment regimens into the pediatric world is evident to anyone who has attempted to order haloperidol—a first-line medication for the treatment of nausea in adults—for a child. Resistance from the pediatric floor team is common because the medication is best known as an antipsychotic.

Despite these challenges and complexities, PPC receives relatively little attention in the academic literature, with only 3% of articles in palliative care journals devoted to pediatrics. Of these, only 8% are focused on new data, with most of the others being opinion and review articles (Kumar, 2011).

Unique Social Contexts and Constructs

In adult medicine, patients generally receive health care either in the hospital, clinic, or their residence (whether home, assisted living, or nursing home). Children, on the other hand, may require health care in other places like school or camp, so they can enjoy life despite chronic illness. The reality of managing care in remote or socially unaccepting environments can create challenges in terms of available medical technology, prompt medical attention, and adherence to an agreed-upon treatment plan. For example, an out-of-hospital Do Not Attempt Resuscitation (DNAR) order takes on a whole new significance when a child experiences cardiopulmonary arrest in a school setting. The staff may not be familiar with the scope of a DNAR order and may not feel qualified to assess the situation. Even if they are, there is often a reluctance to honor the order out of concern for other children present in a school or community setting, who may perceive that nothing is being done for the child in need (American Academy of Pediatrics, 2010; Kimberly, Forte, Carroll, & Feudtner, 2005).

Further, while social relationships are important for all patients, in pediatrics the role of parents and siblings—not to mention grandparents, extended family, teachers, and camp counselors—is especially crucial. A child's developmental needs continue to evolve over time with regard to emotional maturity, intellectual capability, and social

---

1. Children do not all have the same physiology, and thus interaction with medications needs to be evaluated separately for infants, toddlers, children, and adolescents.

relationships. As a result, it really is not accurate to speak of "pediatric palliative care," as this lumps together the neonate and the adolescent with their widely disparate needs and presenting conditions. It would be more appropriate to break up PPC into subcategories— such as prenatal, neonatal, child, and adolescent palliative care—which reflect the unique aspects of each, as this text does in ensuing chapters.

Children Aren't Supposed to Die

The death of any person—whether young or old—is a cause for sadness. But whereas an adult's passing can prompt reflections of a full life well-lived, children who die never had that opportunity. Medical advances have led many to believe that every sick child can be cured. Further, there is perhaps no stronger instinct than a parent's to protect her child. All of these lead to a presumption toward more aggressive treatment in pediatrics than adult medicine, in the face of what is inherently an "unnatural" state of affairs. As some have put it, "When an eighty-year-old gets cancer, you have a conversation. When an eight-year-old gets cancer, you start chemotherapy."

This can lead to a protracted and extremely burdensome course of illness. The combination of aggressive treatment and children's inherent resilience can lead to a child "dying many times," referring to situations where a pediatric patient is pulled back from the brink of death. While understandably a cause of celebration—if only transiently— among the patient's family, it also runs the risks of exacerbating suffering and merely delaying the inevitable.

Given the relative rarity of death in childhood, parents also often feel isolated and alone in their situation, with no one with whom to compare notes. They often report that friends and family withdraw from intense involvement in their searingly painful circumstances; they either "just can't bear to hear it" or feel inadequate to offer support. Thankfully, the Internet has enabled people in far-flung locations to reach out to each other, such as through the Courageous Parents Network (https://courageousparentsnetwork. org) and National Organization for Rare Disorders family support program (https:// rarediseases.org/for-patients-and-families).

The "unnatural" quality of a child's death creates a great burden not only on the child's family but also on his caregivers. Concern for burnout is at least as high in pediatric as in adult palliative care (Liben, Papadatou, & Wolfe, 2008), and even those who have found healthy ways to cope with the death of adults struggle when it comes to children.

End-of-Life Decision-Making in Pediatrics

For all of the reasons noted here, the uniqueness of PPC has increasingly been recognized in recent years. An Institute of Medicine (2003) report raised awareness about the particular complexities, needs, and opportunities inherent in PPC. There has also been growing attention to services provided to children and their families, ranging from the construction of the first freestanding pediatric hospice in the United States that same year to the consistent growth of perinatal hospice programs and increased understanding of the grief support and prolonged bereavement needs of parents (Snaman et al., 2016).

As noted, PPC is not limited to EOL situations, which is especially relevant to pediatrics given the more gradual trajectory of illness and complex family dynamics. Nevertheless, EOL decisions and care still represent an incredibly important aspect of PPC. In recognition of this, pediatric-specific approaches to EOL decision-making have begun to be formulated, and the framework offered by the Royal College of Paediatrics and Child Health is particularly helpful (Larcher et al., 2015).

This framework identifies three situations when forgoing treatment might be considered. The first is limited quantity of life, where death is either imminent (i.e., cannot be delayed) or inevitable (i.e., can be delayed but not prevented). As noted, the types of illnesses often seen in PPC can make it difficult to predict at what point a child—especially one living with a chronic illness—is "dying." Even when it is clear that a child will not survive, the decision to forgo medical intervention can be excruciatingly difficult for parents and families.

The second situation is limited QOL, which necessarily raises the question of how to define QOL and who assesses it. Limited QOL may refer to the burdens of treatment being considered—which include psychological or spiritual suffering, as well as physical pain—as well as to refractory symptoms or functional restrictions. The challenge here is that first-person reports may not be available, especially for younger or developmentally disabled children. External assessments of QOL are susceptible to well-documented biases, whereby physicians consistently underestimate a patient's self-assessed QOL.

In one study, for instance, subjects were asked to assess the QOL of a child who was either blind, deaf, or unable to talk, and required help to walk and do schoolwork, but who was happy and worry-free "most of the time" and whose occasional pain was effectively managed with acetaminophen. The control group—made up of healthy adolescents as well as those who were born prematurely—rated the QOL of this patient as substantially reduced. The other group—comprised of health care professionals—however, went so far as to rate his QOL as worse than death (Saigal et al., 1999).

This underscores the point that people who have lived with limitations all their lives can truly enjoy an existence that others cannot imagine. Even some who are thrust suddenly into chronic illness or disability adapt well, occasionally viewing the new existence as a major growth experience.

The reason for the discrepant perceptions of health care professionals may be that they were answering the wrong question. Subconsciously, they might have been comparing the hypothetical patient's life to their own QOL, which presumably includes far fewer burdens and restrictions. But the real question is whether the hypothetical patient's life is better than *no life* at all.

This is particularly relevant in PPC, where the life-limiting diagnosis is often present from birth in the form of congenital anomalies and many genetic conditions. The significance of this is that many children have never experienced life without illness, so comparing their own QOL to that of a healthy child is unimaginable. There is no "new normal" to become accustomed to, and certain limitations are taken for granted because that is the only life the patient and family have ever known. External observers—especially health care professionals, but even parents themselves, who are often healthy though disproportionately burdened in providing the day to day care—may not fully appreciate this and therefore need to approach QOL estimations with appropriate humility.

The third situation when forgoing treatment might be considered is refusal of treatment by a patient with sufficient decision-making capacity (DMC), which is obviously less common in pediatrics than in adult medicine. But when this is a possibility, the situation is complicated by both statute and case law which address when a minor is permitted to make his own medical decisions. This topic is addressed in detail in chapter 13.

Differences between Pediatric Ethics and Adult Ethics

Many ethical principles apply both to adults and children. These include

- the need to comprehensively analyze an ethical dilemma and balance competing rights and obligations (chapter 2)
- the importance of advance care planning (p. 70)
- the challenges of prognostication (p. 84)
- the need to establish a code status which reflects goals of care (p. 101)
- the role of time-limited trials (p. 118) and no escalation of treatment orders (p. 120)
- the right to obtain optimal symptom management (chapter 7), up to and including complete sedation to unconsciousness (chapter 9)

In areas such as the right to forgo life-sustaining medical treatment, pediatric decision-making is often a logical extension of surrogate decision-making for an adult patient who lacks DMC, with specific emphasis on assessing the benefits and burdens (American Academy of Pediatrics, 2017).

Many other issues, though, have permutations and applications that are unique to pediatrics.

In General, the Patient Is Not the Decision-Maker

Adult patients are generally presumed to possess DMC, in which case they can refuse any treatment, even one that is necessary to sustain life (*In re Quinlan,* 1976). As Justice Cardozo wrote in the famous *Schloendoerff* decision: "Every human being *of adult years and sound mind* has a right to determine what shall be done with his own body" (emphasis added). Adults who lack DMC are the exception, and when this occurs the first step is to attempt to restore capacity, such as by lightening sedation or addressing met-abolic abnormalities. If DMC cannot be restored, the next step is to seek substituted judgment (i.e., what the patient would want, if he still had DMC), either in the form of an advance directive or the input from a surrogate. Only when this is not possible does one move on to the best interest standard for decision-making.

By contrast, in pediatrics the patient is presumed to lack DMC. This is clearly true for very young children, but even teenagers often lack sufficient DMC to make com-plex, serious decisions. (The special case of adolescent palliative care is addressed in chapter 13.) The official standard for pediatric decision-making is, therefore, the best interests of the child as interpreted by the parents or guardian(s).

It is important to note that simply because a child is not the legal decision-maker re-garding his care does not mean that the child has *no* role in reaching decisions. Children should be included in discussions and decision-making to the degree that their age and maturity allow. In cases where the child is old enough to understand what is being considered, it is important to obtain his assent prior to commencing (or withholding) treatment. In contrast to *consent*—which involves sufficient understanding of the infor-mation presented and the application of reason and values in coming to a decision—*assent* requires only that the child agree to the plan presented in basic terms appropriate to his cognitive development and emotional maturity (Miller & Nelson, 2006).

Some treatment plans demand the assent of the child and should be deferred if the child is not presently offering it (or cancelled if the child never does). Other treatment plans, however, have such a positive benefit/burden ratio that the withholding of assent by a child with limited DMC should not stand in the way of implementing it. Examples of this include low-burden treatment of life-threatening infections in otherwise healthy children. In such situations, the child should not be asked for his assent but rather in-formed in developmentally appropriate terms what is going to happen, while being offered control over discretionary aspects of care, such as the setting of care and who will be present when the treatment is provided (American Academy of Pediatrics, 2016). In PPC cases where the complexity of the illness and treatment exceeds the patient's DMC, the tenuous balance of benefit and burden often render the child's assent relevant.

The Decision-Maker Is Not Chosen by the Patient

Adults have the opportunity and authority to delegate decision-making responsibility to someone else—known as a health care proxy or agent—should they become unable to do so for themselves (p. 77). By contrast, decision-making for a child is accomplished by someone the child had no choice about: his parents. Historically this stems from the out-dated view that children were merely property belonging to their parents (Mason, 1994). Put quite simply,

> The *laissez-faire* mentality that dominated much of American life well into the
> 20th century gave adults far greater leeway to use children as they wish than

we can imagine today. . . . children could be required to work in unregulated industries for as long as their parents deemed appropriate. Protecting children from harm was not a public responsibility. (Guggenheim, 2005)

The last hundred years have clearly brought greater recognition of children's rights, but the locus of pediatric decision-making appropriately remains with the parents. They (as well as the child) will have to live with the repercussions of any decision, and parents will (ideally) have the fullest sense of what is best for the child (Buchanan & Brock, 1989). Technically, parents provide "permission" rather than consent—since only patients with sufficient DMC and who meet legal requirements can give informed consent (American Academy of Pediatrics, 1995)—but the same requirements for informed consent still apply: voluntariness, appropriate and accurate information, and sufficient DMC (p. 58).

This, however, does not mean that parents have unlimited authority. While a competent adult may refuse any treatment—even for reasons that not everyone would agree with, including personal religious beliefs—the refusal of appropriate treatment for a child constitutes neglect. In such situations, the state has an obligation to intervene to protect the child from harm (the doctrine of *parens patriae*). As famously stated by the US Supreme Court, "Parents have the right to make martyrs of themselves, but they don't have the right under the same circumstances to make martyrs of their children" (*Prince v. Massachusetts*, 1944). The American Academy of Pediatrics (1997) affirms that children—regardless of their own religious beliefs or those of their parents—deserve effective medical care that is not overly burdensome. To emphasize this, in recent statements the academy has shifted from referring to the parental right of decision-making to parental responsibility (American Academy of Pediatrics, 2016).

Best Interest Standard

For an adult who has lost DMC (and it cannot be restored), ideally substituted judgment can be provided by a surrogate decision maker. By contrast, most children do not "lose" DMC. By virtue of age and developmental level, they never possessed it. Logically, then, it would not make sense to try to "restore" something that was never present. It would also not make sense to explore what a child would have decided if he still possessed DMC, since there was never a point in his life when he did. Nor can one accurately predict what a child would one day decide, upon ultimately developing DMC.

The parents are therefore tasked with making decisions in the child's "best interests," which has been defined as "acting so as to promote maximally the good of the individual" (Buchanan & Brock, 1989). Rather than being the "last resort" as it is in adult ethics, the best interest standard is the official basis of pediatric decision-making (Berlinger, Jennings, & Wolf, 2013; Larcher et al. 2015).

While acting in the child's "best interests" may sound good, it is also profoundly impersonal. The values that drive the treatment plan are not the child-patient's—either directly communicated or inferred by someone close to them—but rather those of someone else. Treatment is based on what the parents *believe* is in the child's best interests, which in some cases is unduly influenced by the parents' own views and may not comport with what the clinical team believes is "best" for the child.

In the real world, however, the best interest standard is not truly representative of how medical decisions are made for pediatric patients. Such decisions generally involve multiple options, whereas "best" interest is, by definition, a superlative. Imagine that there are five possible treatment plans for a patient, involving various combinations of potentially beneficial interventions. And further imagine that the medical staff deem the acceptability of the various options on the following scale:

- Option #1: ideal
- Option #2: almost as good as #1, and acceptable
- Option #3: not quite as good as #2, but begrudgingly acceptable
- Option #4: generally unacceptable by virtue of burden/benefit ratio
- Option #5: entirely unacceptable given lack of potential benefit

According to the best interest standard, the parents would essentially be obligated to choose Option #1. Should they not do so, they would not be acting in the child's *best* interests and this could reasonably lead the physicians to report the parents to the appropriate authorities for medical neglect or abuse. Taking "best" literally, therefore, makes a sham of parental autonomy, in that parents are obligated to do what the physicians prefer.

In practice, parents are offered some degree of latitude. They are not required to do what the physicians feel is best but rather what is generally acceptable (based on factors such as the probability of success, the ratio of benefits and burdens, etc.). A more helpful way, then, to approach decision-making for children is by using the "harm principle," whereby parents are permitted to make choices—even "suboptimal" ones—as long as they are not deemed harmful to their children (Diekema, 2004). Diekema has identified eight conditions which must be fulfilled, in order to justify state interference to prevent harm to the patient (Figure 10.2).

Conditions for Justified State Interference with Parental Decision-making

1 By refusing to consent are the parents placing their child at significant risk of serious harm?
2 Is the harm imminent, requiring immediate action to prevent it?
3 Is the intervention that has been refused necessary to prevent the serious harm?
4 Is the intervention that has been refused of proven efficacy, and therefore, likely to prevent the harm?
5 Does the intervention that has been refused by the parents not also place the child at significant risk of serious harm, and do its projected benefits outweigh its projected burdens significantly more favorably than the option chosen by the parents?
6 Would any other option prevent serious harm to the child in a way that is less intrusive to parental autonomy and more acceptable to the parents?
7 Can the state intervention be generalized to all other similar situations?
8 Would most parents agree that the state intervention was reasonable?

FIGURE 10.2 Criteria of harm to justify potential overriding of parental decision-making (Diekema, 2004)

The Decision-Maker May Have Specific Divided Loyalties

It is not unusual for a surrogate decision-maker to have divided loyalties. Consider the loving spouse of a patient who almost surely will not recover and who has expressed a desire to avoid burdensome treatment. Appropriate substituted judgment should lead to a decision to focus on comfort but the fear of losing one's mate might lead the surrogate to make decisions based on her own emotional needs, rather than what the patient would have wanted.

Divided loyalties are especially common in pediatrics. Studies have shown that parental decisions are influenced by a variety of factors, including emotions, faith, provider relationships, prior knowledge, and changes in a child's health status (Lipstein, Brinkman, & Britto, 2012). In situations where the burdens of treatment outweigh the benefits, parents are asked to put the well-being of their child above their own feelings and needs. It runs contrary to every human instinct, though, to "let your child go," even when it has become clear that cure is not possible. Not surprisingly, serious decisions can cause such significant psychological stress as to interfere with decision-making (Benedict, Simpson, & Fernandez, 2007; Miller, Luce, & Nelson, 2011; Pyke-Grimm, Stewart, Kelly, & Degner, 2006) and may also lead to requests for nonbeneficial and even harmful intervention (which is addressed in chapter 14).

Parental decisions are influenced not only by their own feelings but also by conern for the well-being of other members of the family. This raises its own set of questions, including the degree to which the parents' decisions should be based purely on the best interest of the patient in isolation, or whether they can (or should) take into account the well-being of the family as a whole (Downie & Randall, 1997).

This remains a matter of debate. Ross (1998), for example, has put forth a theory of "constrained parental autonomy," whereby parents are permitted to make "intrafamilial trade-offs" so long as "the basic needs of each child member is secured." Others argue that it violates the principle of justice for two children in equivalent medical situations to receive different treatments, based purely on social or familial considerations (McDougall & Notini, 2014).

The latter argument, however, seems to rely on the impractical best interest standard, rather than the more applicable harm principle. As long as parents choose a treatment option that is not harmful, the clinical team is bound to respect their decisions for whatever reason they made it (whether it be social, financial, spiritual, etc.). But when a decision falls below the harm threshold, societal intervention is necessary even when the basis of the decision is understandable and may even be emotionally compelling.

The Clinical Relationship Is a Triad

Finally, the clinical relationship is more complex in pediatrics. In adult medicine, this relationship is generally between the patient and the physician. The other members of the clinical team are often involved—as ideally is the patient's family—but the fundamental relationship governing decisions is a dyad.

By contrast, in pediatrics the clinical relationship is a triad: patient, parent(s), and physician. This introduces greater complexity, based on who is giving permission (parent) and assent (the child, depending on maturity). Normally a patient would be fully informed about his health status and options, but parents often want to "shield" their child from burdensome knowledge, which developmentally he may not be able to handle. This increased complexity in areas of consent and disclosure can result in significant ethical dilemmas and moral distress (p. 514).

Summary Points

- Pediatric palliative care (PPC) is largely distinct from adult palliative care.
  - Distinct diagnoses and illness trajectories exist in pediatrics, as well as unique aspects of treatment and social contexts.
  - Perhaps most fundamentally, children "aren't supposed to die," leading to a greater tendency toward aggressive treatment than in adult care. Palliative care consultation may come very late in the child's course of treatment.
- Pediatric ethics is also largely distinct from "adult ethics."
  - The decision-maker is not the patient—nor even chosen by the patient—and may have significant divided loyalties.
  - The fundamental paradigm is not respect for autonomy but rather the best interest standard (which in practice is more often actualized as the harm principle).
  - The clinical relationship can be more complex, involving not only the patient and physician but also the patient's parents and perhaps other family members as well.
- Because of these unique qualities, the ethics of PPC merit not merely a passing mention but rather an in-depth analysis.

References

American Academy of Pediatrics. (1995). Informed consent, parental permission, and assent in pediatric practice. *Pediatrics, 95*(2), 314–317.

American Academy of Pediatrics. (1997). Religious objections to medical care. *Pediatrics, 99*(2), 279–281.

American Academy of Pediatrics. (2010). Honoring do-not-attempt-resuscitation requests in schools. *Pediatrics, 125*(5), 1073–1077. doi:10.1542/peds.2010-0452

American Academy of Pediatrics. (2016). Informed consent in decision-making in pediatric practice. *Pediatrics, 138*(2), 1–8.

American Academy of Pediatrics. (2017). Guidance on forgoing life-sustaining medical treatment. *Pediatrics, 140*(3), 1–10.

Benedict, J. M., Simpson, C., & Fernandez, C. V. (2007). Validity and consequence of informed consent in pediatric bone marrow transplantation: The parental experience. *Pediatr Blood Cancer, 49*(6), 846–851. doi:10.1002/pbc.21073

Berlinger, N., Jennings, B., & Wolf, S. M. (2013). *The Hastings Center guidelines for decisions on life-sustaining treatment and care near the end of life* (rev. and expanded 2nd ed.). Oxford: Oxford University Press.

Buchanan, A. E., & Brock, D. W. (1989). *Deciding for others: The ethics of surrogate decisionmaking.* New York: Cambridge University Press.

Burke, K., Coombes, L. H., Menezes, A., & Anderson, A. K. (2017). The "surprise" question in paediatric palliative care: A prospective cohort study. *Palliat Med*, 269216317716061. doi:10.1177/0269216317716061

Burns, J. P., Mitchell, C., Outwater, K. M., Geller, M., Griffith, J. L., Todres, I. D., & Truog, R. D. (2000). End-of-life care in the pediatric intensive care unit after the forgoing of life-sustaining treatment. *Crit Care Med*, 28(8), 3060–3066.

Carter, B. S., Howenstein, M., Gilmer, M. J., Throop, P., France, D., & Whitlock, J. A. (2004). Circumstances surrounding the deaths of hospitalized children: Opportunities for pediatric palliative care. *Pediatrics*, 114(3), e361–e366. doi:10.1542/peds.2003-0654-F

Christakis, N. A. (1999). *Death foretold: Prophecy and prognosis in medical care*. Chicago: University of Chicago Press.

Copnell, B. (2005). Death in the pediatric ICU: Caring for children and families at the end of life. *Criti Care Nurs Clinics N Am*, 17(4), 349–360. doi:10.1016/j.ccell.2005.07.007

Diekema, D. S. (2004). Parental refusals of medical treatment: The harm principle as threshold for state intervention. *Theor Med Bioethics*, 25(4), 243–264.

Downie, R. S., & Randall, F. (1997). Parenting and the best interests of minors. *J Med Phil*, 22(3), 219–231.

Feudtner, C., Kang, T. I., Hexem, K. R., Friedrichsdorf, S. J., Osenga, K., Siden, H., . . . Wolfe, J. (2011). Pediatric palliative care patients: A prospective multicenter cohort study. *Pediatrics*, 127(6), 1094–1101. doi:10.1542/peds.2010-3225

Feudtner, C., Christakis, D. A., Zimmerman, F. J., Muldoon, J. H., Neff, J. M., & Koepsell, T. D. (2002). Characteristics of deaths occurring in children's hospitals: Implications for supportive care services. *Pediatrics*, 109(5), 887–893.

Garros, D., Rosychuk, R. J., & Cox, P. N. (2003). Circumstances surrounding end of life in a pediatric intensive care unit. *Pediatrics*, 112(5), e371.

Guggenheim, M. (2005). *What's wrong with children's rights*. Cambridge, MA: Harvard University Press.

Himelstein, B. P., Hilden, J. M., Morstad Boldt, A., & Weissman, D. (2004). Pediatric palliative care. *N Engl J Med*, 350(17), 1752–1762. doi:10.1056/NEJMra030334350/17/1752

Hunger, S. P., Lu, X., Devidas, M., Camitta, B. M., Gaynon, P. S., Winick, N. J., . . . Carroll, W. L. (2012). Improved survival for children and adolescents with acute lymphoblastic leukemia between 1990 and 2005: A report from the children's oncology group. *J Clin Oncol*, 30(14),1663–1669. doi:10.1200/JCO.2011.37.8018

In re Quinlan. 70 10 (N.J. 1976).

Institute of Medicine Committee on Palliative and End-of-Life Care for Children and Their Families. (2003). *When children die: Improving palliative and end-of-life care for children and their families*. Washington, DC: National Academy Press.

Kimberly, M. B., Forte, A. L., Carroll, J. M., & Feudtner, C. (2005). Pediatric do-not-attempt-resuscitation orders and public schools: A national assessment of policies and laws. *Am J Bioeth*, 5(1), 59–65. doi:10.1080/15265160590900605

Kamal, A. H., Swetz, K. M., Carey, E. C., Cheville, A. L., Liu, H., Ruegg, S. R., . . . Kaur, J. S. (2011). Palliative care consultations in patients with cancer: A Mayo Clinic 5-year review. *J Oncol Pract*, 7(1), 48–53. doi:10.1200/JOP.2010.000067

Kumar, S. P. (2011). Reporting of pediatric palliative care: A systematic review and quantitative analysis of research publications in palliative care journals. *Ind J Palliat Care*, 17(3), 202–209. doi:10.4103/0973-1075.92337

Larcher, V., Craig, F., Bhogal, K., Wilkinson, D., & Brierley, J. (2015). Making decisions to limit treatment in life-limiting and life-threatening conditions in children: A framework for practice. *Arch Dis Child*, 100(Suppl. 2), s3–s23. doi:10.1136/archdischild-2014-306666

Lee, K. J., Tieves, K., & Scanlon, M. C. (2010). Alterations in end-of-life support in the pediatric intensive care unit. *Pediatrics*, 126(4), e859–e864. doi:10.1542/peds.2010-0420

Liben, S., Papadatou, D., & Wolfe, J. (2008). Paediatric palliative care: Challenges and emerging ideas. *Lancet, 371*(9615), 852–864. doi:10.1016/S0140-6736(07)61203-3

Lipstein, E. A., Brinkman, W. B., & Britto, M. T. (2012). What is known about parents' treatment decisions? A narrative review of pediatric decision making. *Med Decis Making, 32*(2), 246–258. doi:10.1177/0272989X11421528

Mason, M. A. (1994). *From father's property to children's rights: The history of child custody in the United States.* New York: Columbia University Press.

McDougall, R. J., & Notini, L. (2014). Overriding parents' medical decisions for their children: A systematic review of normative literature. *J Med Ethics, 40*(7), 448–452. doi:10.1136/medethics-2013-101446

Miller, V. A., Luce, M. F., & Nelson, R. M. (2011). Relationship of external influence to parental distress in decision making regarding children with a life-threatening illness. *J Pediatr Psych, 36*(10), 1102–1112. doi:10.1093/jpepsy/jsr033

Miller, V. A., & Nelson, R. M. (2006). A developmental approach to child assent for nontherapeutic research. *J Pediatr, 149*(1 Suppl.), S25–S30. doi:10.1016/j.jpeds.2006.04.047

Osterman, M. J., Kochanek, K., MacDorman, M. F., Strobino, D. M., & Guyer, B. Annual summary of vital statistics: 2012–2013. *Pediatrics, 135*(6), 1115–1125. doi:10.1542/peds.2015-0434

Pandolfini, C., & Bonati, M. (2005). A literature review on off-label drug use in children. *Eur J Pediatr, 164*(9), 552–558. doi:10.1007/s00431-005-1698-8

Prince v. Massachusetts. (1944). U.S. Supreme Court.

Pyke-Grimm, K. A., Stewart, J. L., Kelly, K. P., & Degner, L. F. (2006). Parents of children with cancer: Factors influencing their treatment decision making roles. *J Pediatr Nurs, 21*(5), 350–361. doi:10.1016/j.pedn.2006.02.005

Ross, L. F. (1998). *Children, families, and health care decision making.* Oxford; New York: Clarendon Press.

Saigal, S., Stoskopf, B. L., Feeny, D., Furlong, W., Burrows, E., Rosenbaum, P. L., & Hoult, L. (1999). Differences in preferences for neonatal outcomes among health care professionals, parents, and adolescents. *JAMA, 281*(21), 1991–1997.

Schloendorff v. Society of New York Hospital (211 NY 125, 105 NE 92 [1914])

Snaman, J. M., Kaye, E. C., Levine, D. R., Cochran, B., Wilcox, R., Sparrow, C. K., . . . Baker, J. N. (2016). Empowering bereaved parents through the development of a comprehensive bereavement program. *J Pain Symptom Manage, 53*(4), 767–775. doi:10.1016/j.jpainsymman.2016.10.359

Stephenson, T. (2005). How children's responses to drugs differ from adults. *Br J Clin Pharmacol, 59*(6), 670–673. doi:10.1111/j.1365-2125.2005.02445.x

Tan, G. H., Totapally, B., Torbati, D., & Wolfsdorf, J. (2006). End-of-life decisions and palliative care in a children's hospital. *J Palliat Med, 9*(2), 332–342. doi:10.1089/jpm.2006.9.332

11

Ethics of Prenatal Palliative Care

Some of the most difficult questions in palliative care begin before the patient is even born. Not even counting those which occur prior to twenty weeks gestation—for which no statistics are kept—over 24,000 fetal demises occur each year in the United States, (Osterman, Kochanek, MacDorman, Strobino, & Guyer, 2015). This number exceeds either infant or child/adolescent deaths.

This has not received as much attention, however, because in many situations the death of the fetus is not preventable and the life-threatening condition is often not identified in advance. These are among the reasons why the development of prenatal palliative care has lagged behind the rest of pediatric palliative care (which, in turn, has lagged behind adult palliative care).

Case Study

A thirty-two-year-old woman is pregnant with her third child. The two previous pregnancies were uneventful, and her two-year-old son and five-year-old daughter are healthy and thriving. This pregnancy's first ultrasound, however, identified features that are strongly suggestive of Trisomy 13 with obstructive hydrocephalus. The patient and her husband request a confirmatory amniocentesis which the obstetrician initially questions the utility of, since the family's religious beliefs do not permit termination of pregnancy.

The obstetrician ultimately agrees, with the result confirming the trisomy. The physician explains that the majority of fetuses with this condition die in utero. Of infants born alive, less than half survive two weeks or more. The parents grasp what he is saying, yet express their hope of savoring any time they may have with their child.

They therefore request that a caesarian section be performed in the event that the fetus is in distress during birth (which is likely, given the enlarged head). The obstetrician, however, is reluctant to subject the pregnant woman to such risks, given that the baby would only survive for a short period of time, if at all.

Historicolegal Background

From a legal standpoint, the primary consideration involving pregnancy-related issues is termination of pregnancy. The best-known court case (*Roe v. Wade*, 1973) established a trimester-based metric for termination. According to this decision in the first trimester the state is not allowed to place any limitations on a woman's right to terminate her pregnancy. In the second trimester, the state may establish limitations only insofar as they are directed to safeguard the life or health of the pregnant woman. (For example, the state could outlaw a specific procedure that it felt was inferior to another procedure.) In the third trimester, the state may place any limitations it wishes on termination of pregnancy, as long as there are exceptions made to safeguard the life or health of the pregnant woman.

When *Roe v. Wade* was decided in 1973, the point of viability was approximately twenty-eight weeks, coinciding with the beginning of the third trimester of pregnancy. As the field of neonatology has advanced, however, the point of viability has been pushed back into the second trimester. It is now generally held to be at twenty-three weeks, although some studies have shown that twenty-two might be a better approximation (Rysavy et al., 2015). As a result, the framework of *Roe* no longer neatly coincides with viability.

Currently, the prevailing national judicial precedent is *Planned Parenthood v. Casey* (1992), which did away with the trimester system of *Roe*. In its place, the Supreme Court held that states may not place an "undue burden" on the right of a pregnant woman to terminate a fetus, up until the point of viability. This, of course, leaves it up to individual states to determine what represents an "undue burden," with contentious state laws ultimately winding their way through the judicial system. Requirements such as waiting periods, compulsory viewing of ultrasounds, methods of termination, scripted explanations of risks that not all professionals recognize, gestational age limits prior to the point of viability, and parental consent for minors have prompted judicial review (Shimabukuro, 2016) and professional commentary (Buchbinder, Lassiter, Mercier, Bryant, & Lyerly, 2016).

One of the challenges of these restrictions on termination is that they are primarily directed at purely elective termination of a healthy fetus. In order to qualify for perinatal palliative care, however, the fetus must be experiencing a serious medical problem. As a result, some of the protective measures put in place to prevent potentially "inappropriate" termination—however one defines that term—of a healthy fetus may represent an obstacle to termination of a pregnancy affected by serious or even lethal anomalies.

Clinical

The emotional impact of a life-limiting fetal diagnosis is profound. At least in planned pregnancies, the news that a woman is pregnant is cause for celebration. Generally, unless there is personal experience of pregnancy-related complications or losses, most pregnant women and their partners anticipate that the pregnancy will go smoothly resulting in the birth of a healthy child. The news that the fetus is not healthy can be among the most devastating that anyone can receive.

Parents[1] in such a situation face more decisions now than ever. Enhanced screening techniques have yielded additional information earlier in pregnancy (Gregg et al., 2013), such as the likelihood of genetic conditions such as Trisomy 21 (Down syndrome). Confirmation of suspected conditions requires invasive diagnostic testing, such as amniocentesis. This, in turn, carries the risk of complications including miscarriage (Akolekar, Beta, Picciarelli, Ogilvie, & D'Antonio, 2015).

If the diagnosis is confirmed, many parents elect not to continue the pregnancy. In the United States, for instance, two out of three fetuses prenatally diagnosed with Down syndrome are terminated, although this percentage seems to be decreasing (Natoli, Ackerman, McDermott, & Edwards, 2012). The fact that the majority of pregnant women elect to terminate may lead clinicians to expect—or even appear to encourage—this decision. Parents of even more severe trisomies have thus reported feeling pressured into terminating or judged for not choosing to do so (Guon, Wilfond, Farlow, Brazg, & Janvier, 2014).

Some conditions identified through prenatal testing have fairly established trajectories, allowing for accurate prognostication and identification of treatment options. Others, however—including many genetic conditions—may have variable expression, which make it difficult to anticipate how severely the fetus will be affected or what the baby's condition will be upon delivery (if the pregnancy is continued). In a sense, the only thing that is certain is uncertainty, which may be helpful to acknowledge to parents in order to validate the emotions that naturally arise from such a situation (Feudtner & Munson, 2009).

---

1. "Parent" refers to the pregnant woman and her partner—if she has one—who may or may not be the biological father of the fetus. This terminology is not meant to comment on whether the fetus is or is not a "person," but is used merely for the sake of convenience as continually repeating "the pregnant woman and her partner if she has one" is cumbersome. It should not be taken as equating the decisional authority of the pregnant woman's partner—if there is one, and even if that person is the biological father of the fetus—before and after delivery, as prior to delivery the locus of decision-making rests entirely with the pregnant woman. Even after delivery, state laws often restrict the other parent's involvement in decision-making unless he or she is married to the mother or the mother has consented to that person's name appearing on the birth certificate.

Decision-making is further complicated by the fact that the fetus is known only indirectly, through ultrasound images and laboratory tests generally done on the pregnant woman (American Academy of Pediatrics, 2009). Decisions made prior to delivery may be reconsidered once the baby is delivered, as additional clinical information becomes available. The emotional context changes, too, as the mother has had to cope with delivery and when presented with her newborn may make different choices than she did prenatally.

Ethical

Invasive Testing

Prenatal screening, for all the remarkable technological advances in recent years, still only generates probabilities. While it can be reassuring to learn that there is a one-in-a-million chance that a baby will be born with a specific condition, this is still not an absolute guarantee that the baby will be healthy. Conversely, an increased risk—say, from one-in-a-thousand at baseline to one-in-ten—is cause for additional concern, but in terms of probabilities the condition in question is still likely *not* to be present.

Once screening has identified a fetus at increased risk, confirmatory testing is offered. When this is invasive, it poses a small but real risk both to the fetus and to the pregnant woman. This brings to mind a famous saying in medicine: "Don't do a test unless it's going to change management." In other words, do not subject a patient to the discomfort, risk, and/or cost of a diagnostic procedure unless the result will be practical and helpful. In light of this, one might reasonably question whether amniocentesis is indicated in this chapter's case if the pregnant woman is not considering termination. Why run the low risk of inducing a miscarriage if a positive result will not affect clinical care?

Such a view, however, overlooks the broader aspects of palliative care which consider not only somatic health but other elements of a person as well: the spiritual, the emotional, and the social. Viewed in this light, "management" becomes a very broad term indeed. The parents may suffer emotionally from not knowing whether the fetus really has the suspected life-limiting diagnosis. If the diagnosis is established, the parents have the opportunity to emotionally prepare for the possibility of an intrauterine fetal demise or (at best) markedly reduced survival after birth.

The parents can also address pressing questions, such as whether the extended family will be present for the delivery (given the short life expectancy of the baby, if born alive), whether a clergyperson will be in attendance to baptize or bless the baby (depending on their faith tradition), and whether the parents should begin grieving now so that they can be fully present for their baby when he is born. "Perinatal hospice" can be invaluable in addressing these concerns (p. 299).

This is not to say that prenatal diagnosis is always the best course of action. Some families might prefer *not* to know whether the fetus is affected, to preserve the possibility of optimism through the rest of the pregnancy. For others, the admittedly remote possibility of causing a miscarriage of a healthy fetus is of such concern that they would prefer to cope with uncertainty rather than risk this "worst-case scenario." Like so many other issues in palliative care, the deeply held personal beliefs of the patient and family will lead them to their own conclusions, which might differ from what others would decide in a similar situation.

The key from a palliative care perspective is providing information in a way that is understandable to the pregnant woman and her partner. Statistics in and of themselves may not be helpful, based on the bias introduced by framing (p. 60) and the different ways people process various representations of information (such as percentages, fractions, and odds). It is more important to identify what the family's hopes, goals, and fears are, inherently recognizing the relevance of nonphysical factors such as emotional burden. Only after such a nuanced conversation is it possible to formulate a thoughtful testing recommendation that reflects the family's overall goals.

Continue or Terminate the Pregnancy?

Once confirmed, the fact that a fetus is affected by a life-limiting condition can be devastating to a pregnant woman and her partner. Many people in that situation opt to terminate the pregnancy, rather than continue it knowing that the fetus might not have survived the pregnancy anyway, and even if it did was likely to suffer from serious limitations (Crider, Olney, & Cragan, 2008). Legal considerations may play a role in this, depending on the gestational age of the fetus and the state of residence (Guttmacher Institute, 2017). Institutional policy and individual clinicians' personal beliefs could also come into play.

A pregnant woman might also choose to continue the pregnancy in the hope that her child will "defy the odds." As noted, uncertainty is an inherent element in many prenatal diagnoses and conditions. Choosing to continue one's pregnancy in such a situation should therefore not be viewed as a sign of "denial." Parents might well accept the reality of the diagnosis and prognosis, yet simultaneously maintain hope for significant meaning for however long their child is able to survive (Kamihara, Nyborn, Olcese, Nickerson, & Mack, 2015).

This approach is not unreasonable, especially given evolving outcome data related to conditions such as Trisomy 13. While earlier studies had suggested that fewer than one in twenty liveborn infants survived six months or more (Lakovschek, Streubel, & Ulm, 2011), newer studies have revealed a significant "tail" to the survival curve. For while half of liveborn patients may die within the first two weeks, recent studies have shown that nearly one in seven can survive for a decade or more (Nelson, Rosella, Mahant, & Guttmann, 2016).

One reason for documented improved survival is the increasing willingness of medical centers to honor families' requests for aggressive treatment, often including cardiac surgery for heart malformations that are common to Trisomy 13 (Peterson, Kochilas, Catton, Moller, & Setty, 2017). While such procedures are certainly high risk, there is increasing recognition of the possibility of benefit. Previously more sobering data may, therefore, have to some degree reflected a "self-fulfilling prophecy," whereby surgery was forgone based on supposedly poor outcomes, thus making early death more likely and further lowering survival statistics.

For parents who request maximal interventions after delivery, the team should be clear with the family about what this means. Such a discussion should examine both the likelihood of success—however that is defined—as well as the burdens inherent in treatment. These include not only pain and suffering on the part of the infant but lost opportunities for emotional connection in the midst of intensive and invasive interventions (Macauley, 2015).

Preliminary plans can be formulated, but these should be reevaluated as additional clinical information becomes available. Expected "waypoints" should also be identified, to prepare the family for developments or events that lend themselves to reevaluation of the appropriateness of the treatment plan.

Up to this point, only two options have been considered in the case of a serious fetal condition: termination of pregnancy or continued pregnancy with maximal treatment if the baby is born alive. This is a false dichotomy, however. Parents may also choose to continue the pregnancy and provide comfort-directed care to the neonate (Feudtner & Munson, 2009). Such a plan might reflect a moral or religious opposition to termination of pregnancy, as in this chapter's case. Or the pregnant woman might acknowledge the burdens of aggressive treatment, while also hoping her baby will be born alive. The possibility of even a short period of time with her child could warrant continuing the pregnancy.

In such situations, it is crucial to formulate a birth plan which reflects the family's goals, including obstetrical management that is consistent with the postnatal plan of care. Some families are content to trust that "what will be, will be," in which case intrapartum monitoring would not be required. Others, though, so desire a live birth that they would want a Caesarian section (or C-section) if the fetus were to experience distress. This would only be detected through intrapartum monitoring, which would therefore be consistent with the patient's goals.

In either case, following delivery the baby should immediately be brought to the mother and all steps taken to maximize the quality of the limited time the parents have with the baby before he dies.

Caesarian Section

One of the most common ethical dilemmas in prenatal palliative care is "maternal-fetal conflict" (i.e., when what is good for the pregnant woman is not good for the fetus, or vice versa). In many ways pregnancy itself is a risk factor to the mother's health, based on complications such as pregnancy-induced hypertension, gestational diabetes, and uterine rupture. A pregnant woman will almost always be healthier once the pregnancy is over.

C-section is not without risks, however. Emergency peripartum hysterectomy is more common than with vaginal births (Machado, 2011), and anesthesia complications in rare cases can be lethal. It also impacts future reproductive capability with an elevated risk of uterine rupture in subsequent pregnancies, potentially precluding vaginal births.

Acknowledging these risks, the standard of care in obstetrics is to proceed with delivery—either by induction of labor or C-section, irrespective of gestational age—if the pregnancy is endangering the life of the pregnant woman and she consents to the intervention. This may place the fetus at risk, but if it is appropriate for an otherwise healthy (although perhaps premature) fetus, it is also appropriate for a fetus who is affected with a life-limiting condition.

The key here is the consent of the pregnant woman, without which induction of labor or C-section cannot proceed. Thus she may also refuse it, even when it is recommended by the medical team. For example, a woman diagnosed with cancer during an early stage of pregnancy might opt to defer treatment that could be harmful to the fetus until after delivery (Han, Mhallem Gziri, Van Calsteren, & Amant, 2013). That, too, is her right, as long as she is fully informed of the risks, benefits, and alternatives. Given the steadily improving outcomes with increasing gestational age, the decision as to precisely when to deliver the baby—as waiting until full term confers proportionately greater risk to the woman than benefit to the fetus—may be complex.

In addition to maternal indications, C-section or induction of labor can also be performed for fetal indications. A fetus might suffer from a condition (such as hydrops fetalis) that becomes more serious as the pregnancy continues or could be experiencing compromised umbilical blood flow from uterine contractions during labor. Intervening to safeguard the fetus is not contentious when an otherwise healthy fetus is at risk, with the pregnant woman's consent being sufficient grounds.

But what if the fetus suffers from a life-limiting condition? Already fragile, such fetuses are less likely to survive the process of vaginal delivery. In some cases—as in this chapter's example of severe hydrocephalus—the physical difficulty of an enlarged head making its way through the birth canal renders vaginal birth especially risky.

The normal justification for C-section for fetal distress (i.e., making possible a hopefully long and healthy life) is not operative here. In the absence of maternal distress, the only benefit of C-section would be whatever importance the parents might place on holding a living child during the child's short life, and whatever meaning the child himself derives from that experience.

Interestingly, the question of whether to perform a C-section in this context has received relatively little attention in the ethics literature. Two recent commentaries, however, have addressed the question, with both authors advocating honoring the patient's request for C-section, based on respect for her autonomy (Mayor, 2015; White, 2015).

This topic is also rarely mentioned in the clinical literature and then generally only as parts of case series of pregnancies affected by a terminal condition (Breeze, Lees, Kumar, Missfelder-Lobos, & Murdoch, 2007). While rigorous studies of obstetricians' opinions on this issue is lacking, anecdotally many physicians—especially senior ones—are reluctant to perform a C-section for fetal distress in the context of serious fetal condition.

Intraoperative complications during C-section may be relatively rare, but experienced clinicians have been practicing long enough to encounter them and thus appreciate the suffering and grief they bring. These physicians often express concern that the pregnant woman may not fully appreciate the risk to her health or the impact on future reproductive options.

Alternatively, clinicians may not appreciate the emotional importance the woman ascribes to holding a live newborn. Pregnant women and their families in that situation report that the experience of holding their living baby—if only for a few hours, or even minutes—can be profound (Breeze et al., 2007). And this assumes that the baby will only live for minutes or hours, which in light of recent studies is far from certain.

Clearly, C-section is offered by some obstetricians for less momentous justification, such as convenience or simply a pregnant woman's desire to forgo vaginal birth. Such "elective primary C-sections" represent as many as 3% of all C-sections in the United States (Gossman, Joesch, & Tanfer, 2006; MacDorman, Menacker, & Declercq, 2008), with the rate associated with maternal affluence and appearing to be growing (Alves & Sheikh, 2005). While the American College of Obstetricians and Gynecologists (2013) officially discourages the practice, its most recent position statement rejects it outright only for pregnancies that have not yet reached full term. Certainly if one grants the ethical permissibility of elective primary C-section, then one should be willing to perform a C-section for fetal distress in the context of a life-limiting condition if the pregnant woman so values a live birth.

But even if one takes a more judicious approach and would decline requests for elective primary C-section, the sacred nature of a parent and newborn having a few moments or hours (or longer) together would seem sufficient justification to perform a C-section for fetal distress in that situation. To refuse a pregnant woman's request is paternalistic,[2] essentially concluding that the woman's expressed heartfelt goals are not sufficient to justify a procedure frequently performed for more conventional "medical indications." If one takes seriously the concepts of total suffering and patient autonomy, then a C-section should be performed for fetal distress if the pregnant woman requests it, even when the fetus is affected by a terminal condition.

Terminalogy

The terminology that professionals use to describe a patient's condition can have significant impact both on treatment decisions that are made, as well as the emotional response of the patient and family. This is particularly true when describing conditions that are associated with imminent or inevitable death, which many would describe as "terminal." The way medical professionals talk about a child and his illness is as important as how

---

2. The term "paternalistic"—rather than the more inclusive "parentalistic"—is appropriate here, reflecting the lack of respect shown to the pregnant woman's goals.

they treat that illness; indeed, it directly affects the way the patient is viewed and cared for (Nickel, Barratt, Copp, Moynihan & McCaffery, 2017).

In the prenatal period a term that is often used is "incompatible with life." This has been used to refer to fetal anomalies that invariably result in miscarriage or death in the first hours, days, or weeks of life (Fleming, Iljuschin, Pehlke-Milde, Maurer, & Parpan, 2016). In a recent study, almost 90% of parents expecting a baby affected with either Trisomy 13 or 18 were told that condition was "incompatible with life" (Janvier, Farlow, & Wilfond, 2012).

This term appears unique to the prenatal period, since it does not make sense to say that an adult or child has a condition "incompatible with life," simply because that patient is currently alive. Affected fetuses, on the other hand, may never experience postnatal life, frequently dying *in utero*.

This term should be avoided. One reason is that it is inaccurate, as its application has broadened beyond conditions inevitably leading to deaths *in utero* to those that could permit live birth but with a likely limited life expectancy. Indeed, some conditions formerly termed "incompatible with life"—such as Trisomy 18—are now recognized to have longer term survivors (Kosho et al., 2006) and thus are no longer included in the list of conditions which justify not offering resuscitation (Kattwinkel et al., 2011).

Further, even if a condition is uniformly fatal in the first weeks or months of life for survivors, it would still be inappropriate to call it *incompatible* with life. To do so demeans the patient who lived—admittedly briefly—as well as the family who loved that child. Understandably, parent and professional groups have begun to highlight the inappropriateness of the term ("Geneva Declaration on Perinatal Care," 2015).

"Lethal anomaly" is another term that is often misapplied. The term itself is imprecise, as it would seem to cover both conditions that will imminently cause the death of the child, as well as those that will inevitably cause death at some point in the perhaps distant future (Larcher et al., 2015). It also does not take into account the degree of quality of life or extent of suffering (if any) the child will experience, however long he lives. As Koogler, Wilfond, and Ross (2003) observe, " 'Lethal anomaly' is not an accurate clinical description; instead, it serves to convey an implicit normative view about quality of life."

Perinatal Hospice

In situations where it becomes clear that a fetus will not be born alive—or a neonate will die soon after birth—perinatal hospice can provide crucial support to the pregnant woman and her family. Because this is not a routine pregnancy, it is especially important to formulate a clear birth plan that includes both medical and nonmedical considerations. From a medical perspective, the birth plan might identify clear treatment goals for both the mother and the fetus (such as addressing the question of C-section for fetal distress, as noted earlier). From a nonmedical perspective, the birth plan could address relevant spiritual beliefs (such as the desire for baptism, should the baby be born alive) as well as specific requests following the death of the baby (which might include being permitted private time to grieve).

Memory-making is also an important part of hospice care. Preparations can be made for creating treasured keepsakes after birth—such as foot or hand impressions—even if the baby is not born alive. Many parents value family photographs, which can be performed before birth as well as after. Particularly in situations where there may be significant physical deformities affecting the fetus (as in the case of delivery after longstanding fetal demise), photos of the pregnant woman with her family can provide comfort. Volunteer professional photographers are often available for this service ("Now I Lay Me Down to Sleep," 2016). When parents are not sure if they would want to ever look at those photos, it is reasonable to encourage them to permit the photos to be taken, preserving the option—should they choose to exercise it—of viewing them at a later date.

Anticipating the birth of a child with life-limiting illness can be a very bittersweet experience. Intermixed with profound sadness and anticipatory grief is the natural excitement that comes with being pregnant, and the measured hopes for meaningful time with one's child. Focusing all attention on grief may detract from this profound experience.

Casual acquaintances may not, however, appreciate the bittersweet balance of the experience. They may, for example, congratulate a pregnant woman with comments like "You must be so excited." Contexts where others are reasonably expecting healthy babies—like birthing classes—can be heartbreaking. Providing support to the pregnant woman and her partner through these difficult times by normalizing their feelings and equipping them with "scripts" to respond to such comments (without making the innocent commenter feel bad) can be very helpful.

It is also important to recognize that pregnant women and their partners experience loss on many levels: a mixture of joy and sadness over a live birth and lost dreams of a healthy, thriving child over many years. Grief occurs at different moments, too, as a diagnosis may require time to become clear. In the case of a miscarriage, sadness comes upon being informed, and there is a pain of a different sort upon giving birth to a baby who has already died.

While the pregnancy is exceptional in many ways, it is not so in others. The expectant mother will experience the same symptoms as any other pregnant woman: nausea, weight gain, possible diabetes and depression. She can often "get lost in the mix," as the bulk of attention is directed to the fetus and planning for delivery. Perinatal hospice attends not only to needs related to the fetus/newborn but also to those of the pregnant woman, both during pregnancy and following delivery.

Return to the Case

In preparation for the baby's birth, the parents asked their pastor to be in attendance in order to baptize the baby immediately, should Rose (her given name) be born alive. They have also had extensive discussions with the obstetrical team, reiterating their hope for a live birth. The team has explained the risks associated with C-section, but the parents wish to proceed. They and the team reach a compromise: there will not be a scheduled C-section, but if during labor the fetus exhibits distress and the team feels that the probability of a live birth would be increased by doing a C-section, they will perform one.

The pregnant woman goes into labor at thirty-six weeks, and Rose remains fairly stable through the early stages of labor. Eventually, though, the fetal heart rate becomes more unstable, and a C-section is performed.

The baby is born alive, and the baby is dried and swaddled and given to the family. The pastor immediately baptizes her, and the medical team offers the family privacy to spend quality time with their child.

Rose lives for approximately three hours. The parents and their other children are immensely grateful for that time with her and for the team's support.

The patient recovers without complication and feels that even if she is not able to have a vaginal delivery in subsequent pregnancies—should there be any—the C-section was worth it for the moments they had with their daughter.

Summary Points

- In the United States, *in utero* deaths outnumber those of children.
- While state laws vary, from the federal perspective a state is not permitted to place an "undue burden" on a pregnant woman's right to terminate a previable pregnancy.
- Even if parents are not considering termination of pregnancy, prenatal testing may be beneficial in order to best prepare them for what is to come and to formulate a birth plan that reflects their goals.
- When a fetus is diagnosed with a life-limiting condition, termination of pregnancy and maximal treatment are not the only two options. Another is to work toward a live birth—which would include fetal monitoring and C-section for fetal distress—at which point comfort care would be provided, allowing the parents to have meaningful time with their child.
- Some of the terminology sometimes used in prenatal care—such as "incompatible with life" and "lethal anomaly"—is inaccurate and unhelpful and should be avoided.
- Perinatal hospice can provide invaluable care to parents of a fetus with a life-limiting condition, both during the pregnancy and after delivery.

References

Akolekar, R., Beta, J., Picciarelli, G., Ogilvie, C., & D'Antonio, F. (2015). Procedure-related risk of miscarriage following amniocentesis and chorionic villus sampling: A systematic review and meta-analysis. *Ultrasound Obstet Gynecol, 45*(1), 16–26. doi:10.1002/uog.14636

Alves, B., & Sheikh, A. (2005). Investigating the relationship between affluence and elective caesarean sections. *BJOG, 112*(7), 994–996. doi:10.1111/j.1471-0528.2005.00657.x

American Academy of Pediatrics. (2009). Antenatal counseling regarding resuscitation at an extremely low gestational age. *Pediatrics, 124*(1), 422–427. doi:10.1542/peds.2009-1060

American College of Obstetricians and Gynecologists. (2013). Cesarean delivery on maternal request. *Obstet Gynecol, 121*(4), 904–907. doi:10.1097/01.AOG.0000428647.67925.d3

Breeze, A. C., Lees, C. C., Kumar, A., Missfelder-Lobos, H. H., & Murdoch, E. M. (2007). Palliative care for prenatally diagnosed lethal fetal abnormality. *Arch Dis Child Fetal Neonatal Ed, 92*(1), F56–F58. doi:10.1136/adc.2005.092122

Buchbinder, M., Lassiter, D., Mercier, R., Bryant, A., & Lyerly, A. (2016). Reframing conscientious care: Providing abortion care when law and conscience collide. *Hastings Cent Rep, 46*(2), 22–30.

Crider, K. S., Olney, R. S., & Cragan, J. D. (2008). Trisomies 13 and 18: Population prevalences, characteristics, and prenatal diagnosis, metropolitan Atlanta, 1994–2003. *Am J Med Genet A, 146A*(7), 820–826. doi:10.1002/ajmg.a.32200

Feudtner, C., & Munson, D. (2009). The ethics of perinatal palliative care. In V. Ravitsky, A. Fiester, & A. L. Caplan (Eds.), *The Penn Center guide to bioethics* (pp. 509–518). New York: Springer.

Fleming, V., Iljuschin, I., Pehlke-Milde, J., Maurer, F., & Parpan, F. (2016). Dying at lifes beginning: Experiences of parents and health professionals in Switzerland when an "in utero" diagnosis incompatible with life is made. *Midwifery, 34*, 23–29. doi:10.1016/j.midw.2016.01.014

Geneva Declaration on Perinatal Care. (2015). Retrieved from http://www.genevaperinatalcare.com/

Gossman, G. L., Joesch, J. M., & Tanfer, K. (2006). Trends in maternal request cesarean delivery from 1991 to 2004. *Obstet Gynecol, 108*(6), 1506–1516. doi:10.1097/01.AOG.0000242564.79349.b7

Gregg, A. R., Gross, S. J., Best, R. G., Monaghan, K. G., Bajaj, K., Skotko, B. G., . . . Watson, M. S. (2013). ACMG statement on noninvasive prenatal screening for fetal aneuploidy. *Genet Med, 15*(5), 395–398. doi:10.1038/gim.2013.29

Guon, J., Wilfond, B. S., Farlow, B., Brazg, T., & Janvier, A. (2014). Our children are not a diagnosis: The experience of parents who continue their pregnancy after a prenatal diagnosis of trisomy 13 or 18. *Am J Med Genet A, 164A*(2), 308–318. doi:10.1002/ajmg.a.36298

Guttmacher Institute. (2017). An overview of abortion laws. Retrieved from https://www.guttmacher.org/state-policy/explore/overview-abortion-laws

Han, S. N., Mhallem Gziri, M., Van Calsteren, K., & Amant, F. (2013). Cervical cancer in pregnant women: Treat, wait or interrupt? Assessment of current clinical guidelines, innovations and controversies. *Ther Adv Med Oncol, 5*(4), 211–219. doi:10.1177/1758834013494988

Janvier, A., Farlow, B., & Wilfond, B. S. (2012). The experience of families with children with trisomy 13 and 18 in social networks. *Pediatrics, 130*(2), 293–298. doi:10.1542/peds.2012-0151

Kamihara, J., Nyborn, J. A., Olcese, M. E., Nickerson, T., & Mack, J. W. (2015). Parental hope for children with advanced cancer. *Pediatrics, 135*(5), 868–874. doi:10.1542/peds.2014-2855

Kattwinkel, J., Bloom, R. S., American Academy of Pediatrics, & American Heart Association. (2011). *Textbook of neonatal resuscitation* (6th ed.). Elk Grove Village, IL: American Academy of Pediatrics.

Koogler, T. K., Wilfond, B. S., & Ross, L. F. (2003). Lethal language, lethal decisions. *Hastings Cent Rep, 33*(2), 37–41.

Kosho, T., Nakamura, T., Kawame, H., Baba, A., Tamura, M., & Fukushima, Y. (2006). Neonatal management of trisomy 18: Clinical details of 24 patients receiving intensive treatment. *Am J Med Genet A, 140*(9), 937–944. doi:10.1002/ajmg.a.31175

Lakovschek, I. C., Streubel, B., & Ulm, B. (2011). Natural outcome of trisomy 13, trisomy 18, and triploidy after prenatal diagnosis. *Am J Med Genet A, 155A*(11), 2626–2633. doi:10.1002/ajmg.a.34284

Larcher, V., Craig, F., Bhogal, K., Wilkinson, D., Brierley, J., Royal College of Paediatrics and Child Health. (2015). Making decisions to limit treatment in life-limiting and life-threatening conditions in children: A framework for practice. *Arch Dis Child, 100 Suppl 2*, s3–23. doi:10.1136/archdischild-2014-306666

Macauley, R. (2015). Turn of phrase. *J Palliat Med, 18*(2), 197–199. doi:10.1089/jpm.2014.0262

MacDorman, M. F., Menacker, F., & Declercq, E. (2008). Cesarean birth in the United States: Epidemiology, trends, and outcomes. *Clin Perinatol, 35*(2), 293–307. doi:10.1016/j.clp.2008.03.007

Machado, L. S. (2011). Emergency peripartum hysterectomy: Incidence, indications, risk factors and out-come. *N Am J Med Sci*, *3*(8), 358–361. doi:10.4297/najms.2011.358

Mayor, M. T. (2015). Case study: "Lethal" fetal anomalies and elective cesarean. Commentary. *Hastings Cent Rep*, *45*(6), 13–14.

Natoli, J. L., Ackerman, D. L., McDermott, S., & Edwards, J. G. (2012). Prenatal diagnosis of Down syn-drome: A systematic review of termination rates (1995–2011). *Prenat Diagn*, *32*(2), 142–153. doi:10.1002/pd.2910

Nelson, K. E., Rosella, L. C., Mahant, S., & Guttmann, A. (2016). Survival and surgical interventions for children with trisomy 13 and 18. *JAMA*, *316*(4), 420–428. doi:10.1001/jama.2016.9819

Nickel, B., Barratt, A., Copp, T., Moynihan, R., & McCaffery, K. (2017). Words do matter: A systematic review on how different terminology for the same condition influences management preferences. *BMJ Open*, *7*(7), e014129. doi:10.1136/bmjopen-2016-014129

Now I Lay Me Down to Sleep. (2016). Retrieved from https://www.nowilaymedowntosleep.org/

Osterman, M. J., Kochanek, K. D., MacDorman, M. F., Strobino, D. M., & Guyer, B. (2015). Annual sum-mary of vital statistics: 2012–2013. *Pediatrics*, *135*(6), 1115–1125. doi:10.1542/peds.2015-0434

Peterson, J. K., Kochilas, L. K., Catton, K. G., Moller, J. H., & Setty, S. P. (2017). Long-term outcomes of children with trisomy 13 and 18 after congenital heart disease interventions. *Ann Thorac Surg*, *103*(6), 1941–1949. doi:10.1016/j.athoracsur.2017.02.068

Planned Parenthood v. Casey. (1992). 505 U.S. 833.

Roe v. Wade. (1973). 410 U.S. 113.

Rysavy, M. A., Li, L., Bell, E. F., Das, A., Hintz, S. R., Stoll, B. J., . . . Human Development Neonatal Research Network. (2015). Between-hospital variation in treatment and outcomes in extremely preterm infants. *N Engl J Med*, *372*(19), 1801–1811. doi:10.1056/NEJMoa1410689

Shimabukuro, J. (2016). Abortion: Judicial history and legislative response. Washington, DC: Congressional Research Service.

White, A. (2015). Case study: "Lethal" fetal anomalies and elective cesarean. Commentary. *Hastings Cent Rep*, *45*(6), 14.

12

Ethics of Neonatal Palliative Care

Case Study

A twenty-eight year old woman is pregnant for the first time. Everything was going well until twenty-four weeks' gestation, when her amniotic membranes spontaneously rupture (i.e., her "water breaks"). She is rushed to the hospital where it is determined that labor has begun and prenatal steroids are instituted. Despite maximal intervention, the doctors feel that delivery is inevitable.

"But it's too early!" she says, upon hearing this news.

The medical team provides a wealth of information about the probabilities of survival and "brain damage" to the infant and asks whether she and her husband want aggressive treatment or "just comfort care."

The parents haven't even prepared the nursery at home—they thought they had several more months to get it ready—and are overwhelmed by profound and complex questions about how to treat their baby once he is born. A palliative care consultation is requested.

Historicolegal Background

The distant history of neonatal ethics is not a pretty one. Plato endorsed infanticide for "the offspring of the inferior and of those of the other sort who are born defective" (Plato & Jowett, 1941). Aristotle followed suit: "As to exposing or rearing the children born let there be a law that no deformed child shall be reared" (Aristotle & Jowett, 1943). In the ancient world this view stemmed from a combination of the belief that full personhood was acquired sometime after birth—and then fully only by those who were emotionally and physically healthy—as well as a sense that children were valued based on their usefulness to their parents, or to society as a whole (Wyatt, 2009).

The Judeo-Christian world view differed from this, however, and after Constantine converted to Christianity, laws throughout the Roman Empire began to change. Infanticide (i.e., the active killing of an impaired newborn) was outlawed in 374 CE (Ferngren, 1987), although it continued to be practiced in many places until the twentieth century (Langer, 1963). Modern commentators—with only rare exceptions (Singer, 2011)—reject it on ethical grounds, viewing it as murder.

Yet even once it was decided that impaired newborns should not be left to die, there was relatively little that could be done to sustain them. This extended into the second half of the twentieth century, as physicians struggled in vain to ventilate immature fetal lungs. As an example, in 1962 President Kennedy's son was born at thirty-four weeks' gestation, which today carries a 98% chance of survival. Yet despite receiving the best medical care available at the time, the child died on the second day of life.

Since that time several seminal discoveries—such as improved mechanical ventilation, steroids for fetal lung maturation, surfactant to replace the protein premature lungs are deficient in, and phototherapy for hyperbilirubinemia—have made it increasingly possible to save extremely premature, critically ill newborns. Such exciting discoveries led to the presumption that everything that could be done *would* be done. These were children, after all, and the smallest and most fragile among them.

As more premature babies were able to survive, the incidence of neurodevelopmental impairment (NDI) began to increase. This prompted some to wonder whether the pendulum had swung too far in the other direction, in favor of maximal treatment in every case. The primary question of neonatology—which once had been whether to euthanize "impaired" newborns—thus turned to how much treatment was "enough" and how much was "too much."

These questions first came to public notice in the 1970s through the well-known "Baby Doe" cases: babies with Trisomy 21 (Down syndrome) who also had atresia of their gastrointestinal tract. Surgical repair of this condition was quite straightforward even then, but in the majority of the Baby Doe cases, the parents declined operative repair, opting instead to let their children die.[1] One mother famously remarked that it would be "unfair to the other children of the household to raise them with a mongoloid" (De Cruz, 2000).

Surveys at the time revealed that the majority of pediatricians (Todres, Krane, Howell, & Shannon, 1977) and the vast majority of pediatric surgeons (Shaw, Randolph, & Manard, 1977) would respect parents' refusal of treatment in such a situation.

---

1. While "provide exclusively palliative care" is more appropriate terminology, "let die" accurately describes how the Baby Does were treated. Palliative care was essentially unknown at that time (especially for children). The ideal set forth in this textbook—of broad-ranging support for a patient and family, attending to physical, social, spiritual, and psychological needs—was not met in those early cases. Some nurses at the hospital where one of the Baby Does died still recall the baby's anguished cries, as she was literally left in a corner to die of dehydration over a period of several days, without symptomatic management.

High-profile cases in other countries, such as the United Kingdom, illustrated similar deference to parental preferences (Brahams & Brahams, 1983).

At approximately the same time, an article in the *New England Journal of Medicine* revealed that 14% of the babies who died in the neonatal intensive care unit (NICU) at Yale-New Haven Hospital were receiving less than maximal treatment (Duff & Campbell, 1973). Publicly calling into question societal assumptions that every baby received maximal treatment, this prompted greater governmental scrutiny.

To ensure that no baby received insufficient treatment, the Justice Department established the "Baby Doe Rules" (Department of Health & Human Services, 1984). According to these rules, infants were required to receive maximal treatment unless one of three conditions applied:

1. The infant was irreversibly comatose; or
2. Treatment was futile (in terms of survival); or
3. Treatment was "virtually futile" (in terms of survival) and inhumane.

Forgoing treatment in other situations was deemed to be discriminatory and a violation of the infant's civil rights (US Rehabilitation Act, 1973). A hotline was set up to accept reports of alleged child neglect, in the form of insufficient treatment to impaired newborns. These rules fundamentally altered the latitude by which pediatricians could formulate individualized treatment plans, leading to maximal treatment in nearly all cases (Kopelman, Irons, & Kopelman, 1988).

The Baby Doe Rules were the administrative response to the question of appropriate treatment of "impaired" newborns. The ethical response came in the form of the President's Commission for the Study of Ethical Problems in Medicine and Biological and Behavioral Research (President's Commission; 1983), which completed its study of this topic at approximately the same time that the Rules were promulgated. In contrast to the three rather stark criteria of the Baby Doe Rules—which paid scant attention to the infant's quality of life—the President's Commission identified several factors that were relevant to treatment decisions for "impaired" newborns and infants. These included amount of suffering, severity of dysfunction, potential for personal satisfaction and enjoyment of life, and the possibility of developing the capacity for self-determination.

Based on these considerations, the President's Commission identified three classifications of treatment: those that were clearly beneficial, those whose benefit was ambiguous, and those that were clearly futile. The President's Commission argued that treatments of the first type were obligatory (and thus parents could not refuse), and that treatments of the third type should not be offered. The second type should be left up to the parents' discretion.

Clearly, the President's Commission felt that the Baby Doe Rules underestimated the importance of quality of life and did not sufficiently respect parental authority (Table 12.1).

TABLE 12.1 Situations where parents may decline maximal treatment for a newborn or infant

Baby Doe Rules	President's Commission
Baby will never achieve consciousness	Treatment is not clearly beneficial when taking into consideration:
Treatment will not save the baby's life	1. amount of suffering
Treatment will almost certainly fail to save the baby's life and would be inhumane	2. severity of dysfunction
	3. potential for personal satisfaction and enjoyment of life
	4. possibility of developing the capacity for self-determination

The US Supreme Court agreed (*Bowen v. American Hospital Association*, 1986), striking down the Rules as being an inappropriate infringement on the parental right of decision-making. The Court felt that the Rules were overly simplistic in ignoring the degree of suffering and disability, which necessarily factors into treatment decisions (Kopelman, 2005).

With the Court having disagreed with the Reagan administration's interpretation of civil rights law, Congress incorporated the Baby Doe Rules as an amendment to the Child Abuse, Prevention, and Treatment Act, tying adherence with the rules to voluntary participation in federal programs to prevent child abuse and neglect (Department of Health and Human Services, 1985). The Baby Doe Rules are therefore not "the law of the land"; they are merely guidelines without legal ramifications if they are not followed.

Physicians are thus not legally required to continue maximal treatment if a child fails to meet the Baby Doe criteria. It would be more appropriate to say that if treatment is forgone in an infant who *does* meet the narrow criteria of the Baby Doe Rules, the physicians would be on very firm legal (and ethical) ground, indeed. But forgoing treatment in infants who do not meet those strict criteria can also be legally and ethically permissible.

Many physicians, however, misunderstand the Baby Doe Rules, believing that they do restrict parental latitude in neonatal decision-making (Kopelman, 2005). This lack of clarity—added to the fairly recent memory of the Justice Department's (temporary) involvement in clinical care—prompted many physicians to implement maximal treatment, even when the parents were ambivalent or even opposed. This led to well-publicized cases where parents were forced to take matters into their own hands in order to spare their children from what they considered inappropriate—and often very burdensome—treatment (Miles, 1989). In other situations, parents brought suit after the fact, not for "wrongful death" as is common in medical malpractice law, but rather for the "wrongful life" of children with neurodevelopmental impairment whose parents felt should have been allowed to die.

One such case is *Miller v. HCA*, where the parents of Baby Miller—born at twenty-four weeks' gestation—refused to give consent for intensive treatment. Instead, they requested purely palliative treatment in light of grim neurological and survival predictions

(*Miller v. HCA*, 2003). The physicians, however, proceeded with resuscitation, based on the fact that the baby girl exceeded the hospital's established minimum weight for mandatory treatment. She ultimately survived but was neurologically devastated.

The Millers sued the hospital, and the trial jury awarded the family $29 million for medical expenses, $17 million in interest, and $13.5 million in punitive damages, reflecting the shift from a "sanctity of life" model to one that respected parental discretion, especially at the limits of viability. The Texas Supreme Court, however, reversed the decision in favor of the hospital, holding that the Millers' refusal could not be considered "informed" because, prior to delivery, they could not have known how the baby would appear or what the outcome would be. The Court concluded that the physicians—when faced with a critical situation—were within their rights to "err on the side of life" by providing maximal treatment. At the same time, the Court supported the Millers' rights to make treatment decisions once the baby was stabilized in the NICU (and when, presumably, the "emergency" situation had passed).

While only a state supreme court decision, the significance of *Miller* should not be underestimated. The case exemplifies the common practice of the medical system of the time to do more rather than less, even over the parents' objections. The jury's conclusions reflect the growing public dissatisfaction with that model, as the parents' right to make decisions in what they consider to be in the best interest of their child is threatened. The final resolution underscores the tension between these views, as well as affirming the basic principle of neonatal ethics that decision-making neither begins nor ends in the delivery room, but rather carries forward into the NICU as additional information becomes available.

This shift toward greater parental latitude in decision-making is evident in the medical literature. Whereas the 1973 *New England Journal of Medicine* study garnered great attention for reporting that one out of seven of babies who died did not receive maximal support, subsequent studies in the 2000s showed that the *majority* of babies in some NICUs were dying without maximal support, to no significant societal outcry. Further, many of these babies were not "moribund" (i.e., imminently dying), but rather suffered from catastrophic yet stable neurologic injury (Singh, Lantos, & Meadow, 2004). Clearly, these babies do not meet the stringent requirements of the Baby Doe Rules for forgoing life sustaining medical treatment (LSMT). This reflects the degree to which much of society has moved from emphasizing the sanctity of life to the quality of life.

This sentiment is not unanimous, however. Over the same time period right-to-life groups grew increasingly concerned about what they considered to be inadequate treatment of newborns, especially at the edges of viability. This prompted the passage of the Born Alive Infant Protection Act (BAIPA) in 2001. BAIPA holds that any infant with a pulse or spontaneous respirations is considered to be "born alive," despite the fact that clearly previable neonates will often exhibit these signs.

Some have attempted to apply the definition set forth in BAIPA to the Emergency Medical Treatment and Labor Act, 1986 (EMTALA). Originally focused on preventing the "dumping" of indigent patients from private to public hospitals, EMTALA requires that any living patient who presents to a hospital must receive a "medical screening examination." If an emergency medical condition exists, the hospital must either admit the patient or appropriately transfer the patient to another facility. By this reasoning, if a twenty-one-week (previable) infant—which could be considered a living person according to BAIPA—"presents to the hospital" by being born there, the hospital must provide resuscitation.

Legally, this reasoning is not sound. There exists strong consensus that EMTALA only applies to outpatients. Indeed, the very purpose of the law is to get patients "into the system" (Final Rule, 1985). By contrast, a baby born in the hospital would be considered an inpatient (Pope, 2008).

Beyond legal details, this interpretation ignores the underlying purpose of EMTALA, namely, to prevent discrimination against patients who are seeking appropriate treatment, not to mandate treatments which have no hope of succeeding. Understandably, attempted applications of BAIPA to EMTALA have not been deemed compelling and have not succeeded in altering clinical practice, or limiting the scope of parental decision-making.

Clinical

A "full-term" pregnancy lasts thirty-nine to forty weeks, with thirty-seven to thirty-eight weeks considered "early term." Deliveries prior to thirty-seven weeks gestation are deemed "preterm" and represent approximately 11% of all pregnancies in the United States (Osterman et al., 2015). Babies born in the "moderate or late" preterm period—from thirty-two to thirty-seven weeks—usually require modest (if any) respiratory support, and usually develop the ability to feed by mouth at around thirty-four weeks. Deliveries prior to thirty-two weeks are considered "very" preterm, and those prior to twenty-eight weeks "extremely" preterm (World Health Organization, 2016).

When a pregnant woman experiences preterm labor, delivery can often be delayed through the use of tocolytics, allowing the fetus to continue to grow and allowing the administration of intravenous steroids to the mother to accelerate fetal lung maturity. (Treatment with steroids for a full forty-eight hours prior to delivery is considered "full treatment.") In the case of ruptured amniotic membranes, however, the risk of infection increases and fetal maturation slows. Thus, the lungs of a fetus after a period of ruptured membranes will be less mature than a fetus of the same gestational age whose membranes remain intact (Hanke et al., 2015).

Over one-third of all pediatric deaths occur in the neonatal period, which encompasses the first twenty-eight days of life. When combined with deaths in infancy—referring to children ages one to twelve months old—this represents the majority of pediatric deaths (Figure 12.1). Not surprisingly, clinical decision-making in the neonatal period is among the most complex.

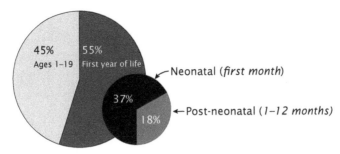

FIGURE 12.1 Deaths in childhood, divided by age (Friebert & Williams, 2015)

There are several reasons for this, which are addressed in the following sections. These include

- inherent uncertainty of gestational age estimates and prognoses drawn from these
- unreliability of conclusions drawn from observations in the delivery room
- lack of correlation of certain radiological findings—such as head ultrasound—on clinical outcomes
- shifting limit of viability
- closing "window of opportunity" as a neonate's respiratory status improves before his prognosis becomes clear
- additional complexity of forgoing medically administered nutrition and hydration (MANH) in this age group

The most difficult clinical decisions used to fall within a fairly narrow time frame. As recently as the 1990s, by the fourth day of life the probability of survival of a patient receiving neonatal intensive care no longer depended on birthweight or gestational age. By that point the sickest babies had usually died, either despite maximal life support or after withdrawal of LSMT. Every four-day-old in the NICU, therefore, had the same chance of survival (Meadow, Lee, Lin, & Lantos, 2004), offering both hope and perspective to those parents who made it that far. But as nonsurvivors have come to live longer—from an average of two days to ten or more (Meadow et al., 2004)—and more treatments have become possible, parents are now faced with gut-wrenching decisions long into the NICU stay.

The NICU is also a "different world," compared to the rest of medicine. Many of the paradigms and terminology (e.g., gestational age, pretreatment with steroids) are not used elsewhere, and many of the interventions (e.g., surfactant and phototherapy) are not applicable outside the newborn period. Even the very size of the patients—which attests to their fragility and make what would be routine procedures in larger patients much more challenging—is unique.

Reasoning by analogy—which is often helpful in applying general concepts to pediatric situations—can therefore be counter-productive. For example, the prognosis for adult patients in the ICU worsens as length of stay increases, which may lead families to consider a shift of goals the longer a hospitalization continues (Moitra, Guerra, Linde-Zwirble, & Wunsch, 2016). By contrast, prognosis *improves* over time for patients in the

NICU, which is one of the reasons why the neonatal ICU is more cost effective than the medical ICU (Lantos, Mokalla, & Meadow, 1997). So rather than giving increasing consideration to forgoing LSMT as a hospitalization continues, parents of critically ill neonates may reasonably take comfort that their child has survived the most dangerous time and continue to request maximal treatment. This, of course, pertains only to survival, leaving open the question of NDI.

Ethical
Prognostic Accuracy and Communication of Information

Because the NICU is such a unique world, parents require a great deal of education as to what the pressing questions are, as well as the potential answers to those questions (American Academy of Pediatrics [AAP], 2007; Rushton, 1994). As the old saying goes, "Good ethics begin with good facts" (Sujdak Mackiewicz, 2016). Establishing the "facts" can be challenging, however, in light of uncertainty about precise gestational age, as well as the likely clinical outcome even if this could be known with certainty. Once all available information is gathered, the optimal way of informing the parents is also unclear (Janvier & Barrington, 2005; Lantos & Meadow, 2006), with the method of communication possessing ethical components of its own.

Gestational age was long thought to be the primary (or perhaps) sole determinant of an otherwise complicated gestation and delivery. Even measuring gestational age, though, involves some degree of uncertainty (Kattwinkel, Bloom, American Academy of Pediatrics, & American Heart Association, 2011; Sladkevicius et al., 2005; Wennerholm, Bergh, Hagberg, Sultan, & Wennergren, 1998). First-trimester ultrasounds are generally deemed the most reliable marker, with less than one week of potential error on either side. Later ultrasounds, though, can vary by as much as two weeks or more in both directions (Butt, Lim, & Society of Obstetricians and Gynaecologists of Canada, 2014). Recollection of last menstrual period shows similar variability, as it is dependent on the woman's memory. So unless a baby is conceived through in vitro fertilization, it is impossible to know exactly what the gestational age is.

Even if gestational age were known for certain, several other variables are relevant to outcome, including the fetus's gender, estimated weight, and administration of prenatal steroids. Whether the fetus is a singleton or part of a multiple birth is also relevant. Taking all these variables into account, the National Institute of Child Health and Human Development (NICHD) database generates probabilities of survival with and without mechanical ventilation, as well as for moderate or severe NDI (Tyson et al., 2008) (Figure 12.2).

While informative, these are still only population-level probabilities. Individual factors also play a role. Location of delivery, for instance, is relevant, as preterm infants born at a perinatal center have better outcomes (AAP, 2009). So rather than relying on national

Outcomes	Outcomes for all infants	Outcomes for mechanically Ventilated infants
Survival	48%	52%
Survival Without Profound Neurodevelopmental Impairment	32%	34%
Survival Without Moderate to Severe Neurodevelopmental Impairment	18%	20%
Death	52%	48%
Death or Profound Neurodevelopmental Impairment	68%	66%
Death or Moderate to Severe Neurodevelopmental Impairment	82%	80%

FIGURE 12.2 Outcome probabilities for a normal-sized male infant at twenty-four weeks' gestation, whose mother received a full course of antenatal steroids (National Institute of Child Health and Human Development, 2017)

data—which may or may not reflect outcomes at the place where the baby will be born— regional or ideally hospital-specific data is best. But even incorporating these, probabilities do not answer the parents' primary question: whether *their* child will survive, and if so, whether he will face significant obstacles from a neurodevelopmental point of view.

Even the terms that are used are open to interpretation. For instance, the "best case scenario" included on the NICHD database is survival without "moderate to severe NDI," which refers to "moderate or severe cerebral palsy, bilateral blindness, or bilateral hearing loss requiring amplification" (Tyson et al., 2008). Clearly, a child could have significant functional limitations and still be considered to have "less than moderate" NDI. Parents, therefore, need to be cautioned that survival without "moderate to severe" impairment is not the same as "unaffected."

The attempt to provide parents with as much information as possible may, in the end, be counterproductive. The NICHD database, for example, provides *twelve* percentage- based predictions for each clinical situation (Figure 12.2). Admittedly, this represents two complementary sets of data points, six framed in terms of survival or the absence of specific impairment and six in terms of death or the presence of specific impairment.

Clinicians might therefore choose to focus only on one set, but the choice of which also has ethical implications given the impact of "framing" on patient decisions (p. 60). Stating that a neonate has a 48% chance of dying (as in this chapter's case study) may make parents more likely to forgo LSMT than stating that there is a 52% chance of sur- vival. This choice may reflect the clinician's unconscious bias, based on what she believes is the appropriate course of action. Recognizing this, the clinician may try to avoid the possibility of framing bias by presenting all the data, but even with written descriptions the sheer abundance of numbers can be overwhelming and make it hard to reach an in- formed decision (Kaempf et al., 2006).

In these situations, it may be worth sacrificing some precision in prognostication for understandability. In place of the (over-)abundance of data provided by the NICHD database, a more graphic representation may help parents appreciate the true chances of

If your baby is an appropriately grown **MALE** singleton who received steroids

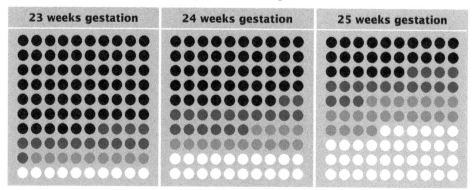

● Baby does not survive

● Baby survives with profound disability including severe
impairment in thinking or movement, or sight, or hearing

● Baby survives with moderate/severe disability including
impairment in thinking or movement, or sight, or hearing

○ Baby survives with no major impairment

FIGURE 12.3 Graphic representation of outcome probabilities for the same infant as described in Figure 12.2, at various gestational ages

the outcome which they are seeking (Figure 12.3). Such a representation also emphasizes the improving probabilities over time, so that parents might be able to understand at what point—if not now—they would want maximal intervention.

Such complexity and ambiguity underscore the importance of identifying what the parents' goals are, to make sure they and the team are using a common language. For instance, if the team is framing outcomes in terms of survival while the parents are focused on survival without NDI, there is a greater chance of misunderstanding and an inappropriate treatment plan. Some studies, for instance, have shown that while survival improves steadily with increasing gestational age from twenty-three to twenty-eight weeks, NDI remains roughly constant at approximately 50% (Andrews, Lagatta, Chu, et al., 2012). Therefore, if the parents' primary goal is to avoid NDI, the most perilous gestational ages for delivery are actually twenty-five to twenty-six weeks, when survival has increased—and maximal treatment may be deemed mandatory (p. 322)—but impairment risk has yet to diminish (Meadow, 2013).

The nature of "disability" should also be clarified, as studies have shown that neonatologists and neonatal nurse practitioners view certain disabilities as more severe than do patients who may suffer from them (Saigal et al., 1999). Medical professionals in neonatology often are unduly pessimistic about outcomes (Blanco, Suresh, Howard, & Soll, 2005), potentially creating a "self-fulfilling prophecy" where LSMT is withdrawn from high-risk patients, negatively impacting survival data which then leads other parents to make the same decision (Gardner et al., 1996; Saigal et al., 1999).

The reason for this may stem from the very human tendency to "remember the catastrophes," such as the twenty-three-weeker who struggled so valiantly—and endured so much—only to die after several months, never getting out of the NICU. Often forgotten are the "victories," like the twenty-three-weeker who had a smooth course and was discharged on schedule, without need for inpatient follow-up. Contrary to popular opinion, former preemies who survive to adolescence have generally the same self-assessed quality of life as control peers (Cooke, 2004; Gray, Petrou, Hockley, & Gardner, 2007; Saigal et al., 2006). A potential explanation is that they have never known any other quality of life to compare theirs to, and thus may not feel deprived or the worse for it.

It is also critical to emphasize to the parents precisely what question they are answering prenatally. It is merely what the *initial* goals of care should be for the baby, once born. Authorizing full resuscitation in the delivery room in no way commits the baby to maximal treatment once in the NICU. As the ethical adage goes, "There is no ethical or legal distinction between withdrawing and withholding" (p. 156). This has been clearly affirmed by the courts in relationship to this precise situation (*Miller v. HCA, Inc.*, 2003). If parents do not appreciate this fact, they might be unduly reticent to authorize full resuscitation for fear of "losing control" over the situation.

In the past, additional relevant information was thought to come very soon after delivery. Parents were given the option of waiting to see how a baby appeared immediately after birth, which some have called a "trial of life." In such cases, a decision as to whether to provide mechanical ventilation and intensive care would depend on the baby's appearance in the delivery room. Babies who appeared "older" (in terms of gestational age) than originally thought—or were more vigorous—were given maximal treatment based on the presumption of an increased chance of a good outcome. Younger-appearing or less responsive babies, on the other hand, were more likely to receive only comfort measures.

This approach promised two important benefits to parents forced to make harrowing decisions. First, it absolved them from having to make a definitive decision prior to delivery (and thus transferred some of the responsibility to the physicians and their assessment in the delivery room). Second, it appeared to offer reassurance that every appropriate treatment would be provided. In cases where the baby seemed younger or less vigorous—and thus comfort became the priority—parents could take solace in believing that they had given their baby "a chance."

The problem with this approach is that it is not reliable. Gestational age is very difficult to assess clinically, especially in a pressure-filled context like the delivery of an extremely premature baby. Standard observational estimations of gestational age often overestimate by up to three weeks (Donovan et al., 1999). And even if a slightly modified gestational age could be known with certainty, it has not been shown to be an appropriate reason to deviate from the original plan (Meadow, 2007).

The degree of "vigorousness" seen in the delivery room also correlates poorly with outcomes. Very active babies in the delivery room often do not survive because of underlying health problems, such as immature lungs. Conversely, seemingly depressed babies may do quite well, especially if their initial unresponsiveness was due to temporary problems such as the effect of maternal opioids or a prolonged delivery. Even the clinical predictions of experienced neonatologists, when provided with a full prenatal history and a detailed video of a premature baby right after birth—as well as at one and five minutes—are no better than chance (Manley et al., 2010).

Predictions of nonsurvival are, however, strongly predictive of significant neurologic impairment (Wood, Marlow, Costeloe, Gibson, & Wilkinson, 2000). In other words, if a neonatologist predicts an extremely premature baby in the delivery room will not survive, this may or may not prove accurate. One can be fairly sure, though, that if that baby does survive, there will be some neurologic impairment.

The appropriate time to reconsider decisions made prior to delivery therefore is not in the delivery room but rather in the NICU, once the team has had a chance to acquire additional information, assuming that the initial signs are not so ominous (e.g., absent heart rate after ten minutes) as to legitimately impact prognosis. This is also the position put forth in the *Miller v. HCA* decision.

Not all subsequently-acquired information, however, is as predictive as once thought. For example, bleeding within the brain (i.e., intraventricular hemorrhage [IVH]) is a common complication in extremely premature babies. Graded on a scale of one to four, the severity of IVH was once thought to be reliable in predicting NDI (Catto-Smith, Yu, Bajuk, Orgill, & Astbury, 1985). Subsequent studies, however, have shown this to not necessarily be so, especially for lower grade IVH (Ann Wy et al., 2015).

In light of this new data, some have wondered if the high mortality associated with IVH might, to some degree, be the result of another "self-fulfilling prophecy." If IVH was thought to inevitably lead to poor neurologic outcomes, parents might be more likely to authorize withdrawal of support. This would lead to death, further worsening outcome data for patients with IVH and leading future parents to forgo LSMT based on the reportedly high risk of death (Patra, 2014).

Armed with a wealth of information of often unclear significance, the medical team should generally take a nondirective approach to questions of treatment in situations where resuscitation is neither contraindicated nor mandated (AAP, 2015). This preserves the parents' freedom to make their own decision based on their personal values.

In critical situations, however, parents may not be able to decide. Until a clear decision is reached, it is appropriate to begin resuscitation in order to preserve future options. This approach has been endorsed by various professional bodies (AAP, 2007; Kattwinkel et al., 2010; Nuffield Council on Bioethics, 2006) as well as by parent surveys (Lee, Penner, & Cox, 1991; Streiner, Saigal, Burrows, Stoskopf, & Rosenbaum, 2001). Interventions that prove to be ineffective or are felt to be inappropriate given the overall plan of care can always be stopped later (Whittall, 2007).

Window of Opportunity

One concept that is important to consider, as parents grapple with often prolonged decisions about whether to continue LSMT, is the "window of opportunity." As noted earlier, the longer a patient in the NICU survives, the greater the probability of eventually being able to go home from the hospital. However, determining the degree of NDI often requires significant time. With early studies previously thought to be definitive for NDI (e.g., cranial ultrasounds) now understood not to be, parents are often faced with ongoing uncertainty in this area.

Even as the neurodevelopmental outcome is becoming clear, other organ systems (particularly the lungs) are improving. By the time neurologic prognosis is established, the neonate may no longer require certain forms of LSMT, such as mechanical ventilation. The option of compassionate extubation—which the parents chose not to exercise when the neurologic prognosis was uncertain but might have wished to do so now—is thus no longer available to them.

This concept is known as the "window of opportunity." Not unique to neonatal intensive care, this term takes a somewhat macabre twist on a term which usually connotes positivity and hope. Used in the context of LSMT, it refers to the period when a patient is temporarily dependent on technological modalities which it would be ethically appropriate to limit, if the legal decision-maker opted to do so. Most commonly this applies to mechanical ventilation, which nearly all extremely premature babies will require, often for days or weeks or even longer. Irrespective of what other challenges a particular infant faces, mechanical ventilation is typically the most invasive, discrete, and limitable intervention they are receiving.

Once a baby no longer requires mechanical ventilation, the only LSMT remaining in use may be medications or MANH (Hack et al., 2002; Saigal, Stoskopf, Streiner, & Burrows, 2001). Forgoing the former may or may not lead to the patient's death, depending on what those medications are. Withdrawing the latter is not associated with the degree of suffering frequently attributed to it (p. 153), but it remains ethically charged for reasons explored in greater detail in the following section. Not receiving MANH can also lead to a rather protracted dying process, and parents may have emotional or religious objections to doing so (p. 494).

Without using the rather macabre term, clinicians need to inform parents about the concept of the "window of opportunity." Without that knowledge, parents cannot appreciate that certain options will cease to be relevant with the passage of time. They will not recognize that for all the emotion of having to decide whether to forgo mechanical ventilation, the decision about whether to forgo MANH may be even harder. Or perhaps it is not an option for them at all—whether for religious or personal reasons—which means that their only choices are to withhold LSMT before all the facts are in hand or to continue on into an uncertain future.

In this respect, neonatal intensive care shares a quality common to all of medicine: not deciding to limit LSMT is essentially a passive decision to continue it. Especially for treatments already in use, repetitive informed consent is not required. A treatment will continue until the appropriate decision maker explicitly declines it, or until that treatment is no longer necessary.

The fact that a baby is no longer dependent on mechanical ventilation does not mean the patient is obligated to live indefinitely in a heavily burdened state, however. Even if the parents opt not to forgo MANH, most patients with severe NDI eventually require other treatments. Subsequent complications are bound to occur, frequently infections such as pneumonia. Antibiotics would then represent a form of LSMT that can be forgone. They are also more easily limited than MANH, based on the absence of emotional or religious significance as well as the clearer prognosis that has been reached by that point.

That is in the indefinite future, however. While the window of opportunity remains open, parents need to understand what their options currently are and which will eventually cease to be considerations.

Medically Administered Nutrition and Hydration

MANH can be administered enterally through an oro-/nasogastric tube—usually as a temporary step—or on a longer term basis through a gastrostomy tube (p. 187). It can also be administered intravenously in the form of total parenteral nutrition, which is more burdensome and requires additional monitoring (p. 192). While food and drink consumed by mouth are basic human care—and it would therefore be unethical to deprive a patient from eating and drinking should she wish to (AAP, 2009)—MANH is a medical treatment like any other (*Cruzan v. Director, Missouri Department of Health*, 1990).

While there exists strong consensus regarding a competent patient's—or his appropriate surrogate's—right to refuse MANH if the burdens outweigh the benefits (Levi, 2003; Meisel, 1992; Truog & Cochrane, 2005), there are several unique aspects of the neonatal period that complicate this issue. One is the instinctual resonance of feeding one's child. Human beings are created with an emotional drive to provide nourishment to their children. This even has physiological manifestations, in the form of a new mother's postpartum "letdown" reflex. Social expectations also play a role, as a well-fed child is taken in many cultures as a sign of good parenting (Frader, 2007; Slomka, 1995). Admittedly, some of the social resonance of feeding is missing in the context of MANH—as there is no appreciation of the taste of food or drink and no sharing of a meal with others—but it is not entirely absent.

Another relevant ethical consideration is *why* a patient is dependent on MANH. Healthy adults are able to consume food and drink orally. While some may need assistance in procuring the food and drink—and, in the case of neurologic or muscular disease, bringing it to their mouths—chewing and swallowing generally occur normally. When this is not the case, it reflects some level of illness. So to withhold MANH from an adult who is unable to eat and drink can be viewed as not intervening in the course of the illness that is preventing him from doing what is required to live (and what he once was able to do).

The situation is somewhat different in neonatology, especially for very premature infants. Healthy term babies have an intact suck reflex, allowing them to nurse or drink from a bottle immediately after birth. Prior to thirty-four weeks, however, nearly all babies will require gavage feeds, since the suck reflex has not yet developed. The fact that extremely premature babies require MANH may, therefore, simply be a result of their current developmental stage (which, by definition, is temporary).

This raises the question of whether prematurity can be considered a "disease," permitting MANH to be withheld on that basis. After all, term neonates are not allowed to go without food or water because developmentally they are unable to obtain it and bring it to their mouths. By similar reasoning, if the only reason that a neonate cannot swallow is his degree of prematurity, it would be inappropriate to withhold MANH on the basis of nonintervention in a "disease process."

Extreme prematurity is, however, often associated with profound NDI. This can independently impede one's ability to feed orally and unlike prematurity may be permanent. There may be situations when a baby is born just past the point of viability, and by the time significant NDI manifests itself, the so-called "window of opportunity" of receiving respiratory support has closed. In such cases, it is appropriate to consider forgoing MANH because the inability eat and drink is clearly the result of neuropathology, not merely a temporary developmental problem (Carter & Leuthner, 2003). This is especially clear after thirty-four weeks' gestation, when unaffected babies should be able to swallow safely and effectively.

It is also appropriate to forgo MANH when a patient is dying. As noted previously (p. 194), MANH does not improve symptoms, quality of life, or survival for patients at the very end of their lives. In that context, the burdens of MANH clearly outweigh any potential benefit (AAP, 2007; Nelson et al., 1995; Porta & Frader, 2007). In those situations, "impaired" newborns are not discriminated against by forgoing MANH. Quite the contrary, it would be discriminatory to compel newborns to endure what incapacitated adults in a similar condition are allowed to avoid, according to the best interest standard (AAP, 2009).

All of the aforementioned considerations involve an extremely limited prognosis or a profoundly diminished quality of life. Additional caution should be used when disability alone is offered as justification for forgoing MANH. As noted earlier (p. 282), external observers tend to severely underestimate quality of life in the context of disability. The AAP (2009) therefore asserts that "disability alone is not a sufficient reason to forgo medically provided fluids and nutrition."

Given the complexity surrounding MANH, it is often helpful to defer definitive decisions until there is greater clarity. When parents are not sure what to do, it is appropriate to provide MANH on a temporary basis in order to provide more time for consideration. Even if the parents opt for longer term MANH—such as via a gastrostomy tube—there is no ethical mandate to continue its use, as withdrawing and withholding are ethically equivalent (p. 156). Parents should also be assured that forgoing MANH need not involve suffering (p. 153) (Cranford, 1995).

This still leaves the matter of the Baby Doe Rules. It would seem a violation of these to forgo MANH for an impaired newborn who is neither unconscious nor inevitably dying. Recognizing this, some have tried to argue that the Baby Doe Rules are actually more flexible than they initially appear (AAP, 1996). For instance, the rules state that "*appropriate* nutrition, hydration, and medication must always be given" (emphasis added) unless one of the three exceptions apply (p. 308). If a clinician deems any of those treatments not "appropriate," so the argument goes, then the Baby Doe Rules permit forgoing it.

The question, then, is not so much whether the patient is irreversibly comatose or the treatment is futile but rather whether MANH is "appropriate" (American Academy of Pediatrics Committee on Bioethics, 2009). Such a determination lies in the eye of the be-holder and could—some would argue *should*—encompass quality of life considerations, essentially reducing the question to one of a balance of benefits and burdens.

This interpretation, however, is clearly not the intention of the Baby Doe Rules, which were implemented precisely to prevent forgoing treatment for quality of life considerations (Reagan, 1986). Indeed, after their adoption the rules were embraced by conservative commentators for accomplishing precisely this (Koop, 1989). The plain lan-guage of the rules seems clear in focusing on consciousness and survival, rather than broader quality of life considerations.

It is more intellectually honest to admit that forgoing MANH in many cases does, indeed, violate the Baby Doe Rules. Given their lack of legal enforceability, however (Nelson et al., 1995)—as well as the ethical consensus that they should not be enforced (Kopelman, 2005)—this should not present a barrier to forgoing burdensome treatment, including MANH. Thus while appropriately taking into account the quality of life of an infant may violate the Baby Doe Rules, it does not break any law. To compel "impaired" newborns to receive a treatment that other patients who lack decision-making capacity are permitted to forgo would be the antithesis—rather than the epitome—of justice.

Are Newborns Treated Differently than Other Patients?

The short answer to this question is "yes." Not only were some newborns—in the after-math of Baby Doe—compelled to receive treatment that adults who lack decision-making capacity are permitted to forgo, the converse situation also occurred: other newborns are deprived of treatments that an incapacitated adult would have had a right to, if the best interest standard (p. 67) were applied.

Consider, for example, an incapacitated, unbefriended (p. 68) adult who has a 50/50 chance of survival, with a nearly even chance of being neurologically intact if he does survive. If a surrogate decision-maker refused LSMT because she did not believe—given those odds—that it was "in the patient's best interests," clinicians would surely question the surrogate's logic and perhaps also her motives. LSMT would likely be maintained until additional information was obtained, or perhaps even an alternate surrogate appointed.

Yet the parents of the twenty-four-weeker in this chapter's case—who has the same outcome probabilities (Figure 12.2, p. 481)—are granted precisely that degree of latitude, even though the baby has many more potential years of life than the hypothetical adult. In some contexts parents are permitted to refuse LSMT up to twenty-five or even twenty-six weeks, when the odds of survival can exceed 80%.

Studies have documented this discrepancy using hypothetical vignettes. In one, a twenty-four-weeker was compared against four other children, as well as three adults ranging in age from thirty-five to eighty years old. None of the other patients had a probability of survival greater than the twenty-four-weeker's, and all had at least the same probability (often greater) of new disability. Only one had a higher probability of a "normal outcome," and that one—a fourteen-year-old with leukemia—had only a 5% chance of survival. Physicians and medical students who responded to the survey were more likely to favor LSMT for each of the other patients—with the exception of the eighty-year-old with severe dementia and a new stroke—over the premature baby, despite their all having worse odds of a good outcome (Janvier, Leblanc, & Barrington, 2008).

There are several potential reasons for this. One is simply that the neonates cannot—and never could—speak for themslves. By contrast, adult patients who are critically ill and incapable of making medical decisions once espoused their own values and beliefs. It is possible to imagine them doing very human things—like eating dinner with friends, holding forth in conversation, engaging in favorite activities—which might lead the family and the team to take all possible steps to give the patient a chance to do those things again. Even a two-month-old baby has fed, smiled, and generally interacted with the world.

By contrast, the neonate never did—and might never, even with LSMT, do—any of those things. No one can point to statements of values or priorities the patient made in the past. And the patient is in no position to object if certain interventions are withheld.

Another reason may be lingering memories of the Baby Doe era, where maximal treatment was mandated for "impaired" newborns without respect for quality of life considerations. The pendulum has gradually swung in the opposite direction, permitting parents in most cases to make discretionary decisions about their newborns. To interfere in this intensely emotional and personal moment in parents' lives may be seen as parentalistic and inappropriate.

A third reason is eminently practical. To compel treatment over parents' objections is extremely difficult from a procedural point of view. As the Baby Doe Rules and their aftermath proved, compulsory treatment is a very provocative concept, leading to significant push-back. Not only might parents sue—and potentially win, as in the jury verdict of *Miller v. HCA*—they might also be subsequently reluctant to care for a potentially severely disabled child who would not be alive had their refusal been respected. This necessarily raises the question of who will care for that child.

But the primary reason why neonates are treated differently—especially compared with adults—is that their parents not only bear the burden of making decisions, they also bear the responsibility of living with them. The twenty-four-weeker mentioned earlier may have a 40% chance of less than moderate NDI should he survive, but that also means that he has a 60% chance of *moderate or worse* NDI. Even patients with less than moderate NDI may still have significant impairments which impact their own quality of life as well as that of the family.[2] Unless the parents are considering relinquishing custody of the child, it seems appropriate that they should be granted some degree of additional latitude in making medical decisions that will impact their entire family.

This discretion is not limitless, however. As the AAP (2007) observes, "The physician's first responsibility is to the patient. The physician is not obligated to provide inappropriate treatment or to withhold beneficial treatment at the request of the parents." There are clearly situations when the neonate's prognosis is so good that comfort measures alone are not appropriate, and thus physicians must understand when overriding parental refusal of LSMT might be justified.

When Parents and Physicians Disagree
Overriding Parental Refusal of LSMT

In responding to parents' refusal of LSMT, the operative ethical question is where to "draw the line" at which point LSMT becomes mandatory (Antommaria, Collura, Antiel, & Lantos, 2015). The AAP describes such situations as having "a high rate of survival and acceptable morbidity," which includes most congenital conditions as well as gestations from twenty-five weeks onward (Kattwinkel et al., 2010). Some other societies draw that line in different places, ranging from twenty-four weeks (Nuffield Council on Bioethics, 2006) to twenty-six weeks (Jefferies, Kirpalani, Albersheim, & Lynk, 2014). Specific regional or institutional outcomes may be taken into consideration in determining what the cut-off is, and often other variables—such as the presence and duration of ruptured membranes, or estimated fetal weight—may be relevant.

One's position on this matter impacts not only response to parental refusal but also what options are presented to the parents in the first place. For if LSMT is deemed mandatory, parents should not be given the option of forgoing it (Peerzada, Richardson, & Burns, 2004).

Treatment before delivery is also affected. As noted, steroids administered to the pregnant woman accelerate lung maturity in the fetus. When the plan is to provide intensive respiratory support to the baby, prenatal treatment with steroids maximizes the probability of a good outcome. But in situations where comfort is the goal and there is no possibility that a baby will survive without respiratory intervention, prenatal steroids

---

2. It is not only parents who bear the burden of a child with significant disability. Neonatologists may also experience a sense of culpability in "creating" a child with significant needs (Janvier & Mercurio, 2013), thus leading them to defer to parental requests for limitation of treatment.

only serve to prolong the dying process. For this reason, steroids should generally be deferred until roughly forty-eight hours prior to the point that either the parents have granted permission for maximal intervention, or this is felt to be warranted based on the likelihood of a good outcome.

The reason for establishing a "higher limit" of gestational age is to offer babies with a favorable prognosis the chance to survive, based on the best interest standard. This is, however, by no means an assurance of a good outcome. Parents must be informed that just because their baby has reached the "higher limit" where intensive care must be provided, this does not guarantee that the baby will survive, let alone be neurodevelopmentally intact. Often clinicians are so focused on the period when there is a legitimate decision to be made (i.e., from the point of viability up to twenty-four to twenty-six weeks) that parents might get the mistaken impression that once the latter is reached, their baby will be fine.

The arbitrariness of any "line in the sand" also has to be acknowledged. A baby's prognosis does not markedly improve at midnight upon the completion of the twenty-fifth week of gestation (or whatever cutoff is selected). The prognosis gradually improves in the days leading up to—and following—that point in time. As a result, it is more appropriate to establish a gradual shift in decision-making than an abrupt one. One could imagine a framework whereby up until twenty-four weeks the decision is left entirely to the parents, and between twenty-four and twenty-five weeks there is increased emphasis on shared decision-making (p. 59).

Past a certain point—such as twenty-five completed weeks of gestation—there is a general expectation of full resuscitation, absent any major confounding variables. All the while the parents are kept fully informed, and reassured that resuscitation in the delivery room does not mandate unlimited intensive care in the hours and days that follow. Should the baby's condition deteriorate in the NICU, the option of shifting goals certainly remains.

Rather than simply refusing to honor the parents' refusal, it is preferable to sensitively explore the reasons for it. Perhaps the parents misunderstood the baby's prognosis, which might have been expressed in confusing or overly technical terms. They could also be afraid of "losing control" if intensive care is instituted, fearing that they will not be able to protect their child from overly burdensome treatment. Their experience with children with disabilities is also relevant, as this could be scary if unfamiliar.

As always, the optimal resolution to an ethical dilemma is to make it "go away," in this case by helping the parents reach a place where they acknowledge the appropriateness of intensive treatment. Sometimes, though, this is impossible, and their refusal must be overridden. This is never comfortable nor simple and should not be undertaken lightly. But the physician's primary obligation is to the patient, whose probability of a good outcome may justify at least a trial of treatment.

To support the physicians in this course of action, it is advisable to have an institutional policy that identifies clinical criteria for mandatory treatment, taking into account factors beyond gestational age and birthweight. Such a policy should also outline procedural steps to ensure equitable treatment, as well as provide parents with resources for both appeal—to ensure due process—as well as emotional support.

Declining Parental Requests for Attempted Resuscitation

For viable infants who do not exceed the upper limit of prematurity, parental decisions regarding resuscitation should generally be respected. Parents could reasonably opt for aggressive treatment in the hopes of a good outcome. By the same token, they might opt to focus on comfort, recognizing the inherent risks and burdens.

Even in the absence of parental refusal, there are two other situations where delivery room resuscitation[3] may be withheld. The first is such a degree of prematurity that the likelihood of survival is low and morbidity is high. The AAP defines this as gestational age less than twenty-three weeks or birthweight of less than 400 grams (Kattwinkel et al., 2010). Decisions based on gestational age must take into account the frequent uncertainty about "dates," especially when they are based on ultrasounds later in the pregnancy (p. 312).

The gestational "lower limit" of resuscitation thus depends on the "point of viability," at which point extrauterine survival becomes possible. As noted (p. 292), this point used to coincide with the third trimester of pregnancy, but technological advances subsequently moved it up into the second trimester. For many years it was acknowledged to be twenty-three weeks gestation, but recent data suggests that twenty-two-weekers have a small but not negligible chance of survival. In one study, nearly one-quarter of babies at this gestational age survived with aggressive treatment. Further, approximately 40% of survivors had less than moderate or severe neurodevelopmental impairment (Rysavy et al., 2015). This raises the question of whether previously documented negligible survival for this age group was yet another "self-fulfilling prophecy": twenty-two-weekers were thought to not survive and thus resuscitation was withheld, effectively assuring their nonsurvival (Mercurio, 2005).

The second situation where delivery room resuscitation may be withheld—even when requested—is where the fetus suffers from a condition that makes extrauterine survival extremely unlikely. In their most recent position statement, the AAP and American Hospital Association identify two such conditions: anencephaly and major chromosomal abnormalities, such as Trisomy 13 (Kattwinkel et al., 2010). Of note, certain conditions previously identified by name no longer appear on this list. Trisomy 18, for instance, was once included in the list of conditions appropriate for nonresuscitation (American Heart Association, 2005; International Liaison Committee on Resuscitation, 2006), but as outcomes with aggressive treatment were shown to be more positive than previously recognized (Kosho et al., 2006), it was subsequently dropped from the list.

---

3. This section focuses on delivery room resuscitation, as that is the aspect of requests for potentially non-beneficial treatment (NBT) that is unique to this age group. Subsequent such requests in the NICU fall under the broader rubric of NBT, which is addressed in detail in chapter 14.

If the clinical team is unwilling to attempt resuscitation, the parents should not be offered this as an option. Doing so while presenting sobering statistics in anticipation that the parents will refuse intervention is disingenuous at best—making a mockery of the informed consent process—and conflict-inciting at worst. A parent could reasonably assume that the physician would not offer something unless it could be helpful. For the physician to refuse to provide something she had just appeared to offer could damage the physician-parent relationship.

Even if the physician does not offer resuscitation, the parents may request it (or assume that it will be provided). In that situation, it is appropriate to explore their reasons for doing so. They might not appreciate the disproportionate burdens of the procedure. They may feel like their obligation as parents is to "do everything" to help their child. They may be afraid of being judged if they "just" provide comfort care to their child.

Each of these positions requires a different response, whether clarification of the medical facts, thoughtful exploration of what it means to be a good parent, or explanation that comfort care can be every bit as intensive as resuscitation, only with a different goal. In some cases the parents will ultimately change their minds, approving a plan to withhold resuscitative efforts.

But what if they continue to demand resuscitation and maximal treatment? Here it is important to note that while withholding resuscitation is ethically justifiable in the context of extreme prematurity, anencephaly, and major chromosomal abnormalities, it is not ethically *required*. This provides some latitude for providers to choose to attempt to resuscitate neonates that have an exceedingly poor prognosis, if the parents are fully informed and the providers feel that they can in good conscience proceed.

One reason for providing aggressive treatment in such cases might be a genuine sense of humility, recognizing the inherent uncertainty is estimating gestational age and the fact that in some cases patients will exceed expectations. Another reason might be to ensure that the parents know that "everything was done" to help their child survive, which can be some consolation even when the treatment is believed to be ineffective (Truog, 2010). Therefore, "in conditions associated with uncertain prognosis, when there is borderline survival and a relatively high rate of morbidity, and where the burden to the child is high, the parent's views on starting resuscitation should be supported" (International Liaison Committee on Resuscitation, 2006).

Two potential misunderstandings may accompany this deference to parental request, however. One is the "What's the worst that can happen?" argument. In other words, if death is inevitable, why not provide aggressive treatment (which will likely be short-lived, anyway)? The problem with this argument is that some extremely high-risk neonates will survive but usually with profound disability. Framing outcomes exclusively in reference to survival, therefore, may not adequately address other parental concerns. Once again, identifying not only what the parents most hope for but also what they most fear will be critical (Bernacki, Block, & American College of Physicians High Value Care Task Force, 2014).

The "Why not try?" approach also assumes that there is no distinction between dying after aggressive treatment and being provided with comfort measures only. Yet the difference is extremely significant both for the neonate—who will be subjected to painful, invasive procedures and might never know life outside the NICU—as well as the parents, who will be separated from their baby and likely be faced with a further series of incredibly difficult decisions. In cases where the ultimate outcome is certain, it is both more honest and more compassionate to be clear about what the parents might lose by opting for aggressive treatment. Rather than framing the decision in terms of survival (which may not be possible), it is preferable to focus on more human goals, such as holding one's child for his entire life (Macauley, 2015).

Groningen Protocol (Netherlands)

As noted in chapter 5, the line between forgoing LSMT and actively hastening death is crisply drawn in the United States. Aggressive symptom management which *conceivably* could hasten death is justified by the Rule of Double Effect (p. 209), and other interventions that may lead to the same result (such as palliative sedation, chapter 9) are only instituted in clearly defined circumstances which make this highly unlikely. The only exception is Physician Assisted Dying (chapter 8) which requires a patient with capacity to choose to hasten his own death, and to do so through his own actions (in the form of ingesting a lethal dose of a pharmaceutical).

In a few other countries, however, physicians are legally permitted to hasten a patient's death in specific circumstances, even without the patient's consent (p. 151). In the context of neonatalogy, the Groningen Protocol from the Netherlands—which permits active euthanasia of some infants—bears specific mention. This protocol came to worldwide attention in 2005 in an editorial in the *New England Journal of Medicine* which attempted to dispel common misperceptions regarding it (Verhagen & Sauer, 2005).

The editorial noted that a medical decision—such as whether to forgo LSMT—preceded most infant deaths in the Netherlands. These infants can be divided into three categories. The first are those who will die despite maximal treatment, and the second are those whose prognosis is poor and are dependent on intensive care. In both of these cases, forgoing LSMT will lead to the child's death and would also be permitted (with the parents' permission) in the United States.

The third category are infants with "a hopeless prognosis who experience what parents and medical experts deem to be unbearable suffering" (Verhagen & Sauer, 2005). The most common diagnosis meeting this criteria in the Netherlands is severe spina bifida. Many of these patients are not dependent on LSMT, and with maximal treatment—including hospital care—could be expected to live a long life. On the calculus of the Groningen Protocol, however, longer life makes euthanasia *more* acceptable because it represents a longer period over which the patient would experience suffering.

To be eligible for the Groningen Protocol, the infant's diagnosis and prognosis must be firmly established. In addition, all attempts to ameliorate suffering must have failed.

The parents must agree, as must the team of physicians (including at least one not directly involved in the patient's care). If all these conditions are met, the infant may be euthanized and the physicians cannot be held criminally liable.

The Groningen Protocol can be criticized in three ways. The first is that the Protocol crosses the bright line between not doing something necessary to sustain life and doing something to hasten death. Palliative care specifically excludes the latter (World Health Organization, 2002), so like any other form of euthanasia the Protocol cannot be considered "palliative care." But beyond its classification, stepping over that line presents all manner of ethical problems including violating the sacred responsibility of a physician, damaging the physician-patient relationship, and imperiling the vulnerable. All the criticisms of active euthanasia noted earlier (p. 150) are applicable to the Groningen Protocol. The fact that it involves vulnerable infants who are, by definition, unable to participate in the process makes it even more unacceptable.

The second criticism involves the variability and inherent subjectivity of quality of life estimations (p. 282). Studies have clearly shown that physicians underestimate the quality of life of formerly premature babies, compared to the patients themselves (Saigal et al., 1999). To be fair, the Protocol requires not only physician estimates of prognosis and suffering but also parental consent. One might respond that parents are the ideal check against quality of life bias, but this potentially overlooks the intertwined nature of suffering that affects families and parental decisions. It may be difficult for parents to separate out their own grief from a patient's suffering as well as the effect the latter might have on other children in the family, if only by virtue of the additional time and energy necessarily devoted to a seriously ill child.

Even if one embraces the concept of "constrained parental autonomy"—whereby parents are permitted to make "intrafamilial trade-offs" as long as each child's "basic needs" are met (p. 287)—to allow that autonomy to extend to active euthanasia is a huge step. What more basic need is there, one might ask, than life itself? The obvious response (particularly in a palliative care context) is that continued existence is not the ultimate good, especially when extreme suffering is involved. But the degree to which infants eligible for the Protocol truly experience "extreme suffering"—and whether the Protocol appropriately addresses the suffering of the infant or the parents—remains unclear.

Third, the Groningen Protocol does not so much increase the risk of sliding down a slippery slope as represent the slope itself. It is not surprising that the Protocol originated in the Netherlands, where active euthanasia has been legal for many years. Studies have shown that a significant proportion of adult patients who are euthanized there did not give their consent (van der Heide et al., 2007). The Protocol is, therefore, basically a logical extension of this practice to a uniformly nonvoluntary population: infants.

But if nonvoluntary euthanasia is permissible for infants severe spina bifida, why limit the practice to this condition? Would not other conditions also involve "unbearable suffering," at least in the eyes of external observers? And if "suffering" is considered in its broadest sense, might that not also include patients whose suffering is nonphysical, such as patients who may be pain-free but "suffer" from disabilities which limit their ability to reach their full potential? Could not isolated developmental delay potentially cause unbearable suffering, if only because of opportunities lost? This might appear extreme were it not for commentators who do not even acknowledge that *healthy* infants are human beings, because they have not yet developed the capacity for language (Singer, 2011).

And why limit the practice to infants? If parents reach the conclusion that their child's suffering is unbearable, why "deprive" the patient of euthanasia simply because his first birthday has passed? The Groningen Protocol is sufficiently far down "the slope of euthanasia" that it seems practically impossible to prevent sliding all the way down, without regard for the wishes or potential of an individual patient.

It is not enough to merely reject active euthanasia for suffering infants, however; that suffering needs to be addressed. All symptomatic treatment must be utilized and options considered, up to and including palliative sedation for truly refractory and intolerable symptoms. Even in the absence of such symptoms, a patient's quality of life may truly be poor. (Just because physicians tend to underestimate quality of life does not mean it cannot be evaluated.) Illness serious enough to thus impact quality of life often requires occasional interventions (such as antibiotics) to sustain that life. Forgoing these can, therefore, provide an "exit ramp" when the burdens of treatment—or of life itself—outweigh the benefits. Rejecting the Groningen Protocol, therefore, neither eliminates the need to make appropriate quality of life estimations, nor condemns the child to maximal treatment and the longest possible life.

Return to the Case

The palliative care team begins by exploring the parents' goals for their child. Obviously, they are hoping for a perfectly healthy baby. At the same time they are willing to accept the risk of neurodevelopmental impairment—which they have little personal experience of—in order to give their baby "a chance."

The parents are also overwhelmed by information, including gestational age, estimated fetal weight, and many probabilities from the NICHD database. The pregnant woman is further burdened by being in active labor. The palliative care team recognizes that there is little chance of enhancing the parents' understanding of the situation, given the pervasive uncertainty. Since the parents are clearly not refusing intervention—and the baby appears to have a reasonable chance of survival (potentially free of neurodevelopmental impairment)—a plan is formulated to provide maximal treatment.

The team is careful not to offer a "trial of life," recognizing its unreliability. They do reassure the parents that everything will be done to help their child in the delivery room, unless it becomes absolutely clear that the baby will not survive (e.g., no heart rate at ten minutes of maximal treatment). The parents are assured that they always have the right to reconsider the treatment plan, especially if the burdens of treatment come to outweigh the benefits. They are also informed that this may not become clear for some time. Discussions of more complex concepts (such as the "window of opportunity" and forgoing MANH) are deferred to a later time when they may be relevant.

The baby is delivered vaginally, resuscitation in the delivery room proceeds according to protocol, and the baby is transferred to the NICU. Early cranial ultrasounds reveal bilateral Grade III intraventricular hemorrhages, with uncertain prognostic implications. The baby weathers the "roller coaster" course that is common in the NICU, with frequent stopping of her gavage feeds because of concerning abdominal exams. Eventually she is extubated but has a lingering oxygen requirement and ultimately is able to tolerate "full feeds" (and thus does not require parenteral nutrition). She is discharged around her original due date with a slightly misshaped head (common to many premature babies) and requiring overnight monitoring for potential desaturations. Her neurologic prognosis remains uncertain.

Summary Points

- Whereas for much of human history the operative question was whether to care for "impaired" newborns at all, over the last several decades the question has shifted to how much care is sufficient and how much is "too much."
- The Baby Doe Rules—which evolved out of concern that "impaired" newborns were receiving insufficient treatment—paid little attention to quality of life and were declared unconstitutional. By contrast, the President's Commission took many factors into account, acknowledging the right of parents to refuse treatment unless it was clearly beneficial.
- It is difficult to prognosticate accurately in neonatology, based on uncertainty of gestational age, the impact of other factors on prognosis, and the variable impact of previously relied-upon findings (such as head ultrasound).
- Forgoing medical administered nutrition and hydration entails more ethical complexity in the neonatal period, but where the burdens outweigh the benefits—and reliance on it is not merely a function of extreme prematurity—parents have the right to refuse it.
- Newborns are often treated differently than adult patients without decision-making capacity. The greater latitude granted to parents appropriately respects the special nature of that relationship, but it is not limitless.
- The "higher limit of resuscitation" refers to the gestational age at which point the likely outcomes are so good that parental refusal of intervention should not

be honored. It is reasonable to draw this line at approximately twenty-five weeks, with a gradual transition toward shared decision-making in the week leading up to that point.

- There also exists a "lower limit" where parental requests for aggressive treatment need not be honored. This includes gestational age of less than twenty-two weeks, anencephaly, and serious chromosomal abnormalities.
  - If an intervention will not be performed, parents should not be given the option of it.
  - If parents nevertheless demand it, some physicians might choose to provide it anyway, in order to reassure the parents that "everything" has been done. It is important to recognize, though, what meaningful experiences would be lost by this course of action.
- The Groningen Protocol refers to active euthanasia of newborns in the Netherlands who are felt to experiencing "unbearable suffering." It is unethical, susceptible to bias, and unnecessary.

References

American Academy of Pediatrics Committee on Bioethics. (1996). Ethics and the care of critically ill infants and children. *Pediatrics, 98*(1), 149–152.

American Academy of Pediatrics Committee on Bioethics. (2009). Forgoing medically provided nutrition and hydration in children. *Pediatrics, 124*(2), 813–822. doi:10.1542/peds.2009-1299

American Academy of Pediatrics Committee on Fetus and Newborn. (2007). Noninitiation or withdrawal of intensive care for high-risk newborns. *Pediatrics, 119*(2), 401–403. doi:10.1542/peds.2006-3180

American Academy of Pediatrics Committee on Fetus and Newborn. (2015). Antenatal counseling regarding resuscitation and intensive care before 25 weeks of gestation. *Pediatrics, 136*(3), 588–595. doi:10.1542/peds.2015-2336

American Heart Association. (2005). 2005 American Heart Association Guidelines for Cardiopulmonary Resuscitation and Emergency Cardiovascular Care. *Circulation, 112*(24 Suppl), IV1–203. doi:10.1161/CIRCULATIONAHA.105.166550

Andrews, B., Lagatta, J., Chu, A., Plesha-Troyke, S., Schreiber, M., Lantos, J., & Meadow, W. (2012). The nonimpact of gestational age on neurodevelopmental outcome for ventilated survivors born at 23–28 weeks of gestation. *Acta Paediatr, 101*(6), 574–578.

Ann Wy, P., Rettiganti, M., Li, J., Yap, V., Barrett, K., Whiteside-Mansell, L., & Casey, P. (2015). Impact of intraventricular hemorrhage on cognitive and behavioral outcomes at 18 years of age in low birth weight preterm infants. *J Perinatol, 35*(7), 511–515. doi:10.1038/jp.2014.244

Antommaria, A. H., Collura, C. A., Antiel, R. M., & Lantos, J. D. (2015). Two infants, same prognosis, different parental preferences. *Pediatrics, 135*(5), 918–923. doi:10.1542/peds.2013-4044

Aristotle, & Jowett, B. (1943). *Aristotle's politics.* New York: Modern Library.

Bernacki, R. E., Block, S. D., & American College of Physicians High Value Care Task Force. (2014). Communication about serious illness care goals: A review and synthesis of best practices. *JAMA Intern Med, 174*(12), 1994–2003. doi:10.1001/jamainternmed.2014.5271

Blanco, F., Suresh, G., Howard, D., Soll, R. (2005). Ensuring accurate knowledge of prematurity outcomes for prenatal counseling. *Pediatrics, 115*(4), e478–87. doi:10.1542/peds.2004-1417

Born Alive Infant Protection Act, Pub. L. No. 107-207 (2001).

Bowen v. American Hospital Association, No. 2101, 106 (S Ct 1986).

Brahams, D., & Brahams, M. (1983). Symposium 1: The Arthur case—a proposal for legislation. *J Med Ethics, 9*(1), 12–15.

Butt, K., Lim, K., & Society of Obstetricians and Gynaecologists of Canada. (2014). Determination of gestational age by ultrasound. *J Obstet Gynaecol Can*, *36*(2), 171–183.

Carter, B. S., & Leuthner, S. R. (2003). The ethics of withholding/withdrawing nutrition in the newborn. *Semin Perinatol*, *27*(6), 480–487.

Catto-Smith, A. G., Yu, V. Y., Bajuk, B., Orgill, A. A., & Astbury, J. (1985). Effect of neonatal periventricular haemorrhage on neurodevelopmental outcome. *Arch Dis Child*, *60*(1), 8–11.

Child Abuse Prevention and Treatment Act, 42 § 5101 (1994).

Cooke, R. W. (2004). Health, lifestyle, and quality of life for young adults born very preterm. *Arch Dis Child*, *89*(3), 201–206.

Cranford, R. E. (1995). Withdrawing artificial feeding from children with brain damage. *BMJ*, *311*(7003), 464–465.

Cruzan v. Director, Missouri Department of Health, 497 261 (S.Ct. 1990).

De Cruz, P. (2000). *Comparative Health Care Law*. New York: Routledge-Cavendish.

Department of Health & Human Services. (1984). Nondiscrimination on the basis of handicap; procedures and guidelines relating to health care for handicapped infants. *Fed Regist*, *48*(8), 1622–1654.

Department of Health and Human Services. (1985). Nondiscrimination on the basis of handicap; procedures and guidelines relating to health care for handicapped infants. *Fed Regist*, *50*(8), 14879–14892.

Donovan, E. F., Tyson, J. E., Ehrenkranz, R. A., Verter, J., Wright, L. L., Korones, S. B., . . . Papile, L. A. (1999). Inaccuracy of Ballard scores before 28 weeks' gestation. National Institute of Child Health and Human Development Neonatal Research Network. *J Pediatr*, *135*(2 Pt 1), 147–152.

Duff, R. S., & Campbell, A. G. (1973). Moral and ethical dilemmas in the special-care nursery. *N Engl J Med*, *289*(17), 890–894. doi:10.1056/NEJM197310252891705

Emergency Medical Treatment and Labor Act. (1986). 42 U.S.C. §1395dd.

Ferngren, G. F. (1987). The status of defective newborns from antiquity to the Reformation. In R. C. McMillan, H. T. Engelhardt, & S. F. Spicker (Eds.), *Euthanasia and the newborn: Conflicts regarding saving lives* (pp. 47–64). Dordrecht; Boston: D. Reidel.

Final Rule, 68 Fed. Reg. at 53,246 (citing H.R. Rep. No. 99-241, pt. 1, at 27 [1985], reprinted in 1986 U.S.C.C.A.N. 579, 605).

Frader, J. E. (2007). Discontinuing artificial fluids and nutrition: Discussions with children' families. *Hastings Cent Rep*, *37*(1), 1 p following 48.

Friebert, S., & Williams, C. (2015). *Pediatric palliative & hospice care in America*. Retrieved from https://www.nhpco.org/sites/default/files/public/quality/Pediatric_Facts-Figures.pdf

Gardner, M. O., Bronstein, J., Goldenberg, R. L., Haywood, J. L., Cliver, S. P., & Nelson, K. G. (1996). Physician opinions of preterm infant outcome and their effect on antenatal corticosteroid use. *J Perinatol*, *16*(6), 431–434.

Gray, R., Petrou, S., Hockley, C., & Gardner, F. (2007). Self-reported health status and health-related quality of life of teenagers who were born before 29 weeks' gestational age. *Pediatrics*, *120*(1), e86–93. doi:10.1542/peds.2006-2034

Hack, M., Flannery, D. J., Schluchter, M., Cartar, L., Borawski, E., & Klein, N. (2002). Outcomes in young adulthood for very-low-birth-weight infants. *N Engl J Med*, *346*(3), 149–157. doi:10.1056/NEJMoa010856

Hanke, K., Hartz, A., Manz, M., Bendiks, M., Heitmann, F., Orlikowsky, T., . . . German Neonatal, N. (2015). Preterm prelabor rupture of membranes and outcome of very-low-birth-weight infants in the German Neonatal Network. *PLoS One*, *10*(4), e0122564. doi:10.1371/journal.pone.0122564

Haywood, J. L., Goldenberg, R. L., Bronstein, J., Nelson, K. G., & Carlo, W. A. (1994). Comparison of perceived and actual rates of survival and freedom from handicap in premature infants. *Am J Obstet Gynecol*, *171*(2), 432–439.

International Liaison Committee on Resuscitation. (2006). The International Liaison Committee on Resuscitation (ILCOR) consensus on science with treatment recommendations for pediatric and neonatal patients: neonatal resuscitation. *Pediatrics*, *117*(5), e978–988. doi:10.1542/peds.2006-0350

Janvier, A., & Barrington, K. J. (2005). The ethics of neonatal resuscitation at the margins of viability: Informed consent and outcomes. *J Pediatr*, *147*(5), 579–585. doi:10.1016/j.jpeds.2005.06.002

Janvier, A., Leblanc, I., & Barrington, K. J. (2008). The best-interest standard is not applied for neonatal resuscitation decisions. *Pediatrics*, *121*(5), 963–969. doi:10.1542/peds.2007-1520

Janvier, A., & Mercurio, M. R. (2013). Saving vs. creating: Perceptions of intensive care at different ages and the potential for injustice. *Journal of Perinatology, 33*(5), 333–335.

Jefferies, A. L., Kirpalani, H., Albersheim, S. G., & Lynk, A. (2014). Counselling and management for anticipated extremely preterm birth. *Paediatr Child Health, 19*(1), 25–26.

Kaempf, J. W., Tomlinson, M., Arduza, C., Anderson, S., Campbell, B., Ferguson, L. A., . . . Stewart, V. T. (2006). Medical staff guidelines for periviability pregnancy counseling and medical treatment of extremely premature infants. *Pediatrics, 117*(1), 22–29. doi:10.1542/peds.2004-2547

Kattwinkel, J., Perlman, J. M., Aziz, K., Colby, C., Fairchild, K., Gallagher, J., . . . American Heart Association. (2010). Neonatal resuscitation: 2010 American Heart Association guidelines for cardiopulmonary resuscitation and emergency cardiovascular care. *Pediatrics, 126*(5), e1400–1413. doi:10.1542/peds.2010-2972E

Koop, C. E. (1989). The challenge of definition. *Hastings Cent Rep, 19*(1), S2–S3.

Kopelman, L. M. (2005). Are the 21-year-old Baby Doe rules misunderstood or mistaken? *Pediatrics, 115*(3), 797–802. doi:10.1542/peds.2004-2326

Kopelman, L. M., Irons, T. G., & Kopelman, A. E. (1988). Neonatologists judge the "Baby Doe" regulations. *N Engl J Med, 318*(11), 677–683. doi:10.1056/NEJM198803173181105

Kosho, T., Nakamura, T., Kawame, H., Baba, A., Tamura, M., & Fukushima, Y. (2006). Neonatal management of trisomy 18: clinical details of 24 patients receiving intensive treatment. *Am J Med Genet A, 140*(9), 937–944. doi:10.1002/ajmg.a.31175

Langer, W. L. (1963). Europe's initial population explosion. *Am Hist Rev, 69*, 1–17.

Lantos, J. D., & Meadow, W. (2006). *Neonatal bioethics: The moral challenges of medical innovation.* Baltimore: Johns Hopkins University Press.

Lantos, J. D., Mokalla, M., & Meadow, W. (1997). Resource allocation in neonatal and medical ICUs: Epidemiology and rationing at the extremes of life. *Am J Respir Crit Care Med, 156*(1), 185–189. doi:10.1164/ajrccm.156.1.9510103

Lee, S. K., Penner, P. L., & Cox, M. (1991). Comparison of the attitudes of health care professionals and parents toward active treatment of very low birth weight infants. *Pediatrics, 88*(1), 110–114.

Levi, B. H. (2003). Withdrawing nutrition and hydration from children: Legal, ethical, and professional issues. *Clin Pediatr (Phila), 42*(2), 139–145.

Manley, B. J., Dawson, J. A., Kamlin, C. O., Donath, S. M., Morley, C. J., & Davis, P. G. (2010). Clinical assessment of extremely premature infants in the delivery room is a poor predictor of survival. *Pediatrics, 125*(3), e559–e564. doi:10.1542/peds.2009-1307

Meadow, W. (2007). Babies between a rock and a hard place—neonatologists vs parents at the edge of infant viability. *Acta Paediatr, 96*(2), 153.

Meadow, W. (2013). Ethics at the margins of viability. *NeoReviews, 14*(12), e588–e591.

Meadow, W., Lee, G., Lin, K., & Lantos, J. (2004). Changes in mortality for extremely low birth weight infants in the 1990s: Implications for treatment decisions and resource use. *Pediatrics, 113*(5), 1223–1229.

Meisel, A. (1992). The legal consensus about foregoing life-sustaining treatment: Its status and its prospects. *Kennedy Inst Ethics J, 2*(4), 309–345.

Mercurio, M. (2005). Physicians' refusal to resuscitate at borderline gestational age. *J Perinat, 25*(11), 685–689.

Miles, S. H. (1989). Taking hostages: The Linares case. *Hastings Cent Rep, 19*(4), 4.

Miller v. HCA, Inc. (2003). 118 S.W.3d 758, 761 (Tex.).

Moitra, V.K., Guerra, C., Linde-Zwirble, W. T., & Wunsch, H. (2016). Relationship Between ICU Length of Stay and Long-Term Mortality for Elderly ICU Survivors. *Crit Care Med, 44*(4), 655–662. doi:10.1097/CCM.0000000000001480

National Institute of Child Health and Human Development. Extremely premature birth outcome data. Rretrieved from https://www1.nichd.nih.gov/epbo-calculator/Pages/epbo_case.aspx

Nelson, L. J., Rushton, C. H., Cranford, R. E., Nelson, R. M., Glover, J. J., & Truog, R. D. (1995). Forgoing medically provided nutrition and hydration in pediatric patients. *J Law Med Ethics, 23*(1), 33–46.

Nuffield Council on Bioethics. (2006). *Critical care and decisions in fetal and neonatal medicine: Ethical issues.* Retrieved from http://nuffieldbioethics.org/wp-content/uploads/2014/07/CCD-web-version-22-June-07-updated.pdf

Osterman, M. J., Kochanek, K. D., MacDorman, M. F., Strobino, D. M., & Guyer, B. (2015). Annual summary of vital statistics: 2012-2013. *Pediatrics, 135*(6), 1115–1125. doi:10.1542/peds.2015-0434

Patra, K. (2014). Severe intraventricular hemorrhage in a new decade: What do we tell parents? *J Perinatol, 34*(3), 167–168. doi:10.1038/jp.2013.165

Peerzada, J. M., Richardson, D. K., & Burns, J. P. (2004). Delivery room decision-making at the threshold of viability. *J Pediatr, 145*(4), 492–498. doi:10.1016/j.jpeds.2004.06.018

Plato, & Jowett, B. (1941). *Plato's The Republic*. New York: Modern Library.

Pope, T. (2008). EMTALA: Its application to newborn infants. *ABA Health eSource, 4* (7). Retrieved from https://www.americanbar.org/newsletter/publications/aba_health_esource_home/pope.html#_ftn11

Porta, N., & Frader, J. (2007). Withholding hydration and nutrition in newborns. *Theor Med Bioeth, 28*(5), 443–451. doi:10.1007/s11017-007-9049-6

President's Commission for the Study of Ethical Problems in Medicine and Biomedical and Behavioral Research. (1983). *Deciding to forego life-sustaining treatment: A report on the ethical, medical, and legal issues in treatment decisions*. Washington, DC: U.S. Government Printing Office.

Reagan, R. (1986). Abortion and the conscience of the nation. In J. D. Butler & D. F. Walbert (Eds.), *Abortion, medicine, and the law* (3rd ed., pp. 352–358). New York: Facts on File.

Rushton, C. H. (1994). Commentary: Guidelines on forgoing life-sustaining medical treatment. *Pediatr Nurs, 20*(5), 522.

Rysavy, M. A., Li, L., Bell, E. F., Das, A., Hintz, S. R., Stoll, B. J., . . . Human Development Neonatal Research Network. (2015). Between-hospital variation in treatment and outcomes in extremely preterm infants. *N Engl J Med, 372*(19), 1801–1811. doi:10.1056/ NEJMoa1410689

Saigal, S., Stoskopf, B. L., Feeny, D., Furlong, W., Burrows, E., Rosenbaum, P. L., & Hoult, L. (1999). Differences in preferences for neonatal outcomes among health care professionals, parents, and adolescents. *JAMA, 281*(21), 1991–1997.

Saigal, S., Stoskopf, B. L., Streiner, D. L., & Burrows, E. (2001). Physical growth and current health status of infants who were of extremely low birth weight and controls at adolescence. *Pediatrics, 108*(2), 407–415.

Saigal, S., Stoskopf, B., Pinelli, J., Streiner, D., Hoult, L., Paneth, N., & Goddeeris, J. (2006). Self-perceived health-related quality of life of former extremely low birth weight infants at young adulthood. *Pediatrics, 118*(3), 1140–1148. doi:10.1542/peds.2006-0119

Shaw, A., Randolph, J. G., & Manard, B. (1977). Ethical issues in pediatric surgery: A national survey of pediatricians and pediatric surgeons. *Pediatrics, 60*(4 Pt 2), 588–599.

Singer, P. (2011). *Practical ethics* (3rd ed.). New York: Cambridge University Press.

Singh, J., Lantos, J., & Meadow, W. (2004). End-of-life after birth: Death and dying in a neonatal intensive care unit. *Pediatrics, 114*(6), 1620–1626. doi:10.1542/peds.2004-0447

Sladkevicius, P., Saltvedt, S., Almstrom, H., Kublickas, M., Grunewald, C., & Valentin, L. (2005). Ultrasound dating at 12-14 weeks of gestation. A prospective cross-validation of established dating formulae in in-vitro fertilized pregnancies. *Ultrasound Obstet Gynecol, 26*(5), 504–511. doi:10.1002/ uog.1993

Slomka, J. (1995). What do apple pie and motherhood have to do with feeding tubes and caring for the patient? *Arch Intern Med, 155*(12), 1258–1263.

Streiner, D. L., Saigal, S., Burrows, E., Stoskopf, B., & Rosenbaum, P. (2001). Attitudes of parents and health care professionals toward active treatment of extremely premature infants. *Pediatrics, 108*(1), 152–157.

Sujdak Mackiewicz, B. N. (2016). Good ethics begin with good facts. *Am J Bioeth, 16*(7), 66–68. doi:10.1080/ 15265161.2016.1180447

Todres, I. D., Krane, D., Howell, M. C., & Shannon, D. C. (1977). Pediatricians' attitudes affecting decision-making in defective newborns. *Pediatrics, 60*(2), 197–201.

Truog, R. D. (2010). Is it always wrong to perform futile CPR? *N Engl J Med, 362*(6), 477–479. doi:10.1056/ NEJMp0908464

Truog, R. D., & Cochrane, T. I. (2005). Refusal of hydration and nutrition: Irrelevance of the "artificial" vs "natural" distinction. *Arch Intern Med, 165*(22), 2574–2576. doi:10.1001/archinte.165.22.2574

Tyson, J. E., Parikh, N. A., Langer, J., Green, C., Higgins, R. D., National Institute of Child, H., & Human Development Neonatal Research, N. (2008). Intensive care for extreme prematurity--moving beyond gestational age. *N Engl J Med, 358*(16), 1672–1681. doi:10.1056/NEJMoa073059

U.S. Rehabilitation Act, 29, USC, Pub. L. No. 93-112 794 (1973).

van der Heide, A., Onwuteaka-Philipsen, B. D., Rurup, M. L., Buiting, H. M., van Delden, J. J., Hanssen-de Wolf, J. E., . . . van der Wal, G. (2007). End-of-life practices in the Netherlands under the Euthanasia Act. *N Engl J Med, 356*(19), 1957–1965. doi:10.1056/NEJMsa071143

Verhagen, E., & Sauer, P. J. (2005). The Groningen protocol—euthanasia in severely ill newborns. *N Engl J Med, 352*(10), 959–962. doi:10.1056/NEJMp058026

Wennerholm, U. B., Bergh, C., Hagberg, H., Sultan, B., & Wennergren, M. (1998). Gestational age in pregnancies after in vitro fertilization: comparison between ultrasound measurement and actual age. *Ultrasound Obstet Gynecol, 12*(3), 170–174. doi:10.1046/j.1469-0705.1998.12030170.x

Whittall, H. (2007). Noninitiation or withdrawal of intensive care for high-risk newborns. *Pediatrics, 119*(6), 1267; author reply 1267–1269. doi:10.1542/peds.2007-0748

Wood, N. S., Marlow, N., Costeloe, K., Gibson, A. T., & Wilkinson, A. R. (2000). Neurologic and developmental disability after extremely preterm birth. EPICure Study Group. *N Engl J Med, 343*(6), 378–384. doi:10.1056/NEJM200008103430601

World Health Organization. (2002). WHO definition of palliative care. Retrieved from www.who.int/cancer/palliative/definition/en/

World Health Organization. (2016). Preterm birth. Retrieved from http://www.who.int/mediacentre/factsheets/fs363/en/

Wyatt, J. (2009). *Matters of life & death: Human dilemmas in the light of the Christian faith* (2nd ed.). Nottingham, UK: InterVarsity Press.

13

Ethics of Child and Adolescent Palliative Care

Preceding chapters have examined the ethics of palliative care prior to, during, and immediately following the birth of a baby. The particular palliative care needs at subsequent developmental stages—infant, toddler, preschool, school age, and adolescent—fall on a spectrum. Earlier on, the issues and needs closely resemble neonatal palliative care. Gradually, as the child develops a greater degree of decision-making capacity (DMC), the issues and needs approach that of an adult. Rather than overly subdivide these analogous and evolving issues, they are addressed under the overall rubric of "child and adolescent palliative care," recognizing that there is significant variability regarding their application depending on the precise age—both in terms of chronology and maturity—of the child, as well as the particular clinical context.

Case Study

A fourteen-year-old girl is diagnosed with acute myeloid leukemia, with five-year survival over 65%. Her parents, concerned that telling her she has "cancer" will take away her hope and cause greater anxiety, forbid the team from informing her of her diagnosis. The team is conflicted, however, wanting the patient to be actively involved in her own care. Up to this point, the patient has asked very few questions about her condition.

Historicolegal Background

For much of human history, children were viewed as the property of their parents (Wyatt, 2009). As such, parents could make whatever decisions they wanted, and special protections for children were essentially unheard of. Children were not entitled to education or protected from harsh work environments, even at young ages. Not surprisingly, under common law patients younger than twenty-one were not granted the right to make their own medical decisions.

This began to change in the nineteenth century, with restrictions placed on child work hours and conditions, as well as safeguards established against mistreatment. These safeguards extended to the medical arena, as well. In the foundational legal case, the US Supreme Court determined that "parents have the right to make martyrs of themselves, but they don't have the right under the same circumstances to make martyrs of their children" (*Prince v. Massachusetts*, 1944).

While the *Prince* case had nothing to do with health care—it involved a minor disseminating religious literature—the court decision has been viewed as limiting the right of parents to refuse beneficial treatment for their children. Obviously, this depends on one's interpretation of what constitutes "beneficial treatment." Generally speaking, parents are granted greater latitude with regard to preventive health care (such as immunizations), but are not permitted to refuse treatment if that will lead to significant harm to the child (p. 286).

At approximately the same time, children began to be allowed to make some of their own medical decisions. The reason was not because their parents were making the "wrong" decisions for them but rather because the parents might simply be unavailable to give permission for high-benefit/low-risk interventions. Why, for example, deprive a sixteen-year-old of the opportunity to be evaluated for strep throat simply because her parents could not accompany her to her appointment?

Gradually the right of a minor to make her own medical decisions was broadened to encompass situations where the parent might be available to participate but could pose an obstacle to the minor getting the treatment that she needed. For example, a minor might be less likely to seek out contraception if her parents needed to approve it.

This shift was prompted by the increased availability of contraception in the 1960s and the legalization of abortion in the 1970s. The reasoning went along these lines: if a minor was "mature" enough to have sexual intercourse, then she should be able to prevent pregnancy that might result from it, or make decisions related to pregnancy if it occurred. Each state developed so-called "minor treatment statutes" that empowered patients under the age of majority to consent to treatment of sexually transmitted infections, addiction to drugs or alcohol, and mental illness.

States also recognized the right of "emancipated minors" to make all of their medical decisions. Individual statutes vary, with pregnancy, parenthood, marriage, and active military service common reasons for a minor's formal emancipation. Absent these automatic qualifications, a minor can also petition the court to become emancipated if she meets certain criteria, often involving a minimum age (such as sixteen), either enrollment in high school or having passed the General Educational Development test, living independently and being self-supporting, and not being in the custody of the child protection or corrections system (State of Vermont, 2009).

The age of majority also decreased during this period, following the passage of the 26th Amendment—which gave eighteen-year-olds the right to vote—in 1971. Prior to that the age of majority had been twenty-one, but a person mature enough to vote was felt to have the right to make other major life decisions, as well. At present forty states set the age of majority at eighteen, with another seven permitting this designation to include persons younger than that as long as they have finished high school. Only three states explicitly set the age of majority higher than that: Delaware and Nebraska at nineteen, and Mississippi at twenty-one (Coleman & Rosoff, 2013).

But what about medical decisions not covered under the minor treatment statutes? The prevailing Supreme Court decision leaves little room for unemancipated "mature minors" to make other decisions. Exploring whether parents have the right to commit their child to a mental institution, the Court declared that "the law's concept of the family rests on a presumption that parents possess what a child lacks in maturity, experience, and capacity for judgment required for making life's difficult decisions" (*Parham v. J.R.*, 1979). The Court's conclusion was blunt: "Most children, even in adolescence, simply are not able to make sound judgments concerning many decisions, including their need for medical care or treatment. Parents can and must make those judgments."

Several state court decisions, however, have affirmed the right of mature minors to make their own medical decisions.[1] The Illinois Supreme Court heard the case of Ernestine Gregory, a 17½-year-old who was refusing blood transfusions for leukemia based on her Jehovah's Witness faith. With transfusions, she was given a 20% to 25% five-year survival, but without transfusions she would likely die within one month. The Court concluded that the age of majority "is not an impenetrable barrier that magically precludes a minor from possessing and exercising certain rights normally associated with adulthood" (*In re E.G.*, 1989). Likely influenced by the fact that Ernestine would reach the age of majority in a matter of months—at which point she would clearly have the right to make all of her own medical decisions—the court endorsed her right to refuse transfusions, which she exercised. She died soon thereafter.

Other state-level decisions have also recognized mature minor doctrine and directed physicians to get input from a minor patient (*Belcher v. Charlestown Medical Center*, 1992). One state court, for instance, explicitly applied what is known as the "rule of sevens," whereby children under seven are thought to definitively lack decision DMC;

---

1.   It is important to recognize that state-level decisions have limited scope. Even a state supreme court decision establishes clear legal precedent only in that individual state.

between seven and fourteen, to have the rebuttable presumption of lacking DMC; and between fourteen and twenty-one, to have the rebuttable presumption of possessing it (*Cardwell v. Bechtol,* 1987).

Approximately one-third of states have developed a specific "mature minor exception," allowing minors who are not emancipated and do not fall under the minor treatment statutes to make their own medical decisions. Three states (Alaska, Delaware, and Louisiana) confer broad authority on minors to consent to treatments if their parents are unavailable or unwilling to do so. Eight states either set specific age requirements (ranging from fourteen to sixteen years of age) or require confirmation of sufficient DMC for consenting to medical treatment. The remaining six states either use some combination of the aforementioned requirements, specify that the mature minor must be a high school graduate, or identify very specific requirements—such as in Maine, which takes into account a minor's prior statements about being maintained in a persistent vegetative state (*In re Chad Swan,* 1990)—for a minor to determine her own course of treatment. It is crucial to note that these mature minor laws generally empower minors to *consent* to treatment rather than to refuse it (Coleman & Rosoff, 2013).

During this period clinical studies were being published (p. 340) which purported to show that a late adolescent's DMC was essentially equivalent to that of an adult.[2] International statements also attested to the right of some minors to make their own decisions. For instance, the UN Convention on the Rights of the Child mandated recognition of the "evolving capacities" of minors and expected signees to grant them decision-making rights (United Nations, 1990). While the United States (along with only Somalia and South Sudan) has not ratified the Convention—ostensibly out of concerns that parental authority in areas like home schooling could be questioned—the degree of respect accorded to minors making their own medical decisions continued to grow.

Some adolescents gained national recognition for their refusal of life-sustaining medical treatment (LSMT). One was Billy Best, who as a sixteen-year-old in 1994 was diagnosed with leukemia. After two months of chemotherapy, he refused any additional treatment. His parents disagreed, so he ran away from home to put his life "in God's hands." He later wrote a memoir defending his decision (Best, 2012), and at the time of this writing is still alive. It is impossible to know whether the conventional chemotherapy he did receive—which fell short of the standard protocol—was nevertheless effective, or whether the alternative therapies he sought out ultimately cured his cancer.

Another patient was Abraham Cherrix, who underwent conventional treatment for Hodgkins Lymphoma at age fifteen but when it recurred, one year later in 2006, opted—with his parents' support—to pursue herbal therapy. His parents were charged

2. *Adolescence* has been defined in various ways, with a starting age ranging from ten (World Health Organization, 2016) to thirteen (Psychology Today, 2017) and ending either at nineteen (World Health Organization, 2016) or "the age of majority" (Merriam-Webster Inc., 2003), which varies from state to state. For the sake of consistency—and recognizing the changing legal rights of patient upon reaching the age of majority, which in the United States is usually eighteen—in this chapter "adolescent" refers to a patient between the ages of thirteen and seventeen.

with medical neglect and eventually reached a settlement whereby he received reportedly low-dose chemotherapy from an oncologist with an interest in naturalistic medicine. He, too, survived.

Responding to this case, the state of Virginia passed "Abraham's Law," which permits parents to refuse medical treatment or choose alternative treatments for children aged fourteen to seventeen with a life-threatening medical condition. The law requires the teenager to be mature, both the parents and the patient to have considered the treatment options available to them, and parents and patient to agree that their choice is in the child's best interest. Ironically, had this law been passed law prior to Abraham's diagnosis, his parents would have been permitted to refuse initial therapy on his behalf and he likely would have died (Mercurio, 2007).

A third famous case involved Daniel Hauser, who suffered from the same disease as Abraham Cherrix. A major difference was that Daniel was only thirteen in 2009 when, after one round of chemotherapy, he refused further treatment. According to the judge Daniel possessed only a "rudimentary understanding at best of the risks and benefits of chemotherapy . . . he does not believe he is ill currently" (Associated Press, 2009b). He was ordered to receive chemotherapy and eventually achieved remission (Associated Press, 2009a).

Billy Best's and Abraham Cherrix's refusal of treatment relied on the claim that an adolescent's DMC is equivalent to that of an adult. This is a two-edged sword, though, for while it might lead to greater autonomy in the medical realm, it also leads to greater culpability in the legal realm. If adolescents are "mature" enough to decide whether to accept LSMT—as asserted in *In re: E.G.* and Abraham's Law—they should also be mature enough to know right from wrong and justifiably be held responsible when they do not. Applying this line of reasoning, the Supreme Court upheld state laws permitting capital punishment for crimes committed as young as sixteen (*Stanford v. Kentucky*, 1989).

At the beginning of the twenty-first century, the pendulum began to swing back in the other direction. The courts increasingly recognized the broad-ranging criminal implications of crediting minors with full-fledged DMC. Could someone who was not even old enough to vote truly appreciate the gravity of her actions, sufficient to justify being executed? This reevaluation coincided with clinical studies (described below) which found that adolescents' DMC can be significantly impaired, especially in highly emotionally, time-pressured situations. The US Supreme Court thus reversed the *Stanford v. Kentucky* decision, holding that capital punishment for crimes committed before age eighteen violated the Eighth Amendment's ban on "cruel and unusual punishment" (*Roper v. Simmons*, 2005). Five years later it also declared unconstitutional a sentence of life without parole for crimes committed at a similarly young age (*Graham v. Florida*, 2010).

Clinical

After long granting minors precious little role in their health care, the last quarter of the twentieth century was marked by great optimism regarding the DMC of adolescents.

Cognitive studies involving hypothetical complex decision-making suggested that mid-adolescents were just as capable of making decisions as adults (McCabe, 1996; Weithorn & Campbell, 1982). Researchers opined that after a "transition period" between the ages of eleven and fourteen, "many minors attain the cognitive developmental stage associated with the psychological elements of rational consent" (Leikin, 1993). Others claimed that there "is little evidence that minors of age fifteen and above as a group are any less competent to provide consent than are adults" (Grisso & Vierling, 1978). Based on these studies Weir and Peters concluded, "The presumption on the part of physicians . . . should be that *all* adolescent patients between 14 and 17 have the capacity to make health care decisions, including end-of-life decisions, *except* when individual patients demonstrate that they do not have the necessary DMC" (Weir & Peters, 1997).

This two-edged sword of autonomy granted to mature minors led to human rights concerns about severe sentences meted out for crimes committed prior to the age of majority. Gradually these concerns acquired empirical support from the cognitive psychology community, which delved deeper into the question of adolescent decision-making in complex situations. By paying additional attention to the pressure-filled context in which these decisions are often made, differences between adolescent and adult decision-making became clearer.

Rather than culminating in mid-adolescence, brain development was recognized as an ongoing process through adolescence and into early adulthood. Early adolescence was notable for the greatest dopaminergic activity in pathways connecting the limbic system (associated with emotions and impulsivity) and the prefrontal cortex (which is the center of more rational thought) (Dahl & Gunnar, 2009; Steinberg, 2010). These connections produce an "emotional reward" for decisions that may not be entirely rational, offering a neurological explanation for long-recognized behaviors of adolescence: impulsivity, sensation-seeking, decreased future orientation, and susceptibility to peer pressure. It also explains why adolescents generally do better with hypothetical situations ("If this were to happen to me . . .") than with actually making decisions about real-life situations (Steinberg, 2005).

This is not meant to suggest that the earlier studies were incorrect. Adolescence is certainly a time of evolving maturity (Cauffman & Steinberg, 2000) when patients are able to process information in an increasingly rational way. The locus of emotional decision-making develops, however, at a faster rate (Figure 13.1).

Brain maturation does not arbitrarily end at the age of majority. Dynamic changes in gray matter volume and myelination continue into the third decade of life (Giedd, 2008; Giedd et al., 1999; Sowell, Thompson, Holmes, Jernigan, & Toga, 1999; Sowell, Thompson, Tessner, & Toga, 2001). This, in turn, prompts more "mature" decision-making. It also provides a neurological explanation for the famous observation attributed to Mark Twain: "When I was a boy of 14, my father was so ignorant I could hardly stand to have the old man around. But when I got to be 21, I was astonished at how much the old man had learned in seven years" (Rasmussen, 1998).

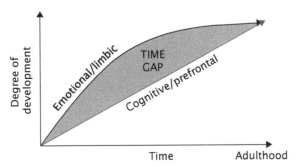

FIGURE 13.1 Dual process model of adolescent brain development

The significance of the "dual-process model" is that adolescents have the ability to understand the facts of a situation, but often decide based on more socioemotional considerations (Diekema, 2011; Silber, 2011). An example would be resisting chemotherapy because of associated hair loss, or refusing limb amputation for bone cancer because of the resultant inability to participate in sports. As Casey, Jones, and Somerville, 2011) observe: "In emotionally salient situations, subcortical systems will win out (accelerator) over control systems (brakes) given their maturity relative to the prefrontal control systems."

This raises the question of how to address complex medical decisions during the "time gap" in the dual process model of brain development (Steinberg, 2005). During this period, adolescents can understand—and likely also be able to apply—relevant information, but the problem arises with the third requirement for DMC (p. 56): the ability to *reason* about the choices in terms of personal goals and values (Appelbaum, Grisso, Frank, O'Donnell, & Kupfer, 1999; President's Commission for the Study of Ethical Problems in Medicine and Biomedical and Behavioral Research, 1982). Such reasoning can be significantly impacted by the strong emotional overlay.

Informed consent not only requires sufficient DMC but also that the decision be reached voluntarily. This is also in question for adolescents because of the influence of the family unit. Even if a patient understands and appreciates the information provided—and is able to manipulate it rationally—she must still have the freedom to make her own voluntary choice in order to be able to give true informed consent. Given the naturally intertwined nature of many families, it may be difficult for an adolescent to separate her own values from her parents'. While in some cases it may lead an adolescent to disagree with her parents' view simply because it is her parents' view, more often in medical situations the adolescent may be unduly positively influenced by the parents' views. This is particularly true with regard to religious or cultural views which may lead to a rejection of allopathic medical care (Scherer & Reppuci, 1988).

It seems clear, then, that adolescents have the ability to make medical decisions in some situations but not all (Canadian Pediatric Society Bioethics Committee, 2004; Levy,

Larcher, & Kurz, 2003; Larcher & Hutchinson, 2010; Michaud, Berg-Kelly, & Macfarlane, 2010). Professional statements provide little concrete guidance, however, in determining what those specific decisions and situations are. The American Academy of Pediatrics (AAP; 2016), for instance, distinguishes between very broad categories. On the one hand is life-saving treatment (such as appendectomy for appendicitis) which "adolescents should not be allowed to refuse." On the other hand, where the prognosis is poor—or the interventions burdensome or unproven—"more consideration should be given by the physician to advocating for the cognitively mature teenager who wants to refuse treatment."

Ethical

Disclosure

One of the most challenging ethical situations encountered in pediatric palliative care is when a sick child's parents ask the medical team not to reveal to her how sick she is, or the likely outcome of the disease. While protective requests for nondisclosure also occur in the adult medical world (p. 478), there is additional complexity in the pediatric realm (Kunin, 1997; Whitney et al., 2006). It is not difficult to understand the parents' desire to protect their child from the additional burden of worry, as well as to nurture hope (Bartholome, 1981; Berger, 2005; Vernick & Karon, 1965). Addressing the issue directly also brings the reality of impending death into the parent's consciousness. As Wolfe (2004) notes, "In telling the child, do we not have to truly hear it ourselves?"

Studies have shown that staff often accede to requests for non-disclosure (Clarke, Davies, Jenney, Glaser, & Eiser, 2005; Clemente 2007), often so as to not create conflict with the parents (Evan & Cohen, 2011). This can, in turn, cause moral distress (p. 514) because the staff do not feel like they can adequately support the child as she explores the reasons why she feels the way she does, and what this might mean going forward (Lee & Dupree, 2008). Being excluded from important discussions can also lead the patient to feel isolated (Faulkner, 1997; Whittam, 1993).

In the past, non-disclosure was the standard of practice. This is reflected in the title of Bluebond-Langner's (1978) groundbreaking work, *The Private Worlds of Dying Children*. The pediatric cancer patients she studied suffered in silence, provided with precious little information about their disease or prognosis. Remarkably, though, every one of those children was aware of their diagnosis, despite the attempts of their families to shield them.

This, in turn, led to "mutual pretense": an unspoken agreement among all participants to act as if the child was not aware. Children played along because that is what they were expected to do and to spare their parents what they knew would be a painful conversation. Parents elected not to explore their suspicion that their children might know more than they were letting on. This made it impossible for parents and children to have open conversations about illness and death.

This is particularly significant because of the potential benefit of such conversations. In a subsequent landmark study, Kreicbergs, Valdimarsdóttir, Onelöv, Henter, and Steineck (2004) interviewed parents after their children had died, specifically asking if they had discussed illness and death in advance. Over half of the parents had not done so, even though the majority of these parents sensed their child had some awareness of their impending death. None of the parents who discussed death with their children later regretted doing so, but over one-quarter of the other parents regretted *not* doing so. Parents who did not speak to their children about death were also more likely to suffer from anxiety at follow-up.

So how should one handle a request from parents for non-disclosure? The first step is to explore the parents' reasons for making the request in the first place. They may want to wait for a particular time in order to tell the child, such as allowing her to have "one more birthday" or school graduation without the burden of the knowledge of the extent of her illness. They may be concerned about what exactly the medical team will tell their child, fearing it may destroy the fragile hope they and their child have for recovery. They may also feel that the child should take the lead in such conversations, interpreting the lack of direct questions on the child's part as representing a desire "not to know."

Each of these positions calls for a specific response. The first might prompt exploration of what time would be better to tell the child, recognizing that for many parents there is no "good time" to break such difficult news. The second might be to paraphrase what information the medical team feels is most important, and then to invite the parents to take part in the conversation too. The team could also share evidence that candidness regarding prognosis does not damage hope, but rather may deepen it (Mack et al., 2007). They might also raise the possibility of regret if parents do not openly discuss the future with their child (Kreicbergs et al., 2004).

Addressing the concern that the patient may not "want to know," the team might wonder aloud if she already does. Information is often gleaned through overheard comments or direct intuition. Identifying subtle ways the child may have already communicated that—such as through gestures or artistic expression—may help the parents recognize this (Bluebond-Langner, 1978; Spinetta, 1974). This could lead the team and parents to brainstorm ways to open the door for conversation, should the child wish to walk through it.

Even if the child does not already know, the practical question of how long that information can be kept "secret" needs to be raised. However difficult it would be for the child to hear that news from a loving parent, it would be far worse to learn of it inadvertently. What a child ends up imagining may be even worse than the actual medical situation (Clarke et al., 2005; Vernick & Karon, 1965), leading to further increase in anxiety (Claflin & Barbarin, 1991; Slavin, O'Malley, Koocher, & Foster, 1982). Candor now generally leads to better adjustment later (Clarke et al., 2005) and may also help with adherence to a treatment regimen once the child understands the necessity of it (Bartholome, 1993).

In some cases parents themselves may not fully appreciate the seriousness of their child's condition. Studies have shown that parents sometimes come to recognize that their child is dying *months* after the medical team has (Wolfe et al., 2000). Of course, this may be because the parents weren't informed of the prognosis, given the emotional challenges involved in doing so. More likely, however, is that they were informed—at least on some level—but were unable to process the information or accept the implications of it. Their reluctance to bring their child into the conversation thus provides an opportunity to enhance the parents' own understanding of the medical situation, which may help them recognize the need for full disclosure.

In some situations, these steps can help bring the parents to a point where they are willing to speak candidly with their child, or at least permit the team to do so. The age of the child is relevant, as studies have shown that parents are more likely to speak to older children about upcoming death (Kreicbergs et al., 2004), reasonably concluding the child is better able to handle the news and may have further questions about it.

The fact that older children will play a more integral role in treatment decisions is not the only reason to disclose diagnosis and prognosis to a child (Cole & Kodish, 2013). Younger children can still grasp the impact of a serious illness, if only in terms of its immediate implications (e.g., inability to go to school, need to stay away from friends who may be sick, etc.). To reduce the obligation of disclosure to one of practicality—in terms of decision-making and adherence to therapy—overlooks the overall well-being of the child, her ability to process information, and her right to it.

But what of situations when parents remain steadfast in their position that the child not be told? There are many valuable sources of guidance for how to communicate with dying children (Beale, Baile, & Aaron, 2005), but far fewer that specifically address this dilemma. An important factor to take into consideration is the imperativeness of the potential disclosure. In some situations, the child's opinion about what is most important in life plays an integral role in larger treatment decisions, some of which may be time-sensitive. In those situations, there is more pressure to decide sooner about whether the child should be informed.

Where decisions are not pressing, the parents may reasonably be afforded more time for reflection and discussion. In the meantime, certain fundamental rules should be identified, including never lying to a child (or any patient, for that matter). It is one thing to not proactively disclose a diagnosis and another to decline to answer a direct question related to it. But it is an entirely different thing to knowingly speak an untruth, especially telling a child who is dying that she is not. Such an action undermines trust, devalues the patient as a person, and is never acceptable.

It is also important to acknowledge the possibility that the child really does not know and does not *want* to know (Leydon et al., 2000). Just as one would with an adult patient, it is reasonable to preface any disclosure with an open-ended question about what the patient is worried and curious about, and how much she wants to know about her illness. In some cases this can be accomplished more effectively without the parents present, so the child does not have to be so concerned about protecting them too.

Even if the child comes right out and asks, "Am I dying?," it may not be entirely clear that she wants to know everything about her illness. In many cases the wisest course of action is to answer a question with another question, as in, "What makes you ask that?" or "What's worrying you?" The child may, in fact, be asking if her increase in symptomatology is a bad sign or if it is treatable, which if nothing else is a clue to the treating team that additional symptomatic treatment is necessary. By asking for more details, the team can better understand what terminology and framework the child is using, in order to answer in a way that is most appropriate and understandable to her.

Ultimately, there may come a time when all attempts at clarification and persuasion have failed, and the child is felt to be suffering from apparently not knowing her diagnosis and prognosis. (It is quite possible that she does know about it but does not feel free to discuss it.) In such situations, it is crucial to recall that for all the family-centeredness of pediatrics, ultimately the child is the patient (AAP, 2012). In situations where the patient—regardless of age—may wish to be informed and her values impact decision-making, disclosure should be considered a professional obligations which protects the interests of the child-patient (Goldberg & Frader, 2008). This is reflected in the AAP's (2016) recent shift from a focus on parental "autonomy" to parental "responsibility."

There may, therefore, be instances when the child's need to know trumps the parents' request for non-disclosure (Goldberg & Frader, 2008; Masera et al., 1999; Hilden, Watterson, & Chrastek, 2000; Himelstein, Hilden, Morstad Boldt, & Weissman, 2004). In those situations, the team should inform the parents of the fact that they have reached that conclusion, as well as the implications of it. Additional services—such as ethics consultation, expanded psychosocial support, and spiritual care—could be utilized to help mediate any potential conflict, time permitting. The parents should also be given the opportunity to influence the context of the disclosure, such as being present (or not).

From a procedural standpoint, it may be helpful to establish clear institutional guidelines affirming the right of children to understand their prognosis (Nitschke et al., 2000). This may pave the way for early discussion of likely outcomes and fuller integration of palliative and potentially-curative therapies (Goldman & Heller, 2000).

Case, Continued

The team explores with the parents their reasons for not wanting to tell their daughter about her diagnosis, which include a desire to protect her and to nurture hope. After thoughtful listening, the team informs the parents that disclosure can actually promote hope, and withholding information can exacerbate anxiety. When asked, they provide data to support these claims, and mention the "mutual pretense" that often surrounds family relationships when children are not told of their diagnosis.

When informed of these, the parents express uncertainty as to whether their daughter might already understand what is going on, given a relative who recently underwent chemotherapy. The team offers to speak with the patient with the parents present and promises to let the child direct the conversation.

In that conversation, it quickly becomes clear that the patient realizes that her diagnosis is serious, and she asks appropriate questions. However, when informed of the side effects of chemotherapy—such as hair loss and nausea—she responds very negatively.

"I'll never do that!" she yells.

Upon leaving her room, the parents ask the team, "So what do we do now?"

Refusal of Medical Treatment

As noted earlier (p. 285), the standard for pediatric decision-making is the permission of the parents and the assent of the child. Rather than *consent*—which implies the ability to comprehend and rationally manipulate information—assent refers to voluntarily agreeing to something that one has a basic understanding of. Instead of expecting a pre-pubescent child to weigh the risks, benefits, and alternatives of chemotherapy, for example, it is much more appropriate to inform the child that she has an illness and this is the medicine for that illness and will (hopefully) make her better.

Assent can be viewed on a spectrum, with the youngest children unable to participate in any meaningful way in medical decision-making, but as they reach school age becoming able to grasp on some level what is being done to them. While not having the ability to consent to treatment, children in this age group still deserve age-appropriate explanations and the right to exert some manner of control of their own bodies. Eventually their DMC will mature to the point where they are able to give true informed consent (or refusal).

In some cases, the benefit/burden ratio of a specific treatment is so overwhelmingly positive that the child is not permitted to decline it. In those situations, it is important to remember core values of pediatrics including "never lie to a child" and also "don't ask a question if you're not going to respect the answer." Therefore, if it is determined that treatment is obligatory, it makes little sense—and can be extremely counterproductive—to ask the child if she is willing to accept that treatment, since a refusal would be overridden. It is far better to explain the reason for that treatment and to offer the child legitimate control over those aspects of her care that she does have the authority to accept, refuse, or dictate, such as the timing of the treatment, who is present during it, what prize she receives following it, and so on. The more discretionary a treatment becomes, however, the more relevant the child's perspective about it is (AAP, 2016).

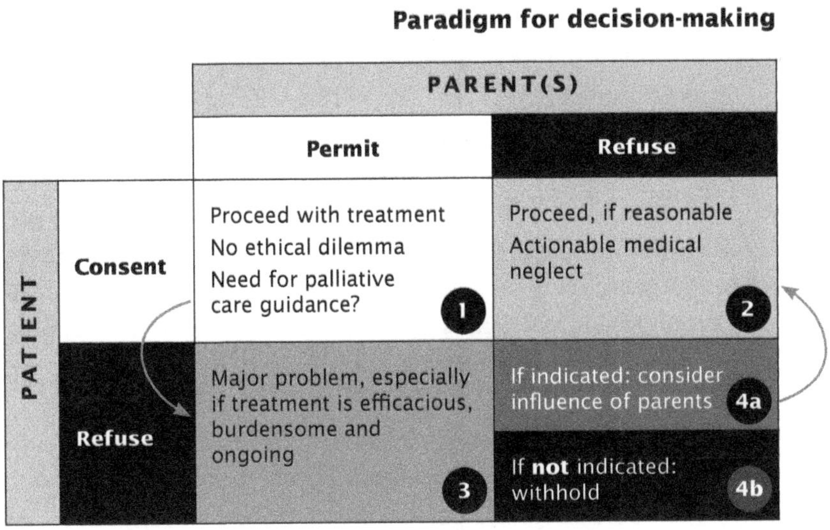

Paradigm for decision-making

FIGURE 13.2 Paradigm for adolescent decision-making, based on whether the patient or parents agree to or refuse treatment

It is also important to consider the imperativeness of the treatment, for even some treatments that are "necessary" can be deferred until such a point as the child is willing to offer her assent. Doing so makes the treatment much less burdensome and also may increase adherence, by virtue of the child's basic understanding and willingness to proceed (Waller, 2001).

Adolescence is an "in-between" state: no longer a child but not quite an adult. An adolescent's cognitive capacity rivals an adult's but is often incompletely utilized in stressful situations and outweighed by a disproportionately strong limbic system that leads to impetuous decisions. Perhaps nowhere else in the practice of medicine is the balance of respect for autonomy and duty of beneficence so tenuous, especially when the legal decision-maker remains the parent.

Given this significant complexity, it is helpful to break down the question of adolescent refusal of treatment into its component parts. Assuming that both the parent(s) and the patient have opinions about potential treatment for a life-threatening disease,[3] there are four basic possibilities (Figure 13.2).

Both Parents and Child Say Yes

Quadrant 1 in Figure 13.2 represents the informed permission of the parents and the assent/consent (depending on developmental stage) of the minor patient. There may need to be thoughtful conversations and perhaps formal palliative care consultation

---

3. If only the parents do—and the adolescent is unable or unwilling to participate in decision-making—then the process would proceed as it would for a younger child. The parents would be tasked with making a decision in the child's best interests, with the state potentially intervening if that decision violates the harm principle.

to ensure the patient and family grasp the benefits and burdens of the treatment. But assuming the treatment in question has been offered by the medical team—and is not a request for inappropriate treatment that has not been offered (chapter 14)—it is hard to imagine the team not providing the treatment.

The only caveat has to do with voluntariness. If the adolescent is merely agreeing because her parents are in favor, this may not represent true concurrence. A classic example of this is the adolescent who realizes that her life is coming to an end but whose parents cannot accept this and continue to advocate for maximal treatment. A person can certainly voluntarily choose to do something she would not otherwise do in order to make someone else happy, but it is important to verify that coercion is not involved.

If it is determined that the adolescent would actually refuse the intervention, then this shifts the conversation to Quadrant 3 (indicated by the arrow on the left) which will be discussed later. This possibility highlights the need to empower the patient to speak for herself and also to engage the parents in a thoughtful discussion of what the child really wants, especially as it may differ from what they want for her.

Parents Say No, Child Says Yes

Quadrant 2 represents the assent/consent of the patient and the refusal of the parents, which would seem to be the least common of the four possibilities. The adolescent is more likely to refuse burdensome treatment for emotional ("limbic") reasons, and as noted the parental instinct toward saving their child's life is incredibly strong. In rare cases where the treatment is deemed to be in the child's best interest, this could represent actionable medical neglect and social services would need to be involved.

The significance of this step should not be underestimated. For even if the parents are not acting in the best interests of the child, they may still be the primary source of support and guidance for that child. The emotional harm done by separating the parents from the child—even if only temporarily, in order to administer the treatment—could be significant. Proceeding with compulsory treatment thus requires significant sensitivity and care (Macauley & Fritzler, 2014).

Parents Say Yes, Child Says No

Quadrant 3 represents the refusal of the patient of a treatment which the parents favor. Admittedly, in some cases the parents might "officially" support the child's refusal in order to maintain relationship with her. An example of this is the case of Billy Best.

The first step in such a situation is to identify the reasons for the patient's refusal, which may include an insufficient appreciation of the risk to her health, a prioritizing of temporal concerns (e.g., keeping her hair) over long-term goals, simple rebellion, or the need to control at least one aspect of her life. Whatever reasons are identified can be addressed through clarification, ongoing discussion, and mediation.

In these discussions it is important to not become wedded to the clinically optimal treatment regimen, as there are important considerations that go beyond somatic benefit. A slightly suboptimal regimen that the patient is willing to accept could in an overall sense be superior to the "standard of care." This approach takes into consideration the burden of imposing treatment on an unwilling patient, as well as the possibility that the patient may not receive *any* treatment if the only option is unpalatable, choosing instead to flee as Billy Best did.

When persuasion and compromise are unsuccessful, two options remain. One is respect for the patient's refusal, which obviously deprives the patient of treatment that could have saved her life. The only other option is parentalism in the form of compulsory treatment. The latter is an unpleasant term, conjuring images of overridden autonomy. But it is accurate in describing the not uncommon response to an adolescent's refusal of treatment (Duncan & Sawyer, 2010).

In deciding which course to pursue, several factors need to be taken into consideration. One is the burdens and benefits of the proposed treatment, with treatable conditions more likely to require compulsory treatment. Indeed, the reason that the cases of Abraham Cherrix and Billy Best are so well known is that they involved cancers with favorable treatment outcomes.

On the other hand, it would be difficult to compel a patient to receive a treatment that entails significant burden and is still unlikely to save her life. In these cases, some adolescents may make an informed choice to defer those aggressive interventions and focus exclusively on palliative care. The AAP (2016) thus recommends additional consideration should be given to "[upholding] an adolescent's assent or refusal for further attempts at curative treatments."

Another relevant factor is the adolescent's burgeoning autonomy, which impacts the "rationality" of her reasons for refusal. A thirteen-year-old like Daniel Hauser—who is concerned about time-limited symptoms after one round of chemotherapy—is a much different patient than an almost-eighteen-year-old, like Ernestine Gregory, who expresses deeply held beliefs which conflict with recommended treatment.

Specifically, the ability of the patient to project into the future—the precise task that is often relatively deficient in the dual process model—is taken into consideration, as is the patient's prior "lived experience with illness." Many patients who have experienced chronic illness and have previously undergone burdensome treatment possess a unique insight into the implications of their illness and the proposed treatments (Diekema, 2011).

The purpose of this nuanced assessment of the degree of DMC is to distinguish between hard and soft paternalism. As noted (p. 125), the former involves overriding the treatment refusal of a patient with intact DMC—and thus is never acceptable—while the latter pertains to a patient with compromised DMC. Soft paternalism, therefore, is only relevant to high-benefit/low-burden decisions which a reasonable person would generally accept. It is not solely applied to adolescents, but the fact that the patient is an adolescent is relevant because this is the basis for concern about diminished DMC in light of recent neurodevelopmental findings.

Another factor is the patient's age and how that relates to the treatment course. Ernestine Gregory, for instance, was only a few months away from her eighteenth birthday. This does not automatically mean that she had full DMC, since there is no "magic age" when this develops. It simply means that from a legal standpoint, she would soon have the authority to refuse treatment (including for religious reasons, as *Prince v. Massachusetts* made abundantly clear). Since her refusal grew out of her deep faith, there was every reason to believe that she would continue to refuse treatment once she had the indisputable legal right to do so. Whatever treatment is being proposed, therefore, should have a high probability of efficacy prior to the patient attaining the age of majority.

If the adolescent's DMC is significantly compromised—and the treatment has a favorable benefit/burden ratio and is likely to achieve its therapeutic goal before the patient reaches the age of majority—then this represents one of the rare situations where a patient's articulated refusal should be overridden. This is primarily based on the principle of beneficence, whereby the patient is protected from herself.

Rather than viewing this as a violation of the patient's autonomy, it is possible to frame it as respecting that very autonomy. The fact that the patient's DMC is compromised means that she is not able to act (fully) autonomously. Some have therefore argued that compulsory treatment protects *future* autonomy, which she would not be able to exercise if her current refusal were respected (Diekema, 2011). Ross (1998) writes, "[A] competent child's short-term autonomy can be morally overridden to promote his lifetime autonomy because of his potential to improve his decision-making skills and broaden his background knowledge."

This is a reasonable ethical position, but clinical ethics also has to be practical. As is evident from the experiences of both Billy Best and Abraham Cherrix, even if the courts mandate treatment, an adolescent may choose not to comply. This may require modifying the "gold standard" treatment to one that is shorter in duration and incurs fewer symptoms, engaging the support of the parents, and articulating a very clear and consistent treatment plan. While it may feel "unprofessional" to some clinicians to advocate for a treatment plan with a lower chance of cure, this may nevertheless be the best available practical option. As such, it may ultimately have a greater chance of leading to a good outcome than demanding the "standard of care."

Both Parents and Child Say No

Quadrant 4 is perhaps the most challenging type of dilemma, with both the patient and the parent(s) opposed to treatment. As in Quadrant 1—where the two parties also appear to agree, only in the other direction—it is important to confirm whether this represents the adolescent patient's true wishes. Is the patient refusing for fear of angering or alienating her parents? If based on a cultural or religious perspective, is the adolescent sufficiently mature to consciously adopt those values for herself, or is she merely emulating the way of life that she is most familiar with? If it is determined that the patient would want to be treated were it not for the influence of her parents (i.e., Quadrant 4a), the dilemma becomes more akin to Quadrant 2 (Figure 13.2, arrow on the right), which was discussed earlier.

But what if the patient is voluntarily refusing and is supported by her parents (i.e., Quadrant 4b)? This is precisely the case with Ernestine Gregory, as well as the more recent case of Abraham Cherrix. There still exists a presumption in favor of treatment with a positive balance of benefits and burdens. As the AAP (2016) observes: "*In general,* adolescents should not be allowed to refuse life-saving treatment even when parents agree with the child" (emphasis added). But the fact that both the patient and her parents are opposed is relevant, and in some cases is sufficient to justify forgoing LSMT.

This in large part depends on whether the treatment could reasonably be refused. Adults with sufficient DMC are, after all, permitted to refuse potentially LSMT. Parents may do the same on behalf of their child if that does not violate the harm principle (p. 286). The same considerations for any parental decision—including the relative balance of benefits and burdens of the treatment, and the increased latitude granted to parents as decision-makers—also apply here.

If parents could ethically forgo a given treatment, then the team would be honoring the refusal of the most uncontroversial decision-maker. The fact that the patient is also refusing would both confirm and strengthen the parents' decision, given the practical obstacles that any compulsory treatment faces.

But what if refusal of treatment is felt to represent potential harm to the child? The same steps recommended for responding to an adolescent's isolated refusal (i.e., Quadrant 3) are relevant here, except they would be applied to both the patient and her parents: exploring the reasons for the refusal, attempting persuasion, and evaluating a moderated course of therapy that the family is willing to accept.

Should the patient and family remain steadfast in their refusal, this creates one of the most complex questions in pediatric ethics. However difficult it was to compel treatment on an unwilling adolescent with the support of her parents, it is much more difficult when the parents are also opposed to treatment.

In exploring the ethical and practical aspects of potential compulsory treatment, it may be helpful to take a casuistical approach (p. 41). The paradigmatic case for overriding a parent's refusal of treatment on behalf of their child is the infant of Jehovah's Witnesses who experiences a serious hemorrhage, perhaps related to trauma (Penson & Amrein, 2004). In such a case, legal precedent is clear (*Prince v. Massachusetts,* 1944), as is the right course of action: override the parents' refusal.

Several aspects of this case are ethically relevant. One is that the patient clearly lacks DMC and is thus not a participant in the decision. The treatment in question is low-risk[4] and only required once, and then over a very short period of time. In this

---

4. At least from a somatic point of view. From a spiritual point of view, a Witness would deem the burdens of blood transfusion—being "disfellowshipped" in this life and not resurrected into the next—to be extreme (Barker, 2000).

	Infant child of Jehovah's Witnesses who is hemorrhaging	Teenager with cancer
DMC	Absent	Evolving
Chance of survival <u>without</u> optimal treatment	0%	20%
Chance of survival <u>with</u> optimal treatment	100%	50%
Risk/burdens of treatment	Minimal	Significant
Duration of treatment	Hours	Months or longer

FIGURE 13.3 Relevant ethical factors for considering overriding refusal of treatment for a minor

hypothetical situation, let us assume that transfusion is necessary for—and essentially guarantees—survival.

All of these factors change when the patient is an adolescent joining her parents in refusing LSMT. Unlike the infant, an adolescent has evolving DMC, as well as her own set of values and beliefs. Treatment—especially for cancer (which all the patients in the relevant legal cases suffered from)—is ongoing, incurs significant burdens, and is not guaranteed to achieve the desired result. Neither is the child certain to die without the treatment, as the examples of Billy Best and Abraham Cherrix attest.

The relevant differences between these two paradigmatic cases are summarized in Figure 13.3, with representative likelihoods of cancer survival.

Applying the methods of casuistry, the more a particular case resembles the infant who is hemorrhaging, the greater the ethical responsibility to intervene. It may not be easy, and the trauma to the family—as well as damage to the physician-patient/parent relationship—may be significant. In such a matter of life and death, however, compulsory treatment is justified.

But as a case more closely approximates the adolescent with cancer, there is no longer an absolute obligation to intervene. When a patient's DMC is significantly greater, the risk/benefit ratio of treatment less clear, and the burdens of treatment—especially if administered over the patient's objections—greater, the ethical balance may tilt in the other direction.

At some point one might conclude that if only from a practical point of view, compulsory treatment (at least with regard to the standard of care) is impossible. Since a basic dictum of ethics is that "ought implies can"—meaning that one cannot say that a person *ought* to do something that they are unable to do (Buckwalter & Turri, 2015)—practical impossibility absolves a person of ethical responsibility.

In some cases where the medical team might deeply wish that the patient receive treatment that would maximize her chance of survival, they may need to reconcile themselves to the impracticality and excessive burden of compulsory treatment, which ultimately might lead to more harm than good. This highlights the importance of fostering trust that might make persuasion possible, as well as the willingness to consider "suboptimal" treatment plans that—if accepted by the patient—are superior to coerced administration of the "standard of care."

Advance Care Planning

The importance of advance care planning (ACP) was noted earlier (p. 70). Most studies of ACP have focused on adults, however. This makes sense because from a strictly legal perspective a patient must have the right to make her own decisions in order to execute a binding advance directive. Unless she is emancipated, an adolescent does not clearly possess the legal right to refuse LSMT. If what she says now is not binding on her current medical care, there is no reason to believe it would be definitive for her future care, should she lose whatever degree of DMC she currently possesses.

It should not come as a surprise, therefore, that much of the literature on pediatric advance care planning (pACP) focuses on *parents* making advance decisions for future eventualities, rather than the patient herself doing so. In a recent study nearly one-third of parents had communicated some advance care guidelines to the medical team, although only 3% had actually created a written advance directive for their child (Liberman, Pham, & Nager, 2014). This reflects understandable parental reluctance to face the possibility their child may become critically ill and ultimately die of her disease.

One might question the value of parental ACP. After all, the purpose of ACP is to allow a patient to express her goals and values, in case at some future point she should lose DMC. When a pediatric patient is critically ill, though, there may not be a need to rely on the parents' ACP since they would presumably still have DMC to make decisions in real time. However, parental ACP crucially allows parents to make decisions in less stressful circumstances, which they usually stick to when anticipated situations present themselves (Hammes, Klevan, Kempf, & Williams, 2005).

The prevailing focus on parental ACP does not mean that adolescents should have no role. Indeed, professional groups recommend that adolescents be involved in end-of-life decision making (AAP, 2000; Field, Behrman, & Institute of Medicine Committee on Palliative and End-of-Life Care for Children and Their Families, 2003; Hinds et al., 2005). This is precisely what adolescents have asked for (Hinds et al., 2005; Lyon, McCabe, Patel, & D'Angelo, 2004; McGrath, 1996), with adolescent cancer survivors indicating that they value the opportunity to decide about—and potentially refuse—specific treatments in advance (Pousset et al., 2009).

The operative question, therefore, is whether an adolescent's advance refusal of treatment would be honored. From a legal standpoint, unemancipated minors have relatively little authority outside the scope of the minor treatment statutes. But from an ethical standpoint, an adolescent has an evolving sense of self which merits respect.

If an adolescent's advance refusal of treatment would be respected, then treatment-directed pACP makes sense just as it does for an adult. Decisions reached in advance may actually be superior to those made in real time, as this bypasses the "dual-process" model of decisional maturation which often leads adolescents to make decisions based on emotional rather than cognitive concerns. Studies have shown that adolescents perform better with hypothetical questions (e.g., "if someone like me was diagnosed with a serious illness. . .") than with direct questions about their own health care, which is more likely to invoke an emotional/limbic response (Steinberg, 2005). pACP also frees adolescents from time pressure, allowing them the opportunity to seek additional counsel and address their own emotional struggles in reaching a conclusion.

By the same token, decisions reached in advance may have less practical impact than those reached in real time. While an adolescent's refusal should be respected if she possesses sufficient DMC, it may also have to be respected if (as noted earlier) compulsory treatment is a logistical impossibility. The very fact of relying on pACP implies that the adolescent is no longer able to participate in decisions (and thus would, at the very least, not be actively resisting treatment). The previous basis for withholding treatment is no longer operative, and thus implementing treatment becomes more practical and less burdensome. This possibility underscores the need to clearly identify the reasons why an adolescent's potential refuse would—or would not—be respected (i.e., legal, ethical, and/or logistical).

But even if advance refusal wouldn't be honored, that does not mean that pACP is not worthwhile. The process of ACP allows patients to express their goals and values, which will influence—although perhaps not determine—the medical treatment they receive. This not only involves treatment decisions but equally profound questions such as how adolescents want to say goodbye and be remembered (Sourkes, 1995). One might say that it carries "moral weight" (Weir & Peters, 1997), even if it is not absolutely binding.

Unfortunately, pACP conversations are not often taking place. Nurses (Feudtner, 2007), doctors (Davies et al., 2008; Morgan & Murphy, 2000), and parents (Steele & Davies, 2006) all report difficulty in engaging in such discussions, for profound emotional reasons. In one study, nearly half of the adolescent subjects with either metastatic cancer or HIV infection hadn't discussed issues such as their goals of care or preferred surrogate with anyone in the previous month (Wiener et al., 2008).

ACP tools may be helpful in fostering such conversations. Some adult tools may be applicable to adolescents, such as "Five Wishes" which allows the patient to answer the following questions:

- Who should make decisions if I can't?
- What kind of treatment do I want?
- How comfortable do I want to be?
- How should people treat me?
- What do I want my loved ones to know? (Wiener et al., 2008)

A newer tool—My Thoughts, My Wishes, My Voice—adapts the Five Wishes approach to younger users, while addressing additional concerns such as spiritual wishes (Wiener et al., 2012). Other pediatric-specific options include Voicing My Choices (Zadeh, Pao, & Wiener, 2015), "child and family wishes" (Kids Health, 2012), and personal resuscitation plans (Wolff, Browne, & Whitehouse, 2011).

One solution to both parental reluctance and adolescent limitation is to engage in facilitated conversations with both the patient and her parents. Even if no written document is produced, the process of communication may foster collaborative and supportive decision making, while also reducing the probability that the family unit is engaging in "mutual pretense." Studies of disease-specific conversations with adolescent and young adult patients and their families have shown significant success in optimizing communication and articulating a clear treatment plan (Lyon et al., 2009).

Return to the Case

The team reassures the parents that the patient's reaction is entirely normal. After giving her some time to process what she has been told, the team invites her to continue the conversation.

"I'm not going to change my mind," she replies, but is also willing to listen.

The team explores the patient's reasons for refusal, which include her having read about "herbal treatments" on the Internet and "just not being able to deal with this right now." Recognizing that she has had no experience with serious illness, they describe the implications of her diagnosis on her present and future life. They also emphasize the importance of her feelings, and that treatment will actually help her achieve her stated goals (which include going to college and becoming a veterinarian).

To give her as much control as possible, they invite her to express her hopes using the My Thoughts, My Wishes, My Voice framework. They do not make any promises they cannot keep, especially involving treatment refusal. Given her prognosis—and in light of her parents' acceptance of treatment—forgoing treatment was never an option.

Over the course of several conversations the patient comes to acknowledge the need for treatment and appreciates the team's sensitive handling of the situation. She begins chemotherapy with significant trepidation but also feeling quite supported.

Summary Points

- For much of human history, children were viewed as their parents' property, with minimal rights of their own.
- Increasing recognition of children's rights occurred in the twentieth century, including granting children the authority to consent to high-benefit/low-risk medical treatments when their parents were not available.

- Medical decision-making authority subsequently expanded under the minor treatment statutes to include contraception, termination of pregnancy, addiction treatment, and mental health care.
- Such expansion was supported by studies which purported to show that a mid-/late adolescent's DMC was essentially equivalent to an adult's. This conclusion was a two-edged sword, however, leading to severe punishment (including capital punishment) of minors convicted of serious crimes.
- Subsequent neurodevelopmental studies have revealed a "dual-process model" of adolescent brain maturation, which leads to more impetuous, emotion-driven decisions than seen in adults. As a result, adolescents came to be granted less latitude in the medical arena and deemed less culpable in the legal arena.
- Parents may resist disclosure of a serious diagnosis or prognosis to their child. Reasons include wanting to wait for a particular time in order to tell the child, concern about what exactly the medical team will tell their child, fear that disclosure may destroy the fragile hope they and their child have for recovery, and feeling that the child should take the lead in such conversations.
  - In these situations, the team should explore the parents' understanding and motivation, while taking into consideration the child's DMC and the imperativeness of the information. Often allaying the parents' concerns and including them in the conversation can lead them to accept the need for disclosure.
  - In certain situations, the obligation to inform the patient outweighs requests to withhold information.
  - At no time should a medical professional ever lie to a child.
- Patient and/or parent refusal of LSMT is a complex ethical dilemma, which can be broken down into four quadrants:
  1. When both parents and patient accept the treatment, no ethical dilemma exists.
  2. When only the parents are refusing, this may represent misunderstanding of the situation or potentially actionable medical neglect.
  3. When only the child is refusing, this may represent immature decision-making driven by emotions rather than rationality. The patient's reasons for refusal should be explored, and she should be granted as much control over the situation as possible. In the context of LSMT, her refusal may need to be overridden to save her life, recognizing logistical limitations that may require a modification of the "standard of care."
  4. When both the parents and child are refusing, it is important to determine whether the child is merely following the parents' lead, or acting independently.
     - If the former, the situation becomes equivalent to Quadrant 2.
     - If the latter, the patient's level of DMC, the chances of survival with and without treatment, and the duration and burden of treatment all need to be taken into account. As with Quadrant 3, a modification of the standard of care may need to be considered. In exceptional circumstances, the logistical

barriers to compulsory treatment may render it unachievable from a practical perspective, and thus not an ethical obligation.

References

American Academy of Pediatrics. (2000). Palliative care for children. *Pediatrics, 106*(2 Pt 1), 351–357.

American Academy of Pediatrics. (2012). Patient- and family-centered care and the pediatrician's role. *Pediatrics, 129*(2), 394–404. doi:10.1542/peds.2011-3084

American Academy of Pediatrics. (2016). Informed consent in decision-making in pediatric practice. *Pediatrics, 138*(2), 136.

Appelbaum, P. S., Grisso, T., Frank, E., O'Donnell, S., & Kupfer, D. J. (1999). Competence of depressed patients for consent to research. *Am J Psychiatry, 156*(9), 1380–1384. doi:10.1176/ajp.156.9.1380.

Associated Press. (2009a). Daniel Hauser done with chemotherapy. Retrieved from http://www.mprnews.org/story/2009/09/04/daniel-hauser-done-with-chemo

Associated Press. (2009b). Judge rules family can't refuse chemo for boy. Retrieved from http://www.nbcnews.com/id/30763438/#.V1GqvUb8coF

Barker, J. (2000). New Watchtower blood transfusion policy. Retrieved from http://www.watchman.org/articles/jehovahs-witnesses/new-watchtower-blood-transfusion-policy/

Bartholome, W. G. (1981). The ethical rights of the child patient. *Front Radiat Ther Oncol, 16*, 156–166.

Bartholome, W. G. (1993). Care of the dying child. The demands of ethics. *Second Opin, 18*(4), 25–39.

Beale, E. A., Baile, W. F., & Aaron, J. (2005). Silence is not golden: Communicating with children dying from cancer. *J Clin Oncol, 23*(15), 3629–3631. doi:10.1200/JCO.2005.11.015

Belcher v. Charleston Area Med. Ctr. 1992.422 S.E.2d 827, 838 (W. Va. 1992).

Berger, J. T. (2005). Ignorance is bliss? Ethical considerations in therapeutic nondisclosure. *Cancer Invest, 23*(1), 94–98.

Best, B. (2012). *The Billy Best story: Beating cancer with alternative medicine.* Sandcastle Memoirs.

Bluebond-Langner, M. (1978). *The private worlds of dying children.* Princeton, NJ: Princeton University Press.

Buckwalter, W., & Turri, J. (2015). Inability and obligation in moral judgment. *PLoS One, 10*(8), e0136589. doi:10.1371/journal.pone.0136589

Canadian Pediatric Society Bioethics Committee. (2004). Treatment decisions regarding infants, children and adolescents. *Paediatr Child Health, 9*, 99–103.

Cardwell v. Bechtol. (1987). 724 S.W.2d 739.

Casey, B., Jones, R. M., & Somerville, L. H. (2011). Braking and accelerating of the adolescent brain. *J Res Adolesc, 21*(1), 21–33. doi:10.1111/j.1532-7795.2010.00712.x

Cauffman, E., & Steinberg, L. (2000). (Im)maturity of judgment in adolescence: Why adolescents may be less culpable than adults. *Behav Sci Law, 18*(6), 741–760. doi:10.1002/bsl.416

Claflin, C. J., & Barbarin, O. A. (1991). Does telling less protect more? Relationships among age, information disclosure, and what children with cancer see and feel. *J Pediatr Psych, 16*(2), 169–191.

Clarke, S. A., Davies, H., Jenney, M., Glaser, A., & Eiser, C. (2005). Parental communication and children's behaviour following diagnosis of childhood leukaemia. *Psychooncology, 14*(4), 274–281. doi:10.1002/pon.843

Clemente, I. (2007). Clinicians' routine use of non-disclosure: Prioritizing protection over the information needs of adolescents with cancer. *Can J Nurs Res, 39*(4), 19–34.

Cole, C., & Kodish, E. (2013). Minors' right to know and therapeutic privilege. Retrieved from http://journalofethics.ama-assn.org/2013/08/ecas1-1308.html.

Coleman, D. L., & Rosoff, P. M. (2013). The legal authority of mature minors to consent to general medical treatment. *Pediatrics, 131*(4), 786–793. doi:10.1542/peds.2012-2470

Dahl, R. E., & Gunnar, M. R. (2009). Heightened stress responsiveness and emotional reactivity during pubertal maturation: Implications for psychopathology. *Dev Psychopathol, 21*(1), 1–6. doi:10.1017/S0954579409000017

Davies, B., Sehring, S. A., Partridge, J. C., Cooper, B. A., Hughes, A., Philp, J. C., . . . Kramer, R. (2008). Barriers to palliative care for children: Perceptions of pediatric health care providers. *Pediatrics, 121*(2), 282–288. doi:10.1542/peds.2006-3153

Diekema, D. S. (2011). Adolescent refusal of lifesaving treatment: Are we asking the right questions? *Adolesc Med*, 22(2), 213–228.

Duncan, R. E., & Sawyer, S. M. (2010). Respecting adolescents' autonomy (as long as they make the right choice). *J Adolesc Health*, 47(2), 113–114. doi:10.1016/j.jadohealth.2010.05.020

Evan, E. E., & Cohen, H. J. (2011). Child relationships. In J. Wolfe, P. S. Hinds, & B. M. Sourkes (Eds.), *Textbook of interdisciplinary pediatric palliative care* (pp. 125–134). Philadelphia: Elsevier/Saunders.

Faulkner, K. W. (1997). Talking about death with a dying child. *Am J Nurs*, 97(6), 64, 66, 68–69.

Feudtner, C. (2007). Collaborative communication in pediatric palliative care: A foundation for problem-solving and decision-making. *Pediatr Clin North Am*, 54(5), 583–607. doi:10.1016/j.pcl.2007.07.008

Field, M. J., Behrman, R. E., & Institute of Medicine Committee on Palliative and End-of-Life Care for Children and Their Families. (2003). *When children die: Improving palliative and end-of-life care for children and their families.* Washington, DC: National Academy Press.

Giedd, J. N. (2008). The teen brain: Insights from neuroimaging. *J Adolesc Health*, 42(4), 335–343. doi:10.1016/j.jadohealth.2008.01.007

Giedd, J. N., Blumenthal, J., Jeffries, N. O., Castellanos, F. X., Liu, H., Zijdenbos, A., . . . Rapoport, J. L. (1999). Brain development during childhood and adolescence: A longitudinal MRI study. *Nature Neurosci*, 2(10), 861–863. doi:10.1038/13158.

Goldberg, A., & Frader, J. (2008). Holding on and letting go: Ethical issues regarding the care of children with cancer. *Cancer Treat Res, 140*, 173–194.

Goldman, A., & Heller, K. S. (2000). Integrating palliative and curative approaches in the care of children with life-threatening illnesses. *J Palliat Med*, 3(3), 353–359. doi:10.1089/jpm.2000.3.353

Graham v. Florida. (2010). 560 U.S. 48.

Grisso, T., & Vierling, L. (1978). Minors' consent to treatment: A developmental perspective. *Prof Psychol*, 9(3), 412–427.

Hammes, B. J., Klevan, J., Kempf, M., & Williams, M. S. (2005). Pediatric advance care planning. *J Palliat Med*, 8(4), 766–773. doi:10.1089/jpm.2005.8.766

Hilden, J. M., Watterson, J., & Chrastek, J. (2000). Tell the children. *J Clin Oncol*, 18(17), 3193–3195.

Himelstein, B. P., Hilden, J. M., Morstad Boldt, A., & Weissman, D. (2004). Pediatric palliative care. *N Engl J Med*, 350(17), 1752–1762. doi:10.1056/NEJMra030334350/17/1752

In re Chad Swan. (1990). 569 A.2d 1202.

In re E.G. (1989). 133 Ill.2d 98.

Hinds, P. S., Drew, D., Oakes, L. L., Fouladi, M., Spunt, S. L., Church, C., & Furman, W. L. (2005). End-of-life care preferences of pediatric patients with cancer. *J Clin Oncol*, 23(36), 9146–9154. doi:10.1200/JCO.2005.10.538

Kids Health. (2012). Child and family wishes. Retrieved from http://www.kidshealth.org.nz/sites/kidshealth/files/images/Child%20%20Family%20Wishes%20advance%20care%20plan_v3.pdf

Kreicbergs, U., Valdimarsdóttir, U., Onelöv, E., Henter, J.-I., & Steineck, G. (2004). Talking about death with children who have severe malignant disease. *N Engl J Med*, 351(12), 1175–1186. doi:10.1056/NEJMoa040366.

Kunin, H. (1997). Ethical issues in pediatric life-threatening illness: Dilemmas of consent, assent, and communication. *Ethics Behav*, 7(1), 43–57. doi:10.1207/s15327019eb0701_4

Larcher, V., & Hutchinson, A. (2010). How should paediatricians assess Gillick competence? *Arch Dis Child*, 95, 301–311.

Lee, K. J., & Dupree, C. Y. (2008). Staff experiences with end-of-life care in the pediatric intensive care unit. *J Palliat Med*, 11(7), 986–990. doi:10.1089/jpm.2007.0283

Leikin, S. (1993). Minors' assent, consent, or dissent to medical research. *IRB*, 15(2), 1–7.

Levy, M., Larcher, V., & Kurz, R. (2003). Informed consent/assent in children: Statement of the Ethics Working Group of the Confederation of European Specialists in Paediatrics (CESP). *Eur J Pediatr, 162*, 629–633.

Leydon, G. M., Boulton, M., Moynihan, C., Jones, A., Mossman, J., Boudioni, M., & McPherson, K. (2000). Cancer patients' information needs and information seeking behaviour: In depth interview study. *BMJ*, 320(7239), 909–913.

Liberman, D. B., Pham, P. K., & Nager, A. L. (2014). Pediatric advance directives: Parents' knowledge, experience, and preferences. *Pediatrics, 134*(2), e436–e443. doi:10.1542/peds.2013-3124

Lyon, M. E., D'Angelo, L. J., Garvie, P. A., Briggs, L., He, J., & McCarter, R. (2009). Development, feasibility, and acceptability of the Family/Adolescent-Centered (FACE) advance care planning intervention for adolescents with HIV. *J Palliat Med, 12*(4), 363–372. doi:10.1089/jpm.2008.0261

Lyon, M. E., McCabe, M. A., Patel, K. M., & D'Angelo, L. J. (2004). What do adolescents want? An exploratory study regarding end-of-life decision-making. *J Adolesc Health, 35*(6), 529 e1–e6. doi:10.1016/j.jadohealth.2004.02.009

Macauley, R., & Fritzler, L. (2014). Parental refusal of pain management: A potentially unrecognized form of medical neglect. *Palliat Med Care, 1*(2), 5–11.

Mack, J. W., Wolfe, J., Cook, E. F., Grier, H. E., Cleary, P. D., & Weeks, J. C. (2007). Hope and prognostic disclosure. *J Clin Oncol, 25*(35), 5636–5642. doi:10.1200/JCO.2007.12.6110

Masera, G., Spinetta, J. J., Jankovic, M., Ablin, A. R., D'Angio, G. J., Van Dongen-Melman, J., . . . Chesler, M. A. (1999). Guidelines for assistance to terminally ill children with cancer: A report of the SIOP Working Committee on psychosocial issues in pediatric oncology. *Med Pediatr Oncol, 32*(1), 44–48.

McCabe, M. (1996). Involving children and adolescents in medical decision making: Developmental and clinical considerations. *J Pediatr Psychol, 21*(4), 505–516.

McGrath, P. A. (1996). Development of the World Health Organization guidelines on cancer pain relief and palliative care in children. *J Pain Symptom Manage, 12*(2), 87–92.

Mercurio, M. R. (2007). An adolescent's refusal of medical treatment: Implications of the Abraham Cheerix case. *Pediatrics, 120*(6), 1357–1358. doi:10.1542/peds.2007-1458

Michaud, P. A., Berg-Kelly, K. & Macfarlane, A. (2010). Ethics and adolescent care: An international perspective. *Curr Opin Pediatr, 22*, 418–422.

Morgan, E. R., & Murphy, S. B. (2000). Care of children who are dying of cancer. *N Engl J Med, 342*(5), 347–348. doi:10.1056/NEJM200002033420510

Nitschke, R., Meyer, W. H., Sexauer, C. L., Parkhusrst, J. B., Foster, P., & Huszti, H. (2000). Care of terminally ill children with cancer. *Med Pediatr Oncol, 34*(4), 268–270.

Parham v. J.R. (1979). 442 U.S. 584.

Penson, R. T., & Amrein, P. C. (2004). Faith and freedom: leukemia in Jehovah Witness minors. *Onkologie, 27*(2), 126–128. doi:10.1159/000076900

Pousset, G., Mortier, F., Bilsen, J., Deliens, L., De Wilde, J., Benoit, Y., . . . Bomans, A. (2009). Attitudes of survivors toward end-of-life decisions for minors. *Pediatrics, 124*(6), e1142–e1148. doi:10.1542/peds.2009-0621

President's Commission for the Study of Ethical Problems in Medicine and Biomedical and Behavioral Research. (1982). Making health care decisions: A report on the ethical and legal implications of informed consent in the patient-practitioner relationship. Washington, DC: U.S. Government Printing Office.

Prince v. Massachusetts. (1944). 321 U.S. 158.

Psychology Today. (2017). Adolescence. Retrieved from https://www.psychologytoday.com/basics/adolescence. Accessed on September 6, 2017

Rasmussen, R. K., ed. (1998). *The quotable Mark Twain: His essential aphorisms, witticisms, and concise opinions.* New York: McGraw-Hill.

Roper v. Simmons. (2005). 543 U.S. 551.

Ross, L. F. (1998). *Children, families, and health care decision making: Issues in biomedical ethics.* Oxford; New York: Clarendon Press.

Scherer, D. G., & Reppuci, N. D. (1988). Adolescents' capacities to provide voluntary informed consent: The effects of parental influence and medical dilemmas. *Law Hum Behav, 12*(2), 123–141.

Silber, T. J. (2011). Adolescent brain development and the mature minor doctrine. *Adolesc Med, 22*(2), 207–212.

Slavin, L. A.,O'Malley, J. E., Koocher, G. P., & Foster, D. J. (1982). Communication of the cancer diagnosis to pediatric patients: Impact on long-term adjustment. *Am J Psychiatr, 139*(2), 179–183. doi:10.1176/ajp.139.2.179

Sourkes, B. M. (1995). *Armfuls of time: The psychological experience of the child with a life-threatening illness.* Pittsburgh: University of Pittsburgh Press.

Sowell, E. R.,Thompson, P. M., Holmes, C. J., Jernigan, T. L., & Toga, A. W. (1999). In vivo evidence for post-adolescent brain maturation in frontal and striatal regions. *Nature Neurosci, 2*(10), 859–861. doi:10.1038/13154

Sowell, E. R., Thompson, P. M., Tessner, K. D., & Toga, A. W. (2001). Mapping continued brain growth and gray matter density reduction in dorsal frontal cortex: Inverse relationships during postadolescent brain maturation. *J Neurosci, 21*(22), 8819–8829.

Spinetta, J. J. (1974). The dying child's awareness of death: A review. *Psychol Bull, 81*(4), 256–260.

Stanford v. Kentucky. (1989). 492 U.S. 361.

State of Vermont. (2009). 12 V.S.A. § 7151.

Steele, R., & Davies, B. (2006). Impact on parents when a child has a progressive, life-threatening illness. *Int J Palliat Nurs, 12*(12), 576–585. doi:10.12968/ijpn.2006.12.12.22544

Steinberg, L. (2005). Cognitive and affective development in adolescence. *Trends Cog Sci, 9*(2), 69–74. doi:10.1016/j.tics.2004.12.005

Steinberg, L. (2010). A dual systems model of adolescent risk-taking. *Dev Psychobiol, 52*(3), 216–224. doi:10.1002/dev.20445

United Nations. (1990). *Convention on the Rights of the Child.* Retrieved from http://www.unicef.org/crc/

Vernick, J., & Karon, M. (1965). Who's afraid of death on a leukemia ward? *Am J Dis Child, 109,* 393–397.

Waller, B. (2001). Patient autonomy naturalized. *Perspect Biol Med, 44,* 584–593.

Weir, R. F., & Peters, C. (1997). Affirming the decisions adolescents make about life and death. *Hastings Cent Rep, 27*(6), 29–40.

Weithorn, L. A., & Campbell, S. B. (1982). The competency of children and adolescents to make informed treatment decisions. *Child Dev, 53,* 1589–1598.

Whitney, S. N., Ethier, A. M., Fruge, E., Berg, S., McCullough, L. B., Hockenberry, M. (2006). Decision making in pediatric oncology: Who should take the lead? The decisional priority in pediatric oncology model. *J Clin Oncol, 24*(1), 160–165. doi:10.1200/JCO.2005.01.8390

Whittam, E. H. (1993). Terminal care of the dying child: Psychosocial implications of care. *Cancer, 71*(10 Suppl.), 3450–3462.

Wiener, L., Ballard, E., Brennan, T., Battles, H., Martinez, P., & Pao, M. (2008). How I wish to be remembered: The use of an advance care planning document in adolescent and young adult populations. *J Palliat Med, 11*(10), 1309–1313. doi:10.1089/jpm.2008.0126

Wiener, L., Zadeh, S., Battles, H., Baird, K., Ballard, E., Osherow, J., & Pao, M. (2012). Allowing adolescents and young adults to plan their end-of-life care. *Pediatrics, 130*(5), 897–905. doi:10.1542/peds.2012-0663

Wolfe, J., Klar, N., Grier, H. E., Duncan, J., Salem-Schatz, S., Emanuel, E. J., & Weeks, J. C. (2000). Understanding of prognosis among parents of children who died of cancer: Impact on treatment goals and integration of palliative care. *JAMA, 284*(19), 2469–2475.

Wolfe, L. (2004). Should parents speak with a dying child about impending death? *N Engl J Med, 351*(12), 1251–1253. doi:10.1056/NEJMe048183

Wolff, A., Browne, J., & Whitehouse, W. P. (2011). Personal resuscitation plans and end of life planning for children with disability and life-limiting/life-threatening conditions. *Arch Dis Child, 96*(2), 42–48. doi:10.1136/adc.2010.185272

World Health Organization. (2016). Adolescent health. Retrieved from http://www.who.int/topics/adolescent_health/en/

Wyatt, J. (2009). *Matters of life & death: Human dilemmas in the light of the Christian faith* (2nd ed.). Nottingham, UK: InterVarsity Press.

Zadeh, S., Pao, M., & Wiener, L. (2015). Opening end-of-life discussions: How to introduce Voicing My CHOiCES, an advance care planning guide for adolescents and young adults. *Palliat Support Care, 13*(3), 591–599. doi:10.1017/S1478951514000054

Other Topics

14

Requests for Nonbeneficial Treatment

Case Study

A fifty-nine-year-old man has worsening multiple sclerosis. Despite maximal medical treatment—including referrals to other centers for second and third opinions—his quality of life has been worsening for many years. Over the last two years he has spent more time in the hospital than at home.

Six months ago he was intubated for respiratory failure and admitted to the intensive care unit (ICU). When he was unable to wean from the ventilator, a tracheostomy was performed. Hemodynamic instability and the challenge of caring for him on a ventilator at home has kept him in the ICU.

He is no longer able to make his own medical decisions. Previously he named his extremely devoted wife as his durable power of attorney for health care, and she states that he told her on many occasions that as long as he could recognize her, he was still "in there" and wanted everything done to help him survive. She, therefore, is requesting maximal treatment, while the staff feel that continued intensive care is not in his best interests. They believe the patient should, at the very least, not undergo CPR for cardiac arrest, as they deem it to be "futile."

The patient's wife, however, continues to demand maximal intervention. Given the impasse, an ethics consult is requested.

Historicolegal Background

According to the Hippocratic tradition, the purpose of medicine is "to do away with the suffering of the sick, to lessen the violence of their diseases, and to *refuse to treat those who are overmastered by their disease, realizing that in such cases medicine is powerless*" (Hippocrates, 1959, emphasis added). In Hippocrates' time—and for nearly 2,500 years afterward—this was not problematic, since beneficence was the overriding ethical principle of medical practice. If a physician felt that a potential intervention would not help a patient, she simply would not mention it, since she was not going to provide it, anyway (p. 4). At a time when most people could not read—let alone surf the Internet in search of medical advice—patients were generally none the wiser that a decision had been made on their behalf.

Medicine has come a long way since the days of Hippocrates. The shift from beneficence to autonomy over the course of the twentieth century—coupled with expanded access to medical information (much of it unreliable)—have combined to make the process of medical decision-making infinitely more complex. No longer do physicians have the practical or professionally approved option of simply not mentioning treatments they feel are inappropriate. Patients expect to be apprised of all relevant options and sometimes demand those which the physician has neglected to mention (and perhaps even failed to consider). Yet even in the modern world of advancing technology, some patients are still "overmatched by their disease." What should a physician do, then, when patients or their families request a treatment which she feels is not appropriate?

This question came to the fore of the ethics world in the 1990s. The recognition of the importance of informed consent in the early to mid-twentieth century (p. 5) and an expanding emphasis on patients' rights in the latter half of the century (Natural Death Act, 1976; *In re Quinlan*, 1976) led some to believe that patients not only had the right to refuse treatment, they also had the right to receive any treatment that they requested. With the explosion of medical technology, it became increasingly possible to institute treatments that held questionable benefit, or that medical professionals felt would not even achieve physiologic goals. Reacting to this, the so-called "futility decade" of the 1990s inverted the focus: instead of empowering patients to say no to treatments physicians favored, the question became whether physicians had the right to forgo treatments that patients were requesting.

Extensive efforts were undertaken to define what constituted "futile" treatment and determine how to respond when a family rejected this determination.[1] For example,

---

1. The term *futile* is set off in quotation marks because although it was commonly used during the debates of the 1990s, as a term it is problematic. It often gives the false impression that the medical team believes that the patient is not *worth* saving, rather than unable to be saved (Berlinger, Jennings, & Wolf, 2013; Gillon, 1997). It can also be defined in many ways, as subsequently described. In the ethical analysis *futile* is used to specifically refer to interventions that cannot achieve their physiologic goal, while the preferable term "potentially nonbeneficial treatment" refers to interventions that were at the heart of the debate during the "futility decade."

Murphy and Finucane (1993) proposed several conditions—such as coma lasting more than forty-eight hours—where ongoing clinical treatment should not be provided. Attempts were also made to define futility in probabilistic terms (Schneiderman, Jecker, & Jonsen, 1990). For instance, Schneiderman and Jecker (2000) suggested that a treatment is "futile" if it has not worked for the last one hundred patients on which it was attempted. One could then predict—with a 95% degree of confidence—that the treatment would be successful in no more than three of the next one hundred cases. Procedural steps were proposed to guide clinicians from the declaration of "futility" to the forgoing of the treatment in question (Texas Advance Directives Act, 1999).

As the 1990s came to a close, though, the focus abated. One reason was that people could not agree on what the term "futile" meant, leading to often conflicting debates over a concept defined in significantly different ways. Even if people had been able to agree on what the term meant, it was not clear where to draw the line in terms of probability of efficacy: 0%, 1%, 5%? Even if they had agreed on where to draw the line, it was often impossible to determine on which side of that line a patient fell, given the uncertainty of prognostication (p. 84). Even if precise prognostication were possible, it was unclear what to do if the patient or family objected to withdrawing or withholding the requested treatment (Helft, Siegler, & Lantos, 2000). In the end, some wondered if the futility debate had itself been "futile," depending on what one meant by that term.

More recently, however, the term has returned to the medical conversation (Figure 14.1). A likely reason is skyrocketing health care costs which necessarily prompt exploration of where money can be saved, with an obvious choice being nonbeneficial treatment (NBT). The degree to which forgoing such treatment would save money is debatable, with some studies showing significant expenditures in this area (Huynh et al., 2013) even as others question the extent of savings that are possible (Truog & White, 2013). There is also risk in limiting *potentially* NBT in order

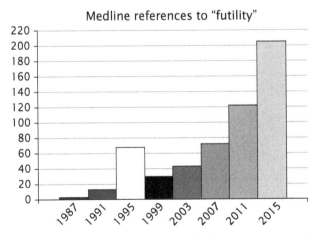

FIGURE 14.1 Annual references in the medical literature to "futility," showing peaks of interest in the mid-1990s and the present

to save money, as this could resurrect the infamous "death panel" controversy that imperiled the Affordable Care Act and delayed reimbursement for advance care planning conversations (p. 510).

In the future, the financial issue may not be as pressing as hospitals move away from fee-for-service and toward an accountable care model (Obama, 2016), removing institutional financial incentives to provide additional treatment. The question remains, however, how to respond to persistent patient or family demands for treatments that clinicians worry will not benefit the patient.

A crucial question related to the "futility" debate is whether it is even legal to forgo requested treatment on this basis. Consideration of unilateral forgoing is actually quite rare, as most such disputes are ultimately resolved through enhanced communication and expert consultation. In the fraction that are not, the courts may come into play (Pope, 2011).

Court involvement may either precede or follow limitation of life-sustaining medical treatment (LSMT). In the former situation, courts often grant temporary injunctions to prevent LSMT from being forgone. This allows more time to hopefully reach consensus about whether treatment is actually beneficial. As the US Supreme Court concluded: "An erroneous decision not to terminate results in maintenance of the status quo . . . An erroneous decision to withdraw . . . is not susceptible of correction" (*Cruzan v. Director, Missouri Department of Health*, 1990).

Undergirding the practical wisdom of the "keep all options open" verdict is a very human motivation. Physicians enter their profession with the full knowledge that they may, one day, have to make difficult decisions which involve discontinuing LSMT. Whatever one's primary motivations for becoming a judge might be, unlikely to be among them is telling a grieving family that they cannot prevent the medical establishment—which likely is not willing to declare that there is absolutely *no* chance of recovery—from withdrawing LSMT from their loved one.

Requests for permanent injunctions, however, are generally refused.[2] This may reflect the hope that consensus among the family and the medical team can ultimately be achieved, as well as a recognition that in some cases medical intervention will do more harm than good.

Plaintiffs also rarely prevail in civil suits brought *after* LSMT has been withdrawn, which is the basis of most "futility" claims. Courts usually find in favor of the health care professionals who exhausted all other avenues and took great pains to document their reasons for forgoing (Boyd et al., 2010; Pope, 2009, 2010). If, however, the medical team used insensitive terminology or coercion in an attempt to get the family to agree to voluntarily forgo LSMT, some courts have subsequently found in favor of the family (*Bernstein v. Sup. Ct. Ventura Cty*, 2009).

---

2. As usual, there are some notable exceptions to this trend (e.g., *Betancourt v. Trinitas Hospital*, 2010).

Despite the fact that courts rarely hold physicians liable for forgoing LSMT over the objections of a patient or their surrogate, physicians—and the health systems in which they work—may be reluctant to take that chance. Unless the family can be persuaded to consent to limitation of treatment, the only other alternative would be to petition the court to replace the surrogate who is requesting that treatment. This is precisely what Hennepin County Medical Center attempted to do in one of the most famous "futility" cases (*In re Helga Wanglie*, 1991).

Helga Wanglie was an elderly woman in a persistent vegetative state whose husband continued to request aggressive treatment based on her previous statement that "If anything happens to me, I want everything done." The hospital, however, felt this was contrary to her best interests and asked the court to appoint an alternate decision-maker. The court denied the request because it believed that her husband was providing accurate substituted judgment, without commenting on the physicians' professional obligations. Mrs. Wanglie died from multisystem organ failure three days after the court's decision (Drane & Coulehan, 1993).

As the *Wanglie* case illustrates, it is difficult to replace a surrogate who has close personal ties to the patient, unless she is clearly acting contrary to the patient's expressed wishes and values. It is also a very confrontational path to take, essentially questioning the surrogate's fitness to serve in that role or even their fidelity to the patient she claims to care for. That being said, in recent years courts have shown greater willingness to either replace a surrogate who is making unreasonable demands (*Bernstein v. Sup. Ct. Ventura Cty*, 2009; *In re Livadas*, 2008) or to place limitations on a surrogate's authority (*Cardoza v. USC University Hospital*, 2008).

These principles pertain to civil actions. In terms of administrative or criminal sanctions, the most relevant court case is that of Baby K, an anencephalic infant whose mother repeatedly requested resuscitation. The local hospital petitioned the court for permission to forgo resuscitation based on its purported "futility" in the context of such a serious illness. The court denied the hospital's request, asserting that "it is beyond the limits of our judicial function to address the moral or ethical propriety of providing emergency stabilizing medical treatment to anencephalic infants. We are bound to interpret federal statutes in accordance with their plain language" (*In re Baby K*, 1994).[3]

However, most patients involved in "futility" disputes are—unlike Baby K—inpatients. As such, they are not subject to Emergency Medical Treatment and Labor Act regulations (p. 310). Criminal prosecution is thus extremely rare when LSMT is forgone on the basis of "futility" (Pope, 2011).

In terms of statute, the majority of states have laws which explicitly permit health care providers to refuse requested treatment that they determine is medically inappropriate.

---

3. The statute in question is the Emergency Medical Treatment and Labor Act (1986), which requires that patients who present with a medical emergency must receive "such treatment as may be required to stabilize the medical condition" before the patient can be transferred to another facility.

However, the safe harbors in most of these statutes are defined by reference to vague standards such as "significant benefit," "medically inappropriate," or "generally accepted healthcare standards." This vagueness results in "chilling" uncertainty because providers are unsure how to satisfy the standard for legal immunity. As a result, they are often reluctant to unilaterally refuse requested treatment (Pope, 2007).

An exception to this general rule is the very explicit Texas Advance Directives Act (TADA). This is also known as the Texas Futile Care Law, even though the act does not include the word "futile," instead focusing on "medically inappropriate" treatment (TADA, 1999). The law mandates a specific multistage review process for situations where a health care professional does not wish to honor a patient or surrogate's request for continued treatment. These stages include a second clinical opinion followed by a multidisciplinary ethics committee meeting—with forty-eight hour's written notice to the patient/family—which allows both clinicians and patients/families to be heard. If the committee concurs that the treatment is nonbeneficial, the health care team must continue to provide the treatment for up to ten days while transfer to another facility is attempted. If, after those ten days, transfer is not accomplished, then the NBT may be withdrawn. (This can also occur prior to that time, if the family withdraws their objections to forgoing.)

Data from TADA is sporadic, but some basic conclusions can be drawn. One is that the number of ethics consults increased after the act was passed, presumably because there was now a potential endpoint to "futility" consults. Most such consults did not proceed all the way to the end, however. In one report, out of 974 such consults, only 65 ten-day letters were generated, suggesting that the combination of a second clinical opinion, outside consultants, and the "threat" of unilateral withdrawal led to consensus before that point. For those patients who received letters, less than half had LSMT unilaterally withdrawn, with the remainder either dying or being transferred within the original time frame, or being granted an extension by the court (Fine, 2009).

It is important to note that, if the TADA process is followed, the ethics committee's decision cannot be appealed to a court. The court can only provide a temporary stay to allow the family more time to find an accepting facility. Providers who follow TADA's prescribed procedures are also immune both from disciplinary action and from civil and criminal liability (Fine, 2000).

Clinical

Studies have shown that NBT occurs frequently in the practice of medicine, involving over a third of patients at the end of life (Cardona-Morrell et al., 2016). It is especially common in ICUs, with one-quarter of European intensivists providing such treatment on any given day (Piers et al., 2011), and one in five ICU patients in the United States receiving at least one day of NBT (Huynh et al., 2013).

Physicians are often willing to provide such treatment at least temporarily, in the hope that patients or families will eventually recognize that it will not achieve the patient's goals (and thus stop requesting it). So while NBT is rather commonplace, true "futility disputes" are relatively rare. Most that arise can be resolved through enhanced communication, such as via ethics or palliative care consultation (Fine & Mayo, 2003; Garros, Rosychuk, & Cox, 2003; Prendergast & Luce, 1997). As noted in the previous section, only the select few require legal adjudication.

In addressing such disputes, one of the challenges—as was the case with "palliative sedation" (p. 252)—is choosing and then precisely defining the terms involved. The word "futile" is derived from the Greek *futilis*, which literally means leaky or untrustworthy, and refers to the failure to achieve an intended goal (Merriam-Webster Inc., 2003). The challenge, though, is identifying what that goal actually is. Generally speaking the patient (or their decision-maker) determines the goal, and it is then up to the medical team to evaluate whether the goal is achievable (i.e., whether or not it is "futile"). Goals of medical treatment can range from mere physiologic effect—such as a pressor increasing blood pressure—to postponing death, extending length of life, and maintaining or improving quality of life (Youngner, 1988).

Clearly, if a treatment will not achieve its physiologic goal, then there is no chance it will lead to any of the more profound goals noted previously. An example would be CPR in the context of cardiac wall rupture, which has no chance of restoring spontaneous circulation. "Physiologic futility," therefore, is the least contentious term used in the debate, and some have gone so far as to call it "value-neutral" (Truog, 1992).

The choice to emphasize a physiologic effect may, however, be itself a matter of values (Schneiderman, 2011). A medication that successfully raises blood pressure would not be considered physiologically futile, but if that merely prolongs the dying process by a few minutes, it would seem not to provide true benefit.

For this reason it is critical—when determining any level of "futility" beyond that of pure physiology—to identify what the precise goal is. Take, for instance, a patient with end-stage chronic obstructive pulmonary disease (COPD) who is in respiratory distress and will not survive without mechanical ventilation. Given the severity of his disease, once intubated he will almost surely never be able to breathe independently again. If the goal is for the patient to ultimately go home and lead an independent life, then intubating the patient cannot achieve the goal. But if the goal is to keep the patient alive for a period of time in order for his loved ones to say goodbye, then this is achievable.

For every potential goal there is also the added consideration of the probability of actually achieving it. Physicians vary widely on where to draw the line of so-called "probabilistic futility," below which a requested treatment is so unlikely to achieve its goal that it will not be provided. A significant portion of physicians state that if there is *any* chance of achieving the patient's goal, the treatment should not be deemed "futile." Another significant subset draw the line between 1% and 5% chance of success (i.e., possible but exceedingly unlikely). The problem, though, lies in the small percentage of physicians who draw the line much higher, in some cases as high as a 40% to 60% chance of success (McCrary, Swanson, Youngner, Perkins, & Winslade, 1994).

It is hard to believe that these physicians truly believe that something with an even chance of success is "futile." It is more likely that they are reasoning backward from conclusion to premise. In other words, there is a procedure that a physician does not wish to provide a patient. A hundred years ago that physician would simply have not mentioned the procedure to the patient or would have summarily declined to provide it if the patient had somehow known to ask for it. But in the era of patient autonomy, the physician now feels obligated to inform the patient of the procedure, while also taking great pains to explain why she does not believe it is indicated.

If the patient persists, the only recourse the physician may feel is open to her is to claim futility given the support of various codes of ethics, including the American Medical Association's (2016), which states that

> Physicians are not required to offer or to provide interventions that, in their best medical judgment, cannot reasonably be expected to yield the intended clinical benefit or achieve agreed-on goals for care. Respecting patient autonomy does not mean that patients should receive specific interventions simply because they (or their surrogates) request them.

Invoking futility thus permits the physician to withhold essentially any treatment she does not believe is indicated, even if it possibly—or even *probably*—would achieve the patient's stated goals. This is one of the reasons that futility is sometimes called "the F-word in medical ethics," as it stifles dialogue (Seattle Children's Hospital, 2007).

Even assuming, though, that a probability can be agreed upon below which interventions are deemed to be "futile," there remains the question of how to know whether a specific case falls above or below that line. While it might make intellectual sense to draw the line at a procedure that was unsuccessful the last hundred times it was attempted (Schneiderman & Jecker, 2000), few institutions actually have one hundred equivalent cases to allow such a comparison. Recognizing this, one might turn to the published literature, but typically this information is either anecdotal in the form of case reports about similar patients—leading one to question the generalizability of the reported results—or it is population-based from larger series which necessarily raises the question of the extent to which the patient in question resembles those in the report. Every patient is unique, and if it is difficult to determine if there is *any* chance of achieving the patient's goals, it is even harder to determine what precisely that chance is.

The analysis becomes so complex that a simple "above-or-below the line" question is essentially unanswerable. So even when the odds of achieving the goal are extremely low, it is often impossible to say with confidence that the odds are lower than the predetermined line, which ultimately leads to the exception becoming the rule. Rather than identifying the cases when treatment can be forgone on the basis of "futility"—which was the intention of the policy in the first place—the debate instead serves to highlight how difficult such a determination is, and why any such determination is fraught with doubt and uncertainty.

This underscores the fact that "all [aspects of futility] except for physiologic futility and an absolutely inability to postpone death . . . also involve value judgments" (Youngner, 1988). These judgments not only pertain to the requisite likelihood of success for a treatment to not be considered "futile" but also to the goals to which this probability refers. Clearly, the physicians who might be willing to deem "futile" an intervention that will probably achieve a specific goal are not basing their estimation on probabilities but rather on the inherent value of the goal itself. A potential example of so-called "qualitative futility" is medically administered nutrition and hydration (MANH) for a patient in a vegetative state, who previously stated that he wanted "everything done" to keep him alive, regardless of the circumstances.

Clearly, without intervention such a patient—who cannot eat or drink—will die of dehydration. MANH, however, can be provided effectively for years or decades. It is therefore neither physiologically nor probabilistically futile, and the only reason to unilaterally withhold it is based on a sense that a vegetative state represents an exceedingly poor quality of life. In other words, the patient (or appropriate surrogate) identified a goal which is clearly achievable but the clinician deemed that goal not *worth* achieving. Critics understandably question whether physicians are in any position to assess overall benefit (Veatch, 1994), especially given the risks of faulty quality of life estimations (Saigal et al., 1999).

Qualitative futility can also be viewed in a more positive light. Also referred to as "normative futility" (Mason & Laurie, 2011), it can shift the focus of the conversation from physiologic efficacy to overall benefit. After all, the real goal of CPR is not temporary return of spontaneous circulation but rather some degree of meaningful recovery that spontaneous circulation permits. When viewed in this light, the concept of normative futility provides a way of broadening the discussion with patients and families beyond mere physiologic effects to their heartfelt goals and whether the intervention in question will help the patient achieve these.

The wide variation on how "futility" is defined is evident in the professional statements about how to respond to it. Some statements use the term in a probabilistic sense ("highly unlikely to result in meaningful survival," American Thoracic Society, 1991), others in a qualitative sense ("no beneficial physiologic effect," Society of Critical Care Medicine, 1997), and still others they do not even define the term at all (Council on Ethical and Judicial Affairs, 1999; TADA, 1999). It is little wonder that the debate rages on when commentators have such a hard time defining the term, let alone applying the concept to clinical medicine.

Ethical

Before analyzing the ethics of "futility"—which is defined in terms of lack of benefit or efficacy—it is important to note that this is not the only potential reason why a patient would not receive a treatment that he is requesting. Excessive risk or burden may also justify forgoing requested treatment. Nearly every medical treatment—and in particular critical care interventions that are often at the heart of the futility debate—entails some degree of burden or risk. This may impact the patient either physically (such as through physical pain from invasive procedures) or emotionally (in the form of false hope or dying an undignified death).

While not determinative, the suffering of others may also contribute to a decision to forgo a treatment of unclear benefit. Families may be harmed by having to watch the patient suffer for prolonged periods of time. Finally, staff may suffer from moral distress (p. 514), feeling like they should be doing something else for the patient but are prevented by family demands for potentially NBT (Meltzer & Huckabay, 2004).

Framing nontreatment debates *only* in terms of inefficacy—as some "futility" discussions tend to do—may give the false impression that there is nothing to lose by trying the treatment. This fails to adequately recognize the potential for harm, a nonmaleficence-based concern. To illustrate this, Kite and Wilkinson (2002) use a lottery analogy. Reasonable people might not buy a lottery ticket because of the extremely poor odds of winning, but most would generally accept a free lottery ticket if someone handed it to them. The chances of winning are still astronomically slim, but now there is nothing to lose (not even the price of the ticket). Framing debates about "inappropriate treatment" only in terms of benefit and not also of burden runs the risk of making it seem like a "no-lose proposition," which it most certainly is not.

In addition to risk of harm, rationing—a justice-based concern—is another reason to forgo requested treatment. There may be an extremely limited supply of a specific treatment (such as organs for transplantation) necessitating rationing in an ethical manner, such as first-come/first-served, degree of need, or a lottery (Persad, Wertheimer, & Emanuel, 2009). It is important to note that rationing presupposes both that the resource in question is quantitatively limited and also would be effective if used. In the ICU—where most futility debates occur—this could refer to modalities such as ventilators or simply bed space. It can also apply to health care spending in general, as clinicians increasingly feel an obligation to be appropriate stewards of precious health care dollars (Cook, 2010).

Some clinicians acknowledge the need to ration treatment and openly admit to doing so (Chevlen, 2009). This involves forging treatment which is expensive or which might have a higher probability of benefitting another patient. Acknowledging that a patient already receiving treatment has a *prima facie* right to continue it (p. 157), forgoing in this case usually involves withholding rather than withdrawing.

Others clinicians deny they ever ration treatment (Strech, Synofzik, & Marckmann, 2008). This is because rationing is a highly charged term, especially in political circles. Prioritizing the common good over individual request seems almost "un-American" (Hoffman, 2012). If futility is the "F-word," then rationing might be considered the "R-word" (Bloche, 2012) in terms of its potential to stifle debate.

This aversion to rationing could lead a clinician who feels that an expensive treatment is a poor use of resources to forgo it by claiming it would not be "beneficial," even though it very well could be in that case. It is imperative, therefore, to determine whether a claim of "futility" is actually covert rationing, which demands a much different analysis and response.

In addition to excessive burden and rationing, "futility" is the third reason to not provide a treatment that the patient or family is requesting.[4] Recognizing the definitional challenges noted previously, the framework set forth by the 2015 consensus statement of several professional societies is extremely helpful (Bosslet et al., 2015). The authors suggest restricting the term "futile" to refer to interventions that "simply cannot accomplish the intended physiologic goal." While physiologic futility may itself be susceptible to some ambiguity, at the very least it is less contentious than other terms such as probabilistic or qualitative futility.

When a physiologically futile intervention is requested, clinicians should decline to provide that treatment while explaining the rationale for their refusal. This includes the obligation to do no harm, as well as the need to safeguard the integrity of the medical profession. The consensus statement appropriately notes that such requests are more the exception than the rule, as most futility debates involve treatments that might—or even might *well*—achieve the physiologic goal. The statement appropriately groups truly futile interventions with those that are legally proscribed, which clinicians should also refrain from providing.

The statement also specifies that a surrogate's request for continued treatment that is not appropriately based on substituted judgment—which can certainly occur in highly emotional situations (Schenker et al., 2012)—should not be honored. If the surrogate persists in demanding that treatment, an alternate decision-maker may need to be identified.[5] The logistical challenges in doing so are discussed earlier (p. 367).

---

4. Often the reason for physician reluctance to provide a requested treatment is a combination of all of these: burden, expense/scarcity, and presumed lack of benefit. Once the first two are included in the discussion, however, the issue is no longer purely one of "futility."

5. It is worth observing that the vast majority of requests for possibly "futile" treatment—especially in the ICU—come from surrogates, rather than from the patient himself. Admittedly, that might be because the patient is too ill at the time to engage in decision-making (and, thus, to request such treatment). Another important reason is that the surrogate will not directly experience the burden of the proposed treatment, and thus might be more accepting of it. If the patient himself were demanding the treatment—and was fully cognizant of the possibility of success and the associated burdens—the physician would probably be much more likely to offer it.

The consensus statement uses the term "potentially inappropriate" to refer to treatments that might achieve a physiologic goal but are either likely not to provide benefit ("probabilistic futility") or that benefit is not thought sufficient to justify the procedure ("qualitative/normative futility"). The modifier "potentially" appropriately stresses that it is only a preliminary judgment which is open to dialogue and review.

In describing the proposed treatment, the authors prefer the term "appropriateness" because it stems from a combination of clinical assessment and values, not merely technical judgment. "Nonbeneficial" is preferable, however. One reason is that it maintains the focus on what will *benefit* the patient. This a net term, balancing overall positive and negative outcomes rather than relying on degree of efficacy. "Benefit" is also a more patient-centered term than the more formal, bureaucratic "appropriate." Further, "inappropriate" often carries a psychotherapeutic (Oz, 1991) or even judgmental connotation that can introduce an adversarial tone into an already tense dialogue.

Before addressing how to respond to requests for potentially NBT, it is worth exploring how to *prevent* them. Many such requests stem from poor communication, misunderstandings, or feelings of not being cared for. There may also be a lack of guidance from the medical team, presenting the family with a range of options without a recommendation grounded in the patient's own values, thus creating fertile ground for a futility dispute to grow. Many potential such disputes can be prevented from occurring in the first place by getting to know the patient and family, conveying recommendations in a clear and compassionate way, and potentially seeking informed assent to limitation of treatment (p. 382), if appropriate.

Once such a dispute arises, many position statements—including the recent consensus statement (Bosslet et al., 2015)—put forth a similar procedural approach. The first response is to optimize communication. There is solid evidence that ongoing communication can assist in resolving these disputes (Garros et al., 2003; Prendergast & Luce, 1997), as can the assistance of expert consultants from ethics or palliative care (Schneiderman et al., 2003).[6] In one study in Texas, a basic ethics consultation resolved 86% of futility cases without needing to resort to the TADA process (Fine & Mayo, 2003). Improved communication which helps the family recognize the lack of treatment benefit may explain the cost savings associated with ethics consultation in the ICU setting (Gilmer et al., 2005; Schneiderman et al., 2003).

If disagreement remains, the surrogates should be notified—verbally as well as in writing—of the next steps in the process, and given adequate time to prepare for committee review. The committee should be interdisciplinary and composed of professionals not directly involved in the patient's care.

In the meantime, a second clinical opinion should be sought to either confirm or critique the initial determination that the requested treatment is not beneficial. This is

---

6. It is important that these consultants be distinct from whatever interdisciplinary committee may ultimately review the claim of lack of benefit, if it reaches the final stage of the process.

particularly important given concerns raised about the variability among physicians as to what constitutes "appropriate care" (Cook et al., 1995; Curtis, Park, Krone, & Pearlman, 1995; Garland & Connors, 2007; Piers et al., 2011; Sprung et al., 2003; Wunsch, Harrison, Harvey, & Rowan, 2005), as well as the documented differences in end-of-life perspectives between patients and ICU clinicians (Gramelspacher, Zhou, Hanna, & Tierney, 1997; O'Donnell et al., 2003; Steinhauser et al., 2000). For instance, studies have shown that cancer patients are more likely to accept treatments with a lower possibility of success than physicians, while also overestimating the chances of those treatments working (Kite & Wilkinson, 2002). In one survey, 70% of patients and families with recent ICU experience were willing to receive intensive care again if it meant as little as one additional month of life (Danis, Patrick, Southerland, & Green, 1988).

If the second opinion concurs with the first, the interdisciplinary committee meets with the clinical team and the family to hear their respective opinions, confirms that required prior steps were completed, and determines whether the treating clinicians' claim of lack of benefit "represents a broadly held judgment within the institution rather than an idiosyncratic view of a few clinicians" (Bosslet et al., 2015). If the initial opinion is affirmed, the family is given the opportunity to transfer the patient to another institution. Unlike under the TADA, the family also has the right to an extramural appeal. If transfer is not possible and the family does not pursue extramural appeal—and no alternative providers within the institution can be found—then after an appropriate period of time (usually on the order of seven to ten days) the contested treatment can be withdrawn. As in Texas, this can occur earlier if the family withdraws the objections to forgoing.

The consensus statement also addresses situations where time does not permit such a comprehensive review. After pausing to confirm the facts and identify any potential blind spots—as well as confer with colleagues to verify consensus—clinicians should "explain to the surrogates the reasons for refusing to administer the requested treatment, with the goal of reaching a mutually agreeable decision." (Bosslet et al., 2015) (It is important to note that the presumption here is in favor of *not* providing the treatment in question.) The authors appropriately admit that the relative lack of procedural safeguards may lead to a "higher degree of legal uncertainty" (Bosslet et al., 2015).

Much of the process put forth by the consensus statement is uncontroversial, including second opinions and enlistment of communication experts. Granted, some have criticized the fairness of the process, especially the role of the interdisciplinary committee—made up, as it likely is, of hospital staff and few (if any) community members—as the final arbiter. In one report on TADA, for instance, the interdisciplinary committee agreed with the physician's assessment of lack of benefit over 90% of the time (Fine & Mayo, 2003). The process also requires a rather specific definition of what constitutes medical benefit, and also what does *not* (a critical point which many procedural policies conspicuously omit). It bears reminding that no physician is ever obligated to activate the NBT review process, if the treatment in question is likely to be short-lived or without excessive burden.

The major point of contention is the conclusion of the process, namely, whether in the absence of agreement treatment should be unilaterally withdrawn. Some commentators feel very strongly that it should be. Randall and Downie (2006), for instance, assert that requiring physicians to do whatever patients demand is a relationship for which no similar or parallel model exists. They argue that not only may clinicians withhold NBT; they *should* withhold it. Roy (2004) concurs, asserting that the "ethically critical question" is not whether physicians are justified in discontinuing treatment but rather what ethical justification exists for *continuing* it. Others reach the same conclusion out of respect for physician autonomy (Berlinger et al., 2013), declaring that honoring requests for "futile" treatment makes the physician merely an extension of the patient's wishes, rather than a moral agent in her own right (Brody, 1994; Paris & Reardon, 1992; Tomlinson & Brody, 1990). The British Medical Association (2001) position statement supports this view: "Unless some other justification can be demonstrated, treatment that does not provide net benefit to the patient may, ethically and legally, be withheld or withdrawn and the goal of medicine should shift to the palliation of symptoms."

Others, though, have questioned whether this is the ethical—or wise—thing to do. Some have argued that the best person to determine whether a treatment will benefit a patient is the patient himself (Lantos et al., 1989), and that physicians—while technically knowledgeable—cannot claim *moral* expertise in this area (Veatch, 1994). Truog (2009), addressing specifically the procedures outlined in TADA, argues that providing NBT to the <3% of futility consults that reach the final "letter stage" is preferable to accepting "a law that effectively terminates these conflicts at the expense of systematically undermining important Constitutional and ethical principles."[7]

Specifically within the palliative care community, some have cautioned against so-called "futilitarianism," which refers to the claim that "futility is a sufficient ethical ground for the unilateral withholding/withdrawing of treatment from patients" (Dunphy, 2000). As Burns and Truog (2007) write, "The best solution—although perhaps the most difficult—is to turn our efforts toward tolerating the demands for care that we believe to be futile, and finding ways to better support the emotional needs of each other in those rare cases where we are called upon to provide this care."

Recognizing this diversity of opinion, it is appropriate for an institution to establish its own policy for potentially NBT, which may include the option of unilateral forgoing after all previous steps are completed. Such a policy should stress that attending clinicians are never obligated to invoke it and thus can choose to continue to provide potentially NBT if they believe that the benefit/burden balance is not overwhelmingly poor. By the time unilateral forgoing is a practical consideration, cost should not be a huge issue, as

---

7. This criticism is directed specifically at TADA, which precludes extramural appeal. By contrast, the approach laid out in the consensus statement specifically includes notification of family of their judicial options and thus is not directly susceptible to this criticism.

the vast majority of potential futility disputes either would have been prevented or resolved by following the steps listed previously (Luce & Rubenfeld, 2002).

Such a policy should also permit judicial review, as the consensus statement does. This is crucial to provide a safeguard against bias or discrimination, especially given the internal nature of the interdisciplinary committee that supports the clinician determination the vast majority of the time (at least in Texas).

A policy should also be explicit about what constitutes a minimal quality of life. While patients and their surrogates have the right to determine what the goals of care are, there may be times when the burden is so great so as to not justify continued treatment. By making this explicit, the organization standardizes the approach and also takes responsibility for the definition it has established. Expanding on the consensus statement—and using its language of "inappropriate" treatment—Kon et al. (2016) offer this definition:

> ICU interventions should generally be considered inappropriate when there is no reasonable expectation that the patient will improve sufficiently to survive outside the acute care setting, or when there is no reasonable expectation that the patient's neurologic function will improve sufficiently to allow the patient to perceive the benefits of treatment.

Appropriately, this sets the bar for "benefit" rather low in order to prevent parentalistic value judgments.

Rather than simply putting a policy in place, institutions should also be transparent about their approach. A truly ethical policy should stand up to criticism and provide a solid rationale for its existence. Members of the interdisciplinary committee require training, not only about the components of the policy but also about the specific role that they are tasked with. Simulation of a review can help identify weaknesses in the process, as well as preparing committee members for the emotionally charged task of adjudicating futility disputes. It is one thing to formulate a policy; it is quite another to implement that policy in a specific case, which may well lead to the death of a patient and cause the family profound grief (Harari & Macauley, 2016).

A policy that does not allow for the option—after all prior steps have been taken—of unilateral forgoing is ill-equipped to address the extreme outlier cases that inflict great distress, not only on patients but also on staff. Being asked to provide a treatment that is felt to be "futile" can be very difficult on medical staff, particularly if the treatment is burdensome to the patient. Even if the interdisciplinary committee does not confirm the finding of lack of benefit, a comprehensive process affords the opportunity for staff to share their concerns, thus hopefully attenuating the effects of moral distress (p. 514).

At the same, invoking such a policy—which necessarily reflects an adversarial relationship with the family and a breakdown of communication—should not be done with the frequency of TADA in Texas. If unilateral forgoing became anything other than the rarest of exceptions, this would likely reflect an absence of sufficient preventive steps to preempt potential futility disputes.

The Special Case of CPR

In any discussion of "futile" or nonbeneficial treatment, CPR deserves special mention. One reason is that CPR, alone among all medical interventions, is assumed to be provided unless there is a specific order that it be withheld. As noted earlier (p. 5), one of the paradigmatic shifts in clinical medicine over the last half of the twentieth century was the requirement for informed consent before performing a procedure on a patient. At first glance, then, it may seem odd that there is one procedure—and a rather common one at that—for which the paradigm is reversed.

The reason for this exception is obvious: CPR is an emergent procedure which addresses the final common pathway to dying. Nothwithstanding the relatively few patients who are declared dead by neurologic criteria, patients die from cardiac arrest. In some cases such arrest is foreseen, such as the end result of multisystem organ failure. But in other cases—such as a previously undiagnosed electrical conduction defect in the heart—it could affect previously healthy people.

While it would seem odd to presume treatment wishes related to, say, dialysis—which is usually foreseen and nonemergent—CPR is a unique case. The only alternative to presuming that patients who did not previously refuse the procedure will receive it would be to presume that those who did not previously consent to the procedure *will not*. Given the challenges in getting patients to engage in advance care planning, the mere absence of prior consent is no guarantee of an informed refusal. And while one might reasonably conclude—based on a benefit/burden analysis—that too many patients are receiving CPR, shifting the paradigm to the traditional "opt-in" model would prevent some patients who might benefit from CPR from receiving it, and subsequently surviving. It would also be inconsistent with surveys that show that the majority of Americans would wish to receive CPR, in the absence of a terminal illness (Marco & Larkin, 2008).

One must also take into account the ritualistic status CPR has attained in Western society, such that it almost seems wrong for a patient to go his whole life without receiving it. To allow a patient to die peacefully without pressing on the chest and counting 1-2-3-4-5 seems unprofessional, or even *unnatural*. This cultural norm underscores the need to thoughtfully address goals of care—and the interventions that may or may not be consistent with them—long before a "code is called."

It is worth mentioning the curious path that led to this point. The first report of "closed-chest massage" was published in 1960, showing significant efficacy (Kouwenhoven, Jude, & Knickerbocker, 1960). Seventy percent of patients with *witnessed intraoperative* arrests survived to discharge. The context here is particularly important, given that the arrests to some degree were anticipated—at least insofar as they were known complications of invasive procedures—and thus the team responding to them was both proximate and prepared.

Without supporting data—indeed, without *replication* of the original highly opti-mistic reports (Schneider, Nelson, & Brown, 1993)—the application of CPR soon ex-panded beyond the operating room to the rest of the hospital. It quickly became apparent, however, that the outcomes were not nearly as good. This prompted the AMA to issue recommendations on both the content of advance planning discussions related to CPR, as well as standards for documentation of these discussions. The AMA acknowledged that CPR was the only procedure requiring a physician's order *not* to occur but specifically recommended against CPR in the case of terminal irreversible illness. "Resuscitation in these circumstances," the AMA (1974) concluded, "may represent a positive violation of an individual's right to die with dignity."

In the same year that the *Quinlan* decision and California Natural Death Act began to codify patients' right to refuse unwanted treatments, reports were published of insti-tutional Do Not Recesitate (DNR) policies that followed the AMA's recommendations (Clinical Care Committee of the Massachusetts General Hospital, 1976). These policies allowed patients—and sometimes their physicians without their knowledge—to prevent CPR from occurring. In cases where the patient demanded CPR and the physician felt that it would not be beneficial, there were reports of "slow" or "show" codes (p. 108). This refers to a widely condemned practice of going through the motions of a code so as not to subject a patient to the burden of a procedure that is anticipated to be ineffective (Gazelle, 1998).

In 1983, the much-awaited President's Commission report affirmed the notion of presumed consent, justifying CPR in nearly all circumstances. It made no mention of lim-iting the application of CPR based on inefficacy, as the AMA statement had (President's Commission for the Study of Ethical Problems in Medicine and Biomedical and Behavioral Research, 1983). Over the course of that decade various states began to pass laws gov-erning the documentation and implementation of DNR orders, generally based on the informed refusal of the patient or family. In 1988 the Joint Commission—then known as the Joint Commission for the Accreditation of Healthcare Organizations—began to require each accredited hospital to have a policy related to DNR orders (Rothschild & Hattis, 1988).

As CPR became a universal expectation, the cumulative probabilities of success di-minished. Individual studies have reported slightly different outcomes based on the pre-cise cardiac nature of the arrest, which of course cannot be known in advance. In the largest data set, the American Heart Association estimates the current rate of survival to discharge for in-hospital arrests to be approximately 25% (Mozaffarian et al., 2015). Roughly two-thirds of survivors are ultimately able to return to their previous level of functioning (Peberdy et al., 2003).

The expansion of CPR was not only from the operating room to other hospitalized patients. It also became the norm in the outpatient setting where nearly 400,000 arrests occur in the United States each year. As is the case with in-hospital arrests, survival rates are better if the patient experiences a "shockable rhythm" such as ventricular fibrillation or pulseless ventricular tachycardia. By virtue of the delay in medical attention, however, the odds of survival in the outpatient context are reduced by more than half (Mozaffarian et al., 2015).

While the data is quite clear—and sobering—public perception is more sanguine. This may be due, in large part, to the depiction of CPR in the media. On television, the vast majority of patients who experience cardiac arrest are young, have no pre-existing heart or lung disease, and make a full recovery (Diem, Lantos, & Tulsky, 1996; Portanova, Irvine, Yi, & Enguidanos, 2015). If this is the basis of a patient's understanding of CPR, it would be entirely reasonable to request maximal treatment, especially when the alternative is certain death. Coupled with the lack of appreciation of the burdens associated with CPR—which include rib fractures, internal organ damage, and potential indignity (Peberdy et al., 2003)—it should be obvious that a patient simply saying that he "wants CPR" falls well short of true informed consent.

In the United States, current American Heart Association recommendations are that CPR should be performed unless there is a DNR order, or it is "physiologically futile" (Mancini et al., 2015). The use of the latter term raises the definitional challenges related to futility in general, as exemplified by Kite and Wilkinson's (2002) assertion that "CPR in patients with advanced, progressive cancer who have poor performance status, and irreversible medical problems, can be classified as physiologically futile according to any definition." This is not true, however, because even a patient with advanced cancer and poor performance status could conceivably experience return of spontaneous circulation (i.e., the physiologic goal of CPR). The point Kite and Williamson are trying to make is that CPR will likely not provide *benefit* to patients in those circumstances. To help the patient see this requires thoughtful and nuanced conversation, with recognition of the patient's goals.

Unfortunately, this does not always happen. Studies have shown that CPR decisions for inpatients generally occur in one of four ways. The first is that CPR is not even discussed and the patient is assumed to be "full code." Clearly this pays insufficient respect to the patient's goals and values.

Alternatively, there may be a succinct question along the lines of "If your heart were to stop, do you want us to restart it?" This is extremely misleading, though, as it presumes that the patient's heart *could* be restarted, which is far from certain given the probabilities noted earlier. For this reason, many have started to use the term DNAR (Do Not Attempt Resuscitation) instead, which emphasizes that all the medical team can promise is to *attempt* resuscitation (Pitcher, Smith, Nolan, & Soar, 2009).[8]

A third way CPR is discussed is as part of a menu of options which includes intubation, medications, dialysis, and so on. Without sufficient context, however, this may

8. An alternative term that has been suggested is "Allow Natural Death," or AND. The advantage of this term is that it does not emphasize what *will not* be done (i.e., CPR) or inaccurately suggest that resuscitation will be achieved, if CPR is provided. It is, however, an imprecise term, as much of end-of-life care (e.g., benzodiazepines and synthetic opioids) is not "natural." In many ways, palliative care is dedicated to *not* allowing patients to die "naturally," if that means suffering from pain, air hunger, and so on (Macauley, 2014) (p. 106).

represent abandonment, leaving the patient and his family to choose between modalities that they do not understand. Not surprisingly, this often leading to nonsensical treatment plans such as permitting CPR but not intubation, which is frequently required during or following CPR.

The fourth way CPR is addressed is through repeated questions from multiple providers, attempting to confirm that the code status in the chart truly reflects the patient's wishes (Anderson, Chase, Pantilat, Tulsky, & Auerbach, 2011; Anderson, Pantilat, et al., 2011). This may, however, feel like "badgering," especially when the patient's wishes do not comport with the team's sense of what is appropriate (Billings, 2012). The team may not be so much "confirming" the patient's wishes as attempting to persuade him to change his mind.

Each of these approaches is clearly substandard, often leading to false assumptions, incomplete understanding, and even patient harm. This is clearly not the intent of physicians, however, who work under demanding time constraints and often do not receive adequate training in conducting these complex discussions (Knauft, Nielsen, Engelberg, Patrick, & Curtis, 2005). The end result is increased family stress, anxiety, decisional regret, depressive symptoms, and treatment plans that may be incongruent with the patient's goals of care (Weiner & Essis, 2006).

So what should be done to determine whether to provide CPR to a patient in the event of a cardiac arrest? Beginning with open-ended questions is generally a good approach, but in this case it runs the risk of relying on an overly optimistic perception on the part of the patient. So rather than opening with a query about CPR, it is better to begin with an exploration of the patient's goals in order to frame the outcomes in meaningful terms.

Recognizing the variability in CPR outcomes in relation to patient goals, a graded approach is optimal (Blinderman et al., 2012). Where the benefits and burdens of CPR are uncertain, it should be presented as a plausible option. Before asking whether the patient wants "CPR," it is important to make sure he understands what that term refers to. Cumulative data as to the overall effectiveness of CPR in hospitalized patients should be modified to fit the precise patient circumstance, in order to ensure the patient understands the choice he is making (Ebell, Jang, Shen, Geocadin, & Get With the Guidelines-Resuscitation, 2013).

When the benefit/burden balance is primarily negative, there should be a recommendation against CPR. Of course, some patients might adopt a "nothing to lose" approach (Randall & Downie, 2006), recognizing that successful CPR is the only chance at survival following cardiac arrest. But viewing failed CPR as equivalent to being made DNAR fails to take into account the burdens associated with the former, including rib fractures and internal organ damage. It also overlooks the risk of "successful" CPR leading to an extremely compromised quality of life, which the patient may not find acceptable.

In some cases, the benefit/burden ratio is overwhelmingly negative. There is reliable data that patients with certain serious conditions—such as metastatic cancer, COPD with oxygen dependence, and advanced heart or liver failure—are exceedingly unlikely to ever leave the hospital after attempted CPR, and essentially are never able to live independently again (Stapleton, Ehlenbach, Deyo, & Curtis, 2014). If that prognosis would not be acceptable to the patient, it may be appropriate to take an "informed assent" approach. This involves the same level of disclosure as informed *consent*, but rather than requiring the decision-maker to explicitly authorize forgoing—which feels to some like they are signing their loved one's (or their own) "death warrant"—the clinician makes a recommendation based on the patient's identified goals.

The clinician then invites the decision-maker to accept the recommendation, perhaps using language along the lines of "unless you disagree, we'll proceed with that plan." This is, therefore, stronger than a recommendation, in that it allows the proffered course of action to become the treatment plan in the absence of dissent from the decision-maker. This may lessen the burden that surrogates subsequently carry after making these decisions, which is increasingly being recognized (p. 65). As Curtis (2007) writes, "As a psychologic proposition, informing the patient or family surrogate that they are entitled to accept those recommendations can convey to them the information that the clinicians are prepared to relieve them of unwanted burdens of making life-or-death decisions."

Lest informed assent be written off as parentalistic, it is important to note that this approach is actually more patient-centered—and requires more time—than a simple listing of options and deferring to the patient or family's choice. The plan suggested in the informed assent process should reflect the patient's values in light of the current treatment situation. While the clinical team is well aware of the latter, it takes time, energy, and thoughtful communication skills to ascertain the former. Only when both are known can a plan be proposed and assent obtained.

But what about situations where the patient "will die imminently or has no chance of surviving CPR to the point of leaving the hospital?" (Blinderman, Krakauer, & Solomon, 2012). Blinderman et al. argue CPR should not even be offered because the burdens will far outweigh the benefits.

This position is not without controversy, however. It is one thing to not offer an esoteric procedure that the patient would not normally expect to receive, but CPR has come to be viewed as a universal right. Even advocates of an informed assent approach concede that patients need to be explicitly informed if CPR is not going to be provided (Curtis & Burt, 2007).

In situations such as this, it is best to be open with the patient and family about the treatment plan, framed in terms of the patient's goals. Too often the focus is on procedures such as CPR, and specifically the withholding of those procedures. Excessive emphasis on what will not be done to the patient—such as CPR or intubation—could well leave him wondering what (if anything) *will* be done for him. Framing forgoing CPR as the norm in that particular context—and avoiding negative terms like "do *not* resuscitate"—has been shown to help the patient and family accept the recommended plan

(Barnato & Arnold, 2013). If they want further explanation, the clinician should be able to articulate the reasons for not attempting CPR.

But what if the patient or family demands CPR, despite strong medical recommendations to the contrary? Here it is important to identify the reason for the continued demand. Perhaps there is lingering misunderstanding about the outcomes of CPR that can be clarified. The patient may simply be afraid of dying, highlighting the need for emotional support rather that informational clarification. Alternatively, patients might be worried that if they consent to a DNR order, they might not receive other therapies—short of attempted resuscitation—which could be helpful.

To this, palliative care clinicians often reassure patients that DNR does not mean "Do Not Respond." Studies have shown, however, that patients who are DNR are less likely to receive care that has nothing to do with resuscitation, such as laboratory studies, x-rays, blood transfusions, and even chart entries and physician visits (Beach & Morrison, 2002). A more honest response to patients concerns might be that DNR *should not* mean "Do Not Respond," but occasionally it does. This underscores the need to educate staff on precisely what DNR means and what it does not (Macauley, 2014).

If even after optimal clarification the patient continues to request CPR, Blinderman et al. (2015) suggest referring the case to the ethics committee, for which the previously described model of responding to requests for potentially NBT may be relevant. Yet if the "menu approach" constitutes patient abandonment by its lack of guidance and perspective, then a unilateral DNR approach—especially one where the patient is not even informed that CPR will not be provided—is abandonment of a different sort. It undermines patient trust and may lead down the slippery slope to discrimination based on perceived insufficient quality of life (Mercurio, Murray, & Gross, 2014). It may also place staff in difficult positions, feeling like the patient's or family's wishes are not being respected (Anderson-Shaw, 2003).

The alternative would be to proceed with seemingly "futile" CPR. Some have recommended this, arguing that it may provide reassurance to the family that everything had been done (Truog, 2010). Knowing he was "full code" could also offer comfort to a patient for whom it was important to "go down fighting" (Macauley, 2011).

This proposal can be critiqued on several grounds. Some view it as improperly prioritizing the family's needs over that of the patient (Hanto & Ladin, 2010). Others question whether a patient in cardiac arrest is truly "beyond suffering" (Truog, 2010) and therefore may experience additional burden (Fine, 2010). Futile—or what some might call "sham"—CPR could also feed into public misperceptions about the efficacy of the procedure, as well as call into question physicians' professionalism for doing something they know will not be successful (Gelbman & Gelbman, 2010).

Faced with the choice of either unilaterally withholding CPR—thus damaging one's relationship with the patient and family and potentially heightening their emotional suffering—or engaging in futile CPR, the most can hope for is identifying the "least bad option" (p. 26). In rare cases of true physiologic futility, CPR should not be offered as an option and requests for it met with an explanation for why it has no possibility of benefit.

Further, in exceptional situations where an institution's NBT policy is invoked and the multidisciplinary committee confirms lack of benefit, it would be illogical to unilaterally withhold all LSMT *except* CPR (given the high burden and low probability of success of the latter). The purpose of such a policy is to permit a patient to die in peace, and instituting CPR at the very end would not be consistent with that purpose.

In situations short of "true physiologic futility" or confirmation of NBT—where all attempts to persuade the patient and family to accept DNAR status have been unsuccessful—it can be appropriate to administer CPR that the team feels is highly unlikely to be beneficial. This reflects humility with regard to outcomes, which can never be known with absolute certainty. It also shows respect for the patient's values, even if they differ from the team's own.

The qualifiers noted earlier in relationship to "fast" or "tailored" codes (p. 109) are crucial here. A team may be willing to undertake futile CPR, but once their sense of inefficacy is confirmed by lack of response, resuscitative efforts should immediately cease (Lantos & Meadow, 2011). This will hopefully minimize any risk of additional suffering while still providing the family solace in knowing the patient's wishes were respected.

Return to the Case

While acknowledging the deep devotion of the patient's wife—and the credible evidence that she was offering appropriate substituted judgment—the physicians caring for the patient come to believe that he will never leave the ICU. Consultation with palliative care, clinical ethics, and spiritual care fail to resolve the impasse. The institution's NBT policy deems a minimal quality of life to be "the ability to survive outside the acute care setting," and the physicians elect to initiate the stepwise approach outlined in the policy.

The patient's wife is notified of the process, which underscores the profound concerns of the medical staff. She subsequently relinquishes her demand for "full code" status, and the medical team is willing to continue to provide intensive care based on their perception that the patient is so ill as to no longer be suffering. A few weeks later the patient dies (relatively) peacefully with his wife as it side, without undergoing CPR.

Summary Points

- Whereas the "right to die" movement focused on a patient's right to refuse treatment that the physician might feel obligated to provide, the "futility" movement focused on the physician's right to withhold treatment that a patient is requesting.

- The futility movement was dogged by challenges in definition and implementation. After a flurry of interest in the 1990s, the concept has recently received increasing attention because of escalating health care spending.
- The term "futile" should be reserved for cases of true physiologic futility, where a procedure is incapable of achieving its physiologic goal. Yet even when a procedure might achieve its physiologic goal, this may not bring net benefit to the patient.
- Determining whether a patient will benefit from a procedure requires identification of the patient's goals and values. In situations where a patient is requesting treatments that do not appear consonant with his expressed goals, deeper exploration and expert consultation can often lead to clarity.
- Physicians have an obligation to make treatment recommendations based on the patient's goals. When a procedure is highly unlikely to further those goals, an "informed assent" approach may spare the patient or his surrogate decision-maker additional emotional suffering.
- Institutions should formulate a standardized approach for responding to patient or family requests for treatment that is potentially nonbeneficial. This would involve obtaining a second opinion, consultation with other services, exploring options for transfer, and convening a multidisciplinary committee to assess the degree of benefit.
- There is no obligation to unilaterally withhold treatment that is deemed to be nonbeneficial. Cases in which this is done should be exceedingly rare, and only when the burden to the patient is extreme.
- In situations where CPR is deemed to be physiologically futile, it should not be offered as an option and the patient informed why it will be withheld. If the patient persists in his request for it, the institution's nonbeneficial treatment policy may be invoked.
- In some situations, CPR that is anticipated to be ineffective may still be ethically permissible, out of respect for the patient's values. Resuscitative efforts should continue only so long as to confirm the initial sense that they will not provide benefit.

References

American Medical Association. (1974). Standards for cardiopulmonary resuscitation (CPR) and emergency cardiac care (ECC). *JAMA*, *227*(7 Suppl.), 864–868.

American Medical Association. (2016). Code of medical ethics, annotated current opinions. Chicago: American Medical Association.

American Thoracic Society. (1991). Withholding and withdrawing life-sustaining therapy. *Ann Intern Med*, *115*(6), 478–485.

Anderson-Shaw, L. (2003). The unilateral DNR order—one hospital's experience. *JONAS Healthc Law Ethics Regul, 5*(2), 42–46.

Anderson, W. G., Chase, R., Pantilat, S. Z., Tulsky, J. A., & Auerbach, A. D. (2011). Code status discussions between attending hospitalist physicians and medical patients at hospital admission. *J Gen Intern Med*, *26*(4), 359–366. doi:10.1007/s11606-010-1568-6

Anderson, W. G., Pantilat, S. Z., Meltzer, D., Schnipper, J., Kaboli, P., Wetterneck, T. B., . . . Auerbach, A. D. (2011). Code status discussions at hospital admission are not associated with patient and surrogate satisfaction with hospital care: Results from the multicenter hospitalist study. *Am J Hosp Palliat Care,* *28*(2), 102–108. doi:10.1177/1049909110374352

Barnato, A. E., & Arnold, R. M. (2013). The effect of emotion and physician communication behaviors on surrogates' life-sustaining treatment decisions: A Randomized simulation experiment. *Crit Care Med,* *41*(7), 1686–1691 doi:10.1097/CCM.0b013e31828a233d

Beach, M. C., & Morrison, R. S. (2002). The effect of do-not-resuscitate orders on physician decision-making. *J Am Geriatr Soc, 50*(12), 2057–2061.

Berlinger, N., Jennings, B., & Wolf, S. M. (2013). *The Hastings Center guidelines for decisions on life-sustaining treatment and care near the end of life* (rev. and expanded 2nd ed.). Oxford: Oxford University Press.

Bernstein v. Sup. Ct. Ventura Cty, B212067 (Cal. Ct. App. 2009).

Betancourt v. Trinitas Hospital, No. UNN-C-12-09 (2010).

Billings, J. A. (2012). Getting the DNR. *J Palliat Med, 15*(12), 1288–1290. doi:10.1089/jpm.2012.9544

Blinderman, C. D., Krakauer, E. L., & Solomon, M. Z. (2012). Time to revise the approach to determining cardiopulmonary resuscitation status. *JAMA, 307*(9), 917–918. doi:10.1001/jama.2012.236

Bloche, M. G. (2012). Beyond the "R word"? Medicine's new frugality. *N Engl J Med, 366*(21), 1951–1953. doi:10.1056/NEJMp1203521

Bosslet, G. T., Pope, T. M., Rubenfeld, G. D., Lo, B., Truog, R. D., Rushton, C. H., . . . Society of Critical Care Medicine. (2015). An official ATS/AACN/ACCP/ESICM/SCCM policy statement: Responding to requests for potentially inappropriate treatments in intensive care units. *Am J Respir Crit Care Med,* *191*(11), 1318–1330. doi:10.1164/rccm.201505-0924ST

Boyd, E. A., Lo, B., Evans, L. R., Malvar, G., Apatira, L., Luce, J. M., & White, D. B. (2010). "It's not just what the doctor tells me:" Factors that influence surrogate decision-makers' perceptions of prognosis. *Crit Care Med, 38*(5), 1270–1275. doi:10.1097/CCM.0b013e3181d8a217

British Medical Association. (2001). *Withholding and withdrawing life-prolonging treatment.* London: BMJ Books.

Brody, H. (1994). The physician's role in determining futility. *J Am Geriatr Soc, 42*(8), 875–878.

Burns, J. P., & Truog, R. D. (2007). Futility: A concept in evolution. *Chest, 132*(6), 1987–1993. doi:10.1378/chest.07-1441

Cardona-Morrell, M., Kim, J., Turner, R. M., Anstey, M., Mitchell, I. A., & Hillman, K. (2016). Non-beneficial treatments in hospital at the end of life: A systematic review on extent of the problem. *Int J Qual Health Care, 28*(4), 456–469. doi:10.1093/intqhc/mzw060

Cardoza v. USC University Hosp., B195092 (Cal. Ct. App. 2008).

Chevlen, R. (2009). Confessions of a health care rationer. First Things. Retrieved from https://www.firstthings.com/web-exclusives/2009/08/confessions-of-a-health-care-rationer

Clinical Care Committee of the Massachusetts General Hospital. (1976). Optimum care for hopelessly ill patients. *N Engl J Med, 295*(7), 362–364. doi:10.1056/NEJM197608122950704

Cooke, M. (2010). Cost consciousness in patient care—what is medical education's responsibility? *N Engl J Med, 362*(14), 1253–1255. doi:10.1056/NEJMp0911502

Cook, D. J., Guyatt, G. H., Jaeschke, R., Reeve, J., Spanier, A., King, D., . . . Streiner, D. L. (1995). Determinants in Canadian health care workers of the decision to withdraw life support from the critically ill. Canadian Critical Care Trials Group. *JAMA, 273*(9), 703–708.

Council on Ethical and Judicial Affairs. (1999). Medical futility in end-of-life care. *JAMA, 281*(10), 937–941.

Cruzan v. Director, Missouri Department of Health, 497 261 (S.Ct. 1990).

Curtis, J. R., & Burt, R. A. (2007). Point: The ethics of unilateral "do not resuscitate" orders: The role of "informed assent." *Chest, 132*(3), 748–751; discussion 755–746. doi:10.1378/chest.07-0745

Curtis, J. R., Park, D. R., Krone, M. R., & Pearlman, R. A. (1995). Use of the medical futility rationale in do-not-attempt-resuscitation orders. *JAMA, 273*(2), 124–128.

Danis, M., Patrick, D. L., Southerland, L. I., & Green, M. L. (1988). Patients' and families' preferences for medical intensive care. *JAMA, 260*(6), 797–802.

Diem, S. J., Lantos, J. D., & Tulsky, J. A. (1996). Cardiopulmonary resuscitation on television. Miracles and misinformation. *N Engl J Med, 334*(24), 1578–1582. doi:10.1056/NEJM199606133342406

Drane, J. F., & Coulehan, J. L. (1993). The concept of futility. Patients do not have a right to demand medically useless treatment. Counterpoint. *Health Prog, 74*(10), 28–32.

Dunphy, K. (2000). Futilitarianism: Knowing how much is enough in end-of-life health care. *Palliat Med*, *14*(4), 313–322.

Ebell, M. H., Jang, W., Shen, Y., Geocadin, R. G., & Get With the Guidelines–Resuscitation Investigators. (2013). Development and validation of the Good Outcome Following Attempted Resuscitation (GO-FAR) score to predict neurologically intact survival after in-hospital cardiopulmonary resuscitation. *JAMA Intern Med*, *173*(20), 1872–1878. doi:10.1001/jamainternmed.2013.10037

Emergency Medical Treatment and Labor Act, 42 U.S.C. 1395dd § 1867 (1986).

Fine, R. L. (2010). Is it always wrong to perform futile CPR? *N Engl J Med*, *362*(21), 2035; author reply 2036–2037.

Fine, R. L. (2000). Medical futility and the Texas Advance Directives Act of 1999. *Proc (Bayl Univ Med Cent)*, *13*(2), 144–147.

Fine, R. L. (2009). Point: The Texas Advance Directives Act effectively and ethically resolves disputes about medical futility. *Chest*, *136*(4), 963–967. doi:10.1378/chest.09-1267

Fine, R. L., & Mayo, T. W. (2003). Resolution of futility by due process: Early experience with the Texas Advance Directives Act. *Ann Intern Med*, *138*(9), 743–746.

Garland, A., & Connors, A. F. (2007). Physicians' influence over decisions to forego life support. *J Palliat Med*, *10*(6), 1298–1305. doi:10.1089/jpm.2007.0061

Garros, D., Rosychuk, R. J., & Cox, P. N. (2003). Circumstances surrounding end of life in a pediatric intensive care unit. *Pediatrics*, *112*(5), e371.

Gazelle, G. (1998). The slow code—should anyone rush to its defense? *N Engl J Med*, *338*(7), 467–469. doi:10.1056/NEJM199802123380712

Gelbman, B. D., & Gelbman, J. M. (2010). Is it always wrong to perform futile CPR? *N Engl J Med*, *362*(21), 2035; author reply 2036–2037.

Gillon, R. (1997). "Futility"—too ambiguous and pejorative a term? *J Med Ethics*, *23*(6), 339–340.

Gilmer, T., Schneiderman, L. J., Teetzel, H., Blustein, J., Briggs, K., Cohn, F., . . . Young, E. (2005). The costs of nonbeneficial treatment in the intensive care setting. *Health Aff (Millwood)*, *24*(4), 961–971.

Gramelspacher, G. P., Zhou, X. H., Hanna, M. P., & Tierney, W. M. (1997). Preferences of physicians and their patients for end-of-life care. *J Gen Intern Med*, *12*(6), 346–351.

Harari, D. Y., & Macauley, R. C. (2016). The effectiveness of standardized patient simulation in training hospital ethics committees. *J Clin Ethics*, *27*(1), 14–20.

Hanto, D. W., & Ladin, K. (2010). Is it always wrong to perform futile CPR? *N Engl J Med*, *362*(21), 2034–2035; author reply 2036–2037. doi:10.1056/NEJMc1002983

Helft, P. R., Siegler, M., & Lantos, J. (2000). The rise and fall of the futility movement. *N Engl J Med*, *343*(4), 293–296. doi:10.1056/NEJM200007273430411

Hippocrates. (1959). *The art* (Vol. 2). Cambridge, MA: Harvard University Press.

Hoffman, B. R. (2012). *Health care for some: Rights and rationing in the United States since 1930.* Chicago: University of Chicago Press.

Huynh, T. N., Kleerup, E. C., Wiley, J. F., Savitsky, T. D., Guse, D., Garber, B. J., & Wenger, N. S. (2013). The frequency and cost of treatment perceived to be futile in critical care. *JAMA Intern Med*, *173*(20), 1887–1894. doi:10.1001/jamainternmed.2013.10261

In re Baby K (4th Cir. 1994).

In re Helga Wanglie. Fourth Judicial District, PX-91-283. Minnesota, Hennepin County (1991).

In re Livadas, 080370/30 (NY Supr. Ct. 2008).

In re Quinlan, 70 10 (N.J. 1976).

Kite, S., & Wilkinson, S. (2002). Beyond futility: To what extent is the concept of futility useful in clinical decision-making about CPR? *Lancet Oncol*, *3*(10), 638–642.

Knauft, E., Nielsen, E. L., Engelberg, R. A., Patrick, D. L., & Curtis, J. R. (2005). Barriers and facilitators to end-of-life care communication for patients with COPD. *Chest*, *127*(6), 2188–2196. doi:10.1378/chest.127.6.2188

Kon, A. A., Shepard, E. K., Sederstrom, N. O., Swoboda, S. M., Marshall, M. F., Birriel, B., & Rincon, F. (2016). Defining futile and potentially inappropriate interventions: A policy statement from the Society of Critical Care Medicine Ethics Committee. *Crit Care Med*, *44*(9), 1769–1774. doi:10.1097/CCM.0000000000001965

Kouwenhoven, W. B., Jude, J. R., & Knickerbocker, G. G. (1960). Closed-chest cardiac massage. *JAMA*, *173*, 1064–1067.

Lantos, J. D., & Meadow, W. L. (2011). Should the "slow code" be resuscitated? *Am J Bioeth*, *11*(11), 8–12. doi:10.1080/15265161.2011.603793

Lantos, J. D., Singer, P. A., Walker, R. M., Gramelspacher, G. P., Shapiro, G. R., Sanchez-Gonzalez, M. A., . . . Siegler, M. (1989). The illusion of futility in clinical practice. *Am J Med*, *87*(1), 81–84.

Luce, J. M., & Rubenfeld, G. D. (2002). Can health care costs be reduced by limiting intensive care at the end of life? *Am J Respir Crit Care Med*, *165*(6), 750–754. doi:10.1164/ajrccm.165.6.2109045

Macauley, R. (2011). Patients who make "wrong" choices. *J Palliat Med*, *14*(1), 13–16. doi:10.1089/jpm.2010.0318

Macauley, R. (2014). You keep using that term. *J Palliat Med*, *17*(7), 747–748. doi:10.1089/jpm.2014.0059

Mancini, M. E., Diekema, D. S., Hoadley, T. A., Kadlec, K. D., Leveille, M. H., McGowan, J. E., . . . Sinz, E. H. (2015). Part 3: Ethical issues: 2015 American Heart Association guidelines update for cardiopulmonary resuscitation and emergency cardiovascular care. *Circulation*, *132*(18 Suppl. 2), S383–396. doi:10.1161/CIR.0000000000000254

Marco, C. A., & Larkin, G. L. (2008). Cardiopulmonary resuscitation: Knowledge and opinions among the U.S. general public. State of the science-fiction. *Resuscitation*, *79*(3), 490–498. doi:10.1016/j.resuscitation.2008.07.013

Mason, J. K., & Laurie, G. T. (2011). *Mason and McCall Smith's law and medical ethics* (8th ed.). Oxford; New York: Oxford University Press.

McCrary, S. V., Swanson, J. W., Youngner, S. J., Perkins, H. S., & Winslade, W. J. (1994). Physicians' quantitative assessments of medical futility. *J Clin Ethics*, *5*(2), 100–105.

Meltzer, L. S., & Huckabay, L. M. (2004). Critical care nurses' perceptions of futile care and its effect on burnout. *Am J Crit Care*, *13*(3), 202–208.

Mercurio, M. R., Murray, P. D., & Gross, I. (2014). Unilateral pediatric "do not attempt resuscitation" orders: The pros, the cons, and a proposed approach. *Pediatrics*, *133*(Suppl. 1), S37–S43. doi:10.1542/peds.2013-3608G

Merriam-Webster Inc. (2003). *Merriam-Webster's collegiate dictionary* (11th ed.). Springfield, MA: Merriam-Webster, Inc.

Mozaffarian, D., Benjamin, E. J., Go, A. S., Arnett, D. K., Blaha, M. J., Cushman, M., . . . Turner, M. B. (2015). Heart disease and stroke statistics—2015 update: A report from the American Heart Association. *Circulation*, *131*(4), e29–322. doi:10.1161/CIR.0000000000000152

Murphy, D. J., & Finucane, T. E. (1993). New do-not-resuscitate policies: A first step in cost control. *Arch Intern Med*, *153*(14), 1641–1648.

Natural Death Act, 7, California Health and Safety Code § 7185-95, 1 Stat. (1976).

O'Donnell, H., Phillips, R. S., Wenger, N., Teno, J., Davis, R. B., & Hamel, M. B. (2003). Preferences for cardiopulmonary resuscitation among patients 80 years or older: The views of patients and their physicians. *J Am Med Dir Assoc*, *4*(3), 139–144. doi:10.1097/01.JAM.0000064464.85732.45

Obama, B. (2016). United States health care reform: Progress to date and next steps. *JAMA*, *316*(5), 525–532. doi:10.1001/jama.2016.9797

Oz, F. (1991). *What about Bob?* Burbank, CA: Touchstone Pictures.

Paris, J. J., & Reardon, F. E. (1992). Physician refusal of requests for futile or ineffective interventions. *Camb Q Healthc Ethics*, *1*(2), 127–134.

Peberdy, M. A., Kaye, W., Ornato, J. P., Larkin, G. L., Nadkarni, V., Mancini, M. E., . . . Lane-Trultt, T. (2003). Cardiopulmonary resuscitation of adults in the hospital: A report of 14,720 cardiac arrests from the National Registry of Cardiopulmonary Resuscitation. *Resuscitation*, *58*(3), 297–308.

Persad, G., Wertheimer, A., & Emanuel, E. J. (2009). Principles for allocation of scarce medical interventions. *Lancet*, *373*(9661), 423–431. doi:10.1016/S0140-6736(09)60137-9

Piers, R. D., Azoulay, E., Ricou, B., Dekeyser Ganz, F., Decruyenaere, J., Max, A., . . . Benoit, D. D. (2011). Perceptions of appropriateness of care among European and Israeli intensive care unit nurses and physicians. *JAMA*, *306*(24), 2694–2703. doi:10.1001/jama.2011.1888

Pitcher, D., Smith, G., Nolan, J., & Soar, J. (2009). The death of DNR: Training is needed to dispel confusion around DNAR. *BMJ*, *338*, b2021. doi:10.1136/bmj.b2021

Pope, T. M. (2007). Medical futility statutes: No safe harbor to unilaterally refuse life-sustaining treatment. *Tenn Law Rev*, 1–81.

Pope, T. M. (2009). Legal briefing: Medical futility and assisted suicide. *J Clin Ethics, 20*(3), 274–286.

Pope, T. M. (2010). Legal update. *J Clin Ethics, 21*(1), 83–85.

Pope, T. M. (2011). Legal briefing: Futile or non-beneficial treatment. *J Clin Ethics, 22*(3), 277–296.

Portanova, J., Irvine, K., Yi, J. Y., & Enguidanos, S. (2015). It isn't like this on TV: Revisiting CPR survival rates depicted on popular TV shows. *Resuscitation, 96*, 148–150. doi:10.1016/j.resuscitation.2015.08.002

Prendergast, T. J., & Luce, J. M. (1997). Increasing incidence of withholding and withdrawal of life support from the critically ill. *Am J Respir Crit Care Med, 155*(1), 15–20. doi:10.1164/ajrccm.155.1.9001282

President's Commission for the Study of Ethical Problems in Medicine and Biomedical and Behavioral Research. (1983). *Deciding to forego life-sustaining treatment: A report on the ethical, medical, and legal issues in treatment decisions.* Washington, DC: U.S. Government Printing Office.

Randall, F., & Downie, R. S. (2006). *The philosophy of palliative care: Critique and reconstruction.* Oxford; New York: Oxford University Press.

Rothschild, I. S., & Hattis, P. A. (1988). JCAHO: Accreditation requires DNR policy. *Health Law Vigil, 11*(3), 3.

Roy, D. (2004). Euthanasia and withholding treatment. In D. Doyle (Ed.), *Oxford textbook of palliative medicine* (3rd ed., pp. 84–97). Oxford; New York: Oxford University Press.

Saigal, S., Stoskopf, B. L., Feeny, D., Furlong, W., Burrows, E., Rosenbaum, P. L., & Hoult, L. (1999). Differences in preferences for neonatal outcomes among health care professionals, parents, and adolescents. *JAMA, 281*(21), 1991–1997.

Schenker, Y., Crowley-Matoka, M., Dohan, D., Tiver, G. A., Arnold, R. M., & White, D. B. (2012). I don't want to be the one saying "we should just let him die": Intrapersonal tensions experienced by surrogate decision makers in the ICU. *J Gen Intern Med, 27*(12), 1657–1665. doi:10.1007/s11606-012-2129-y

Schneider, A. P. 2nd, Nelson, D. J., & Brown, D. D. (1993). In-hospital cardiopulmonary resuscitation: A 30-year review. *J Am Board Fam Pract, 6*(2), 91–101.

Schneiderman, L. J. (2011). Defining Medical futility and improving medical care. *J Bioeth Inq, 8*(2), 123–131. doi:10.1007/s11673-011-9293-3

Schneiderman, L. J., Gilmer, T., Teetzel, H. D., Dugan, D. O., Blustein, J., Cranford, R., . . . Young, E. W. (2003). Effect of ethics consultations on nonbeneficial life-sustaining treatments in the intensive care setting: A randomized controlled trial. *JAMA, 290*(9), 1166–1172. doi:10.1001/jama.290.9.1166

Schneiderman, L. J., & Jecker, N. S. (2000). *Wrong medicine: Doctors, patients, and futile treatment.* Baltimore, MD: Johns Hopkins University Press.

Schneiderman, L. J., Jecker, N. S., & Jonsen, A. R. (1990). Medical futility: Its meaning and ethical implications. *Ann Intern Med, 112*(12), 949–954.

Seattle Children's Hospital. (2007). Using the "F" word—when parents and doctors disagree. Retrieved from http://www.prnewswire.com/news-releases/using-the-f-word---when-parents-and-doctors-disagree-52733972.html

Society of Critical Care Medicine. (1997). Consensus statement of the Society of Critical Care Medicine's Ethics Committee regarding futile and other possibly inadvisable treatments. *Crit Care Med, 25*(5), 887–891.

Sprung, C. L., Cohen, S. L., Sjokvist, P., Baras, M., Bulow, H. H., Hovilehto, S., . . . Ethicus Study Group. (2003). End-of-life practices in European intensive care units: The Ethicus Study. *JAMA, 290*(6), 790–797. doi:10.1001/jama.290.6.790

Stapleton, R. D., Ehlenbach, W. J., Deyo, R. A., & Curtis, J. R. (2014). Long-term outcomes after in-hospital CPR in older adults with chronic illness. *Chest, 146*(5), 1214–1225. doi:10.1378/chest.13-2110

Steinhauser, K. E., Christakis, N. A., Clipp, E. C., McNeilly, M., McIntyre, L., & Tulsky, J. A. (2000). Factors considered important at the end of life by patients, family, physicians, and other care providers. *JAMA, 284*(19), 2476–2482.

Strech, D., Synofzik, M., & Marckmann, G. (2008). How physicians allocate scarce resources at the bedside: A systematic review of qualitative studies. *J Med Philos, 33*(1), 80–99. doi:10.1093/jmp/jhm007

Texas Advance Directives Act § 166.046 (1999).

Tomlinson, T., & Brody, H. (1990). Futility and the ethics of resuscitation. *JAMA, 264*(10), 1276–1280.

Truog, R. D. (1992). Beyond futility: Commentary. *J Clin Ethics, 3*(2), 143–145.

Truog, R. D. (2009). Counterpoint: The Texas Advance Directives Act is ethically flawed: Medical futility disputes must be resolved by a fair process. *Chest, 136*(4), 968–971; discussion 971–963. doi:10.1378/chest.09-1269

Truog, R. D. (2010). Is it always wrong to perform futile CPR? *N Engl J Med, 362*(6), 477–479. doi:10.1056/NEJMp0908464

Truog, R. D., & White, D. B. (2013). Futile treatments in intensive care units. *JAMA Intern Med, 173*(20), 1894–1895. doi:10.1001/jamainternmed.2013.7098

Veatch, R. M. (1994). Why physicians cannot determine if care is futile. *J Am Geriatr Soc, 42*(8), 871–874.

Weiner, B. K., & Essis, F. M. (2006). Patient preferences regarding spine surgical decision making. *Spine, 31*(24), 2857–2860; discussion 2861–2852. doi:10.1097/01.brs.0000245840.42669.f1

Wunsch, H., Harrison, D. A., Harvey, S., & Rowan, K. (2005). End-of-life decisions: A cohort study of the withdrawal of all active treatment in intensive care units in the United Kingdom. *Intensive Care Med, 31*(6), 823–831. doi:10.1007/s00134-005-2644-y

Youngner, S. J. (1988). Who defines futility? *JAMA, 260*(14), 2094–2095.

15

Neuropalliative Care

Rather than employ the historicolegal, clinical, and ethical format of other chapters, the diversity of illness within neurology prompts a more condition-based format, with each of the aforementioned considerations addressed in the context of specific conditions. Before proceeding, some basic clinical background is necessary.

Clinical

Perhaps no other field of medicine illustrates the ethical dilemmas occasioned by the explosion of technology more than neurology. Prior to the widespread use of ventilators and medically administered nutrition and hydration (MANH), there was no reason to debate the definition of death or professional obligations toward patients in a so-called "vegetative state." But in the present day, such debates are the basis of court cases, news headlines, and ethical pontification. Diagnostic capability has also greatly expanded, from computerized tomography (CT) to magnetic resonance imaging (MRI) to positron emission tomography (PET) scans. The wealth of clinical information afforded by neuroradiological studies has logically prompted the question of what to *do* with all that information.

Several characteristics of neurologic diseases make providing palliative care somewhat unique. One is their prolonged and variable course, often leading to significant prognostic uncertainty (Oliver & Silber, 2013). Unlike the more predictable trajectory of cancer—which often allows for high functioning through most of the disease course (Teno, Weitzen, Fennell, & Mor, 2001)—neurological illnesses (especially dementia) are often "characterized by unexpected declines and gradual accumulation of impairments" (Dallara & Tolchin, 2014) (Figure 15.1). This demands specific preparation for patients and families alike, as well as grief support in light of the frequent losses they experience.

Some neurological conditions—such as Huntington's disease (HD)—are inherited, making family dynamics more complicated and raising questions about confidentiality

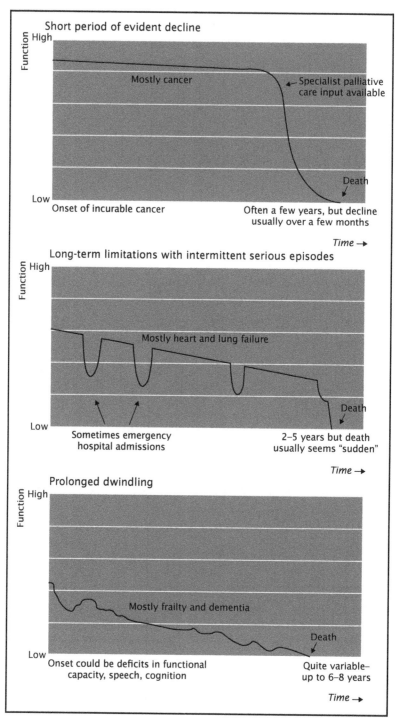

FIGURE 15.1 Typical illness trajectories for people with progressive illness (Murray, Kendall, Boyd, & Sheikh, 2005)

and the duty to warn/inform. Many neurological illnesses also have both cognitive and physical symptoms: dementia in multiple sclerosis (MS), amyotrophic lateral sclerosis (ALS, or Lou Gehrig's disease), and Parkinson's disease (PD), cognitive changes in HD, and hallucinations and other psychological changes in PD. These create specific care needs while simultaneously impairing the patient's ability to communicate and make decisions.

Symptom management is especially challenging, not in the least because certain symptoms often go unrecognized. For instance, the pain burden in PD is equivalent to that in cancer, with 42% of patients experiencing moderate to severe pain in the last month of life. Despite this, over one-quarter of these patients receive no pain medication (Miyasaki et al., 2012). The same is true of ALS, with over half of patients suffering from significant pain, yet nearly one in five receive no analgesia (Goy, Carter, & Ganzini, 2008). Overall, pain is the most common presenting symptom requiring neurological evaluation (Foley & Carver, 2001).

Studies have shown that non-motor symptoms are among the most impacting (Cheon, Ha, Park, & Kim, 2008; Fruehwald, Loeffler-Stastka, Eher, Saletu, & Baumhackl, 2001; Simmons, Bremer, Robbins, Walsh, & Fischer, 2000). ALS, for instance, leads to more frequent demoralization, hopelessness, and suicidal ideation in patients than does metastatic cancer (Clarke, McLeod, Smith, Trauer, & Kissane, 2005).

Despite the frequency of symptoms such as depression, fatigue, and sleep disorders, neurologists often fail to diagnose them. For example, up to half of PD patients with depression are not treated for it (Chen & Marsh, 2013; Lemke et al., 2004). A potential reason is that neurologists' focus is more on the "primary" manifestations of the disorder (Attarian, 2009; Inelmen et al., 2012; Maass & Reichmann, 2013), rather than symptoms that are not specifically neurological.

The complexity of neuropalliative care is not limited to the patient's symptoms. Some conditions create distinctive social work needs (Phillips, Shannon, & Barker, 2008), such as placing a patient with HD—who is often quite young when additional assistance is required—in a nursing home (Dawson, Kristjanson, Toye, & Flett, 2004). Patients' families also have significant emotional and practical needs, such as the increased sense of burden experienced by caregivers of patients with ALS (Clarke et al., 2005). Families caring for patients with dementia report similarly decreased quality of life (Clipp & George, 1993). They also exhibit elevated risk of complicated bereavement after the patient's death (Schulz, Boerner, Shear, Zhang, & Gitlin, 2006).

Advance care planning (ACP) could also be improved. Despite the fact that patients suffering from neurological illness seek assistance in ACP, it often comes too late (Tuck, Brod, Nutt, & Fromme, 2015). Only 20% of patients with advanced dementia, for example, have advance directives (ADs) (Mitchell, Kiely, & Hamel, 2004). The lack of ACP—especially related to foreseeable complications—results in a very high number of patients dying in the hospital. In a recent British study, the majority of patients with MS and nearly half of patients with PD died in the hospital, with only 2.5% and 0.6% of them, respectively, receiving hospice care (Sleeman et al., 2013).

Despite the frequency of neurological illness—over five million Americans suffer from Alzheimer's disease and another one million from PD—palliative care options are slim. The relative dearth of clinicians formally trained in palliative care is addressed later (p. 508), but arguably nowhere does the supply fall so short of the demand than in neurology. Less than 1% of neurologists are board-certified in palliative medicine (American Board of Psychiatry and Neurology, 2016), and <2% of palliative medicine physicians are trained neurologists (Dallara & Tolchin, 2014). Even where palliative care and neurology specialty services are both available, there is often a mismatch in services provided leading to gaps in care (van Vliet et al., 2016).

This would seem the ideal situation for implementation of "generalist palliative care" (Quill & Abernethy, 2013). Given the intensity and chronicity of the patient's illness—as well as internists' decreased comfort managing neurologic disease compared to others, such as cancer (Manu et al., 2012)—neurologists often end up functioning as the primary care physician for the patient (Boersma, Miyasaki, Kutner, & Kluger, 2014). For this reason, the American Academy of Neurology (AAN) recommends that all neurologists "understand, and learn to apply, the principles of palliative medicine" (AAN Ethics and Humanities Subcommittee, 1996). This is especially critical given the complex—and occasionally unique—treatments employed, including monocolonal antibodies for MS or deep brain stimulation for PD.

Yet many neurologists lack adequate education and experience to provide even generalist palliative care (Borasio, 2013; Turner-Stokes et al., 2007). The situation is not likely to improve with barely half of neurology residency programs offering didactic training in palliative care and only 8% offering an elective (Creutzfeldt, Gooley, & Walker, 2009). More promising are recent advances toward integrating palliative care into neurocritical care (Tran, Back, & Creutzfeldt, 2016).

Dementia
Case Study

A fifty-four year old woman is suffering from Alzheimer's disease. Long before she developed dementia, she completed an AD refusing medical intervention if she lost the ability to recognize her family and friends. Now, though, she often wanders out aimlessly at night, constantly rereads the same book passage, draws the same painting every day, and takes great pleasure in eating peanut butter and jelly sandwiches.

This is the sort of life she always dreaded, but now she does not seem sad or depressed. To the contrary, she appears to be remarkably happy. She is also quite amenable to receiving health care.

Should the patient's AD be honored, or does her current level of contentment indicate that at least basic medical care should be provided?

Prior Advance Directives

One of the primary reasons for the emphasis on ACP is the high likelihood of a patient losing decision-making capacity (DMC) by the time critical medical decisions need to be made. In some cases a patient may have possessed DMC right up until the acute illness that prompted her hospitalization, but in others the patient lost DMC long before. One example of the latter is dementia, which can impair DMC in its moderate stages and eliminate DMC in its advanced stages.

The question of how to best prepare in advance for dementia—and address in real time the decisions or values previously voiced—is becoming more pressing with its increased prevalence. In the United States, for instance, one out of nine patients over sixty-five suffers from dementia, and the rate rises to one in three patients over eighty-five. In nursing homes, over half of elderly patients suffer from it (Kamble, Chen, Sherer, & Aparasu, 2009).

The primary effect of dementia is impairment of memory, ultimately leading patients to be unable to recognize their loved ones, have difficulty speaking, experience loss of spatial/temporal orientation, and suffer from incontinence and gait instability (Provinciali et al., 2016). They may also experience neuropsychiatric symptoms such as paranoia, restlessness, insomnia, and delusions. Significant dysphagia may also occur, which necessarily raises the question of MANH (addressed later). Because of the usual age of onset of dementia, patients may also suffer from other conditions such as heart failure and lung disease.

As with any other patient who lacks DMC, the standard approach is to attempt to determine what the patient would have wanted when she did have capacity, relying on ADs, prior statements, or the impressions of loved ones. This may, however, be a challenge, given the low percentage of patients who complete an AD or engage in ACP at all (p. 71).

If the patient did complete an AD at a time of capacity, the appropriate course of action would seem clear. If she refused burdensome life-sustaining medical treatment (LSMT), then it should be withheld out of respect for her autonomy. But what if the patient in her demented state now demonstrates what many would consider an acceptable quality of life? The patient may even be expressing goals and values distinct from those articulated over the course of a lifetime. Specifically, a person who once said (at a time of capacity) that she would never want LSMT if she became unable to recognize her loved ones might in fact appear rather content to live a life that she previously considered unthinkable.

For while the initial stages of dementia—when the patient retains sufficient memory and perspective to recognize what she is losing—can be traumatic, the advanced stages are not necessarily so. A patient with severe dementia may be unaware of what her life is lacking and how it conflicts with the dreams she once had. Some commentators have gone so far as to refer to such patients as the "contented demented" (Orr, 2009).

Firlik (1991) describes just such a patient (whom he refers to as Margo) on whom this section's case is based. There would seem to be two options: either honor Margo's AD and withhold LSMT based on her prior autonomy or provide interventions—especially high-benefit/low-burden interventions, such as antibiotics—that seem consistent with her current best interests. The choice between these two stems from one's view of the relationship of the earlier, competent Margo (who might be called "Margo 1") and "Margo 2," who now suffers from severe dementia.

Margo 2 clearly has impaired DMC, but in contrast to many patients with advanced dementia who are visibly suffering—such as from paranoia or agitation—she is quite happy. And while she cannot offer informed consent for treatment, it would seem wrong to withhold potentially beneficial interventions based on the statements she made in the distant past, perhaps unable to conceive of the possibility that she could be happy in such a state. Viewed in this way, Margo 2 almost seems like an entirely different person than Margo 1, and it would make as little sense to enforce Margo 1's AD on her as it would a stranger's. One might go so far as to claim that doing so would "enslave" Margo 2 to the wishes of Margo 1 (Defanti, 2004).

Precedent exists for honoring incapacitated requests for treatment. Imagine, for example, an elderly patient with underlying lung disease who decides she would rather die than be put on a ventilator, but upon experiencing respiratory distress—and facing death square in the eye—requests to be intubated after all. Certainly, if she retained DMC she would have the right to authorize this. But even if she clearly lacked capacity, it is difficult to imagine a physician declining to do something that the patient is requesting and would clearly be beneficial, based on a previously expressed wish (Dresser, 1995).

At the same time, changing goals based on incapacitated declarations—or merely intimations—would seem to undercut the primary purpose of ACP: to avoid circumstances that are inconsistent with one's values (Newton, 1999). The very reason a patient might have requested limitation of treatments is because she wanted to be remembered as she was at her capacitated best, not in an altered state where she might well be a significant logistical and financial burden on her loved ones. While Margo 2 appears content, for many people—especially those who take active steps to plan their medical future—the thought of reading the same page over and over again, not recognizing one's family, and taking delight in inconsequential things (like peanut butter and jelly sandwiches) might not only be distasteful but even horrifying. Some might even describe it as "worse than death."

So how might one defend enforcing Margo 1's AD? One possibility is to deny that Margo 2 is even a person at all and therefore does not have the rights normally associated with personhood. The basis for this argument is the dependence of personhood on memory (or "psychological continuity") which was proposed as long ago as John Locke (1970): "[A person] is a thinking intelligent being, that has reason and reflection, and can consider itself as itself, the same thinking thing at different times and places." Margo 2 is not only incapable of remembering the values that led her to complete the AD—or even completing it all—she is also unable to build new, sustainable memories, leading some to question whether she should be considered a person in the first place.

Advocates of this view argue that personhood is not an all-or-nothing phenomenon but rather a matter of degree which diminishes consequent to the loss of memory and intentions. The emphasis here is not merely on the persistence of direct psychological connections over time ("connectedness") but rather *continuity*, which implies the persistence of overlapping chains of direct connections that permit a patient to hold stable values and act according to them (Parfit, 1984).

The claim that Margo 2 is not a person—but rather a "surviving non-person" (Defanti, 2004)—certainly yields an elegant conclusion, as there is no longer any autonomy at risk of compromise. Precedent autonomy would be determinative, and treatments could be withheld based on previously stated wishes.

This is an extreme claim, though. It contravenes many religious traditions, which view personhood as inherent in humanity and not dependent on psychological continuity. Advocates for the disabled also note that such a definition could also render patients with severe intellectual disability—not to mention newborns—"non-persons." As such, it seems like a classic case of reasoning from conclusion to premise: if one does not want to honor Margo 2's acceptance of medical treatment, what sort of argument could be devised to support that position?

A less extreme argument for defending the primacy of Margo 1's AD is put forth by Dworkin (1993) in his seminal book, *Life's Dominion*. Autonomy is based on a patient's integrity, which he defines as the expression of "one's own character—values, commitments, convictions, and critical as well as experiential interests—in the life one leads."[1] Once a patient suffers sufficiently profound dementia that her choices are self-contradictory and reflect no "coherent sense of self," the patient is no longer able to act autonomously and the only obligation remaining to that patient is one of beneficence. Dworkin concludes that goals expressed at a time of capacity are determinative, because "it is no kindness to allow a person to take decisions against [her] own interests in order to protect a capacity [she] does not and cannot have." On Dworkin's view, beneficence demands adherence to the previously stated wishes, based on the critical interests the patient once espoused (even if she is no longer able to do so). On this view, allowing Margo 2 to trump Margo 1 would constitute "an unacceptable form of moral paternalism."

Here it is important to note that situations such as the one Firlik (1991) raises and Dworkin (1993) addresses are quite rare. Not all patients with advanced dementia are as contented as Margo 2 is, thus lessening the chasm between previously expressed wishes and what is currently deemed in her best interests. And even if a patient is that contented, it is unlikely—based on population studies—that she filled out an AD, let alone one so specific about refusal of LSMT (Tulsky et al., 2011). If she did, she might well have

---

1. "Experiential" interests—such as enjoying peanut butter and jelly sandwiches—are shared with all sentient creatures, but "critical" interests are inherently human and add coherence and meaning to one's life.

included a caveat permitting her health care proxy to modify the treatment directives based on subsequent developments, such as unforeseen contentment in the context of dementia (Sehgal et al., 1992).

But granting that Margo is one of those exceptional cases, a more even-handed approach to the dilemma is to acknowledge Margo 2 is, indeed, a person. She may be the same person as Margo 1 only now with different values or an at least slightly different person, yet a person nonetheless. Her values have changed, but even if she lacks Dworkin's "critical interests," there remains the obligation to respect her basic human rights. This involves applying either the values the current Margo is expressing, or if these cannot be identified then furthering her best interests. Both approaches lead to the same conclusion in this case: providing basic health care.

This clearly does not mean maximal treatment without concern for burden and outcome. Even defenders of demented patients' right to treatment acknowledge that there may well be instances where best interests dictate limitation of LSMT (Callahan, 1995). But where a patient's apparent quality of life is good, she is acting in such a way as to suggest she would like to continue living that life, and the treatments in question have a positive balance of benefit and burden, these treatments should be provided.

Ultimately, the question of what to do when a person changes in the context of dementia may reflect the understandable fear of many that they may be remembered much differently than how they have spent their entire competent lives. But responding too firmly to this fear of the unknown—such as by denying that patients like Margo 2 are even *persons*—risks "stigmatizing the condition all the more" (Callahan, 1995). Without glamorizing dementia, it is important to recognize the brave humanity of the patients who suffer from it:

> [Dementia patients] are generally more authentic about what they are feeling and doing; many of the polite veneers of earlier life have been stripped away. They are clearly dependent on others, and usually come to accept that dependence; where many "normal" people, living under the ideology of extreme individualism, strenuously deny their dependency needs. They live largely in the present, because certain parts of their memory function have failed. We often find it very difficult to live in the present, suffering constant distraction; the sense of the present is often contaminated by regrets about the past and fears about the future. (Kitwood & Bredin, 1992)

Treating dementia as distinct from other serious illnesses risks both overestimating the burden of dementia—which can be great, although not in cases like Margo's—and also minimizing the possibility that even if someone cannot express "critical interests," they nevertheless can be engaged with the world, in relationships, contented. As Floely (1992) writes, "We too often assume that the absence of emotional display means that no emotion is being experienced. We too often assume that because communication is absent, internal mental process has stopped." Rather than minimizing a patient's worth by virtue of a supposed lack of "critical interests"—or, even worse, denying their very humanity—a more nuanced approach balances previously expressed values with the reality (and possible goodness) of their current life.

Spoon-Feeding

Patients with very advanced dementia often are not able to feed themselves, thus requiring assistance if they are going to take in sufficient nutrition and hydration orally. This typically involves "spoon-feeding" either by loved ones or nursing home staff, which can be an extremely time-consuming process. For this reason, some nursing homes prefer that patients have feeding tubes inserted, even though this has not been shown to prolong survival in advanced dementia (see following section).

Patients, too, may recoil at the thought of being spoon-fed, recognizing it as a signal that their disease has advanced to the point where they lack the ability to make thoughtful decisions about their health care. Since absence of DMC eliminates certain end-of-life options—such as physician-assisted dying (Hertogh, de Boer, Droes, & Eefsting, 2007)—for a patient not dependent on LSMT, forgoing nutrition and hydration represents the only "exit ramp" left, as otherwise the patient could live for a prolonged period. This has prompted some patients to specify in their AD that they do not wish to be spoon-fed.

But what if, once experiencing severe dementia, such a patient no longer actively refuses spoon-feeding? To the contrary, when food is brought to her lips she swallows it, perhaps even showing pleasure in doing so. Should her prior refusal be honored?

Those who believe it should offer arguments similar to those in favor of Margo 1's right to refuse medical treatment. A life spent pursuing one's "critical interests" should not be prolonged if the patient is unable to perform even the most basic activities of daily living. A willingness to chew and swallow food placed in one's mouth is not seen as evidence that she *wants* to eat but merely a primitive reflex akin to that of a newborn baby's. There is no conscious choice, and certainly not one that recognizes one's current quality of life and the respective benefits and burdens of various treatment plans. Dependence on spoon-feeding stands in stark contrast to Margo 2's love of peanut butter and jelly sandwiches, reflecting a quality of life which may not justify intervention based on the patient's best interests. Some take this even further in arguing that not only should patients not be offered spoon-feeding if they previously refused it, but that they should not even be *exposed* to food or drink which might lead them—even if only instinctually—to seek it out.

The request not to be spoon-fed raises the fundamental question of whether feeding is a medical treatment or basic human care. Patients with sufficient DMC—or their surrogates if that is absent—have the right to refuse any *medical* treatment, even one that is life-sustaining (*Cruzan v. Director, Missouri Department of Health*, 1990). But patients (and certainly not their surrogates) are generally not permitted to refuse basic human care, in the form of respect, dignity, cleaning up after having soiled oneself, and so on.

It is a moral obligation to provide such care to a person, especially when that person—although incapacitated—appears to be accepting of it.

To argue that spoon-feeding should be withheld thus requires a claim that it is a medical treatment. Admittedly, it is often provided by medical personnel. And if it is a medical treatment—and the patient has refused it—then provision could constitute battery, or nonconsensual touching (Cantor, 2007; *Morton v. Wellstar Health Sys., Inc.,* 2007).

Yet while spoon-feeding *can* be provided by medical personnel, it does not have to be. It happens each day between a parent and an infant, and not infrequently between nonprofessional caregivers and the elderly. And if spoon-feeding is not deemed a medical treatment, then *failure* to provide it could constitute neglect. As such, it would violate both case law (*Bentley v. Maplewood Seniors Care,* 2014; *In re Conroy,* 1985) and state statutes.

But this is only the case when the person is seeking it. While a demented patient may appear to be voluntarily accepting spoon-feeding, in severe cases she may only be *reflexively* accepting it. To attribute volition to a primitive reflex is to posit a thoughtful assessment of spoon-feeding that may be absent. It is often unclear, then, whether volition is involved in a patient's accepting of spoon-feeding.

It is precisely because of this uncertainty that advance proscriptions on spoon-feeding should not automatically be honored, without thoughtful evaluation. To do so risks falling down the slippery slope, especially given the inherent vulnerability of patients with dementia. Recalling the warning against assuming that because "communication is absent, internal mental process has stopped" (Foley, 1992), might it be that the patient actually enjoys eating but is simply not able to express it? And if one asserts an obligation to forgo spoon-feeding for demented patients who previously refused it in an AD, is it that great a leap to do the same for patients without an AD who "surely would have refused" it if they had engaged in ACP? And how much might the labor-intensiveness—which incurs a burden on caregivers, whether family or staff—contribute to a conclusion that spoon-feeding is not really ethically required?

Ultimately, as was the case with prior ADs requesting limitation of treatment, the context is determinative. To say that a patient with dementia is unable to feed herself provides no context as to whether that patient seems to experience any pleasure in eating and drinking, or in any other aspect of life. A patient who requires prompting to eat but then seems to enjoy it might still value some degree of human interaction, as well as the life she is currently living.

Conversely, a patient who is not responsive in any way and for whom only a primitive oral reflex allows the opening of one's mouth and swallowing of whatever is placed within it is expressing no such value in eating (or perhaps any other aspect of life). Compelling such a patient to eat or drink—especially when she previously expressed values deeming such a life of insufficient quality—could be considered invasive and unwanted.

Striking this balance both honors the right of patients to receive basic human caring and also spares them the indignity and invasiveness of being maintained on the basis of only a primitive reflex. So while it would be imprudent to promise a patient that her advance refusal of spoon-feeding will automatically be honored, she can be assured that her overall quality of life will be taken into consideration, and she will not be fed if swallowing is merely a reflex absent—as is the rest of her life—any pleasure.

For those who would not want to be fed even when they evidence pleasure in the process (akin to the Margo 2 of the LSMT example), it is important to note that there are other "exit ramps"—admittedly, somewhere in the distance—to living in such a compromised state. These include forgoing burdensome LSMT such as CPR and mechanical ventilation, which even the staunchest advocates of Margo 2 likely could not justify.

Medically Administered Nutrition and Hydration in Dementia

The last issue to address in relation to dementia is MANH. Some patients—even with the option of spoon-feeding—are unable to effectively and safely take in sufficient nutrition and hydration to survive. It would appear logical to simply insert a nasogastric or gastrostomy tube in order to provide this, which would seem to address the problems of dehydration and starvation, thus making possible prolonged survival. This also spares the patient's caregivers the time- and labor-intensive task of spoon-feeding.

The primary issue here is clinical rather than ethical: patients whose dementia is so advanced as to prevent safe oral intake do not derive benefit from MANH. The likely reason that oral feeding was deemed insufficient and unsafe was that the patient was aspirating either directly (i.e., food or liquid went directly into her lungs, rather than stomach) or indirectly (i.e., food or liquid was regurgitated from her stomach back up and into her lungs). While MANH might reduce the volume or severity of direct aspiration of food or drink, it does nothing to prevent the patient from directly aspirating oral secretions (McClave & Chang, 2003), nor from indirectly aspirating (which would likely be worsened by increased volume infused into the stomach).

In addition, enteral MANH incurs a symptom burden and risk of complications. A temporary nasogastric tube is unpleasant both when it is being inserted as well as while it is maintained (Farrington, Bruene, & Wagner, 2015). This discomfort might naturally prompt a patient—especially one whose dementia prevents her from appreciating the "need" for the tube—to attempt to remove it, thus necessitating physical restraint. The ongoing risk of aspiration—either indirectly or perhaps also directly if the tube were to become displaced—then requires the use of pulse oximetry to permit timely response to any aspiration event (p. 189). So not only is the patient not permitted to eat; she is restrained in bed and not permitted to move around.

While a gastrostomy tube does not incur the same level of ongoing discomfort or risk of becoming dislodged, there are other risks associated with it. The surgical procedure required to place it may cause complications related to anesthesia, infection, and incorrect placement. Patients with memory deficits may not even recall it having been placed, leading them to attempt to remove it (which is much more serious than pulling out a nasogastric tube).

In other cases, such an increase in symptom burden and risk of complications might be offset by significant benefits. But for patients with severe dementia, MANH does not improve nutritional status nor prevent pressure ulcers. Most importantly—and rather counterintuitively—it also does not prolong life.

This has been clearly documented by multiple studies (Finucane, Christmas, & Travis, 1999; Sampson, Candy, & Jones, 2009; Teno et al., 2012) and can partly be explained by the heightened risk of complications. It is also important to recognize that dementia is a terminal illness, and by the time it has become so severe as to preclude oral feeding, the patient has reached the last stage of her life.

Despite the overwhelming empirical evidence, however, physicians still frequently overestimate the potential benefit of MANH in conditions such as dementia (Hanson et al., 2008). Recent professional position statements have attempted to address this (Mitchell et al., 2009). In particular, the "Choosing Wisely" campaign has highlighted interventions whose burdens outweigh their benefits, among them MANH in the context of severe dementia (American Academy of Hospice and Palliative Medicine, 2013). In such cases, "oral assisted feeding" is the recommended alternative, which should be evaluated thoughtfully as previously described.

When faced with a patient who cannot safely and effectively eat—and after being informed that MANH does not confer a survival benefit—families may wonder what choice is left to them. Here it is important to reassure them that, properly managed, forgoing MANH is not painful or uncomfortable (Pasman et al., 2005). Reviewing the importance of optimal oral care and the evolutionary protective mechanisms associated with dehydration (p. 186) may also be helpful. It is also important to clarify that MANH is classified as a medical treatment, which ethically and legally may be limited like any other medical treatment (*Cruzan v. Director, Missouri Department of Health*, 1990).

Despite the clinical ineffectiveness of MANH in the context of dementia—and the ethical permissibility of forgoing it—there may yet be instances when the patient's family requests it. Perhaps they do not accept the counterintuitive conclusion that it does not prolong life, which should prompt further discussion of the clinical impact of feeding tubes.

Alternatively, religious views may be involved that seem to mandate the use MANH. For instance, the Ethical and Religious Directives of the Roman Catholic Church state that "in principle, there is an obligation to provide patients with food and water, including medically assisted nutrition and hydration for those who cannot take food orally" (United States Conference of Catholic Bishops, 2009). The context in which this statement was made is crucial, however. Ideally the clinician will be able to engage the family in discussion from within their religious tradition, exploring ways that they can remain faithful both to the Church and to the patient.

The family may also be understandably reluctant to do anything that might even resemble "starving" their loved one, or simply not doing everything possible to keep her alive for another day. Exploring cultural bases for their request may identify worthy avenues of exploration (p. 481). Reframing language—such as to avoid use of the heavily connotative term "feeding tube"—may also be helpful.

Ultimately, the family may simply need some time to come to grips with the situation, forcing the medical team to choose whether to "take a stand" and decline to insert a gastrostomy tube or accede to the family's request. Here the determining factors include the potential burden of the procedure incurred by the patient as well as the subsequent likelihood that the family will consent to withdrawing treatment. An appropriate middle ground may to offer a time-limited trial of MANH in order to gauge efficacy and burden (p. 118). Before proceeding, it is important to acknowledge the often greater emotional burden involved in withdrawing rather than withholding, despite their ethical equivalence (p. 156).

Return to the Case

While not disputing that Margo's current DMC is severely compromised and that she is espousing radically different goals than she once did, the fact remains that she is a person with basic human rights. These extend to high-benefit/low-burden medical interventions, such as antibiotics for infection. To administer these is not a violation of her autonomy; to the contrary, forgoing them would amount to a denial of her humanity.

A DNAR order is placed in Margo's chart to spare her excessive burden, but less invasive modalities—such as antibiotics—are used, as necessary.

Over the next two years, her condition declines to the point where she no longer engages in favorite activities and can no longer feed herself.

The nursing home where she resides recommends placement of a gastrostomy tube, but recognizing the pleasure Margo takes in eating, the family chooses to emphasize spoon-feeding. Although it is labor intensive, Margo seems to enjoy it.

Gradually, though, her pleasure seems to lessen, and swallowing food placed in her mouth appears more reflexive than voluntary. The nursing home again raises the option of a gastrostomy tube, and the family again refuses, but this time for a different reason. Whereas before they opted for a more pleasurable method of providing nutrition and hydration, they now recognize that Margo has reached the end of her life. A gastrostomy tube would add burden rather than time to her life, and thus they opt for forgo nutrition and hydration altogether.

Margo does not appear to notice this shift, and with optimal oral care provided by hospice, she dies comfortably approximately ten days later, with her family at her side.

Disorders of Consciousness
Case Study

A twenty-four-year-old woman experiences cardiac arrest, and by the time circulation is reestablished she has experienced significant oxygen deprivation to her brain. Her clinical exam is consistent with unresponsive wakefulness syndrome, commonly referred to as a vegetative state. As less than thirty days have passed, it is not yet classified as "persistent."

Her prognosis is nevertheless grim, with minimal probability of meaningful neurological recovery. She is currently dependent on the ventilator but is likely to wean from it over the next several days.

The team meets with the family to discuss the goals of care. The patient did not complete an AD, which is not uncommon for someone her age. The family does not recall her saying anything about what she would want in such a situation.

When the team raises the possibility of limiting LSMT, the family responds very negatively. They mention how young she is, and how she seems to be getting better because she's opening her eyes more frequently.

The team is unsure how to proceed.

Consciousness has two primary components: arousal (also called alertness) and awareness (which includes cognition, memory, and intention). In most physiologic states, these two are positively correlated, as noted in Figure 15.2. However, there are certain situations when this is not so, such as "vegetative" and minimally conscious states.

A vegetative state is defined as a "clinical condition of complete unawareness of the self and environment, accompanied by sleep-wake cycles with either complete or partial preservation of hypothalamic and brainstem autonomic functions" (Multi-Society Task Force on PVS, 1994). In other words, the patient can open her eyes but will not track objects, respond to stimuli, or in any other sense be aware of her surroundings.

Such states are subclassified based on the duration a patient has been in one. "Persistent" is a diagnosis, specifying that the patient has been vegetative for at least thirty days. "Permanent," on the other hand, is a prognosis, predicting that the patient will always be in such a state. To meet this criterion, following a nontraumatic (e.g., anoxic) brain injury a patient must be in a vegetative state for at least three months. Given the increased likelihood of improvement after a traumatic injury, twelve months is required in such cases to justify the declaration of permanence.

The term "PVS" is often used as an abbreviation for persistent vegetative state, but this is problematic on several levels. In the first place, in practice it is often applied indiscriminately to describe a vegetative state of any duration. It is also imprecise, given that "P" could stand for either persistent or permanent. Third, there remains a

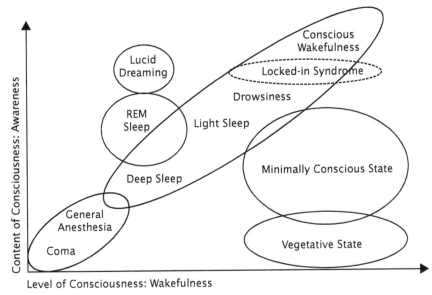

FIGURE 15.2 Stages of consciousness based on levels of awareness and wakefulness (Gosseries et al., 2011)

possibility—however slim—that a patient in a "permanent" vegetative state may yet recover. The AAN consensus statement acknowledges that over 6% of patients who qualify for a diagnosis of "permanent vegetative state" after traumatic injury—and a lower percentage after nontraumatic injury—eventually recover consciousness (Multi-Society Task Force on PVS, 1994). Finally, any term that uses the adjective "vegetative" is viewed by many as pejorative, as if the patient were being called a *vegetable*.[2]

For all these reasons, a more preferable term is "unresponsive wakefulness syndrome" (UWS) (Laureys et al., 2010). It avoids any inaccurate modifiers or negative connotations and better describes the wakefulness that can lead some to falsely infer awareness.

UWS has garnered significant public attention. The famous case of Terri Schiavo (p. 11) brought the condition into the national spotlight, as her parents contested the medical opinion that she was truly unaware of her surroundings (and produced edited video recordings to "prove" this). There have also been many reports of patients "recovering fully" for prolonged unresponsive wakefulness (Andrews, 1993), some of which may represent initial misdiagnoses.

More fundamentally, application of newly developed radiological techniques has called into question the fundamental belief that patients diagnosed with UWS are entirely unaware (Cruse et al., 2011; Laureys et al., 2010). Despite meeting clinical criteria for UWS, some patients were shown on functional MRI to manifest small

---

2. The actual derivation of the term is from Aristotelian categories, whereby vegetables were acknowledged to have the abilities of growth and reproduction, animals the additional abilities of locomotion and decision-making, and only humans capable of higher rational thinking.

increases in regional brain blood flow after being asked to imagine favorite activities, such as playing tennis (Chennu et al., 2014). Awareness was thus not entirely absent, despite the patients' inability to display this to others. This suggests these patients might have actually been in a minimally conscious state (MCS), which describes "a condition of severely altered consciousness in which minimal, but definite, behavioral evidence of self or environmental awareness is demonstrated" (Cranford, 2002).

The presence of awareness may not, however, be good news. A state of unresponsive wakefulness is clearly tragic, but at least it does not involve active suffering. The fact that the patient is not aware of what she has lost in life could be a "blessing in disguise." By contrast, a patient in MCS is aware—at least on some level—of what is going on around her yet is unable to interact or even process all that information. The patient could therefore be actively suffering, but the medical team has no way to verify, measure, or ensure adequate treatment of that suffering. The impetus to forgo LSMT may therefore be *greater* in MCS than UWS.

Another ethical issue is the role of pain management in UWS. According to the AAN, patients in a "vegetative" state are unable to experience pain, which requires some level of consciousness and cortical integration (Multi-Society Task Force on PVS, 1994). This conclusion influences acute management because opioids themselves can depress level of consciousness. Withholding them can, therefore, make neurological examination more straightforward, avoiding their confounding effects on the patient's awareness. Yet given the patient's inability to report suffering, it is impossible to know precisely what she is experiencing.

Such uncertainty impacts the overall plan of care. Upon diagnosing a patient with UWS, physicians may well recommend forgoing LSMT. The patient's quality of life is essentially absent, given that the patient is thought not to be able to interact with—or even perceive—the world around her. She cannot experience pleasure, after all, or even pain.

But what if the family disagrees with the recommendation? Perhaps they are concerned about misdiagnosis or are hoping for a miracle (p. 490). Or maybe they just cannot bear to "let her go today," and thus defer the decision for another day, and then another. As noted earlier (p. 191), not making decision to withdraw a treatment already in use is practically equivalent to deciding to continue it. There is no way to know how long the family will continue to defer that decision.

In response, rather than focusing on absent quality of life, clinicians may cite the negative aspects of continued survival, framed in terms of suffering. Certainly the inability to interact with others is deeply unfortunate, but if the AAN's position is accepted, the patient is not actively suffering because she has no awareness of her current condition. Shifting the emphasis from lack of awareness to unnecessary pain may be an example of "playing both sides against the middle," with the underlying goal being to convince the family to withdraw support.

Rather than being manipulative, concern for suffering may reflect the physician's legitimate uncertainty. Studies have shown that the majority of physicians believe patients in UWS can experience pain, or at least are concerned that they might (Demertzi et al.,

2009). This may explain the use of standard symptomatic treatment (such as opioids) at the end of life, despite the logical conclusion from the AAN's statement that this is unnecessary.

The most that can be said with certainty is all available evidence points to an inability to experience pain. So rather than standing on principle—which, as is evident from recent functional MRI studies, can be modified over time—it is reasonable to act out of caution and proper humility as to whether the patient truly can experience pain (or even whether the diagnosis of UWS is correct). In the end, it is better to overtreat some patients who are not able to suffer than undertreat even one who is. Concern for pain should not be used to induce families to withdraw support, though. The appropriate immediate response to potential pain is analgesia, not forgoing LSMT.

The concept of the "window of opportunity" (p. 317) is also relevant to UWS. Often the insult leading to UWS renders the patient critically ill and initially dependent on mechanical ventilation. Forgoing this would therefore quickly lead to the patient's death. This is also, however, a time of diagnostic and prognostic uncertainty, often leading the family to continue treatment until greater clarity is achieved.

By the time this has occurred, patients are often able to breathe on their own, dependent only on MANH. The question, then, is whether to forgo MANH, which even though it is clearly considered a medical treatment (*Cruzan v. Director, Missouri Department of Health*, 1990) may be emotionally very difficult for families to forgo. With provision of MANH, patients in UWS—especially younger patients, as in the landmark case of Karen Ann Quinlan (*In re Quinlan*, 1976)—can survive for very long periods. This decision may also be influenced by the family's religious beliefs (p. 494).

As always, the appropriate approach to a situation where the patient lacks DMC is to apply substituted judgment. Ideally, the patient would have filled out an AD specifying her wishes, or at least specifically authorized an agent to make decisions regarding MANH. Here it is important to recall that while the *Cruzan* case deemed MANH a medical treatment that may be limited, it also supported states' rights to require "clear and convincing evidence" that the patient would not want to receive it.

In all probability, though, the patient has not completed an AD. Some have, therefore, argued that—based on population surveys showing that the majority of people would not want MANH in UWS (Blendon, Benson, & Herrmann, 2005)—treatment may be forgone based on the best interest standard. Others taken it even further, asserting that there should be a *presumption* against providing LSMT, unless there is clear evidence the patient would have wanted it (Davis, 1993).

This takes the matter too far, however. Especially when a patient is thought not to be suffering, it is appropriate to grant additional time and latitude to families in decision-making. The presumption toward more treatment rather than less preserves options. Intermediate steps—such as a DNAR order—can help address staff moral distress and concerns for utilization of scarce resources. As the family comes to accept the patient's condition and prognosis, they will hopefully be able to apply her goals and values to the decision at hand.

If the family continues to request maximal treatment that does not appear in keeping with the patient's wishes, an institution's nonbeneficial treatment policy (chapter 14) may need to be utilized.

Return to the Case

The team is well aware of how grim the patient's prognosis is, which the family is struggling to accept. The team should also acknowledge the uncertainty about the patient's prognosis, and the fact that the patient was up until recently a perfectly healthy young woman. That the family needs to time to come to grips with the situation is far from surprising.

It is clear that forgoing all LSMT is not an option at this time. But that does not mean that maximal treatment is appropriate, and thus the team broaches the possibility of withholding CPR in the event of cardiac arrest. Even though—given her UWS—she should not "suffer" from receiving CPR, it would certainly be difficult for the family to watch and the staff to administer. Even if CPR is "successful," it would likely result in even more compromised brain function. The family agrees to a DNAR order.

The team also sensitively identifies the "window of opportunity," without using the macabre term. The family acknowledges that limiting treatment later might be more difficult than doing so now—as eventually this will involve forgoing MANH—but cannot bring themselves to withhold LSMT at this time.

Over the next few days the patient weans from the ventilator. As a young, previously healthy person, she is hemodynamically stable. In the absence of a decision to forgo MANH, a gastrostomy tube is placed. No longer requiring hospital care, the patient is transferred to a nursing home, where discussions continue about how long to administer MANH.

Amyotrophic Lateral Sclerosis
Case Study

After experiencing weakness for several months, a sixty-three-year-old woman is diagnosed with ALS. She has always been fiercely independent and is extremely realistic. She tells her family that she would never want to rely on machines or devices. In conversations with her neurologist she expresses a wish to live "on her own terms" for as long as she can, but at whatever point she cannot breathe or eat independently, she requests only comfort measures.

Her quality of life at this point is so good, however, that her physician feels that it is too early to have an end-of-life conversation. A palliative care consultation is requested.

ALS—better known as Lou Gehrig's disease or motor neurone disease—is an incurable, progressive disorder. It affects both upper motor neurons (causing spasticity, slowed movements, poor dexterity, pseudobulbar affect, and pathologic reflexes) as well as lower (causing weakness, atrophy, fasciculations, reduced tone, and hyperreflexia) (Elman et al., 2007). Five thousand new cases are diagnosed each year in the United States, with a likely survival of three to five years from diagnosis (Strong & Rosenfeld, 2003).

ALS was the focus of the earliest neuropalliative care literature (Kristjanson, Nelson, & Henteleff, 1987). This included an exploration of how to break the news of the diagnosis to the patient as well as symptomatic treatment for respiratory insufficiency, dysphagia, impaired communication, depression, spasticity, pain, and pseudobulbar affect. Given the complexity of the condition, palliative care is now recommended for all patients from the time of diagnosis (Oliver et al., 2016).

From an ethics perspective, ALS represents a specific application of ACP related to declines in respiratory and swallowing function. With regard to the former, thoughtful exploration of the use of both non-invasive (e.g., bilevel positive airway pressure) and invasive ventilation (i.e., via tracheostomy) needs to occur early on in the course of the illness. This topic should also be revisited frequently, as patients not uncommonly are willing to accept more intensive modalities later in the illness than they had originally predicted, as they adapt to a less independent life and understandably wish to delay death.

In anticipation of impaired swallowing function, the use of MANH must also be explored. Unlike patients with dementia for whom a gastrostomy tube does not prolong life, ALS patients can often be sustained for long periods on MANH.

In many ways, the same approach to breaking bad news and establishing goals of care for any other terminal illness is also applicable to ALS. Is noninvasive ventilation a bridge to recovery from a temporary respiratory illness or to tracheostomy if that becomes necessary? Will MANH be used to minimize the risk of aspiration while still allowing eating for pleasure, as the sole source of hydration and nutrition once dysphagia becomes severe, or not at all?

ALS is rather unique in one respect: unlike many other neurological conditions which entail some cognitive involvement—such as PD and dementia—patients with ALS remain largely cognitively intact, even as they watch their condition deteriorate along a well-defined and inexorable course.[3] This predictability allows for specific ACP based on the anticipated trajectory. For instance, if a patient is willing to accept a gastrostomy tube, it may be wiser to move ahead with this sooner rather than later, in order to optimize nutritional status and preserve respiratory function (Tsou, Karlawish, McCluskey, Xie, & Long, 2012). Both practical and emotional considerations must also be discussed, as tracheostomy and mechanical ventilation require significant ongoing care and

---

3. Some recent studies, however, have begun to note increased incidence of cognitive and behavioral impairments in ALS patients (Khin, Minor, Holloway & Pelleg, 2015), underscoring the need for a thoughtful evaluation of DMC and providing maximal supports in decision-making.

monitoring, ultimately raising the question of when—if ever—compassionate extubation might occur.

Physician-assisted dying (PAD, p. 348) is also a consideration for many patients with ALS. In a recent Dutch study nearly one-third of ALS patients requested either euthanasia—which is legal in the Netherlands—or PAD, and over two-thirds of those who did ended up dying by this method (Maessen et al., 2014). In the United States, the percentage of patients with ALS who request PAD exceeds that of cancer patients (Oregon Health Authority, 2017; Wang et al., 2016). However, by the time a patient's life expectancy qualifies her for PAD she may be too weak to "self-administer" the lethal dose, as required by law.

Return to the Case

When it comes to end of life conversations, "It's always too early until it's too late" (Byock, 2012). The palliative care consultant delves deeply into the patient's goals and values, actively listening to the patient's hopes and fears. The consultant finds that she is addressing her diagnosis straightforwardly and courageously, which is admirable. ALS is a terminal disease, and the patient clearly has sufficient DMC to refuse LSMT.

At the same time, the gradual and largely predictable course of ALS may permit additional discoveries, and also perhaps a change of heart. What she could never imagine living without may—when the alternative becomes not living at all—take on less importance.

Rather than questioning her current decision, the palliative care consultant opts to keep the lines of communication open. Given the balance of benefits and burdens in attempting CPR, a DNAR order is instituted with the patient's consent. But rather than a blanket Do Not Intubate order, the consultant recommends focusing on context. Clearly the patient would not want to be intubated if she will never regain her ability to breathe independently, but the consultant asks if she would be willing to accept it for a short period to remedy a transient problem, such as pneumonia. The patient had not foreseen that possibility and said she is willing to let her agent (her husband) make that decision when the time comes.

The question of MANH is similarly complex. There may come a point where she is still able to eat and drink but not in sufficient quantities as to maintain her nutritional status. If she would consider the option of a gastrostomy tube in that situation, earlier intervention may help maintain a higher quality of life over time. At the same time, ceasing to use an indwelling gastrostomy tube would be a very emotional decision.

Since currently the patient is able to eat and drink safely, the consultant does not press for an answer. He and the patient make a plan to revisit that question at her next visit, and she is appreciative for the opportunity to express herself and be heard.

Acute Spinal Cord Injury
Case Study

A thirty-four-year-old woman suffers a high spinal cord injury in a diving accident, leading to quadriplegia and temporary need for mechanical ventilation. At first she seems withdrawn, in a state of shock over what has happened to her. Over the next forty-eight hours, though, she appears increasingly angry and frustrated. Her family notes that she has always been an avid athlete and probably cannot conceive of a life where she cannot use her arms or legs.

She unable to speak because of the endotracheal tube. But whenever the team attempts to engage her in discussion, she mouths what appears to be "Let me go!" over and over again.

Her family is grief-stricken and has attempted to buoy her spirits, but to no avail. They want her to survive, but they also want to respect her wishes.

A palliative care consultation is requested.

One of the most challenging situations in neuroethics is that of a patient who sustains a high spinal cord injury (SCI), leading to quadriplegia. In many cases, the patient may have been extremely healthy prior to the injury. Suddenly faced with a life of extreme—perhaps complete—dependence on others, with so many dreams now seeming unachievable, it is difficult hard to understand why a patient might refuse treatment aimed at prolonging her life. This dilemma has even been addressed in popular media (Amenabar, 2004; Eastwood, 2004).

Palliative care is necessary at extremely difficult times like this, to support both the patient and her loved ones. Acknowledging and normalizing the patient's response—and being willing to enter into the intense grief the patient must be feeling at that time—are imperative. Explaining (often repeatedly) what is being done to the patient and the reasons behind it can lessen the sense of powerlessness the patient is feeling. Placing the patient's injury in context—and walking the fine line between realistic expectations and false hopes—is critical.

But what if despite optimal palliative care the patient expresses a strong desire to forgo LSMT? Patients with sufficient DMC clearly have the right to refuse any treatment, including one that is life-sustaining (p. 9). This logically raises the question of whether a patient who just incurred SCI possesses sufficient DMC to make this irrevocable decision. This would require that she understand her condition and prognosis, appreciate the consequences of her decision, and reason from the question to the conclusions (p. 58).

There are many reasons why these necessary components may not be present. Grief and reactive depression are natural responses to such a catastrophic event (Patterson, Miller-Perrin, McCormick, & Hudson, 1993). Medical factors—such as electrolyte abnormalities or hemodynamic instability—may compromise a patient's ability to assimilate and apply information. Even the ICU environment itself—with attendant sensory overload and sleep deprivation—has been shown to compromise DMC (Gelling, 1999).

Given the acute change in her condition and the profound limitations on her function, the patient may not be able to fully appreciate the potential for recovery or acceptable quality of life (Caplan, Callahan, & Haas, 1987). She might assume that patients suffering from paralysis are likely to get divorced or are unable to continue working. She might anticipate that whatever depression she is currently experiencing will continue to worsen, perhaps even leading to suicidal ideation.

Studies, however, have debunked assumptions about increased divorce rates (El Ghatti & Hanson, 1975) and inability to work (Siegel, 1969). And while it is true that rates of depression (Frank, Elliott, Corcoran, & Wonderlich, 1987) and suicide (Bombardier, Richards, Krause, Tulsky, & Tate, 2004) are increased in the SCI population, the vast majority of these patients suffer from neither. In fact, in one study, 90% of patients with SCI reported that they were glad to be alive (Whiteneck, Carter, & Charlifue, 1985).

Just as acceptance of CPR based on television depiction falls short of informed consent (p. 380), so too may rejection of LSMT after SCI—if based on an unrealistically negative sense of one's future quality of life—fall short of informed refusal. Physicians may not recognize this, however, because many might feel that the choice is logical. Moreover, they might anticipate making the same choice themselves in similar circumstances. In a recent study, only 18% of emergency department personnel thought they would feel "glad to be alive" after suffering a SCI (Gerhart, Koziol-McLain, Lowenstein, & Whiteneck, 1994). This prompts concern that physician bias may unduly influence the decisions a patient with recent SCI makes, especially in the acute setting.

Even assuming the patient has been provided with accurate information, the degree to which she comprehends that information may be unclear. DMC is very challenging to assess in an intubated patient (Scanlon, 2003). The endotracheal tube prevents her from speaking, and her SCI makes it impossible for her to write or make hand gestures. Likely she will be limited to nodding or shaking her head. While it might be tempting to interpret certain actions—such as repeatedly mouthing "No"—as indications of a thoughtful choice, it may be impossible to verify that the patient truly appreciates the implications of the sentiments she is expressing (p. 123).

The AAN (1993) recognizes the complexity of balancing all these factors in its position statement on forgoing LSMT after SCI. In addition to reasserting the right of competent patients to refuse treatment, it includes the following caveats:

> Physicians have the duty to ascertain that the patient's decision to refuse treatment has been reached with full knowledge of the consequences and with appropriate consideration of treatment alternatives, the patient has had a consistently held position over time, and the decision is not merely an impulsive or transient decision to his or her severe illness.

It may take time to confirm each of these requirements, prompting some to argue that patients should not be permitted to refuse treatment in the immediate—or even inter-mediate—aftermath of an SCI. Many authors have suggested a time-limited trial (TLT, p. 118) of treatment in order to address the underlying factors that may be driving the patient to initially refuse it (Kirschner et al., 2011). This provides the patient time to grasp—both emotionally and intellectually—the complexities and possibilities of her new situation. The offer can be framed as an invitation and a pledge for future respect for autonomy (once restored), along the lines of, "I promise that we will honor your request to discontinue treatment, but for the time being would you be willing to continue so we can make sure your choice is informed?" Suggested durations of the TLT range from two weeks (Taub, Keune, Kodner, & Schwarze, 2014) to two years (Patterson et al., 1993), with the latter involving significant neurorehabilitation.

This waiting period reflects concern that the patient may be refusing LSMT be-cause she is asking the wrong question. For instance, surrogates will often report—when patients are unable to speak for themselves—that the patient previously said, "I never want to live in that condition." But spoken at a time of able-bodiedness, the statement likely reflects the patient's preference to live in her baseline state of health rather than as a quadriplegic. Following an SCI, though, the operative choice is whether the patient would prefer to live as a quadriplegic or not live at all. It is unlikely the patient was able to grasp the import of that question when death and quadriplegia were both hypothet-ical states, but now that she is experiencing the latter, it behooves her—and her family as well as the medical team—to allow her time to understand what living in that state truly amounts to.

But what happens if the patient is unwilling to undergo a TLT? From a purely phys-ical point of view, it is easier to compel a quadriplegic patient to accept treatment simply by virtue of her physical inability to resist. But the emotional toll this would take on the patient—who is completely disempowered at that point—as well as the medical team would be substantial. As always, persuasion is far superior to coercion, but given the lit-erally mortal stakes involved—and the significant likelihood that the patient's opinion might change over time—it is reasonable to consider a compulsory TLT even if the pa-tient does not agree to it. Here it would be important to specify the time involved in the trial, which should be sufficient to allow for whatever clinical improvement may occur, as well as reestablishment of emotional equilibration.

The latter, however, is thought to take six to twenty-four months (Powell & Lowenstein, 1996). Therefore, a TLT of days or even weeks may not be sufficient to afford the patient a reasonable chance to fully grasp her situation. By the same token, compel-ling treatment for extended periods—which may not yield additional clinical or emo-tional improvement—is an inappropriate infringement on the patient's autonomy. In the end, a compromise may need to be reached, compelling the patient to accept more treatment than she (initially) was willing to and also potentially forgoing that treatment before her DMC has fully returned to its pre-injury level.

Return to the Case

This is clearly a tragic situation. The patient is obviously in great distress, dealing with immense grief and fear. She has lost control of nearly everything in her life, and compelling her to continue LSMT seems like it takes away the last thing she can decide for herself.

Compassion would seem to compel the team to honor her refusal, but it also risks loss of perspective. A very high percentage of patients with SCI achieve what they consider to be an acceptable quality of life. The very grief and fear that are eliciting such a compassionate response in the team also call into question the patient's current level of DMC. It is, therefore, prudent to defer decisions concerning LSMT until her immediate grief has subsided, her DMC has been maximized, and she has a fuller understanding of what her life might look like.

The team engages in empathic listening with the patient's family and attempts to build rapport with the patient (who cannot speak). They try to maximize her sense of control by expressing their respect for her right to refuse treatment, while asking her to "give it a little time" so they can optimize her condition and confirm that her decision truly reflects her values.

She is steadfast in her refusal of treatment. The team sensitively informs her that they cannot honor that request at the present time, but they will in the future if she remains consistent in her request and all steps have been taken to support her. When pressed for a definitive time frame, they demur so as not to make any promises they cannot keep. Privately, they anticipate waiting approximately two weeks before reassessing.

The family is grateful for the decision, and that they didn't have to make it themselves. They use the reprieve to care for and support the patient, who remains withdrawn but is able to be extubated. Gradually she seems to regain a sense of hope, and her requests for withdrawal of LSMT become less frequent. They have stopped altogether by the time the team is prepared to revisit the issue.

The patient consents to gastrostomy placement and is discharged to home.

Stroke
Case Study

An eighty-four-year-old woman with a previously good quality of life suffers an ischemic stroke to her nondominant hemisphere. She had previously expressed her wish to avoid burdensome treatment and thus already had a DNAR order in place. She is currently intubated and unable to participate in decision-making.

Her loving family is acutely grieving and also wants to respect her wishes. The patient's husband died several years earlier after a long hospitalization following a massive stroke. On several occasions, the patient clearly stated that she did not want to "die that way." They feel obligated, therefore, to withdraw support.

The neurology team recognizes that the patient will likely wean from the ventilator, and her residual neurological deficit may be quite mild. A palliative care consultation is requested.

Stroke is the third leading cause of death in the United States—trailing only heart disease and cancer—and 6% of hospice patients are admitted with this diagnosis (Center for Medicare and Medicaid Services, 2013). It is also very heterogeneous, encompassing distinct mechanisms (hemorrhagic or ischemic) as well as locations within the brain (Hademenos & Massoud, 1997). Given how common and varied it is—and the frequent uncertainty of prognosis, especially in the immediate aftermath—clinicians must be prepared to deal with the ethical issues that may arise.

The primary issue involves the determination of prognosis, which necessarily will influence medical decision-making. At first, the patient and her family may be overwhelmed by the acute change in the patient's condition. Over half of stroke patients experience significant dysphagia, for instance, and one in fifteen hospitalized stroke patients also require mechanical ventilation (Huttner, Kohrmann, Berger, Georgiadis, & Schwab, 2006; Roch et al., 2003).

After such a significant decompensation, the family may find it difficult to imagine the patient ultimately regaining her ability to breathe and eat and drink independently, prompting discussion of forgoing LSMT. The patient herself, confronted with such an acute change and unable to envision a life of sufficient quality—and perhaps also fearing that the longer treatment is continued the harder it will become to refuse it—might also make early requests for limitation of treatment (Quill, 1993).

This tendency may be reinforced by prognostic models showing poor outcomes. These models are aggregate, however, and not necessarily applicable to the patient's specific condition (Ariesen, Algra, van der Worp, & Rinkel, 2005). For instance, such models frequently cannot distinguish between death despite provision of LSMT and death following its withdrawal (Mayer & Kossoff, 1999). For instance, studies have shown that a DNAR order is associated with higher risk of short-term mortality (Creutzfeldt et al., 2011). But was the DNAR a reflection of imminent death, or did it accompany withdrawal of currently effective LSMT?

Such "withdrawal bias" (Creutzfeldt & Holloway, 2012) may account for as much as 40% of the observed mortality in ischemic strokes (Kelly, Hoskins, & Holloway, 2012). This, in turn, may result in a "self-fulfilling prophecy" (Becker et al., 2001): based on high mortality data patients opt to forgo LSMT, which in turn reinforces the mortality data.

In reality, initial impressions are often unreliable. Aside from specific conditions with known high mortality—such as basilar artery infarct with coma and apnea and malignant middle cerebral artery infarct (Holloway et al., 2014)—many patients exhibit significant recovery after strokes. Mortality is admittedly quite high for the subset of patients who initially require mechanical ventilation, but as many as one-third of these patients ultimately have no or minimal disability (Rabinstein & Wijdicks, 2004). Similarly, half of dysphagic patients will recover their ability to swallow safely within two weeks (Holloway et al., 2014), but it is extremely difficult to predict *which* half (Martino et al., 2005).

Instead of attempting to apply aggregate data to specific cases, some clinicians rely on their personal experience. This, however, can vary substantially (Racine, Dion, Wijman, Illes, & Lansberg, 2009) and is susceptible to both optimistic and pessimistic biases (Finley Caulfield et al., 2010). Clinicians—as well as families—may also be susceptible to "cognitive bias" (Holloway et al., 2014), which underestimates the quality of life of patients who suffer cognitive deficits. Such bias fails to recognize the "disability paradox," whereby people with disabilities actually rate their quality of life higher than non-disabled persons (Albrecht & Devlieger, 1999). Stroke patients consider long-term functional outcome and quality of life as the most important considerations related to health care decisions, as these can often be satisfying even with significant functional deficits (Benejam et al., 2009; Weil, Rahme, Moumdjian, Bouthillier, & Bojanowski, 2011).

Given the heterogeneity of stroke, the inherent uncertainty early on in the disease course, and the potential for several types of bias, accurate prognostication requires thoughtful interpretation of available data to confirm applicability and avoid the self-fulfilling prophecy. Personal experience can be helpful, but because of its inherent idiosyncrasies, second opinions are extremely important (Christakis & Lamont, 2000; Glare & Sinclair, 2008). With the exception of types of stroke known to have very poor outcomes, it may be more appropriate to defer definitive decision-making in order to better gauge the possibility of recovery (Jauch et al., 2013).

Given the frequency of dysphagia and the importance of optimal nutrition for maximal recovery, MANH is often required in the immediate aftermath of a stroke. While gastrostomy tube placement optimizes safety of administration—especially for long-term use—it should usually be delayed. Not only has early gastrostomy tube placement been shown to increase the risk of death and poor outcomes (Dennis, Lewis, Warlow, & Collaboration, 2005), it may be emotionally taxing on the family to discontinue using the gastrostomy once inserted.

While acknowledging the inherent uncertainty, it is important to resist the temptation to avoid prognostication entirely. There are certain situations when at least some elements of the patient's future condition can be known with a level of certainty, and these should be shared with the family. Even when the patient's precise condition cannot be foreseen, it may be helpful to sketch the "reasonable best case scenario" (i.e., a slightly optimistic but not entirely unrealistic sense of what the patient might ultimately achieve). As long as this is not presented to the patient or family as a promise or firm prediction, it may help them appreciate what is possible. If this clearly falls short of the minimal quality of life the patient is willing to accept—such as permanent nursing home placement for a patient who never wanted to be in a nursing home—goals may need to be clarified and care perhaps redirected. If the "reasonable best case scenario" is acceptable, however, then further discussion about what probability of achieving that goal is sufficient to justify continued treatment—and what burdens would be incurred in the process—would logically follow.

It is also helpful, especially with stroke patients, to identify future decision points that may be determinative. For instance, for a ventilated patient who is expected to make some recovery, the initial days may represent a "window of opportunity" (p. 317) when withdrawal of mechanical ventilation would lead to the patient's death. After that point, the only LSMT the patient may be relying on could be MANH, which carries strong emotional significance (p. 185). Families should also be informed that should they decide to forgo MANH, the resulting dehydration—in addition to ultimately causing the patient's death—may initially cause some clinical improvement by virtue of decreased intracranial pressure. This should not be taken as a sign of recovery, however.

Another decision point is tracheostomy, which is generally performed no longer than two to three weeks after initiation of mechanical ventilation. As such, it represents a logical opportunity to reassess goals of care in light of clinical progress. In many cases this will have allowed sufficient time to pass for the patient's prognosis to become clearer. If uncertainty remains, framing tracheostomy placement as a TLT (p. 118) may make it easier for a family to subsequently consider not continuing it, if the patient's overall goals are not met.

Return to the Case

The palliative care team meets with the family, empathizes with their situation, and tries to learn more from them about the patient. Along with the neurologist, they try to clarify the patient's current condition and prognosis, uncertain as it is.

"I'm worried we've already done more than she wanted," the patient's daughter says. "She has a DNR."

The clinician clarifies that a DNAR order only applies to situations of cardiac arrest (p. 104) and also inquires as to what the patient might have meant when she said she did not want to die the same way her husband had.

"The doctors just kept going!" the daughter says. "They wouldn't listen to us."

Sensing that the family is concerned about losing control of the situation—as seems to have happened in the case of the patient's husband—the clinician reassures the family that they are the patient's voice and their wishes will be respected. He also emphasizes that the patient's DNAR order remains in place, while also expressing tempered optimism about the patient's recovery.

"The next few days will tell us a lot," he says.

When framed as a TLT (p. 118), continued mechanical ventilation is acceptable to the family. They also appreciate the promise of frequent meetings to update them and reevaluate the plan in light of recent developments. By the end of the initial meeting they are able to appreciate this situation is much different than what happened to their father and are eager to see how their mother progresses.

The patient is extubated three days later, and after some temporary dysphagia—requiring supplemental nutrition and hydration—she is cleared to eat again. She has some mild speech and cognitive deficits related to the stroke but is able to return home.

Summary Points

- Patients suffering from neurological illness have profound palliative care needs that often go unaddressed.
- Dementia
  - Patients with advanced dementia may espouse different values than they did when they possessed DMC. Rather than automatically honoring or disregarding previously expressed wishes, it is important to assess the benefits and burdens of proposed treatment.
  - Patients with dementia who can no longer feed themselves may benefit from spoon-feeding. It is important to distinguish between voluntarily engaging in eating and reflexively responding to food placed in one's mouth.
  - MANH does not improve life expectancy or symptomatology in patients with severe dementia.
- Unresponsive wakefulness (or "vegetative") syndrome
  - By virtue of having sleep/wake cycles, patients in a vegetative state may appear alert, even though they are not. For this and other reasons, the term "unresponsive wakefulness syndrome" is preferable.
  - Patients in a UWS are believed not to be able to experience pain, but given recent neuroradiological discoveries—as well as the potential for misdiagnosis—clinicians should "err on the side of safety" and provide standard symptomatic management.
  - While most people would not opt to be maintained in a UWS, some patients might. Consideration of forgoing LSMT should therefore involve the standard evaluation of respective benefits and burdens, with recognition of a "window of opportunity" in many cases for respiratory support.
- ALS (or Lou Gehrig's disease)
  - ALS is somewhat unique among neurological diseases, by virtue of leaving cognition largely intact.

- The well-known trajectory of ALS permits thoughtful ACP, which should recognize the possibility of the patient changing her mind over time.
- Spinal cord injury leading to quadriplegia often prompts requests for limitation of treatment. Given the likelihood of compromised DMC—as well as the high prevalence of acceptable quality of life among survivors—such decisions should be deferred for a brief period to permit optimizing support for the patient and maximizing of her DMC.
- Stroke is a common and heterogeneous condition. Prognostication is susceptible to multiple biases, including withdrawal bias and cognitive bias. As a result, it is often helpful to sketch out the "reasonable best case scenario," and if this would potentially be acceptable to the patient, the likelihood of achieving it.

References

Albrecht, G. L., & Devlieger, P. J. (1999). The disability paradox: High quality of life against all odds. *Soc Sci Med*, *48*(8), 977–988.

Amenabar, A. (2004). *Mar Adentro* (The Sea Inside). Fine Line Pictures.

American Academy of Hospice and Palliative Medicine. (2013). Percutaneous feeding tubes in patients with dementia. Retrieved from http://www.choosingwisely.org/clinician-lists/american-academy-hospice-palliative-care-percutaneous-feeding-tubes-in-patients-with-dementia/

American Academy of Neurology. (1993). Position statement: Certain aspects of the care and management of profoundly and irreversibly paralyzed patients with retained consciousness and cognition. Report of the Ethics and Humanities Subcommittee of the American Academy of Neurology. *Neurology*, *43*(1), 222–223.

American Academy of Neurology Ethics and Humanities Subcommittee. (1996). Palliative care in neurology. *Neurology*, *46*(3), 870–872.

American Board of Psychiatry and Neurology. (2016). Facts and statistics. Retrieved from http://www.abpn.com/about/facts-and-statistics/

Andrews, K. (1993). Recovery of patients after four months or more in the persistent vegetative state. *BMJ*, *306*(6892), 1597–1600.

Ariesen, M. J., Algra, A., van der Worp, H. B., & Rinkel, G. J. (2005). Applicability and relevance of models that predict short term outcome after intracerebral haemorrhage. *J Neurol Neurosurg Psychiatry*, *76*(6), 839–844. doi:10.1136/jnnp.2004.048223

Attarian, H. (2009). Importance of sleep in the quality of life of multiple sclerosis patients: A long under-recognized issue. *Sleep Med*, *10*(1), 7–8. doi:10.1016/j.sleep.2008.02.002

Becker, K. J., Baxter, A. B., Cohen, W. A., Bybee, H. M., Tirschwell, D. L., Newell, D. W., . . . Longstreth, W. T., Jr. (2001). Withdrawal of support in intracerebral hemorrhage may lead to self-fulfilling prophecies. *Neurology*, *56*(6), 766–772.

Benejam, B., Sahuquillo, J., Poca, M. A., Frascheri, L., Solana, E., Delgado, P., & Junque, C. (2009). Quality of life and neurobehavioral changes in survivors of malignant middle cerebral artery infarction. *J Neurol*, *256*(7), 1126–1133. doi:10.1007/s00415-009-5083-9

Bentley v. Maplewood Seniors Care (2014). 2015 BCCA 91.

Blendon, R. J., Benson, J. M., & Herrmann, M. J. (2005). The American public and the Terri Schiavo case. *Arch Intern Med*, *165*(22), 2580–2584. doi:10.1001/archinte.165.22.2580

Boersma, I., Miyasaki, J., Kutner, J., & Kluger, B. (2014). Palliative care and neurology: Time for a paradigm shift. *Neurology*, *83*(6), 561–567. doi:10.1212/WNL.0000000000000674

Bombardier, C. H., Richards, J. S., Krause, J. S., Tulsky, D., & Tate, D. G. (2004). Symptoms of major depression in people with spinal cord injury: Implications for screening. *Arch Phys Med Rehabil*, *85*(11), 1749–1756.

Borasio, G. D. (2013). The role of palliative care in patients with neurological diseases. *Nat Rev Neurol*, *9*(5), 292–295. doi:10.1038/nrneurol.2013.49

Byock, I. (2012). *The best care possible: A physician's quest to transform care through the end of life.* New York: Avery.

Callahan, D. (1995). Terminating life-sustaining treatment of the demented. *Hastings Cent Rep*, *25*(6), 25–31.

Cantor, N. L. (2007). On hastening death without violating legal and moral prohibitions. *Spec Law Dig Health Care Law*, *338*, 9–31.

Caplan, A. L., Callahan, D., & Haas, J. (1987). Ethical & policy issues in rehabilitation medicine. *Hastings Cent Rep*, *17*(4, Suppl.), 1–20.

Center for Medicare and Medicaid Services. Medicare hospice data trends: 1998–2009. (2013). Retrieved from https://www.cms.gov/Medicare/Medicare-Fee-for-Service-Payment/Hospice/Medicare_Hospice_Data.html

Chen, J. J., & Marsh, L. (2013). Depression in Parkinson's disease: Identification and management. *Pharmacotherapy*, *33*(9), 972–983. doi:10.1002/phar.1314

Chennu, S., Finoia, P., Kamau, E., Allanson, J., Williams, G. B., Monti, M. M., . . . Bekinschtein, T. A. (2014). Spectral signatures of reorganised brain networks in disorders of consciousness. *PLoS Comput Biol*, *10*(10), e1003887. doi:10.1371/journal.pcbi.1003887

Cheon, S. M., Ha, M. S., Park, M. J., & Kim, J. W. (2008). Nonmotor symptoms of Parkinson's disease: Prevalence and awareness of patients and families. *Parkinsonism Relat Disord*, *14*(4), 286–290. doi:10.1016/j.parkreldis.2007.09.002

Christakis, N. A., & Lamont, E. B. (2000). Extent and determinants of error in doctors' prognoses in terminally ill patients: Prospective cohort study. *BMJ*, *320*(7233), 469–472.

Clarke, D. M., McLeod, J. E., Smith, G. C., Trauer, T., & Kissane, D. W. (2005). A comparison of psychosocial and physical functioning in patients with motor neurone disease and metastatic cancer. *J Palliat Care*, *21*(3), 173–179.

Clipp, E. C., & George, L. K. (1993). Dementia and cancer: A comparison of spouse caregivers. *Gerontologist*, *33*(4), 534–541.

Cranford, R. E. (2002). What is a minimally conscious state? *West J Med*, *176*(2), 129–130.

Creutzfeldt, C. J., Becker, K. J., Weinstein, J. R., Khot, S. P., McPharlin, T. O., Ton, T. G., . . . Tirschwell, D. L. (2011). Do-not-attempt-resuscitation orders and prognostic models for intraparenchymal hemorrhage. *Crit Care Med*, *39*(1), 158–162. doi:10.1097/CCM.0b013e3181fb7b49

Creutzfeldt, C. J., Gooley, T., & Walker, M. (2009). Are neurology residents prepared to deal with dying patients? *Arch Neurol*, *66*(11), 1427–1428. doi:10.1001/archneurol.2009.241

Creutzfeldt, C. J., & Holloway, R. G. (2012). Treatment decisions after severe stroke: Uncertainty and biases. *Stroke*, *43*(12), 3405–3408. doi:10.1161/STROKEAHA.112.673376

Cruse, D., Chennu, S., Chatelle, C., Bekinschtein, T. A., Fernandez-Espejo, D., Pickard, J. D., . . . Owen, A. M. (2011). Bedside detection of awareness in the vegetative state: A cohort study. *Lancet*, *378*(9809), 2088–2094. doi: 10.1016/S0140-6736(11)61224–5

Cruzan v. Director, Missouri Department of Health, 497 261 (S.Ct. 1990).

Dallara, A., & Tolchin, D. W. (2014). Emerging subspecialties in neurology: Palliative care. *Neurology*, *82*(7), 640–642. doi:10.1212/WNL.0000000000000121

Davis, D. S. (1993). Shifting the burden of proof. *Second Opin*, *18*(3), 31–36.

Dawson, S., Kristjanson, L. J., Toye, C. M., & Flett, P. (2004). Living with Huntington's disease: Need for supportive care. *Nurs Health Sci*, *6*(2), 123–130. doi:10.1111/j.1442-2018.2004.00183.x

Defanti, C. A. (2004). Personal identity and palliative care. In R. Voltz (Ed.), *Palliative care in neurology* (pp. 327–334). New York: Oxford University Press.

Demertzi, A., Schnakers, C., Ledoux, D., Chatelle, C., Bruno, M. A., Vanhaudenhuyse, A., . . . Laureys, S. (2009). Different beliefs about pain perception in the vegetative and minimally conscious states: A European survey of medical and paramedical professionals. *Prog Brain Res*, *177*, 329–338. doi:10.1016/S0079-6123(09)17722-1

Dennis, M. S., Lewis, S. C., Warlow, C., & Collaboration, F. T. (2005). Effect of timing and method of enteral tube feeding for dysphagic stroke patients (FOOD): A multicentre randomised controlled trial. *Lancet*, *365*(9461), 764–772. doi:10.1016/S0140-6736(05)17983-5

Dresser, R. (1995). Dworkin on dementia: Elegant theory, questionable policy. *Hastings Cent Rep*, *25*(6), 32–38.

Dworkin, R. (1993). *Life's dominion: An argument about abortion, euthanasia, and individual freedom* (1st ed.). New York: Knopf.

Eastwood, C. (2004). *Million dollar baby*. Burbank, CA: Warner Bros.

El Ghatti, A. Z., & Hanson, R. W. (1975). Outcome of marriages existing at the time of a male's spinal cord injury. *J Chronic Dis*, *28*(7–8), 383–388.

Elman, L. B., Houghton, D. J., Wu, G. F., Hurtig, H. I., Markowitz, C. E., & McCluskey, L. (2007). Palliative care in amyotrophic lateral sclerosis, Parkinson's disease, and multiple sclerosis. *J Palliat Med*, *10*(2), 433–457. doi:10.1089/jpm.2006.9978

Farrington, M., Bruene, D., & Wagner, M. (2015). Pain management prior to nasogastric tube placement: Atomized lidocaine. *ORL Head Neck Nurs*, *33*(1), 8–16.

Finley Caulfield, A., Gabler, L., Lansberg, M. G., Eyngorn, I., Mlynash, M., Buckwalter, M. S., . . . Wijman, C. A. (2010). Outcome prediction in mechanically ventilated neurologic patients by junior neurointensivists. *Neurology*, *74*(14), 1096–1101. doi:10.1212/WNL.0b013e3181d8197f

Finucane, T. E., Christmas, C., & Travis, K. (1999). Tube feeding in patients with advanced dementia: A review of the evidence. *JAMA*, *282*(14), 1365–1370.

Firlik, A. D. (1991). A piece of my mind. Margo's logo. *JAMA*, *265*(2), 201.

Foley, J. M. (1992). The experience of being demented. In R. H. Binstock, S. G. Post, & P. J. Whitehouse (Eds.), *Dementia and aging: Ethics, values, and policy choices* (pp. 30–43). Baltimore: Johns Hopkins University Press.

Foley, K. M., & Carver, A. C. (2001). Palliative care in neurology. *Neurol Clin*, *19*(4), 789–799.

Frank, R. G., Elliott, T. R., Corcoran, J. R., & Wonderlich, S. A. (1987). Depression after spinal cord injury: Is it necessary? *Clin Psychol Rev*, *7*, 611–630.

Fruehwald, S., Loeffler-Stastka, H., Eher, R., Saletu, B., & Baumhackl, U. (2001). Depression and quality of life in multiple sclerosis. *Acta Neurol Scand*, *104*(5), 257–261.

Gelling, L. (1999). Causes of ICU psychosis: the environmental factors. *Nurs Crit Care*, *4*(1), 22–26.

Gerhart, K. A., Koziol-McLain, J., Lowenstein, S. R., & Whiteneck, G. G. (1994). Quality of life following spinal cord injury: Knowledge and attitudes of emergency care providers. *Ann Emerg Med*, *23*(4), 807–812.

Glare, P. A., & Sinclair, C. T. (2008). Palliative medicine review: Prognostication. *J Palliat Med*, *11*(1), 84–103. doi:10.1089/jpm.2008.9992

Gosseries, O., Vanhaudenhuyse, A., Bruno, M., Dermetzi, A., Schnakers, C., Boly, M., . . . Laureys, S. (2011). Disorders of consciousness: Coma, vegetative, and minimally conscious states. In D. Cvetkovic & I. Cosic (Eds.), *States of consciousness: Experimental insights into meditation, waking, sleep, and dreams* (pp. 29–56). Heidelberg: Springer.

Goy, E. R., Carter, J., & Ganzini, L. (2008). Neurologic disease at the end of life: Caregiver descriptions of Parkinson disease and amyotrophic lateral sclerosis. *J Palliat Med*, *11*(4), 548–554. doi:10.1089/jpm.2007.0258

Hademenos, G. J., & Massoud, T. F. (1997). Biophysical mechanisms of stroke. *Stroke*, *28*(10), 2067–2077.

Hanson, L. C., Garrett, J. M., Lewis, C., Phifer, N., Jackman, A., & Carey, T. S. (2008). Physicians' expectations of benefit from tube feeding. *J Palliat Med*, *11*(8), 1130–1134. doi:10.1089/jpm.2008.0033

Hertogh, C. M., de Boer, M. E., Droes, R. M., & Eefsting, J. A. (2007). Would we rather lose our life than lose our self? Lessons from the Dutch debate on euthanasia for patients with dementia. *Am J Bioeth*, *7*(4), 48–56. doi:10.1080/15265160701220881

Holloway, R. G., Arnold, R. M., Creutzfeldt, C. J., Lewis, E. F., Lutz, B. J., McCann, R. M., . . . Council on Clinical Cardiology. (2014). Palliative and end-of-life care in stroke: A statement for healthcare professionals from the American Heart Association/American Stroke Association. *Stroke*, *45*(6), 1887–1916. doi:10.1161/STR.0000000000000015

Huttner, H. B., Kohrmann, M., Berger, C., Georgiadis, D., & Schwab, S. (2006). Predictive factors for tracheostomy in neurocritical care patients with spontaneous supratentorial hemorrhage. *Cerebrovasc Dis*, *21*(3), 159–165. doi:10.1159/000090527

In re Conroy (N.J. 1985).

In re Quinlan, 70 10 (N.J. 1976).

Inelmen, E. M., Mosele, M., Sergi, G., Toffanello, E. D., Coin, A., & Manzato, E. (2012). Chronic pain in the elderly with advanced dementia. Are we doing our best for their suffering? *Aging Clin Exp Res*, 24(3), 207–212. doi:10.3275/8020

Jauch, E. C., Saver, J. L., Adams, H. P., Jr., Bruno, A., Connors, J. J., Demaerschalk, B. M., . . . Council on Clinical, C. (2013). Guidelines for the early management of patients with acute ischemic stroke: A guideline for healthcare professionals from the American Heart Association/American Stroke Association. *Stroke*, 44(3), 870–947. doi:10.1161/STR.0b013e318284056a

Kamble, P., Chen, H., Sherer, J. T., & Aparasu, R. R. (2009). Use of antipsychotics among elderly nursing home residents with dementia in the US: An analysis of National Survey Data. *Drugs Aging*, 26(6), 483–492. doi:10.2165/00002512-200926060-00005

Kelly, A. G., Hoskins, K. D., & Holloway, R. G. (2012). Early stroke mortality, patient preferences, and the withdrawal of care bias. *Neurology*, 79(9), 941–944. doi:10.1212/WNL.0b013e318266fc40

Khin, E., Minor, D., Holloway, A. & Pelleg, A. (2015). Decisional capacity in amyotrophic lateral sclerosis. *J Amer Acad Psychiatr Law*, 43(2), 210–217.

Kirschner, K. L., Kerkhoff, T. R., Butt, L., Yamada, R., Battaglia, C. C., Wu, J., . . . Bahr, E. (2011). "I don't want to live this way, doc. Please take me off the ventilator and let me die." *PM R*, 3(10), 968–975. doi:10.1016/j.pmrj.2011.09.001

Kitwood, T., & Bredin, K. (1992). Towards a theory of dementia care: Personhood and well-being. *Ageing Soc*, 12, 269–287.

Kristjanson, L. J., Nelson, F., & Henteleff, P. (1987). Palliative care for individuals with amyotrophic lateral sclerosis. *J Palliat Care*, 2(2), 28–34.

Laureys, S., Celesia, G. G., Cohadon, F., Lavrijsen, J., Leon-Carrion, J., Sannita, W. G., . . . European Task Force on Disorders of Consciousness. (2010). Unresponsive wakefulness syndrome: A new name for the vegetative state or apallic syndrome. *BMC Med*, 8, 68. doi:10.1186/1741-7015-8-68

Lemke, M. R., Fuchs, G., Gemende, I., Herting, B., Oehlwein, C., Reichmann, H., . . . Volkmann, J. (2004). Depression and Parkinson's disease. *J Neurol*, 251(Suppl. 6), VI/24–27.

Locke, J. (1970). *An essay concerning human understanding, 1690*. Menston: Scolar Press.

Maass, A., & Reichmann, H. (2013). Sleep and non-motor symptoms in Parkinson's disease. *J Neural Transm (Vienna)*, 120(4), 565–569. doi:10.1007/s00702-013-0966-4

Maessen, M., Veldink, J. H., Onwuteaka-Philipsen, B. D., Hendricks, H. T., Schelhaas, H. J., Grupstra, H. F., . . . van den Berg, L. H. (2014). Euthanasia and physician-assisted suicide in amyotrophic lateral sclerosis: A prospective study. *J Neurol*, 261(10), 1894–1901. doi:10.1007/s00415-014-7424-6

Manu, E., Marks, A., Berkman, C. S., Mullan, P., Montagnini, M., & Vitale, C. A. (2012). Self-perceived competence among medical residents in skills needed to care for patients with advanced dementia versus metastatic cancer. *J Cancer Educ*, 27(3), 515–520. doi:10.1007/s13187-012-0351-2

Martino, R., Foley, N., Bhogal, S., Diamant, N., Speechley, M., & Teasell, R. (2005). Dysphagia after stroke: Incidence, diagnosis, and pulmonary complications. *Stroke*, 36(12), 2756–2763. doi:10.1161/01.STR.0000190056.76543.eb

Mayer, S. A., & Kossoff, S. B. (1999). Withdrawal of life support in the neurological intensive care unit. *Neurology*, 52(8), 1602–1609.

McClave, S. A., & Chang, W. K. (2003). Complications of enteral access. *Gastrointest Endosc*, 58(5), 739–751.

Mitchell, S. L., Kiely, D. K., & Hamel, M. B. (2004). Dying with advanced dementia in the nursing home. *Arch Intern Med*, 164(3), 321–326. doi:10.1001/archinte.164.3.321

Mitchell, S. L., Teno, J. M., Kiely, D. K., Shaffer, M. L., Jones, R. N., Prigerson, H. G., . . . Hamel, M. B. (2009). The clinical course of advanced dementia. *N Engl J Med*, 361(16), 1529–1538. doi:10.1056/NEJMoa0902234

Miyasaki, J. M., Long, J., Mancini, D., Moro, E., Fox, S. H., Lang, A. E., . . . Hui, J. (2012). Palliative care for advanced Parkinson disease: An interdisciplinary clinic and new scale, the ESAS-PD. *Parkinsonism Relat Disord*, 18(Suppl. 3), S6–S9. doi:10.1016/j.parkreldis.2012.06.013

Morton v. Wellstar Health Sys., Inc., 653 S.E.2d 756, 757 (Ga. Ct. App. 2007).

Multi-Society Task Force on PVS. (1994). Medical aspects of the persistent vegetative state (1). *N Engl J Med*, 330(21), 1499–1508. doi:10.1056/NEJM199405263302107

Murray, S. A., Kendall, M., Boyd, K., & Sheikh, A. (2005). Illness trajectories and palliative care. *BMJ*, *330*(7498), 1007–1011. doi:10.1136/bmj.330.7498.1007

Newton, M. J. (1999). Precedent autonomy: Life-sustaining intervention and the demented patient. *Camb Q Healthc Ethics*, *8*(2), 189–199.

Oliver, D., & Silber, E. (2013). End of life care in neurological disease. In D. Oliver (Ed.), *End of life care in neurological disease* (pp. 19–32). London: Springer-Verlag.

Oliver, D. J., Borasio, G. D., Caraceni, A., de Visser, M., Grisold, W., Lorenzl, S., . . . Voltz, R. (2016). A consensus review on the development of palliative care for patients with chronic and progressive neurological disease. *Eur J Neurol*, *23*(1), 30–38. doi:10.1111/ene.12889

Oregon Health Authority. (2017). Death with Dignity Act: 2016 data summary. Retrieved from http://www.oregon.gov/oha/PH/PROVIDERPARTNERRESOURCES/EVALUATIONRESEARCH/DEATHWITHDIGNITYACT/Documents/year19.pdf.

Orr, R. D. (2009). *Medical ethics and the faith factor: A handbook for clergy and health-care professionals.* Grand Rapids, MI: William B. Eerdmans.

Parfit, D. (1984). *Reasons and persons*. Oxford: Clarendon Press.

Pasman, H. R., Onwuteaka-Philipsen, B. D., Kriegsman, D. M., Ooms, M. E., Ribbe, M. W., & van der Wal, G. (2005). Discomfort in nursing home patients with severe dementia in whom artificial nutrition and hydration is forgone. *Arch Intern Med*, *165*(15), 1729–1735. doi:10.1001/archinte.165.15.1729

Patterson, D. R., Miller-Perrin, C., McCormick, T. R., & Hudson, L. D. (1993). When life support is questioned early in the care of patients with cervical-level quadriplegia. *N Engl J Med*, *328*(7), 506–509. doi:10.1056/NEJM199302183280712

Phillips, W., Shannon, K. M., & Barker, R. A. (2008). The current clinical management of Huntington's disease. *Mov Disord*, *23*(11), 1491–1504. doi:10.1002/mds.21971

Powell, T., & Lowenstein, B. (1996). Refusing life-sustaining treatment after catastrophic injury: Ethical implications. *J Law Med Ethics*, *24*(1), 54–61.

Provinciali, L., Carlini, G., Tarquini, D., Defanti, C. A., Veronese, S., & Pucci, E. (2016). Need for palliative care for neurological diseases. *Neurol Sci*, *37*(10), 1581–1587. doi:10.1007/s10072-016-2614-x

Quill, T. E. (1993). Doctor, I want to die. Will you help me? *JAMA*, *270*(7), 870–873.

Quill, T. E., & Abernethy, A. P. (2013). Generalist plus specialist palliative care—creating a more sustainable model. *N Engl J Med*, *368*(13), 1173–1175. doi:10.1056/NEJMp1215620

Rabinstein, A. A., & Wijdicks, E. F. (2004). Outcome of survivors of acute stroke who require prolonged ventilatory assistance and tracheostomy. *Cerebrovasc Dis*, *18*(4), 325–331. doi:10.1159/000080771

Racine, E., Dion, M. J., Wijman, C. A., Illes, J., & Lansberg, M. G. (2009). Profiles of neurological outcome prediction among intensivists. *Neurocrit Care*, *11*(3), 345–352. doi:10.1007/s12028-009-9225-9

Roch, A., Michelet, P., Jullien, A. C., Thirion, X., Bregeon, F., Papazian, L., . . . Auffray, J. P. (2003). Long-term outcome in intensive care unit survivors after mechanical ventilation for intracerebral hemorrhage. *Crit Care Med*, *31*(11), 2651–2656. doi:10.1097/01.CCM.0000094222.57803.B4

Sampson, E. L., Candy, B., & Jones, L. (2009). Enteral tube feeding for older people with advanced dementia. *Cochrane Database Syst Rev*(2), CD007209. doi:10.1002/14651858.CD007209.pub2

Scanlon, C. (2003). Ethical concerns in end-of-life care. *Am J Nurs*, *103*(1), 48–55; quiz 56.

Schulz, R., Boerner, K., Shear, K., Zhang, S., & Gitlin, L. N. (2006). Predictors of complicated grief among dementia caregivers: A prospective study of bereavement. *Am J Geriatr Psychiatry*, *14*(8), 650–658. doi:10.1097/01.JGP.0000203178.44894.db

Sehgal, A., Galbraith, A., Chesney, M., Schoenfeld, P., Charles, G., & Lo, B. (1992). How strictly do dialysis patients want their advance directives followed? *JAMA*, *267*(1), 59–63.

Siegel, M. S. (1969). The vocational potential of the quadriplegic. *Med Clin North Am*, *53*(3), 713–718.

Simmons, Z., Bremer, B. A., Robbins, R. A., Walsh, S. M., & Fischer, S. (2000). Quality of life in ALS depends on factors other than strength and physical function. *Neurology*, *55*(3), 388–392.

Sleeman, K. E., Ho, Y. K., Verne, J., Glickman, M., Silber, E., Gao, W., . . . Higginson, I. J. (2013). Place of death, and its relation with underlying cause of death, in Parkinson's disease, motor neurone disease, and multiple sclerosis: A population-based study. *Palliat Med*, *27*(9), 840–846. doi:10.1177/0269216313490436

Strong, M., & Rosenfeld, J. (2003). Amyotrophic lateral sclerosis: A review of current concepts. *Amyotroph Lateral Scler Other Motor Neuron Disord*, *4*(3), 136–143.

Taub, A. L., Keune, J. D., Kodner, I. J., & Schwarze, M. L. (2014). Respecting autonomy in the setting of acute traumatic quadriplegia. *Surgery, 155*(2), 355–360.

Teno, J. M., Gozalo, P. L., Mitchell, S. L., Kuo, S., Rhodes, R. L., Bynum, J. P., & Mor, V. (2012). Does feeding tube insertion and its timing improve survival? *J Am Geriatr Soc, 60*(10), 1918–1921. doi:10.1111/j.1532-5415.2012.04148.x

Teno, J. M., Weitzen, S., Fennell, M. L., & Mor, V. (2001). Dying trajectory in the last year of life: Does cancer trajectory fit other diseases? *J Palliat Med, 4*(4), 457–464. doi:10.1089/109662101753381593

Tran, L. N., Back, A. L., & Creutzfeldt, C. J. (2016). Palliative care consultations in the neuro-ICU: A qualitative sutdy. *Neurocrit Care, 25*(2), 266–272.

Tsou, A. Y., Karlawish, J., McCluskey, L., Xie, S. X., & Long, J. A. (2012). Predictors of emergent feeding tubes and tracheostomies in amyotrophic lateral sclerosis (ALS). *Amyotroph Lateral Scler, 13*(3), 318–325. doi:10.3109/17482968.2012.662987

Tuck, K. K., Brod, L., Nutt, J., & Fromme, E. K. (2015). Preferences of patients with Parkinson's disease for communication about advanced care planning. *Am J Hosp Palliat Care, 32*(1), 68–77. doi:10.1177/1049909113504241

Tulsky, J. A., Arnold, R. M., Alexander, S. C., Olsen, M. K., Jeffreys, A. S., Rodriguez, K. L., . . . Pollak, K. I. (2011). Enhancing communication between oncologists and patients with a computer-based training program: A randomized trial. *Ann Intern Med, 155*(9), 593–601. doi:10.7326/0003-4819-155-9-201111010-00007

Turner-Stokes, L., Sykes, N., Silber, E., Khatri, A., Sutton, L., & Young, E. (2007). From diagnosis to death: Exploring the interface between neurology, rehabilitation and palliative care in managing people with long-term neurological conditions. *Clin Med (Lond), 7*(2), 129–136.

United States Conference of Catholic Bishops. (2009). *Ethical and religious directives for Catholic health care services* (5th ed.). Washington, DC: USCCB Pub.

van Vliet, L. M., Gao, W., DiFrancesco, D., Crosby, V., Wilcock, A., Byrne, A., . . . Neuro, O. (2016). How integrated are neurology and palliative care services? Results of a multicentre mapping exercise. *BMC Neurol, 16*, 63. doi:10.1186/s12883-016-0583-6

Wang, L. H., Elliott, M. A., Henson, L. J., Gerena-Maldonado, E., Strom, S., Downing, S., . . . Weiss, M. D. (2016). Death with dignity in Washington patients with amyotrophic lateral sclerosis. *Neurology 87*, 2117–2122.

Weil, A. G., Rahme, R., Moumdjian, R., Bouthillier, A., & Bojanowski, M. W. (2011). Quality of life following hemicraniectomy for malignant MCA territory infarction. *Can J Neurol Sci, 38*(3), 434–438.

Whiteneck, C. G., Carter, R. E., & Charlifue, S. W. (1985). *A collaborative study of high quadriplegia.* Washington, DC: National Institute of Handicapped Research.

16

Death and Organ Donation

Case Study

A fifty-three-year-old man is involved in a motor vehicle accident, causing a massive intracranial hemorrhage and subsequent brain swelling requiring a craniectomy. Despite maximal measures to control the swelling, his neurologic condition deteriorates and clinical examination—including apnea test—confirm death by neurological criteria ("brain death"). His family, though, is unwilling to accept the diagnosis, observing that he does not appear different than many other patients in the intensive care unit (ICU), who also are motionless and dependent on ventilators to breathe. The family notes that he is a "fighter," and they want to give him every opportunity to "pull through," which includes continuing mechanical ventilation.

The critical care team is unsure what to do, as it seems profoundly wrong to continue to ventilate a dead patient. An ethics consultation is requested.

Historicolegal Background

One would think that among the questions related to the death of a person, whether or not he is actually dead would be among the simplest. And it was for most of human history, because mechanical ventilation was not available. Without sufficient brain function a patient would not breathe, and lack of oxygen would cause cardiac arrest. Cardiorespiratory failure—what is now known as "circulatory death"—was therefore the final common pathway of both neurological as well as non-neurological causes of death.

With the discovery and implementation of invasive mechanical ventilation in the 1950s, however, it became possible to physiologically sustain a patient, even in the absence of brain function. The scientific community initially struggled to classify patients in such a state, with initial reports referring to "death of the nervous system" and *coma dépassé*, or "a state beyond coma" (Forbess et al., 1995; Jouvet, 1959). This prompted deeper reflection on what obligations remained toward a person in that state, given that the right of competent patients to refuse life-sustaining medical treatment (LSMT) had yet to be established. If the patient were dead, however, ventilators and feeding tubes and the like would not represent "*life-supporting* medical treatment" and nothing would prevent their withdrawal.

In addition to withdrawing mechanical ventilation—which was not generally done to living patients in the pre-Quinlan era (*In re Quinlan*, 1976)—there is one other thing that can only be done to dead patients: retrieve vital organs[1] for transplantation to another patient. The line between life and death, therefore, needs to be crisply drawn, because even though surrogates now definitively have the right to refuse interventions when a patient's prognosis is poor—even if he is clearly still alive—the opportunity for retrieval of vital organs only exists for dead patients.

Prior to the advent of mechanical ventilators—and the possibility of declaring heartbeating patients dependent on them as dead—organs were generally procured through "uncontrolled donation after circulatory death" (uDCD), such as after the sudden death of a patient in the emergency department (Kootstra, 1997). The demand for transplantable organs outstripped supply from uDCD, though, leading to further exploration of whether patients without absent brain function might also qualify as organ donors.

In 1968 a Harvard University committee released a landmark article which made a bold claim: patients with absent brain function are actually *dead*, even if their hearts and lungs continue to function with assistance (Ad Hoc Committee of the Harvard Medical School to Examine the Definition of Brain Death, 1968). The committee laid out criteria for the clinical determination of brain death and also explored how ethical obligations would change upon such a determination.

This concept of brain death was not universally embraced. Noting the growing waiting lists of hopeful organ recipients—and the increased number of potential donors that recognition of brain death would create—some feared that this was a semantic ruse to increase the pool of available organs. The concept gained increasing traction within the scientific community, though, culminating in the President's Commission which defined death as the "irreversible cessation of function of either circulatory and respiratory functions, or all functions of the entire brain, including the brain stem" (President's Commission for the Study of Ethical Problems in Medicine and Biomedical and Behavioral Research, 1981). The latter came to be known as "death by neurological criteria" or, more colloquially, "brain death."

---

1.   "Vital organs" refer to organs that are necessary for the donor to live.

This definition was included in a model statute, the Uniform Determination of Death Act (National Conference of Commissioners on Uniform State Laws, 1981), and soon affirmed by both the American Medical Association as well as the American Bar Association. Forty-five states have subsequently passed laws with a definition of death that is either identical or substantially similar to the UDDA's (Beresford, 2001). Those states without specific laws rely on precedent-setting court cases, some of which cite the UDDA (President's Council on Bioethics, 2009).

Even with the addition of brain-dead organ donors, a great many patients were still suffering (and dying) on transplant lists. Meanwhile, the societal consensus over the right of competent patients to refuse treatment was leading not only to the withholding of burdensome treatment but also the withdrawing of LSMT in the ICU. Typically, this took the form of "compassionate extubation" when the burdens were felt to outweigh the benefits. The death of these patients was anticipated, creating the possibility of "controlled donation after circulatory death" (cDCD),[2] with greater organ viability than uDCD due to reduced ischemic time.

The first protocol for cDCD was put forth by the University of Pittsburgh (Zawistowski & DeVita, 2003), and the general approach remains the same today. For a patient who is critically ill—generally suffering from neurological injury—and ventilator-dependent, once the family decides to forgo LSMT, the hospital notifies its local organ procurement organization (OPO) as required by the "conditions of participation" set by the Center for Medicare and Medicaid Services (Health Care Financing Administration, 1998). If the OPO determines that the patient is a potential DCD donor, a "designated requestor" approaches the family to discuss organ donation. If the family gives consent, the patient is taken to the operating room for compassionate extubation with standard end-of-life (EOL) care provided by the treating team.

Once the patient becomes pulseless, there is a predetermined waiting period—ranging from ninety seconds to five minutes—to confirm that the patient is, indeed, dead. Once the required duration of pulselessness has elapsed, the organ retrieval team enters the operating room and procures the organs. If the patient has not died within a maximum allotted time (usually one hour), organ retrieval is cancelled and he is taken back to the ICU for continuation of comfort-directed care.

Controlled DCD is not without ethical controversy. Studies have shown, for instance, that EOL care changes during cDCD. Not every hospital allows the family to be present for extubation and/or for declaration of death (Antommaria, Trotochaud, Kinlaw, Hopkins, & Frader, 2009), as is standard for EOL care outside of the operating room. No protocols permit the family to remain after declaration of death, because at that point the

---

2. This procedure was initially termed "non-heart-beating donation" to differentiate it from procurement from a brain-dead donor (whose heart was beating). That was subsequently changed to "donation after cardiac death," which became problematic in light of heart transplants following declaration of death by cardiorespiratory criteria (p. 440). Ultimately, "donation after circulatory death" emerged as the preferred term.

retrieval team takes over and begins the procurement. Other deviations from standard EOL care—such as large bore cannulation and administration of medications to optimize organ viability—are addressed later (p. 441).

Controlled DCD also has not resolved the crisis of a lack of organs for transplantation. Over 30,000 transplants were performed in 2015, but more than 120,000 patients remained on transplant waiting lists (Organ Procurement and Transplantation Network, 2017). As a result, increased attention has returned to uDCD, both in the United States (Reed & Lua, 2014) as well as Europe (Dominguez-Gil et al., 2016).

Neither did the UDDA eliminate controversy related to brain death, which once again made headlines in 2014 with two very high-profile cases (Gostin, 2014). Late the previous year, Jahi McMath—a thirteen-year-old with severe sleep apnea—underwent a tonsillectomy and adenoidectomy. Massive postoperative blood loss led to cardiac arrest and ultimately a determination of brain death. Her family, however, refused to accept this diagnosis, claiming since her heart was beating that she was still alive. Their attorney argued that the UDDA represented an inappropriate infringement on their constitutional religious and privacy rights.

Even though the coroner issued a death certificate and multiple courts of appeal refused to compel the hospital to continue treatment—which over the long term would require tracheostomy and gastrostomy tube insertion—the hospital reached a settlement with the family whereby Jahi's body would be released to them. They subsequently secured the services of physicians who were willing to perform those procedures, prompting calls for an investigation by the California state medical board (Pope, 2014). With the help of like-minded organizations—such as the Terri Schiavo Life and Hope Network—the family then transferred Jahi to a facility in New Jersey.

That choice was significant, as New Jersey is one of four states which do not follow the UDDA. According to New Jersey law,

> the death of an individual shall not be declared upon the basis of neurological criteria. . . . when the licensed physician authorized to declare death, has reason to believe . . . that such a declaration would violate the personal religious beliefs of the individual. In these cases, death shall be declared . . . solely upon the basis of cardio-respiratory criteria. (New Jersey Declaration of Death Act, 1991)

Jahi's parents invoked the religious exception in state law, and thus she could not be declared dead by neurological criteria in New Jersey.

The other well-known outlier is state of New York. Its law is broader than New Jersey's—encompassing moral as well as religious objections—but also less demanding. While New Jersey's law precludes a declaration of death by neurological criteria, New York's merely requires hospitals to "establish written procedures for the reasonable accommodation of the individual's religious or moral objections to use of the brain death standard" (New York State Department of Health, 2011). California also requires "a reasonably brief period of accommodation" (Uniform Determination of Death Act, 1982), while Illinois law requires hospitals to "take into account the patient's religious beliefs concerning the patient's time of death" (Hospital Licensing Act, 2008).

The other high-profile case was that of Marlise Muñoz, a thirty-three-year-old woman who at fourteen weeks of pregnancy suffered a cardiac arrest, likely due to a pulmonary embolism. She was subsequently declared brain dead and her husband requested discontinuation of mechanical ventilation. The hospital refused, though, citing the Texas Advance Directive Act—better known for its role in adjudicating requests for potentially nonbeneficial treatment (p. 368)—which specifically disallows withdrawing or withholding LSMT from a pregnant patient (Texas Advance Directives Act, 1999, Section 166.049).

Subsequent appeal sided with Mr. Muñoz. The court did not weigh in on the constitutionality of the law—which eleven other states have versions of (Greene & Wolfe, 2012)—instead simply noting that it did not apply to Ms. Muñoz. The law dealt with *life-sustaining* medical treatment, which it is not possible to administer to a patient who is not alive. The ventilator was ultimately discontinued, leading to the death of the fetus as well.

Palliative care has a critical role in the care of both patients who are—or may be—declared dead by either neurological or circulatory criteria. Empathetic listening, establishing goals of care, and maximizing psychosocial/spiritual support are all essential in these situations (Prommer, 2014). For patients who have not been declared dead but are approaching that point, expert symptom management is critical (Rady, Verheijde, & McGregor, 2006). And it is crucial to support families and loved ones through the bereavement process (Kesselring, Kainz, & Kiss, 2007).

Clinical

Death by Neurologic Criteria

Much has been written about what brain death is and how to confirm its presence. Three clinical criteria have been determined: coma, absence of brainstem reflexes, and apnea (Goila & Pawar, 2009). Testing for these criteria involves several steps. First, coma (i.e., total unresponsiveness) must be confirmed and a serious and irreversible cause identified. Any confounding variables—such as electrolyte, acid-base, or endocrine abnormalities, or effects of sedating or paralytic medications—must be excluded. Blood pressure and body temperature must be normalized, and a comprehensive neurologic exam must show complete absence of brain stem reflexes. Spinal cord reflexes—what some have called "Lazarus signs" in this context (Jain & DeGeorgia, 2005)—do not preclude a diagnosis of death by neurological criteria, as they do not require brain involvement.

Typically an "apnea test" is then performed. The patient is preoxygenated with 100% oxygen, arterial blood gases are drawn, and then the ventilator is discontinued while the patient is observed for any evidence of respiratory effort. Approximately eight minutes later, blood gases are drawn again. $PaCO_2$ of greater than 60 mm Hg—or

20 mm higher than the initial measurement—confirms lack of response to rising $PaCO_2$ and absence of brain stem function. The ventilator is reinitiated after repeat blood gases are drawn, or earlier if oxygen saturations drop below 85% for more than thirty seconds.

In situations where confounding factors cannot be removed—or apnea testing cannot be accomplished or is inconclusive—confirmatory tests such as electroencelphalogram (EEG) or cerebral flow study can be performed. These can also be problematic, however, as *any* activity on EEG (even "background noise") precludes confirmation of brain death. A flow study can also be misleading, for while lack of blood flow to the entire brain clearly indicates brain death, a positive finding does not preclude the diagnosis because it is possible to perfuse dead tissue. Diagnosis is even more complex for pediatric patients, as serial confirmatory exams/tests are required over increasing periods of time for extremely young patients.

Whether patients who "rule in" for brain death are actually dead is an ethical question, addressed later. From a clinical standpoint, however, contrary to reports of "recovery" following a diagnosis of brain death (Furness, 2012), a comprehensive meta-analysis of available data found no such cases (Wijdicks, Varelas, Gronseth, & Greer, 2010).

Death by Circulatory Criteria

Compared with the ethical debates about whether brain death is a reliable concept, diagnosing death by circulatory criteria might seem rather straightforward. At least on television, all that is required is placing one's finger on a patient's carotid or radial artery, feeling no pulse for a few seconds, and declaring him dead.

In reality, however, it is more complicated because circulatory death requires "*irreversible* cessation of function of . . . circulatory and respiratory functions" (italics added). Pulselessness and lack of respiratory effort indicate cessation of these functions, but it is not entirely clear at what point this becomes irreversible. After all, the default response to finding a patient without pulse or respiratory effort is to perform CPR, and while the outcomes of this procedure are much worse in real life than on television (Diem, Lantos, & Tulsky, 1996), it is effective in a significant number of cases. Since the patient had been in full arrest, this is classified as resuscitation. But if the patient had been "dead," this would technically be *resurrection*, which is quite a claim indeed.

So how can one know whether cessation of cardiorespiratory function is "irreversible," especially given documented cases of autoresuscitation where a patient's heart resumes functioning in the absence of intervention? Assuming the patient has a Do Not Attempt Resuscitation (DNAR) order—or else resuscitation would have been initiated immediately—the most reliable method is to wait long enough that autoresuscitation is no longer possible. Studies have shown that two minutes is sufficient to preclude the possibility of autoresuscitation (Sheth, Nutter, Stein, Scalea, & Bernat, 2012). But if external resuscitation has been declined and organ retrieval is not part of the plan of care, there is no reason not to wait longer to obtain definitive reassurance that the patient is dead. The

Institute of Medicine (2009), for example, recommends waiting five minutes from the onset of pulselessness before declaring death.

But when organ retrieval *is* a concern—as in the case of cDCD—there are countervailing reasons to not wait any longer than necessary, as prolonged warm ischemic time negatively impacts organ viability (Hosgood, Shah, Patel, & Nicholson, 2015). This creates the ethical dilemma of balancing certainty that the patient is dead while also honoring the needs of patients in need of transplantation.

Ethical

A clinician's obligations fundamentally change once a patient is declared dead. Prior to that point, beneficence, non-maleficence, and especially respect for autonomy are fundamental principles. Once a patient dies, though, he is technically no longer a "patient" (*Douglas v. Janssen Funeral Homes*, 2011). From that point on the hospital is merely the custodian of a dead body (Miller & Steiner, 2014). As such, declaration of death—including by neurological criteria—identifies a "hard stop" where medical interventions exceed their proper scope of practice (Clarke, Remtema, & Swetz, 2014). Indeed, continuing to use them might represent mistreatment of the newly dead (Anderson, Vernaglia, Morrigan, & Bard, 2007).

This does not mean, of course, that clinicians have *no* obligations toward newly dead persons. Different obligations are in place, namely reverence and respect, as well as care and concern for the family.

It is clear, then, that the line separating being alive and dead is distinct and crucial. Moving from one side to the other alters obligations and opportunities. This highlights the importance of accurately determining whether a patient is dead, either based on neurological or circulatory criteria.

Death by Neurologic Criteria
Controversies about Brain Death

Since originally put forth by the Harvard Ad Hoc Committee in 1968, the concept of brain death has become generally accepted within the medical community. It justifies not only shifting obligations and goals after its declaration—from those of a living patient to those of a dead person—but also the retrieval of vital organs.

The basis of this is the "Dead Donor Rule," a fundamental component of transplant ethics. This rule states that "donors must not be killed to obtain their organs" (Robertson, 1999) or, alternatively, that "persons must be dead before their organs are taken" (Arnold & Youngner, 1993). From the perspective of organ procurement, therefore, there is a sharp distinction between a living patient with severe neurological injury (such as in a coma) and a patient declared dead by neurological criteria. Given that transplant can literally be a life-saving procedure—and provide the family of the donor with some solace in their grief—it is imperative to accurately make this distinction.

Brain death is not without its critics, however. As a concept, it is difficult for some laypeople—and even some physicians—to accept (Siminoff, Burant, & Youngner, 2004). Contrary to the conventionally accepted understanding of death as the heart no longer beating and the patient not breathing, brain-dead patients often resemble other (living) patients in the ICU. Their chests rise and fall with each ventilator-assisted breath, and a regular tracing appears on the EKG monitor.

The term "brain dead" itself may perpetuate the misconception that such a patient is not truly dead. It can suggest that while the patient's brain is not currently functioning, there remains hope for some measure of recovery of the whole person. The reason for specifying a patient is brain dead is obvious: a physician's assertion that a patient with a beating heart is merely "dead" would likely provoke looks of incredulity. But the clarification also seems to dilute the power of the determination, as one would not pronounce a pulseless patient "heart/lung dead."

Brain death has been criticized not only for being counterintuitive but also for being philosophically inconsistent. Some have questioned the basic premise that the brain—as the purported primary integrator of bodily functions (Bernat, Culver, & Gert, 1981)—is necessary for a person to be alive. Shewmon (2001), for instance, presents a list of "non-brain-mediated somatically integrative functions," such as filtering of toxins and maintenance of body temperature. By this argument, cessation of function of the brain does not necessarily mean the patient is dead.

Others have argued that the brains of patients declared dead by neurological criteria have not ceased functioning entirely. Specifically, they point to continued neurohormonal regulation in the presence of a flat EEG (Halevy & Brody, 1993). If the entire brain has ceased to function—and the hypothalamus is part of the brain—how can the latter continue to participate in the negative feedback loop of the endocrine system?

If some question whether a patient who meets the accepted clinical criteria for brain death is truly dead, others have argued that even patients who *do not* meet those blanket criteria could, in fact, also be dead. Why, they ask, is cessation of function of the "entire brain, *including the brain stem*" (emphasis added) required for a determination of death? After all, what is truly unique about each person is not his brain stem—and other autonomic brain function—but rather his beliefs, memories, feelings, and so on, which reside in the cortex. Adopting this "higher brain" definition of death would allow patients with brain stem (but no cortical) function to be declared dead (Veatch, 1993), significantly expanding the pool of organ donors.

However, if patients who currently meet the criteria for brain death do not "seem" dead, then patients declared dead on the higher brain criteria *really* do not seem dead. For example, a patient with no cortical function could still breathe independently, if his brain stem were intact. And while it might seem bizarre to procure essential organs from a spontaneously breathing patient, an even greater quandary occurs with the more common response to a person's death (i.e., burial or cremation). Are we really prepared to bury a breathing person, based on the medical establishment's reassurance that the patient is dead by virtue of irreversible cessation of cortical function? This could prompt reconsideration of so-called "safety coffins," eighteenth-century devices with ventilation pipes and signaling devices to protect against misdiagnosis of death and premature burial (Cascella, 2016).

There is also the concern for the slippery slope if the blanket requirements of the UDDA are softened. What does it mean, after all, to say that there is "no cortical function"? Certainly, complete absence of cerebral flow to the cortices would prove this. But what of patients whose neurons continue to be perfused and discharge electric signals, yet are not able to perform basic functions associated with higher brain activities, such as interacting with others and forming memories? On this revised definition, a breathing, conscious patient with severe dementia might not merely be deemed impaired but potentially qualify as *dead* (and thus appropriate for burial).

Others have sought to increase the pool of essential organs for transplantation not by revising the definition of death but by questioning the requirement of death itself. They argue that what is most important is not so much that the patient already be dead but rather that adequate informed consent for donation be provided and that disproportionate harm be avoided (Truog & Robinson, 2003). After all, is there such a huge difference between two ventilator-dependent patients for whom the decision has been made to remove physiologic support—if both have previously given consent for organ donation—if one has a few neurons still functioning while the other does not? The end result (i.e., death) is the same, including for patients without any neurological injury who are about to be compassionately extubated. Why eliminate willing candidates simply because they do not meet the UDDA definition of brain death, or risk compromising the viability of organs by having to wait the required time period of the cDCD protocol?

There are two primary reasons why focusing solely on informed consent is a dangerous step. The first has to do with what limits—if any—are placed on the organ donation process. If the only thing that matters is the patient's informed consent, why limit this to patients who are imminently dying? A patient given a terminal diagnosis—especially if he has decided to forgo LSMT, or even take the further step of physician-assisted dying—would seem a logical donor. He is going to die anyway, so why not offer someone else the benefit of his organs?

And why require terminal illness at all? A patient who is *chronically* ill but dissatisfied with life might want to make a positive impact as he is liberated from a life he does not want. The ultimate extension of donation criteria would be an "altruistic donor," a term now generally applied to a living patient who donates one of his two kidneys or a portion of his liver. But if informed consent were the only relevant consideration, then the "ultimate altruist" could choose at any point to save the lives of seven other people—by donating two lungs, two kidneys, heart, liver, and pancreas—at the price of his own life. And is it that great a step to reach nonvoluntary donation, involving patients who "obviously" have no quality of life, beginning with those with unresponsive wakefulness syndrome and moving on to the developmentally disabled and persons with other disabilities?

The second reason to not focus exclusively on informed consent is the potential negative impact on public trust in organ donation. Unlike many other countries which use an "opt-out" approach to organ donation—whereby consent to donate is presumed unless a person has taken active steps to refuse (Rudge, Matesanz, Delmonico & Chapman, 2012)—the United States uses an "opt-in" system which is dependent on public trust that organs are procured (as well as subsequently allocated) in a just manner. Misperceptions about cDCD when it was first introduced (Kolata, 1997) highlight the need to safeguard the public trust to avoid discouraging patients (or their families) from consenting to organ donation. Viewed in this light, focusing entirely on informed consent may represent an example of winning the battle but losing the war.

Requests for Continued Physiologic Support after Diagnosis of Brain Death

In most cases, upon a determination of brain death families are ultimately able to grasp the fact that their loved one is really dead. It may take some time, and even if they do not fully accept it, they will at least recognize that there is no possibility of meaningful recovery and authorize discontinuation of mechanical ventilation on that basis. In rare cases, however, a family may remain resolute in demanding continued treatment.

There are three situations where continued support is well-accepted. The first is in the case of organ donation, where time is often required to convene the retrieval teams as well as to stabilize the patient hemodynamically. The second is when continued physiologic support offers benefit other than to an organ recipient, such as the case of a brain-dead pregnant woman who is sustained until her fetus can be safely delivered (Esmaeilzadeh et al., 2010). The last is when the family requires a little more time in order to "say goodbye." (It is hard to imagine a medical team refusing to temporarily delay compassionate extubation so as to allow a distant, beloved relative to reach the patient's bedside.)

Requests for longer delays in terminating physiologic support are problematic, however. One reason is based on distributive justice, given that an ICU bed is being taken up by a patient who cannot conceivably benefit from that level of care (and, indeed, is not even alive). In situations where ICU beds are scarce, depriving needy living patients of their required level of treatment is particularly troublesome.

There is also the matter of reimbursement. Third-party payers generally do not reimburse the hospital for medical treatments which fall outside the standard of care. (Mechanical ventilation for a dead patient would certainly fall into that category.) The hospital is then faced with either absorbing the costs of continued critical care or passing them along to the grieving family.

Finally, there is concern for moral distress of the staff (p. 514). Providing critical care can be emotionally exhausting, given the acuity of the situation and the increased likelihood of a poor outcome. This is especially a concern when staff are asked to continue to care for a dead patient as if that patient were still alive: drawing blood, turning the patient, consoling the family. Basic assumptions of clinical care for a living person—such as local anesthesia prior to invasive procedures—no longer hold for a patient who is incapable of feeling pain. Understandably, most discussions of moral distress comes out of the nursing literature; in contrast to physicians who spend a little time each day with a great many patients, ICU nurses typically care for only one or two patients at a time in prolonged shifts often over a protracted period of time.

When a family requests continued cardiorespiratory support for a brain-dead patient, it is important to identify the reason for their request. It may be rooted in strained communication or mistrust of the medical team. Clearly this is a very emotional time for the family, and if they feel disrespected or disempowered they may "dig in their heels." In such cases, optimized communication—often through consultation with other services such as palliative care or ethics—can be helpful.

Such a request may also stem from cultural objections to the concept of brain death, which is not universally acknowledged. Romania and Pakistan, for instance, generally do not recognize the concept (Japan Organ Transplant Network, 2017).

If the opposition to withdrawing physiologic support is rooted in religious views, clarification can be helpful, generally from within the family's religious tradition. Orthodox Jews are perhaps best known for "denying" brain death. While physical decapitation is accepted as death even if there is still some muscle twitching (Mishna, Oholot 1:6), Orthodox Jews generally are not willing—as progressive Jews often are—to extend this analogy to brain death. They cite rabbinical sources which state that as long as the heart is beating and the lungs are breathing, a patient is not dead (Teshuvot Chacham Tzvi, no 77; Teshuvot Chatam Sofer, Yoreh De'ah, no 338). While this is the standard interpretation within Orthodox Judaism (Rosner, Bleich, & Brayer, 2000), recent position statements have offered some degree of latitude on whether an individual rabbi may endorse—or Jewish patient or family accept—a diagnosis of brain death (Rabbinical Council of America, 2010).

Even if an Orthodox Jewish family refuses to accept a diagnosis of brain death, this is not equivalent to demanding maximal treatment. Continuous monitoring and intravenous antibiotics need not be continued, for instance (Inwald, Jakobovits, & Petros, 2000). Even if physiological functioning can be maintained for a period of time, eventually cardiac arrest will occur leading to a condition that the family accepts as death.

But what of a family who—for religious or other reasons—demands maximal treatment with no clear end point? This would include not only antibiotics, but also endocrine monitoring and supplementation, as well as medically administered nutrition and hydration. With such treatment a brain-dead patient could be physiologically maintained for weeks, months, or even years, as exemplified by Jahi McMath (p. 428). The problems of distributive justice, reimbursement, and moral distress will only worsen over time.

As with many other ethical dilemmas, the best way to respond to this one is to prevent it from occurring in the first place. One might start with the terms often used, including "brain death" itself. If one does not declare a patient whose heart has irreversibly stopped working as being "heart/lung dead," neither should one say that a patient whose brain has irreversibly stopped working is "brain dead." Rather, it is appropriate to say that the patient is "dead," while also explaining why he may resemble living patients on ventilators.

Similarly, one should not talk about "life support" for the patient, since it is logically impossible to support the "life" of a person who is dead. (Newspaper accounts do not help in this regard, as they often speak of a patient being declared brain dead and then "life support" being withdrawn [Buck, 2016]). Finally, using colloquialisms such as "feeding tube" (p. 185) may heighten rather than clarify the emotional challenges of the family's decision.

Asking permission to withdraw mechanical ventilation is also inviting disagreement. In general, clinicians should not ask questions unless they are ready to hear the patient's or family's answer. In this case, professional obligations, expert consensus, and legal opinion—except in a handful of states, particularly New Jersey—are clear: there is no obligation to maintain physiologic support of a person who is brain dead. Thus it is entirely appropriate to approach the family by saying, "We're very sorry to have to inform you that your loved one has died. Is there anyone who wants to spend a few minutes with him before we discontinue the ventilator?"

If the family remains adamant despite this thoughtful approach, there would be seem to be three possible responses. One would be to honor the family's request out of deference to their grief and not wanting to provoke conflict. The patient in this case would not be suffering, and as such this would represent an extreme form of the well-accepted practice of treating the patient "for the benefit of the family," if there is a sense that the patient would have wanted to continue (Hardwig, 1991). Such an approach, however, would have a substantial negative impact on other patients in need of critical care, professional ethics, staff morale, and potentially the family's financial well-being.

The second option is time-limited trial (TLT, p. 118) of continued physiologic support, at least in terms of mechanical ventilation. It would certainly be reasonable to consider decreased monitoring as well as a Do Not Attempt Resuscitation order—which could legitimately be called a *cannot* resuscitate order—in case of cardiac arrest. To the degree that this middle ground could lead to a mutually acknowledged death of the patient without additional conflict and suffering, it resembles a Do Not Escalate Treatment order (p. 120).

The purpose of continued mechanical ventilation is not to determine if it will benefit the patient—which it logically cannot because he is dead—but to determine if the family will come to accept the diagnosis of death over that time. Ideally, such a step will build rapport with the family by showing respect for their beliefs. As a middle ground between two extremes, it moderates the drawbacks of each. For instance, distributive justice and moral distress are still concerns, but not as much as if support continued over the long term.

By the same token, if there is a sense that unilateral withdrawal is intended at the end of the TLT, this may undercut the rapport with the family that the team is attempting to build. Ultimately, this approach will either build consensus (if the family accepts the diagnosis), defer to the inevitable (if the patient's heart stops during the TLT), or simply "kick the can down the road," delaying a definitive decision.

The final option is to unilaterally discontinue physiologic support. This violates neither professional norms nor the vast majority of state laws, while also sparing the staff ongoing moral distress and respecting the needs of other patients in need of critical care. And while it may appear "heartless" in the face of the grieving family's desperate pleas, others might view it as being "cruel only to be kind" (Shakespeare, 1970), sparing the family ongoing suffering by taking the decision out of their hands.

The practical implications of such an action need to be considered. A family that does not accept that their loved one is truly dead is likely to strenuously object to any attempt to discontinue respiratory support. This may take the form of seeking a temporary restraining order against extubation (Burkle, Schipper, & Wijdicks, 2011), or even physical resistance. In the case of families with well-established religious objections, attempted withdrawal may be viewed as disrespecting their faith tradition. And at least in the short term, it may exacerbate an already crippling grief.

Ultimately, the correct approach largely depends on one's sense of the family and their reasons for rejecting the patient's diagnosis. The first option (full capitulation) is rarely right, as it represents an abdication of professional responsibility and an invitation to greater conflict in the future. The second option is moderate and reasonable, especially when there is a sense that the family over time will come to accept the diagnosis. Even if that is not currently apparent, deepening rapport may help them reach this point.

Unilateral discontinuation of respiratory support is a last resort. This is in some ways an extreme example of forgoing nonbeneficial treatment (NBT, chapter 14), for clearly *none* of the treatments in use have any chance of benefitting the patient. But neither can the patient suffer, thus allowing some room for discretion. If the family persists in their demand for maximal treatment even after the TLT has concluded, the process recommended for potentially NBT could be utilized, including a second opinion and consultations with ethics, palliative care, spiritual care, and risk management (although these likely would already have occurred). It may also be possible to transfer the patient to an accepting facility, as occurred with Jahi McMath.

Ultimately, though, this runs the risk of disrespecting the patient as a person. Granted, a brain-dead patient cannot perceive suffering in real time, but if continued interventions violate the patient's values, this could be viewed on inflicting harm on his personhood, his legacy. Rather than transferring the patient to a willing facility—and further prolonging the family's grief—it is usually more appropriate to take a principled stand after the family has been given sufficient time to come to terms with the diagnosis. The question of precisely how much time that is, however, remains.

Palliative care is especially critical in conflictual situations such as these. Expert communication and conflict mediation skills are necessary, especially in an emotionally fraught context. As a consulting service not tasked with the "ultimate decision" of whether to withdraw support, the palliative care team can hopefully be a bridge between the primary team and the family. As specialists comfortable discussing death and familiar with the ambiguities of values-laden decisions, the team is ideally situated to provide support to both the family and the staff, while always keeping the patient's dignity and values paramount in the discussion.

Deciding Whether Even to Test for Brain Death

There is an old saying in medicine: "Don't do a test unless it will change management." Many tests are invasive and painful, and some may cause unnecessary harm or suffering, as in the case of an amniocentesis for a genetic condition if the parents are not considering termination (p. 294). The results could also be misleading, especially if the prior probability of the tested-for condition is sufficiently low. In that case, a positive result is more likely to be a false positive than a true one. A clinical test should, therefore, only be performed if it will generate reliable information that is sufficiently relevant to future decisions to justify any inherent risk.

Take, for example, a patient who has suffered a serious brain injury and whose family has decided to withdraw LSMT. The only reason to pursue a determination of brain death in such a situation is if the patient might wish to be an organ donor, recognizing that the viability of organs from a heart-beating donor will be greater than from a cDCD donor.[3] If the patient did not wish to be an organ donor, LSMT can be withdrawn without having to go through the process of determining whether the patient is actually brain dead. Of course, if the family was uncertain whether to forgo continued treatment, determining that the patient is already dead would remove this burden from them.

The other situation where it may not be reasonable to test for brain death is if the family has made it abundantly clear that they would not accept such a diagnosis, and the clinical team is not currently willing to unilaterally withdraw ventilatory support. As noted earlier, third-party payers will not reimburse the hospital for physiologic support of a brain-dead patient, thus forcing the hospital to either absorb the cost or (more likely) pass it on to the family. For ICU care over a period of days or even weeks, this can result in a massive bill. Some families may therefore withhold consent for apnea testing, fearing the legal and ethical ramifications of a confirmatory test.

It may seem disingenuous to cast a blind eye at what seems obvious (Bliss & Macauley, 2015). But what seems obvious may not be true, especially given the strenuous requirements of the "whole brain definition" of death. It is also important to recall that there are many situations in medicine where confirmation of suspicions is not sought, such as the cachectic patient with a lung mass found on x-ray who does not want to know if it is cancer and would not accept treatment even if it was. Not only would performing

---

3. Assuming that the patient is even a candidate for cDCD donation, which he might not be if he is likely to be able to breathe independently for more than one hour after extubation.

such a biopsy violate the patient's autonomy; it also would not produce results that would change management.

The norm should remain performing an apnea test in cases of suspected brain death. Absent a strong sense that the family is unalterably opposed to withdrawal of support if the diagnosis is confirmed, an apnea test is likely to provide valuable clinical information. But when the family has made it abundantly clear that forgoing mechanical ventilation is not an option, it may be more prudent to defer the test and focus on ongoing dialogue with the family and attending to their emotional needs, which also avoids saddling them with crippling medical bills.

Death by Circulatory Criteria

DCD presents a distinct set of ethical issues. Whereas much of the brain death controversy revolves around whether a patient is truly dead—and whether his family is willing to accept that he is—patients who die during the DCD protocol meet the conventional expectations of death: their hearts are no longer beating and lungs no longer breathing. It is not entirely clear, however, how long one's heart and lungs must go without functioning to meet the UDDA's requirement of "irreversibility." Neither is it obvious what modifications to standard EOL care are permissible, in order to maximize the benefit to another patient (i.e., the organ recipient). Finally, one might reasonably inquire whether the involvement of palliative care clinicians in organ donation risks conflating the latter with EOL care, thereby harming the mission of palliative through inaccurate assumptions.

Irreversibility and Permanence

The UDDA defines circulatory death as the irreversible cessation of heart and lung function. In situations where a patient has a DNAR order and is not a potential DCD donor, the question of what constitutes "irreversibility" is not pressing. There is no rush to declare the patient dead; indeed, taking one's time assures that this is not done prematurely.

For a patient who is not DNAR, irreversibility matters because once a certain amount of time has passed, CPR will not be effective and thus should not be instituted. Conversely, in the context of DCD the time to irreversibility represents a minimum waiting period following pulselessness, to ensure that the Dead Donor Rule is not violated (American Academy of Pediatrics, 2013).

This time pressure creates an inherent trade-off: the longer one waits to declare death, the more certain of the diagnosis but also the longer the "warm ischemia time" of the organs, negatively affecting their viability. On the other hand, a shorter waiting period maximizes organ viability but creates uncertainty as to whether the retrieval might violate the Dead Donor Rule. In an attempt to balance these considerations, the Institute of Medicine (2000) has suggested a five-minute waiting period. Some hospital protocols, though, use as little as ninety seconds (Boucek et al., 2008), running the risk of precluding the possibility of autoresuscitation.

The criteria used for declaring death were the focus of a recent debate concerning pediatric heart transplantation following cDCD (Boucek et al., 2008). It may initially seem contradictory to speak of heart donation after *cardiac death*, as the practice was known at the time. But in this small case series three critically ill infants were compassionately extubated, and ninety seconds after onset of pulselessness, death was declared. The infants' hearts were then procured and transplanted into other babies who were suffering cardiac failure, at which point external resuscitation was applied and the hearts began to function again.

Some have criticized this as a violation of the Dead Donor Rule, since clearly those three hearts did not "irreversibly" cease to function (Veatch, 2008). Defenders of the procedure, however, draw a distinction between "'permanent' (will not reverse) and 'irreversible' (cannot reverse) cessation of functions" (Bernat, 2010). They argue that the transplanted hearts did not function in the donors—as external resuscitation was not offered—but *could* still function in the recipients, with medical assistance. The cessation of function was therefore permanent, although not irreversible.

This distinction is also applied (at least implicitly) in other areas of clinical practice. There have been documented cases of survival—admittedly, often with significant impairment—when CPR has been instituted as long as *fifteen* minutes after the onset of asystole (Joffe et al., 2011). Yet physicians do not generally feel the need to wait such a long period of time after onset of pulselessness to declare death. Asystole just beyond the time limit of possible autoresuscitation is not irreversible but for a patient who is DNAR it is permanent (and thus justifies declaration of death).

The Institute of Medicine definition of death also implicitly appeals to permanence, since pulselessness of greater than five minutes' duration has been reversed in some cases. Raising the bar for declaration of death to require true irreversibility would have a significant negative impact on organ viability in even the most conservative DCD protocols.

The operative question, then, is not whether asystole *can* be reversed but will it be. And if it will not—whether based on impossibility (i.e., irreversibility) or refusal of treatment that could reverse it (i.e., permanence)—then the patient can legitimately be declared dead.

While thoughtful and reasoned, this permanent/irreversible distinction can be lost on many observers, especially given the context of cDCD. In light of these nuanced distinctions, it is not surprising that most pediatricians in a recent survey were not confident that cDCD donors were truly dead (Joffe, Anton, & deCaen, 2008). Even if death is acknowledged, the ethical propriety of cDCD could be questioned (i.e., "Isn't that just killing the patient to get his organs?"). This potential for misunderstanding highlights the need for clinicians—and palliative care clinicians, in particular—to be able to effectively articulate the ethical justification for cDCD.

Treating One Patient for the Benefit of Another

Organ donation creates several scenarios that may appear to violate Kant's (1981) Categorical Imperative, which clearly states that one should never treat another person "merely as a means to an end, but always at the same time as an end." For instance, a living donor incurs significant burden—in the form of pain, as well as increased risk of morbidity or even mortality—in order to provide the recipient with a functioning kidney. But the donor was not treated *merely* as a means to an end; rather, the altruistic act of donating organs reflected his goals and values, thus providing comfort and meaning to both him and (hopefully) his family.

Controlled DCD also involves tradeoffs. Rather than dying surrounded by potentially many relatives in the hospital room that has come to seem familiar, the patient dies in a sterile operating room with only a few family members allowed to be present, who cannot stay with the body after the confirmatory period of pulselessness has elapsed. Clearly there is loss, but hopefully the benefit of offering life to another person is enough to compensate for it. Ultimately, cDCD is an act of respect for an altruistic patient's autonomy.

There is risk, however, that the needs of the organ recipient could take precedence over those of the donor, potentially exposing the latter to unnecessary harm or burden. One such risk involves the consent process, during which it is crucial that the team caring for a potential donor focus exclusively on the care of that patient. Standard practice is that the decision to withdraw LSMT should be made without consideration of possible donation. Only *after* this decision is made should the OPO make contact with the family to discuss donation. This is clearly articulated in policies from both the United Network of Organ Sharing (2011) as well as the Organ Procurement and Transplant Network (OPTN, 2016), which states: "Prior to the OPO initiating any discussion with the legal next of kin about organ donation for a potential DCD donor, the OPO must confirm that the legal next of kin has elected to withdraw life-sustaining medical treatment." The palliative care community also endorses this requirement (Lustbader & Goldstein, 2015).

Once consent is obtained, certain interventions may be considered to optimize organ viability, including heparin and vasodilators to minimize the risk of clotting, as well as placement of a large-bore catheter to administer fluids and medications. These are not generally components of EOL care, and in some cases could conceivably cause harm to the patient (such as by increasing the chance of hemorrhage). Such actions are being taken for the well-being of another patient (i.e., the recipient).

But they are not *merely* being done for the recipient. They should reflect the altruistic values of the donor, which makes obtaining informed consent—and confirming that the donor would have been willing to accept additional interventions—crucial. It is also important to recognize that these interventions are not the cause of the patient's death, given that the decision to withdraw support should have been made prior to the OPO's involvement.

The third area where the needs of the donor and the recipient may seem to be in conflict pertains to the time limit (generally one hour) in the operating room. Past that point, organ viability is sufficiently compromised to justify cancelling the procurement and taking the intended donor back to the ICU to continue comfort care. This may create a sense of pressure to expedite the process within the one-hour time frame in order to fulfill the donor's last wish, as expressed by his family.

This is precisely the reason the organ procurement team is not permitted in the operating room until death is declared. There have been case reports of violations of this rule, with the procurement team supposedly perceiving suffering—which the ICU team did not—and on that basis urging administration of additional opioids, which in one case the surgeon unfortunately referred to as "candy" (McKinley, 2008). This engendered suspicion that the transplant surgeon was attempting to expedite the donor's death to ensure that organ procurement proceeded.

Egregious examples such as this underscore the need to provide the standard of care in EOL treatment. This can be challenging, though, depending on the personnel involved. For instance, an anesthesiologist—whose "domain" is the operating room—might be called upon to care for the donor until death is declared. But unless the anesthesiologist also practices critical care, she may not possess expertise in symptom management at the end of life. This not only impacts the provision of clinical care but could also have repercussions if there are insinuations that the patient's death was hastened in order to procure the organs. Even if upward dose titration conformed to the standard of care, an anesthesiologist—unlike a physician who routinely provides EOL care—would not be able to defend herself by pointing to the equivalent treatment she had provided to other EOL patients (because there would not be any). It is therefore important to consult the palliative care service, if they are not already involved in the care of such a seriously ill patient (Kelso, Lyckholm, Coyne, & Smith, 2007).

Antemortem Retrieval of Vital Organs

Another controversial area where death could be hastened—or at least *perceived* to be hastened—is by stretching the limits of (without technically violating) the Dead Donor Rule, in order to optimize organ viability. For instance, some have suggested that rather than waiting for a cDCD donor to become pulseless for a set period of time—thus risking ischemic damage to the organs—some vital organs could be retrieved before death (Morrissey, 2012). One example is bilateral nephrectomy, for while kidneys are necessary to sustain life, they are not *imminently* necessary (i.e., a patient can survive for days without his kidneys). The rationale is that the patient will die from respiratory failure following compassionate extubation long before he would die of renal failure, thus technically abiding by certain formulations of the Dead Donor Rule.[4]

---

4. In this case, the patient is not killed by the removal of vital organs, but neither is he already dead when they are removed.

However, given the importance of public trust in the process of organ donation, removing vital organs in this way—while likely not actually hastening the patient's death—could negatively impact the overall mission of organ donation. It also creates a slippery slope where other organs might be removed antemortem, anticipating that the patient will die within an hour following extubation (or very soon thereafter). It is often extremely difficult to predict with certainty, however, how long a patient will live (p. 166), even after compassionate extubation. Such a practice therefore risks compromising the fundamental rule of organ donation, for the sake of only modest increases in organ viability.

Blurring the Line between Organ Donation and End of Life Care

As noted, professional and ethical bodies support the position that cDCD be raised by the designated requestor only after the decision has been made to withdraw support. There is concern, however, that in an attempt to increase the number of organs available for transplantation, this requirement may not be adhered to. For instance, recent modifications in OPTN guidelines allow for great individual variation in hospital organ donation policies. An example is a recent media report where OPO representatives were reportedly "introduced to families early, not as organ procurement organizations but as end-of-life care specialists" (National Public Radio, 2013). This may lead to situations where the lines between organ donation and EOL care are blurred.

It is extremely important to be clear with the family about each person's role and primary obligations. Not doing so risks depriving families of the palliative care they need and deserve—by falsely identifying OPO representatives as experts in EOL care—as well as tainting the field of palliative care with misleading associations.

At the same time, one can reasonably wonder whether the requirement that organ donation only be discussed *after* the family has decided to withdraw LSMT is sacrosanct. The underlying premise is obvious and worthy: no patient or family should be pressured to withdraw support in order to donate, which would clearly violate the Categorical Imperative. But is it so hard to imagine a patient whose likelihood of recovery is extremely poor and whose level of consciousness is so depressed that he is thought incapable of suffering, and whose family decides to continue with LSMT—at least temporarily—because "there is nothing to lose"? Imagine further that the patient was a passionate advocate of organ donation, having specified in his advance directive that he very much wanted to be a donor. There might be situations where continued treatment could render the organs less viable for ultimate transplantation, or even disqualify the patient as a donor altogether. If so, wouldn't the fact that organ donation might cease to be an option be a relevant consideration that the family has a right to know about, as they attempt to apply the patient's values to the decision?

Clearly, this is something of an unusual—if not exceptional—circumstance. As such it represents a potential "exception to the rule," rather than a justification for changing the rule itself. Concern for divided loyalties and subtle coercion are more than sufficient to support the standard position that *OPO staff*—whose mission is to foster organ donation—should not raise the issue before the decision to withdraw LMST has been made.

But given that the palliative care team is likely involved in the care of such a critically ill patient, in the course of a comprehensive discussion about the patient's goals and values—perhaps transitioning into dignity therapy (Thompson & Chochinov, 2008) as it becomes clear the patient will not survive—a personal dedication to organ donation may become apparent. If so, it is appropriate for the palliative care team to explore how that might fit into the overall values of the patient, and ultimately to the goals of care. After all, competent patients are permitted to refuse LSMT for essentially any reason; the hope of giving life to another person is surely a worthy one.

Return to the Case

Unfortunately, several of the preparatory steps advised in this chapter—such as not using the term "brain death" and not asking permission from the family to withdraw ventilatory support—were not taken, which may have contributed to the impasse. Recognizing the family's adamant opposition to withdrawal of support, the team decides to take a middle ground by suggesting a TLT of seventy-two hours, at which time another family meeting will be held. The team promises to monitor the patient for any signs of life, which would void the diagnosis of brain death. The family agrees to the plan.

Over that period of time the team continues to support the family, inviting them to take part in serial clinical exams and explaining the significance—or lack of significance—of vital signs and other measurements.

The palliative care team is consulted for additional support, sensitively inquiring about the patient's goals and values. His family relates how important relationships are to him, as well as a sense of independence. Rather than focusing on the disagreement over brain death, the palliative care team reframes the situation in terms of the patient's prognosis, which his family admits is grim.

Through thoughtful and empathetic listening, the family comes to acknowledge that the patient will never recover, which allows them to consent to withholding any escalation of treatment (p. 120). A DNAR order is placed on the patient's chart.

At the conclusion of the TLT, there has been no improvement in the patient's condition. The family thus agrees to withdrawing the ventilator, without explicitly admitting the patient is dead. The team is obligated by law to contact the local OPO, who contacts the family. Having already decided to "let him die," they are grateful for the opportunity to "share him" with others in need. Organ procurement proceeds smoothly and benefits several patients on the transplant waiting list.

Summary Points

- Prior to the use of mechanical ventilators, there was no need to define death, as a patient whose brain was not functioning also would not breathe, and thus his heart would inevitably stop.
- The concept of "brain death" was developed in the 1960s and ultimately came to be incorporated into the UDDA which defined death as the "irreversible cessation of function of either circulatory and respiratory functions, or all functions of the entire brain, including the brain stem."
- The Dead Donor Rule is a foundational principle of transplant ethics, stating that a donor should be dead before vital organs are retrieved.
- Death by neurological criteria:
  - Some have questioned whether patients who meet the criteria for brain death are actually dead (by virtue of continued neuroendocrine function), and others have questioned whether cessation of function of the whole brain is necessary for death. The UDDA definition remains standard, though.
  - When a family rejects the diagnosis of brain death and demands continued ventilatory support, often the wisest response is to offer a TLT of continued support with an agreement not to escalate the current level of treatment.
  - In extreme circumstances, extubation over the family's objections may be necessary.
  - Where it is clear that the family will not accept a diagnosis of brain death, consideration should be given to temporarily deferring apnea testing if it will not change management.
- Death by circulatory criteria:
  - The duration of pulselessness required to determine death by circulatory criteria must exclude the possibility of autoresuscitation and in the context of DCD impacts organ viability.
  - With regard to pulselessness, permanence is a more helpful concept than irreversibility and is generally applied in clinical situations other than transplantation.
  - An organ donor may undergo certain interventions for the benefit of the recipient, but only with explicit informed consent and with the assurance that the standard of treatment for EOL care will be maintained.
  - Antemortem retrieval of vital organs is not consistent with certain formulations of the Dead Donor Rule and endangers public trust in the organ donation process. It should therefore be rejected.
  - While they often collaborate, a crisp line should be drawn between organ procurement representatives and palliative care professionals. The former should never raise the prospect of organ donation before a decision has been made to withhold LSMT. If, however, the family raises that subject with palliative care professionals as part of a general discussion of overall goals of care, it is appropriate to explore acceptable options.

References

Ad Hoc Committee of the Harvard Medical School to Examine the Definition of Brain Death. (1968). A definition of irreversible coma. *JAMA, 205*(6), 337–340.

American Academy of Pediatrics. (2013). Ethical controversies in organ donation after circulatory death. *Pediatrics, 131*(5), 1021–1026. doi:10.1542/peds.2013-0672

Anderson, J. A., Vernaglia, L. W., Morrigan, S. P., & Bard, T. R. (2007). Refusal of brain death diagnosis. *JONAS Healthc Law Ethics Regul, 9*(3), 87–94. doi:10.1097/01.NHL.0000287971.21182.22

Antommaria, A. H., Trotochaud, K., Kinlaw, K., Hopkins, P. N., & Frader, J. (2009). Policies on donation after cardiac death at children's hospitals: A mixed-methods analysis of variation. *JAMA, 301*(18), 1902–1908. doi:10.1001/jama.2009.637

Arnold, R. M., & Youngner, S. J. (1993). The dead donor rule: Should we stretch it, bend it, or abandon it? *Kennedy Inst Ethics J, 3*(2), 263–278.

Bernat, J. L. (2010). How the distinction between "irreversible" and "permanent" illuminates circulatory-respiratory death determination. *J Med Philos, 35*(3), 242–255. doi:10.1093/jmp/jhq018

Bernat, J. L., Culver, C. M., & Gert, B. (1981). On the definition and criterion of death. *Ann Intern Med, 94*(3), 389–394.

Beresford, H. R. (2001). Legal aspects of brain death. In E. F. M. Wijdicks (Ed.), *Brain death* (pp. 151–169). Philadelphia: Lippincott Williams & Wilkins.

Bliss, S. E., & Macauley, R. C. (2015). The least bad option: Unilateral extubation after declaration of death by neurological criteria. *J Clin Ethics, 26*(3), 260–265.

Boucek, M. M., Mashburn, C., Dunn, S. M., Frizell, R., Edwards, L., Pietra, B., ... Denver Children's Pediatric Heart Transplant Team. (2008). Pediatric heart transplantation after declaration of cardiocirculatory death. *N Engl J Med, 359*(7), 709–714. doi:10.1056/NEJMoa0800660

Buck, C. (2016). Brain-dead toddler taken off life support in Los Angeles. *Sacramento Bee.* Retrieved from http://www.sacbee.com/news/local/article97861097.html

Burkle, C. M., Schipper, A. M., & Wijdicks, E. F. (2011). Brain death and the courts. *Neurology, 76*(9), 837–841.

Cascella, M. (2016). Taphophobia and "life preserving coffins" in the nineteenth century. *Hist Psychiatry, 27*(3), 345–349. doi:10.1177/0957154X16650100

Clarke, M. J., Remtema, M. S., & Swetz, K. M. (2014). Beyond transplantation: Considering brain death as a hard clinical endpoint. *Am J Bioeth, 14*(8), 43–45. doi:10.1080/15265161.2014.925166

Diem, S. J., Lantos, J. D., & Tulsky, J. A. (1996). Cardiopulmonary resuscitation on television: Miracles and misinformation. *N Engl J Med, 334*(24), 1578–1582. doi:10.1056/NEJM199606133342406

Dominguez-Gil, B., Duranteau, J., Mateos, A., Nunez, J. R., Cheisson, G., Corral, E., ... Matesanz, R. (2016). Uncontrolled donation after circulatory death: European practices and recommendations for the development and optimization of an effective programme. *Transpl Int, 29*(8), 842–859. doi:10.1111/tri.12734

Douglas v. Janssen Funeral Homes. (2011). Alaska Super. Ct.

Esmaeilzadeh, M., Dictus, C., Kayvanpour, E., Sedaghat-Hamedani, F., Eichbaum, M., Hofer, S., ... Ahmadi, R. (2010). One life ends, another begins: Management of a brain-dead pregnant mother-A systematic review. *BMC Med, 8,* 74. doi:10.1186/1741-7015-8-74

Forbess, J. M., Cook, N., Roth, S. J., Serraf, A., Mayer, J. E. Jr., & Jonas, R. A. (1995). Ten-year institutional experience with palliative surgery for hypoplastic left heart syndrome: Risk factors related to stage I mortality. *Circulation, 92*(9 Suppl.), II262–II266.

Furness, H. (2012, April 25). "Miracle recovery" of teen declared brain dead by four doctors. *Telegraph.*

Goila, A. K., & Pawar, M. (2009). The diagnosis of brain death. *Indian J Crit Care Med, 13*(1), 7–11. doi:10.4103/0972-5229.53108

Gostin, L. O. (2014). Legal and ethical responsibilities following brain death: The McMath and Munoz cases. *JAMA, 311*(9), 903–904. doi:10.1001/jama.2014.660

Greene, M., & Wolfe, L. (2012, August). Pregnancy exclusions in state living will and medical proxy statutes. Retrieved from http://www.centerwomen policy.org/programs%5Chealth/statepolicy/documents/REPRO_PregnancyExclusionsin StateLivingWillandMedicalProxyStatutesMeganGreeneandLeslieR.Wolfe.pdf, archived at http://perma.cc/384Q-74K3

Halevy, A., & Brody, B. (1993). Brain death: Reconciling definitions, criteria, and tests. *Ann Intern Med*, *119*(6), 519–525.

Hardwig, J. (1991). Treating the brain dead for the benefit of the family. *J Clin Ethics*, *2*(1), 53–56.

Health Care Financing Administration. (1998). Hospital Conditions of Participation; Identification of Potential Organ, Tissue, and Eye Donors and Transplant Hospitals' Provision of Transplant-Related Data. 63 FR 3386.

Hosgood, S. A., Shah, K., Patel, M., & Nicholson, M. L. (2015). The effect of prolonged of warm ischaemic injury on renal function in an experimental ex vivo normothermic perfusion system. *J Transl Med*, *13*, 207. doi:10.1186/s12967-015-0571-4

Hospital Licensing Act. (2008). Illinois Public Act 095-0181.

In re Quinlan, 70 10 (N.J. 1976).

Institute of Medicine. (2000). *Non-heart-beating organ transplantation: Practice and protocols*. Washington, DC: National Academies Press.

Inwald, D., Jakobovits, I., & Petros, A. (2000). Brain stem death: Managing care when accepted medical guidelines and religious beliefs are in conflict. Consideration and compromise are possible. *BMJ*, *320*(7244), 1266–1267.

Jain, S., & DeGeorgia, M. (2005). Brain death-associated reflexes and automatisms. *Neurocrit Care*, *3*(2), 122–126. doi:10.1385/NCC:3:2:122

Japan Organ Transplant Network. (2017). Views on brain death. Retrieved from https://www.jotnw.or.jp/english/05.html

Joffe, A. R., Carcillo, J., Anton, N., deCaen, A., Han, Y. Y., Bell, M. J., . . . Garcia-Guerra, G. (2011). Donation after cardiocirculatory death: A call for a moratorium pending full public disclosure and fully informed consent. *Philos Ethics Humanit Med*, *6*, 17. doi:10.1186/1747-5341-6-17

Joffe, A. R., Anton, N. R., & deCaen, A. R. (2008). Survey of pediatricians' opinions on donation after cardiac death: Are the donors dead? *Pediatrics*, *122*(5), e967–e974. doi:10.1542/peds.2008-1210

Jouvet, M. (1959). [Electro-subcorticographic diagnosis of death of the central nervous system during various types of coma]. *Electroencephalogr Clin Neurophysiol*, *11*, 805–808.

Kant, I. (1981). *Grounding for the metaphysics of morals*. Indianapolis: Hackett.

Kelso, C. M., Lyckholm, L. J., Coyne, P. J., & Smith, T. J. (2007). Palliative care consultation in the process of organ donation after cardiac death. *J Palliat Med*, *10*(1), 118–126. doi:10.1089/jpm.2006.0118

Kesselring, A., Kainz, M., & Kiss, A. (2007). Traumatic memories of relatives regarding brain death, request for organ donation and interactions with professionals in the ICU. *Am J Transplant*, *7*(1), 211–217. doi:10.1111/j.1600-6143.2006.01594.x

Kolata, G. (1997, April 13). Controversy erupts over organ removals. *New York Times*.

Kootstra, G. (1997). The asystolic, or non-heartbeating, donor. *Transplantation*, *63*(7), 917–921.

Lustbader, D., & Goldstein, M. J. (2015). Organ donation after cardiac death. Retrieved from http://www.mypcnow.org/blank-b9ix3

McKinley, J. (2008, February 27). Surgeon accused of speeding a death to get organs. *New York Times*. Retrieved from http://www.nytimes.com/2008/02/27/us/27transplant.html

Miller, R. D., & Steiner, J. (2014). *Problems in health care law: Challenges for the 21st century* (10th ed.). Burlington, MA: Jones & Bartlett Learning.

Morrissey, P. E. (2012). The case for kidney donation before end-of-life care. *Am J Bioeth*, *12*(6), 1–8. doi:10.1080/15265161.2012.671886

National Conference of Commissioners on Uniform State Laws. (1981). The Uniform Determination of Death Act 1981.

National Public Radio. (2013). Proposed changes in organ donation stir debate. Retrieved from http://www.npr.org/blogs/health/2013/06/24/194275901/proposed-changes-in-organ-donation-stir-debate

New Jersey Declaration of Death Act, Pub. L. No. 6A, 26 Stat. 5 (1991).

New York State Department of Health. (2011). Guidelines for determining brain death. Retrieved from https://www.health.ny.gov/professionals/hospital_administrator/letters/2011/brain_death_guidelines.pdf

Organ Procurement and Transplant Network. (2016). Policies. Retrieved from https://optn.transplant.hrsa.gov/media/1200/optn_policies.pdf

Organ Procurement and Transplantation Network. (2017). Retrieved from https://optn.transplant.hrsa. gov/

Pope, T. M. (2014). Medical board of California should investigate McMath clinicians. Retrieved from https://medicalfutility.blogspot.com/2014/01/medical-board-of-california-should.html

President's Commission for the Study of Ethical Problems in Medicine and Biomedical and Behavioral Research. (1981). *Defining death: A report on the medical, legal and ethical issues in the determination of death.* Washington, DC: U.S. Government Printing Office.

President's Council on Bioethics. (2009). *Contoversies in the determination of death.* Washington, DC: U.S. Government Printing Office.

Prommer, E. (2014). Organ donation and palliative care: Can palliative care make a difference? *J Palliat Med, 17*(3), 368–371. doi:10.1089/jpm.2013.0375

Rabbinical Council of America. (2010). Halachic issues in the determination of death and in organ transplantation. Retrieved from http://www.rabbis.org/pdfs/Halachi_%20Issues_the_Determination.pdf

Rady, M. Y., Verheijde, J. L., & McGregor, J. (2006). Organ donation after circulatory death: The forgotten donor? *Crit Care, 10*(5), 166. doi:10.1186/cc5038

Reed, M. J., & Lua, S. B. (2014). Uncontrolled organ donation after circulatory death: Potential donors in the emergency department. *Emerg Med J, 31*(9), 741–744. doi:10.1136/emermed-2013-202675

Robertson, J. A. (1999). The dead donor rule. *Hastings Cent Rep, 29*(6), 6–14.

Rosner, F., Bleich, J. D., & Brayer, M. M. (2000). *Jewish bioethics* (Augm. ed.). Hoboken, NJ: KTAV Publishing.

Rudge, C., Matesanz, R., Delmonico, F. L., & Chapman, J. (2012). International practices of organ donation. *Br J Anaesth, 108*(Suppl. 1), i48–i55. doi:10.1093/bja/aer399

Shakespeare, W. (1970). *Hamlet.* Richard L. Coe Theater Programs Collection. Washington, DC: Library of Congress.

Sheth, K. N., Nutter, T., Stein, D. M., Scalea, T. M., & Bernat, J. L. (2012). Autoresuscitation after asystole in patients being considered for organ donation. *Crit Care Med, 40*(1), 158–161. doi:10.1097/CCM.0b013e31822f0b2a

Shewmon, A. D. (2001). The brain and somatic integration: Insights into the standard biological rationale for equating "brain death" with death. *J Med Philos, 26*(5), 457–478. doi:10.1076/jmep.26.5.457.3000

Siminoff, L. A., Burant, C., & Youngner, S. J. (2004). Death and organ procurement: Public beliefs and attitudes. *Kennedy Inst Ethics J, 14*(3), 217–234.

State of New York, Pub. L. No. 16, 400 Stat. (1987).

Texas Advance Directives Act § 166.046 (1999).

Thompson, G. N., & Chochinov, H. M. (2008). Dignity-based approaches in the care of terminally ill patients. *Curr Opin Support Palliat Care, 2*(1), 49–53. doi:10.1097/SPC.0b013e3282f4cb15

Truog, R. D., & Robinson, W. M. (2003). Role of brain death and the dead-donor rule in the ethics of organ transplantation. *Crit Care Med, 31*(9), 2391–2396. doi:10.1097/01.CCM.0000090869.19410.3C

Uniform Determination of Death Act. (1982). CAL. HEALTH & SAFETY CODE § 1254.4.

United Network of Organ Sharing. (2011). Critical pathway for donation after cardiac death. Retrieved from https://www.unos.org/wp-content/uploads/unos/Critical_Pathway_DCD_Donor.pdf

Veatch, R. M. (1993). The impending collapse of the whole-brain definition of death. *Hastings Cent Rep, 23*(4), 18–24.

Veatch, R. M. (2008). Donating hearts after cardiac death—reversing the irreversible. *N Engl J Med, 359*(7), 672–673. doi:10.1056/NEJMp0805451

Wijdicks, E. F., Varelas, P. N., Gronseth, G. S., & Greer, D. M. (2010). Evidence-based guideline update: Determining brain death in adults: Report of the Quality Standards Subcommittee of the American Academy of Neurology. *Neurology, 74*(23), 1911–1918. doi:10.1212/WNL.0b013e3181e242a8

Zawistowski, C. A., & DeVita, M. A. (2003). Non-heartbeating organ donation: A review. *J Intensive Care Med, 18*(4), 189–197. doi:10.1177/0885066603253314

17

Research in Palliative Care

Case Study

A sixty-two-year-old woman with metastatic cancer is admitted to hospice. Living at home, she has reduced oral intake leading to mild dehydration. She is also experiencing some side effects of her opioid medications, including sedation and myoclonus. The standard treatment for these side effects is parenteral hydration, but this also carries risks such as increased urination (with issues of dignity and skin breakdown) and increased oral secretions leading to possible aspiration.

Some researchers have proposed a randomized controlled trial to determine whether such hydration is indeed beneficial. Others, however, question the appropriateness of such a trial, given the vulnerability of hospice patients—who are approaching the end of their lives—and the potential for worsening pain or discomfort. A trial has been approved and the patient would qualify for it, but the clinical team is unsure whether to mention it to her, or simply proceed with treatment based on the current standard of care.

Historicolegal Background

Clinical research has been responsible for countless discoveries that have improved and transformed the practice of medicine. What began as comparative trials of fruit to determine its efficacy against scurvy (Lind, 1757) and the discovery of quinine's activity against malaria (Robertson, 1807) has evolved over time to include more nuanced approaches, utilizing advanced statistical concepts such as randomization (Fibiger, 1898), patient blinding (Amberson, McMahon, & Pinner, 1931), multicenter studies (Medical Research Council, 1934), and placebo controls (Diehl, Baker, & Cowan, 1938).

Along the way patient rights were sometimes sacrificed at the altar of medical progress. In the last decade of the nineteenth century, healthy patients were injected—without their informed consent—with live bacteria to document the natural progression of infection (Jordan, 1897) prompting condemnation by luminaries such as William Osler, who called this "criminal" (Sternberg, 1898). This prompted further examination of how research is carried out, with the identification of fundamental ethical principles including the need for informed consent and the requirement for self-experimentation if there was significant risk (Reed & Carroll, 1901).

It was not until the Nuremberg Trials, however, that research ethics were fully fleshed out. Responding to heinous examples of unethical research perpetrated by Nazi physicians as well as basic scientists, the Nuremberg Code identified "certain basic principles [that] must be observed in order to satisfy moral, legal, and ethical concepts." The first and longest of these principles demands "the voluntary consent of the human subject" (Annas & Grodin, 1992). The Code goes on to include other requirements including that benefits should outweigh risks, subjects can always withdraw from a study, and the result must be for the greater good of society.

It soon became apparent that while the Nuremberg Code was an important step, there was still a long way to go. For instance, focusing so much on informed consent overlooked the overwhelmingly negative risk/benefit ratio of the Nazi experiments. In addition, requiring the informed consent of the subject would necessarily preclude the participation of populations who lack decision-making capacity (DMC)—including young children, as well as adults with significant developmental disability or mental illness—who might ultimately benefit from research discoveries.

This led in 1964 to the formulation of the Declaration of Helsinki—since revised seven times—to serve "as a guide to every physician in biomedical research involving human subjects" (World Medical Association, 2013). Attempting to address some of the shortcomings of the Nuremberg Code, the Declaration focused on ensuring a favorable risk/benefit ratio as well as mandating independent review—which in the modern context is the institutional review board—while also making accommodations for proxy consent (Vanderpool, 1996). The need for such explicit requirements was highlighted two years later when Henry Beecher (1966) published his famous twenty-two examples of clinical research studies published in preeminent journals in which "patients never had the risks satisfactorily explained to them."

The major impetus to developing research ethics in the United States was the Tuskegee syphilis study, which was initiated in 1932 but only came to public attention in 1972. The purpose of the study was to track the natural course of syphilis. The "control" group of infected patients was comprised of four hundred African American men who were monitored for "bad blood." Even after penicillin came to be used to treat syphilis in 1943, investigators failed to inform subjects of their true diagnosis and the possibility of curative treatment. Subjects continued to be monitored as their now-treatable disease progressed, often leading to their death. The study was reapproved by the Centers for Disease Control as recently as 1969, but when it became public knowledge in 1972, there was an understandable outcry and the study was discontinued (White, 2002).

This prompted the formation of the Belmont Commission, whose seminal eponymous report was published in 1978. It identified three basic principles of research ethics: respect for persons, beneficence, and justice (National Commission for the Protection of Human Subjects of Biomedical and Behavioral Research, 1978). This also led to the development of the Code of Federal Regulations and the "Common Rule" (Department of Health and Human Services, 1981), which mandated the formation of institutional review boards to oversee federally funded research (and also established requirements for their membership). At the same time, international guidelines were also being formulated with specific attention to preventing exploitation of patients in developing nations (Council for International Organizations of Medical Sciences, 2002).

Clinical

According to the Common Rule, "clinical research" refers to a systematic investigation designed to develop or contribute to generalized knowledge (Department of Health and Human Services, 1981). Unlike clinical medicine—whose ultimate goal is to benefit a specific patient—clinical research aims to expand understanding in order to benefit many patients in the future, even if it means providing half the subjects in a placebo-controlled trial with a physiologically inert substance. Unlike "innovative therapy"—which involves using a treatment approved for one indication in a different situation (i.e., "off-label") where the clinician feels a patient might respond to it—clinical research is planned, structured, and monitored to ensure that whatever knowledge it generates is generalizable and reliable. And unlike quality improvement—where established interventions/methods are instituted for the benefit of all patients—clinical research seeks to determine whether a certain intervention is, in fact, beneficial (Casarett, 2005).[1]

There are many kinds of clinical research (including in palliative care), and not all present significant ethical dilemmas. Epidemiologic research, for instance, tracks trends and observes outcomes, without specific interventions. Similarly, survey-based research about general patient preferences is ethically contentious only to the extent that it represents a time burden to patients, and certain subtypes (such as bereavement research) can be emotionally painful. Self-reported distress, however, may have as much to do with subject characteristics as the nature of the survey (Takesaka, Crowley, & Casarett, 2004).

These studies may also provide some measure of benefit, such as by offering participants an opportunity to express their thoughts and feelings (Cook & Bosley, 1995;

1. Admittedly, the line between clinical research and quality improvement can be unclear at times (Lynn et al., 2007).

Dyregrov, 2004). Descriptive studies might also identify poorly treated pain (Parmelee, Smith, & Katz, 1993) or undetected symptoms like depression (Derogatis et al., 1983).

The gold standard of clinical research is the randomized controlled trial (RCT) where subjects are randomized into two (or more) groups, one of which functions as a control group receiving either currently-accepted therapy in an equivalence trial, or a placebo in a placebo-controlled trial. This structure reflects the purpose of research: not to benefit an individual research subject but rather to produce generalizable knowledge. Many subjects do not appreciate this, however, falling victim to the so-called "therapeutic misconception," which refers to "[denying] the possibility that there may be major disadvantages to participating in clinical research that stem from the nature of the research process itself" (Appelbaum, Roth, Lidz, Benson, & Winslade, 1987). A classic example is patients' frequent expectation of benefit from participation in Phase I clinical trials (Meropol et al., 2003; Weinfurt, Sulmasy, Schulman, & Meropol, 2003), even though studies have shown that only 5% to 10% of patients actually derive any benefit (Horstmann et al., 2005).

A patient is much more likely to misunderstand the nature of proposed research when a clinician—especially her own clinician—is involved in the trial, as the distinctions between patient-and-subject and clinician-and-investigator become blurred. For this reason, it is important to distinguish between a clinician treating a patient—where the clinician's only concern is the well-being of that particular patient—and an investigator enrolling a subject in a research trial (when the obligations are fundamentally different) (Peppercorn, Weeks, Cook, & Joffe, 2004).

This role distinction can also be blurred in the other direction too. For while a researcher's primary task is to produce generalizable knowledge, this does not mean that he is indifferent to the needs of individual research subjects. For instance, a palliative medicine researcher might identify suboptimal symptom management through epidemiologic surveys. If so, the researcher could suggest to subjects that they might wish to discuss with their clinicians how to be better manage those symptoms (Casarett & Karlawish, 2000).

Some of the risks inherent in clinical research are exacerbated in the field of palliative care. Any interventional study of symptomatic treatment involves the risk that an experimental treatment could worsen suffering, or simply be less effective than the control arm of a study. This is of particular concern in palliative care because of its focus on optimal symptom management and the potentially limited life expectancy of many of the patient-subjects. A "crossover design" permits those subjects receiving placebo (or the current standard of care) to potentially benefit from the intervention at a later time, but for many patients receiving palliative care there may not *be* a later time.

Palliative care's focus on quality of life also presents a conceptual challenge. Unlike fields that emphasize objective measures such as tumor size or cardiac function, most of the measures in palliative care research are subjective. As noted later, to fulfill the ethical requirements for clinical research a study needs to have "scientific validity," such that outcome measures are both relevant and reliable. Palliative care has faced challenges in objectively identifying what constitutes quality palliative care (Dy et al., 2015), let alone determining what will improve these measures. Thus Hallenbeck (2008) writes, "The fundamentally subjective nature of quality and personhood should give us pause for reflection."

This presents methodological challenges (such as how to measure the symptom or situation being studied) as well as conceptual ones. In some cases, a "good outcome" is obvious, as in the reduction of tumor size. In other cases, however, the overall effect of an intervention may not be a net positive because of side effects of a treatment. For instance, decreased pain is generally a good thing, but not for some patients if the price is decreased lucidity (Steinhauser et al., 2000). Dying at home is another example of an outcome that could be good for some patients but not for others. A majority of people in the United States say that this is their wish (Kaufman, 2005), but it is not everybody's wish. So even if this were established as a goal—and was achieved—this would overlook (and thwart) the desire of some people *not* to die at home.

There are also infrastructural problems in performing palliative care research, which takes place in a variety of domains. Systems-based research often has clearly defined contexts, such as heart failure research done with subjects suffering from cardiac disease. However, common topics in palliative care research—such as communication, symptom management, and prognostication—span disease boundaries, involving extremely diverse subject populations. The degree to which principles established in one population carry over to another can be unclear, and the challenge of coalescing palliative care research occurring in such a broad range of contexts can be daunting.

That being said, there is a critical need for palliative care research. Less than 1% of all National Institutes of Health grants support research on palliative care aspects of diseases such as cancer, dementia, and diseases of the heart, brain, lung, or kidney (Gelfman & Morrison, 2008). This hampers development of the field and, out of necessity, forces researchers to seek private sector support.

It is important to recall that the field of palliative care (in the modern sense) began not with heartfelt calls for improved care of the dying but with scientifically rigorous studies documenting the effectiveness of opioids in treating suffering at the end of life (Saunders, 1960). While it may be true that some elements of palliative care would simply have been called "good doctoring" 150 years ago (p. 3), the field would not have been recognized as a medical subspecialty without a substantial evidence base.

Going forward, further rigorous research is necessary so as not to fall back on anecdote and personal experience. Commonly accepted practices—perhaps supported only by preliminary research—also need to be reexamined with greater rigor, so as to identify initial errors or erroneous conclusions which are startlingly common in the practice of medicine (Prasad, Gall, & Cifu, 2011). Viewed in this light, to maintain the credibility of the field—and to further improve the quality of life of patients facing life-threatening illness—clinical research in palliative care is not only advisable; it is absolutely necessary.

Ethical

The evolution of Western research ethics has been largely episodic, arising in specific contexts (e.g., in response to Nazi atrocities) to address particular concerns. As a result, various ethical codes are not entirely consistent in their stated requirements. There are, however, certain requirements that they—as well as relevant professional statements—have in common (Emanuel, Wendler, & Grady, 2000). These include

1. Social or scientific value (sufficient to justify the risks of the research)
2. Fair subject selection (to prevent exploitation of vulnerable populations)
3. Favorable risk/benefit ratio
4. Informed consent
5. Scientific validity (in order to ensure that whatever data is generated is clinically useful and relevant)
6. Independent review (i.e., an institutional review board)
7. Respect for potential and enrolled subjects (including confidentiality and the right to withdraw from the study at any time)

The last three of these are relatively standard across the research spectrum. It would be unethical to perform research that is not scientifically valid, since this would undermine the fundamental goal of producing generalizable knowledge (Freedman, 1987b). Acknowledging the research abuses that prompted various codes and responses (e.g., Nazi atrocities, Beecher's examples), the Declaration of Helsinki demanded independent review (World Medical Association, 2013) and the Code of Federal Regulations took this one step further in mandating not only the role but also the composition of institutional review boards (Department of Health and Human Services, 1981). The last requirement stresses the rights of potential and enrolled subjects, both in terms of the privacy of their information as well as their ongoing option of withdrawing from the research.

The first four requirements, however, are particularly relevant to palliative care research and thus demand additional analysis (Duke & Bennett, 2010).

Informed Consent

Informed consent is the fundamental ethical requirement of any research study. Potential subjects must be informed of the known risks, benefits, and alternatives of enrolling in any study. More than merely reciting these facts, the potential subject must appreciate the significance of these various factors in her life and be able to reason from this understanding and appreciation to a conclusion about whether to enroll (p. 58). For potential subjects who lack sufficient DMC (such as young children or those with severe developmental disabilities), an appropriate proxy must offer consent and additional protections must be established for these vulnerable populations. Lastly, consent must be voluntary, free of coercion and manipulation.

This has particular relevance to palliative care because a disproportionate percentage of palliative care patients have diminished DMC. Between 10% and 40% of patients in the final months of life—and up to 85% of patients in the last week—suffer cognitive impairment (Breitbart, Bruera, Chochinov, & Lynch, 1995). Similarly, clinical depression can affect up to 25% of patients near the end of life (Kathol, Mutgi, Williams, Clamon, & Noyes, 1990). Severe symptoms frequently encountered in palliative care (such as pain and dyspnea) can also impair a patient's ability to process information, which makes consenting to studies involving treatment of such severe symptoms problematic (Eisenach, DuPen, Dubois, Miguel, & Allin, 1995). The fact that some studies occur over prolonged periods—when DMC can wax and wane—makes ongoing consent problematic (Casarett, 2005). And given the low probability of benefit of Phase I trials in particular, concern for misunderstanding and exploitation have led some commentators to argue that hospice patients should not even be offered the chance to participate in them (Ross, 2006).

These factors underscore the need to confirm that the subject has sufficient DMC to enroll in a study. For studies involving only minimal risk—defined as risks encountered in the patient's usual care, or everyday life (Department of Health and Human Services, 1981)—such as questionnaires, an informal capacity assessment should be sufficient (Miller, O'Donnell, Searight, & Barbarash, 1996). But for studies involving greater risk—especially where there is a stronger possibility the subject might be suffering from cognitive impairment—a more in-depth assessment of capacity should be used, such as the MacArthur Competency Assessment Tool for Research (Appelbaum, Grisso, Frank, O'Donnell, & Kupfer, 1999).

In situations where the potential subject cannot give consent, surrogate consent is appropriate based on substituted judgment, a topic which has been explored in detail related to emergency research (Karlawish & Hall, 1996) and research on patients with cognitive impairment (Melnick, Dubler, Weisbard, & Butler, 1984). If the potential subject is able to participate in decisions to some degree, her assent should be sought (High, Whitehouse, Post, & Berg, 1994). In situations where subsequent incapacity can be anticipated, consideration should be given to obtaining consent in advance (Breitbart et al., 1996).

Informed consent not only requires that the subject (or surrogate) have sufficient DMC to consent but also to do so voluntarily (Beauchamp & Childress, 2009). Voluntariness can be placed at risk when a specific study represents the *only* way that a patient might be able to receive appropriate treatment, which has specific implications for palliative care. For instance, what if the only chance to receive a specific treatment is in the context of a clinical trial?[2] With no other options, a patient's informed consent for the trial might not be truly "voluntary."

---

2. Which, it should be noted, in a two-arm placebo-controlled RCT represents only a 50% of chance of actually receiving it.

One response to this quandary is to restrict palliative care research to established centers, where treatments may be available outside trials as well. This, however, might limit the options of patients who live at a distance from such centers. A less severe option would be to include a "lead-in phase" where symptom management is optimized prior to recruitment (Broomhead et al., 1997).

The potential for coercion also exists in the context of the subject's right to withdraw (otherwise considered under the principle of "respect for enrolled subjects"). If the only reason a subject is receiving treatment at an established palliative care center is because she is enrolled in a trial there, withdrawal from a study could imperil her access to appropriate monitoring and treatment. This is particularly relevant in trials of symptom management, especially in areas where expertise in prescribing—and availability of—analgesics may be limited. In the context of a national epidemic of abuse and diversion, it is incumbent upon investigators to ensure that subjects who withdraw from research continue to have access to appropriate treatment.

This concern may become less pressing over time, as palliative care becomes more fully accepted as the standard of care (Smith et al., 2012). As such, not offering basic palliative care in both control and intervention arms may fail to meet clinical equipoise, which requires that there exist genuine uncertainty within the medical community as to which arm of the trial will prove superior (Freedman, 1987a). The question then would no longer be whether palliative care is an effective intervention but rather what form of palliative care provides the greatest benefit.

While there are legitimate concerns about informed consent in the palliative care population, these should not prevent patients receiving it from participating in clinical research. Some patients strongly desire to do so, not only in the hope of potentially benefitting from experimental therapies but also out of a desire to help future generations by contributing to subsequent discoveries related to their disease or to palliative care in general. Precluding such participation out of concern for compromised autonomy risks minimizing that very autonomy, by preventing patients from acting based on their personal goals.

In addition, the aforementioned challenges related to informed consent are not specific to palliative care; patients *not* receiving palliative care are also confronted with complex situations, where they are forced to weigh complex options and make difficult choices (Casarett & Karlawish, 2000). The risk and complexity is simply heightened in certain palliative care situations, demanding additional attention and possibly added safeguards. As a palliative care research work group concluded, "There [are] very few genuine threats to voluntariness that are unique to patients at the end of life" (Fine, 2004).

Scientific and Social Value

Research priorities reflect cultural values. Put another way, the questions we ask determine the answers we get. And for quite some time, not many people were asking questions about palliative care.[3] The focus was on curing disease not "merely" ameliorating it,

---

3. Even now that those questions are being asked, relatively few investigators are getting funded to answer them.

as evidenced by the overabundance of studies on chemotherapy-related nausea and the dearth of those on opioid-related nausea (Hallenbeck, 2008). In fact, the "bible of evidence-based medicine" does not even mention the concept of suffering (Sackett, Strauss, & Richardson, 2000).

These priorities may reflect a primitive understanding of what palliative care is. To reduce palliative care to merely a pleasant bedside manner combined with an empathetic disposition is to belittle the science behind it. Indeed, the only reason that palliative care was finally recognized as a medical subspecialty in 2006 was because it had developed an evidence base that filled multiple professional journals and a knowledge base sufficient to justify a board examination. Compassion and presence are necessarily attributes of palliative care, but not sufficient ones. As Hardy (1997) writes, "If palliative care is to be taken seriously as a medical speciality in its own right it has to be seen to be able to justify what it does and show that it can perform high-quality research."

There should be no debate about the social value of palliative care research. In an aging population more and more people are suffering from chronic or serious illness and thus are in desperate need of quality palliative care: always generalist, sometimes specialist (Quill & Abernethy, 2013). To put it bluntly, everyone will ultimately die. Especially at the end of life, symptomatic management, psychosocial support, and respected autonomy become even more important. In an era of expanding health care costs, palliative care represents a high-benefit/low-cost intervention (Morrison et al., 2011).

One area where palliative care research is especially important is in reframing the questions in order to generate more valuable answers. Many studies, for instance, understandably use survival time as the primary endpoint. But by focusing on quality in addition to duration of life, palliative care research can distinguish between adding years to one's life on the one hand and life to one's years (or months or days or hours) on the other (Rahimzadeh et al., 2015). Distinct endpoints—such as time spent at home or the ability to resume a regular diet—are just as important to some patients as "how much time I have left" (Casarett, 2005). Given the relative dearth of empirical palliative care studies—which is beginning to be addressed as the field gains greater acceptance—and the importance of the issues that need to be addressed, it is imperative that palliative care formulate the most crucial questions and have the wherewithal and support to answer them (Casarett, Karlawish, & Moreno, 2002).

Fair Selection

One of the basic principles of research ethics is that if a vulnerable population—such as children, pregnant women, and prisoners—is to be used for research, there needs be clear justification. For example, it would not be ethical to test a new pharmaceutical intervention on a destitute population simply because this group might be more likely to respond to a modest financial stipend for participation. One might understandably wonder whether palliative care patients are similarly vulnerable.

There are several potential reasons for additional vulnerability. One is potentially compromised DMC, as noted earlier (de Raeve, 1994). Palliative care patients also often have limited life expectancy, and thus participation in research represents precious time that might be devoted to other pursuits. In addition, one of the standard credos of research ethics is that the subject population should have the potential to benefit from the findings of the research. This notion of "fair benefit" is based on the principle of justice (National Commission for the Protection of Human Subjects of Biomedical and Behavioral Research, 1978) and is one of the reasons that after the conclusion of a study with a positive finding subjects in the control arm are usually provided access to the beneficial treatment (Participants in the Conference on Ethical Aspects of Research in Developing Countries, 2002). By virtue of limited life expectancy, however, subjects receiving palliative care often do not experience this direct benefit (Casarett, Karlawish, Sankar, Hirschman, & Asch, 2001).

There are two ways to respond to this concern. One is to call into question the assumption that palliative care patients are inherently vulnerable. Some are, to be sure, given the factors noted previously. But it would be a mistake to label all patients at the end of life as "vulnerable," as this could devalue their personhood and prevent them from acting upon their beliefs and altruistic motives (Mount, Cohen, MacDonald, Bruera, & Dudgeon, 1995). It would also be a mistake to equate that supposed vulnerability with an inability to voluntarily participate in research (Fine, 2004), as noted in the examination of informed consent. To preclude this population from research on the basis of vulnerability condemns future similar patients to an equivalent level of suffering.

The other response is to admit that many (though not all) palliative care patients are, indeed, vulnerable. They are not unique in this respect, though. Many patients who may not be nearing the end of life—and who may not be receiving palliative care—face the same challenges in terms of research participation, and singling out palliative care patients seems unjustified. If palliative care is really about helping all patients live fully until the very end—whenever that comes—then they should be allowed to participate in research that has the possibility of benefitting others, and potentially also themselves (Gysels, Shipman, & Higginson, 2008).

The Common Rule does not say that vulnerable patients cannot participate in research; it simply says that there needs to be sufficient justification for them to participate and added safeguards put in place. The justification should be clear: suffering at the end of life is all too common (SUPPORT Principal Investigators, 1995). And just as advanced research on pregnancy-related complications logically needs to utilize pregnant subjects, so also research on critically important aspects of end-of-life care requires subjects who are approaching the end of life.

Risk/Benefit Ratio

There are risks involved with participating in any research, and these can be magnified for patients requiring palliative care. Given potentially limited life expectancy, should a patient enroll in a trial and be randomized to the arm ultimately proven to be inferior, she may not subsequently have the opportunity to benefit from the superior intervention. Patients with limited life expectancy might wish to focus their remaining time on loved ones rather than on research, which involves informed consent conversations and documentation, ongoing monitoring, and possibly additional diagnostic interventions to measure efficacy. There may also be distress on the part of loved ones, as new therapies are tried out at this "ultimate" time in the relationship (Randall & Downie, 1999).

To be ethically sound, a research study must carry with it a reasonable risk/benefit ratio for potential subjects. Here the concept of "clinical equipoise" is relevant, as the prevailing scientific evidence should not have already shown that one intervention in a study is superior to the other(s). To be sure, the investigator likely *believes* that the intervention is better than the control—if not, why do the study?—but that is a personal belief, not a measured conclusion from currently available evidence.

Clinical equipoise has specific application to placebo-controlled studies, which are less expensive and complicated than equivalence studies because they generally require fewer subjects to detect a statistically significant difference. However, because they risk depriving a patient of beneficial treatment, placebo-controlled studies are generally not acceptable when a proven therapy already exists.

The caveat *generally* is important, in light of an intense debate in the 1990s over research practices in the developing world. Specifically, placebo-controlled studies were performed that evaluated the efficacy of a newer (and easier to administer) treatment for HIV infection, where an established treatment already existed but was generally unavailable in the country where the subjects lived. Some commentators castigated the researchers for unethical practices (Angell, 2000), while others came to their defense (Wilkinson, Karim, & Coovadia, 1999). Ultimately the World Health Organization issued a clarification to the Declaration of Helsinki that established what some consider to be a middle ground on the placebo question: it is generally unacceptable when a proven treatment exists, except "where for compelling and scientifically sound methodological reasons the use of any intervention less effective than the best proven one, the use of placebo, or no intervention is necessary to determine the efficacy or safety of an intervention" (World Medical Association, 2013).

The word *proven* in the previous sentence should be stressed, because many generally accepted treatments (not only in palliative care) have never been proven in a scientific study. Instead, they came into use based on logical extrapolation and biological plausibility, and the perception soon became that they were effective. But there is no way of knowing for sure whether the patients would have improved without (or despite) those interventions unless an appropriate study is performed.

It is possible that the intervention was not pharmacologically effective but rather led to improvement through the well-established placebo effect, which is widely variable (McQuay, Carroll, & Moore, 1996) but can, for instance, improve pain in up to 30% of subjects (Turner, Deyo, Loeser, Von Korff, & Fordyce, 1994). Indeed, patients who are anxious and dependent—which could describe many palliative care patients, especially at the end of life—have been shown to experience a stronger placebo effect (Chaput de Saintonge & Herxheimer, 1994). In such a context, additional physician attention and concern could influence the perception of suffering, rather than some direct physiologic effect of the administered treatment (Shapiro & Shapiro, 1984).

Or perhaps there was no placebo effect at all, but the condition resolved on its own through what is known as "natural history and regression to the mean" (Ernst & Resch, 1995). Some conditions wax and wane, and thus an intervention administered just before an upswing in that cycle might be misperceived as causally effective. By the same token, some conditions (such as opioid-induced nausea) are transient in nature and will resolve with time irrespective of treatment.

To be sure, in any RCT there is a risk that a subject could be randomized into the group that is ultimately shown to be inferior. And while it is natural to want to be protective about patients at the end of life, if we are to improve palliative care in a thoughtful and rigorous fashion, evidence is required. So, too, is humility in the face of uncertainty and the willingness to critically analyze what we only believe—without empirical proof—to be true.

The Limits of Evidence-Based Medicine

The discussion up to this point has focused on ethical issues related to clinical research, with particular attention to palliative care. To be sure, the evidence base in palliative care is expanding in important directions, which is necessary to answer important questions and allay common misperceptions. For instance, assertions that end-of-life discussions take away hope (Mack et al., 2007), palliative care leads to shortened life expectancy (Temel et al., 2010), and parents regret openly talking with their children about impending death (Kreicbergs, Valdimarsdottir, Onelov, Henter, & Steineck, 2004) have been laid to rest through rigorous studies. Evidence-based medicine (EBM) is a precondition for acceptance as a legitimate medical specialty, as establishing an evidence base is a requirement for recognition by American Board of Medical Specialties.

EBM—defined as "the conscientious, explicit, and judicious use of best evidence in making decisions about the care of individual patients" (Sackett, Rosenberg, Gray, Haynes, & Richardson, 1996)—first came into vogue in the early 1990s and now forms the basis of both micro- and macro-level health care decisions. It has a great many benefits, including increasing efficiency through data collection and application, greater uniformity in clinical practice, better-informed patients and clinicians, and an empirical method for establishing organizational priorities and making public policy decisions. Public reporting of evidence-based outcomes has become the norm (Dartmouth Institute for Health Policy and Clinical Practice, 2016).

It is possible, however, to take the emphasis on empirical evidence too far. Some outcomes are very difficult to measure, and attempts to do so may be amenable to multiple interpretations. The degree to which societal values—and funding sources—impact the questions that are asked was already noted. As Bradley and Field (1995) note, "it is a short step from 'without substantial evidence' to 'without substantial value.'" Especially in areas where methodologically and ethically sound research can be difficult to accomplish—as is often the case in palliative care—the lack of clear evidence for a treatment does not necessarily mean that treatment is not effective or worthwhile. Put simply, "the absence of evidence is not evidence of absence" (Altman & Bland, 1995).

Even when evidence is available, it may be complicated to interpret and apply. The way the research question is framed—and the manner in which the data is reported (if it is reported at all) and interpreted—sometimes skew the official results in favor of the desired conclusions (Song et al., 2010). As the famous saying goes: "There are three kinds of lies: lies, damned lies, and statistics."[4]

Some have argued that overreliance on EBM minimizes the "art" of medicine by attempting to apply population-based outcomes to individual patient situations. It may "de-skill" practitioners by fostering a reliance on what some call "cookbook medicine." It could serve as a disincentive to individual innovation by requiring adherence to rigid protocols (Greenhalgh, Howick, Maskrey, & Evidence Based Medicine Renaissance Group, 2014).

The inherent subjectivity of much palliative care research also potentially limits generalizability. By virtue of its emphasis on the experience of patients and families—and the inescapably subjective nature of quality-of-life assessments—palliative care must rely on indirect measures of what it seeks to study. But estimates or measures of suffering are not the same as suffering itself (Hallenbeck, 2008). In this respect, reliability of measurement is easier to achieve than the *validity* of measurement (i.e., the importance of that measurement in the clinical care of patients).

For all these reasons, EBM may not be the holy grail that it initially appeared to be, at least in terms of palliative medicine. As Hallenbeck (2008) observes, "To the extent that the subjective experiences of patients and families are the object of palliative care, we must proceed cautiously [with EBM]."

Many of the ethical reservations related to palliative care research—which can be overcome through thoughtful evaluation and establishment of appropriate safeguards—primarily pertain to the RCT, the acknowledged "gold standard" of clinical evidence (Figure 17.1). Beyond the ethical complexities noted earlier, this model poses other challenges, especially in the palliative care population. Sometimes it is difficult to recruit sufficient patients to complete a trial, whether because of "trial fatigue"—by virtue of multiple trials the patient could choose to participate in—or reluctance on the part of the patient or family (Faithfull, 1996). Unless a trial has a crossover design, half of the

---

4. In an ironic example of false attribution of causation—in this case, authorship—this phrase has been inaccurately attributed to Mark Twain. Twain (1906) did repeat the saying, attributing it at the time to Benjamin Disraeli. In reality, however, Disraeli never said it (Velleman, 2008).

Levels of Evidence for Therapy Question	
Level of Evidence	Type of Study
l a	Systematic reviews of randomized controlled trials (RCTs)
l b	Individual RCTs with narrow confidence interval
2a	Systematic reviews of cohort studies
2b	Individual cohort studies and low-quality RCTs
3a	Systematic reviews of case-control studies
3b	Case-control studies
4	Case series and poor quality cohort and case-control studies
5	Expert opinion

FIGURE 17.1 Levels of evidence based on type of study

patients will generally be deprived of whichever intervention is ultimately deemed superior (if a statistically significant difference is even found).

An RCT also requires a very clear set of enrollment and exclusion parameters, potentially limiting generalizability to other populations. This specificity even limits the utility of systematic reviews of RCTs. As Wee, Hadley, and Derry (2008) write,

> [Systematic] reviews in palliative care are well performed, but fail to provide good evidence for clinical practice because the primary studies are few in number, small, clinically heterogeneous, and of poor quality and external validity. They are useful in highlighting the weakness of the evidence base and problems in performing trials in palliative care.

There are other forms of valid and valuable research, however, which may not be susceptible to similar methodological limitations and ethical criticisms (Fine, 2003). Observational studies, for example, often include patients with coexisting illnesses and a wide spectrum of disease severity, with treatment focused on the individual patient (Hannan, 2008). N-of-1 trials—where subjects receive both intervention and control treatments, in varying orders—not only require a smaller sample size than an RCT but also assure that each patient has the potential to benefit from both interventions. Such trials can be invaluable in tailoring individualized recommendations based on what worked better for that particular patient (Bruera, Schoeller, & MacEachern, 1992).

Admittedly, only an RCT can "prove" causality, and other studies often come with the caveat with that "association does not prove causation" (Hopayian, 2000). That being said, other factors can lead to inferences of causality, based on the Hill (1965) criteria: strength, consistency, specificity, temporality, dose response, plausibility, coherence, experimental evidence, and analogy. In this respect, "the design and ultimate conduct of the study is the principal criterion to consider, not the type of study per se" (Concato, Shah, & Horwitz, 2000). Clinical research projects beyond RCTs may, despite their lower "level of evidence," be easier to perform and less ethically charged, as well as ultimately more beneficial. As Kirkham and Abel (1997) write, "The placebo-controlled trial may provide a gold standard: let us not forget that steel and wood are often more suitable materials than gold."

Clinical Trials and Hospice Enrollment

Patients receiving palliative care are not only potential subjects for research involving "palliative" interventions such as symptom management and enhanced communication and goal-setting. They may well also be seeking potentially curative—or, at the very least, life-prolonging—treatment of their primary condition. This is especially true for cancer, which is the most common diagnosis among adult patients receiving palliative care.

The National Comprehensive Cancer Network (2014) strongly supports clinical trial enrollment, stating that "the best management of any cancer patient is in a clinical trial." While only 5% to 10% of subjects will benefit from a Phase I clinical trial (Agrawal & Emanuel, 2003), this still represents a chance for personal benefit. Patients may also value the opportunity to contribute to the understanding of their disease and the future treatment of other patients.

The decision to enroll in a clinical trial has profound implications on other aspects of care, however, including hospice enrollment. Despite the extremely low response rate, a Phase I clinical trial is still considered "treatment" and thus may appear to preclude hospice enrollment (Byock & Miles, 2003).[5] Indeed, a recent study revealed that 11% of potential subjects chose not to participate in a clinical trial because they chose hospice instead (Fu et al., 2013). The end result is that patients who are desperately seeking a cure would not be able to benefit from hospice services, and patients enrolled in hospice could not contribute to greater understanding of the disease that will take their lives and the lives of countless others in the future. They are also deprived of the admittedly small chance of directly benefitting from the treatment under study.

This situation may be changing. Studies have shown that a majority of clinical investigators and hospice officials feel that patients should be able to enroll in hospice and simultaneously participate in a Phase I trial (Casarett, Karlawish, Henry, & Hirschman, 2002). Concerns about Medicare reimbursement—especially given increased regulatory scrutiny (Whoriskey & Keating, 2014)—may, however, still give representatives of

---

5. It should be noted that this is not the case for children. The Affordable Care Act mandates that pediatric patients with a life expectancy of six months or less are eligible for hospice and can simultaneously receive disease-modifying therapy, which would include eligibility for clinical trials (Keim-Malpass, Hart, & Miller, 2013).

both sides pause. Here it is important to note that hospice enrollment requires a life expectancy of six months or less if the disease runs its normal course. Receiving proven life-prolonging treatment might then disqualify a patient from enrolling, but accepting *experimental* treatment would not definitively impact prognosis (and, thus, eligibility).

Regulatory considerations are not the only limiting factor in enrolling hospice patients in clinical trials. There may also be profound philosophical differences between the two models. Studies have shown that clinical trial participation is often associated with increased probability of aggressive medical care near death (Enzinger, Zhang, Weeks, & Prigerson, 2014). Hospice, on the other hand, emphasizes quality of life over interventions, with a goal of *not* dying in the hospital while receiving intensive care. However ideal it would be to combine the altruism/possibility of benefit of a clinical trial with the comprehensive supportive care of hospice, these two philosophies might take patients in opposite directions, even if regulatory concerns could be assuaged.

One solution to this conundrum is to provide exquisite palliative care in the context of clinical trials, without enrolling in hospice (with its associated regulatory requirements and rather clear philosophy). This would require the jettisoning of stereotypes, including those equating palliative care with "giving up" (Gawande, 2014) as well as those which attribute to oncologists an overzealousness for chemotherapy at the end of life (Behl & Jatoi, 2010). It would also require a nuanced conversation about which of many priorities is the most important, in order to determine the right balance of altruism, possibility of improvement, and overall quality of life for a particular patient.

The Ethics of Compassionate Use

But what of patients who are not enrolled in hospice and who are seeking anything that might prolong their lives? In order to make sure that drugs are effective for their stated indications and have an acceptable safety profile, the Food and Drug Administration (FDA) drug approval process is understandably systematic, and thus also time-consuming. For patients suffering from a condition for which no approved treatment exists, the only possible hope for benefit is a clinical trial.

Investigational new drugs (INDs) undergoing Phase I trials have not yet been proven safe or effective, although there is often great optimism about their potential. Relevant ethical issues include the possibility of the therapeutic misconception and the impact of trial participation on hospice enrollment, as discussed earlier.

By the time an IND has reached Phase III, however, at least some measure of efficacy and safety have been proven. The remaining criterion prior to FDA approval is efficacy compared to current treatment or—if no current treatment exists—placebo. Particularly in the latter case, a patient facing life-threatening disease may well be willing to "take her chances" on an unproven IND, feeling like she has no other alternative.

Not all potential subjects are accepted into a clinical trial, however, as some may have contraindications or otherwise not have access to a relevant trial. And even if a patient does enroll, she may not be randomized to the intervention arm. Especially when the IND holds out significant promise of benefit—news of which is often available through the Internet and social media (Harmon, 2010a)—a patient dying of a potentially treatable disease understandably would want access to the IND now, rather than wait until FDA approval (by which time the patient may no longer be alive).

At first it might seem obvious that an IND should be provided to such terminally ill patients on a "compassionate use" basis since they surely will die without it, thereby justifying the unclear risks of complications. But there are several reasons why this is not typically done. One is that INDs are often very expensive to produce—if only because they are new and unproven—which means there may be inadequate supply outside the context of the clinical trial. In addition, if an adverse event befalls a patient taking an IND, it may not be clear (for lack of comprehensive monitoring) whether it was the IND that caused it. This may have financial and regulatory implications for the pharmaceutical company attempting to bring the IND to market. It is also possible that the IND could worsen the patient's condition or even hasten her death. This is precisely the reason, after all, that the IND is still undergoing trials and has not yet received FDA approval.

Perhaps most importantly, if INDs were made available to all patients suffering from a specific disease, none of those patients would have any reason to enroll in a clinical trial for that IND. Doing so would reduce their chance of getting the pharmacologically active compound by half. This would undercut or delay the clinical trials process, with the end result being continued uncertainty as to whether the IND was actually superior to current treatment, potentially preventing FDA approval. For these reasons, the courts have held that pharmaceutical companies have no obligation to release an IND on a compassionate use basis (*Abigail Alliance v. von Eschenbach*, 2007).

One possible solution is "expanded access programs," which must be FDA approved. These programs permit the pharmaceutical company to dispense an IND to patients who have a physician's prescription. The pharmaceutical company collects some clinical data, although without the randomization and statistical power of an RCT. Any conclusions based on patient outcomes would thus be modest and clearly insufficient to justify FDA approval. But if such a program is not in place—or cannot accommodate all patients who are interested—then terminally ill patients are left to die for wont of a drug that could save their lives (or, to be clear, could also make their condition worse).

Recognizing this dilemma, several states have passed so-called "right-to-try laws," which allow patients battling fatal illness to legally obtain medications that have yet to be approved by the FDA. The practical problem with these laws is that while they make it *legal* for pharmaceutical companies to dispense these medications, those companies are under no obligation to do so. For this reason, Caplan (2015) refers to these laws as "right to beg" laws. In addition, should the company release the medication, the cost to the patient could be exorbitant, since insurance companies are unlikely to pay for an IND that is not FDA approved.

Confronted with these obstacles—and facing their own impending death or that of a loved one—patients and their families often take matters into their own hands. In the era of social media, patients who share a common disease often form tight on-line communities and are thus able to track the progress of others receiving certain treatments. This also permits rapid, widespread advocacy efforts to compel pharmaceutical companies to provide INDs on a compassionate use basis, many of which prove effective. The negative publicity associated with refusing a request for compassionate use can be significant for a pharmaceutical company, impacting stock prices and even involving death threats toward the company's leaders (Harmon, 2010b). This practice has inevitably led to justice-based concerns that patients and families of means—whether financial or technological—will gain access by virtue of being able to exert social and po-litical pressure, while disadvantaged families will not (Caplan & Moch, 2014).

When it comes to the ethics of compassionate use, the first thing to acknowledge is how understandable it is that patients or families would do everything in their power to gain access to a promising IND (especially when no proven therapy exists). The FDA rarely stands in the way of such requests. Pharmaceutical companies would therefore be legally permitted to dispense the IND on a compassionate use basis, if they chose to do so.

Not doing so can cause a company to appear unsympathetic to the needs of ter-minally ill patients. The general public distrust of the pharmaceutical industry (Gallup, 2015) can also contribute to this perception. Some may infer that reluctant companies are acting based solely out of concerns for future profits, seeking to accelerate FDA approval and minimize any risks (especially those that might come from clinical complications of uncertain cause, occurring outside the context of an RCT).

But here it is important to remember that despite public perception and word-of-mouth, unless a medication is proven effective, safe, and superior to alternatives, there is no way to know whether it will benefit patients in need (or, conversely, whether it might actually be harmful). There are well-known recent examples of medications that were felt based on personal and anecdotal experience to be effective against a certain condition, only to be shown through rigorous research to be no better than placebo (Ranieri et al., 2012).

The mere fact that a pharmaceutical company declines to make available an IND based on compassionate use is, therefore, not necessarily a sign of corporate greed or heartlessness. It might stem from a collective sense of societal obligation, looking beyond the heart-wrenching case of an individual patient suffering from a specific disease now to the countless patients who will suffer and possibly die from that disease in the future unless a treatment is proven both safe and effective. It could also stem from realistic lim-itations, such as on the capacity of a small pharmaceutical company to produce sufficient quantities of a complex IND or to remain solvent while waiting for FDA approval.

This is a classic ethical dilemma of competing interests, and provocative solutions have been proposed. Pharmaceutical companies have pledged "to help ensure that there are appropriate and targeted regulatory approaches to accelerate the development and availability of innovative new medicines for patients" (PhRMA, 2015). Another option is modifying research design—including the standard 1:1 randomization—to maximize the probability that subjects will receive the intervention being studied (Farrar, Cleary, Rauck, Busch, & Nordbrock, 1998). One pharmaceutical company—whether in a quest for greater justice or public relations cover—has formed what it calls the Compassionate Use Advisory Committee to determine which compassionate use requests should be granted, in a manner designed to level the playing field and shield the company from undue public pressure (NYU Medical Center, 2015).

Given multiple competing concerns and the risk of suffering and injustice, it is imperative to establish clinical and ethical criteria for compassionate use. The first should be an inability to participate in a clinical trial for that IND. This might be because the patient fails to meet inclusion criteria for a relevant trial or because no such trial is currently open and available. This criterion would allay concerns that the option of compassionate use will compromise trial enrollment and thereby delay or prevent subsequent FDA approval.

Another criterion would be the expected health outcome for the patient if compassionate use were not offered. To be sure, an IND could hasten the death of a terminally ill patient, but that is different from causing the death of a patient who could conceivably survive for a very long time on conventional treatment. The risk/benefit balance for INDs for symptomatic conditions might then tilt against compassionate use, at least compared to INDs that could be life-saving.

A fair and equitable process for evaluating requests for compassionate use—as the CompAC model is attempting to do—must also be established. Well-defined and transparent criteria need to be established, which can then be applied impartially. This will serve to minimize favoritism toward patients and families of means and influence.

Ultimately, one's position on compassionate use will likely depend on one's role. A physician treating a patient for whom the only possible life-prolonging treatment is in the investigational stage would be a zealous advocate for obtaining a promising IND through compassionate use. On the other hand, a pharmaceutical company executive might have to make the very difficult decision to decline such a request if he felt that it would imperil the approval process of a drug that could benefit a great many people.

In the end, perhaps the one thing everyone can agree on is the need for humility in the face of empirical uncertainty. Is the physician advocating for his patient to receive an unproven treatment because he is unwilling to confront his own helplessness? How confident is he that the IND will make his patient better (or at the very least have no meaningful effect and not make the patient worse)? And at what point does the desperate search for cure—or even just more time—detract from the quality of the time that is left?

Return to the Case

In reviewing the data supporting use of supplemental hydration to treat opioid side effects, the team determined that the practice was based on some retrospective studies (Bruera, Franco, Maltoni, Watanabe, & Suarez-Almazor, 1995; de Stoutz,

Bruera, & Suarez-Almazor, 1995) and one preliminary trial (Bruera et al., 2005). While recommended as the standard of care (Dalal, 2014; Gagnon, Allard, Masse, & DeSerres, 2000), it had never been confirmed by a multicenter, definitive RCT. Practices varied, as hospitalized patients with advanced cancer almost always received parenteral hydration, while patients in hospice did not (Bruera et al., 2013).

There existed, therefore, clinical equipoise about the relative benefits of supplemental hydration, and the initiation of an RCT was considered ethical. Recognizing that patients suffering from such side effects often had impaired DMC and limited life expectancy, additional safeguards were put in place to be sure that informed consent was obtained and that the risk/benefit ratio was as favorable as possible.

After reviewing these factors, the patient's clinician realizes that his practice of providing supplemental hydration is not really evidence-based. He is aware of the recommendation that "the best management of any cancer patient is in a clinical trial" (National Comprehensive Cancer Network, 2014), and so he advises the patient and her family to consider the placebo-controlled trial to assess the overall benefit of supplemental hydration.

The patient is eligible for the study, and enrollment clearly does not affect her hospice eligibility because the study focuses on symptom management rather than potentially curative treatment. Consent is obtained from her appropriate surrogate, who is assured that the patient can withdraw at any time. The intervention is one liter of normal saline per day—which is consistent with current practice—while the control arm is only 100 ml, infused subcutaneously in response to dehydration symptoms (including fatigue, myoclonus, sedation, and hallucinations).

Since the study is double-blinded, neither the patient nor her caregivers know how much fluid she is receiving. The patient dies comfortably approximately two weeks later, with her symptoms expertly managed by the hospice team.

The study ultimately finds that hydration does not improve any of the measured symptoms, nor does it impact overall survival (Bruera et al., 2013). This leads to a significant clinical practice change, as patients are no longer provided a potentially burdensome treatment without reasonable prospect of benefit, as a result of these valuable research findings.

Summary Points

- Violations of research ethics—such as the Nazi experimentation and the Tuskegee syphilis study—led to codification of basic professional obligations, including respect for persons, beneficence, and justice.
- Subjects enrolled in clinical research protocols often suffer from the "therapeutic misconception," believing that unproven treatments will be beneficial.

- Several basic tenets of research ethics are consistent across position statements: scientific validity, independent review, and respect for potential and enrolled subjects.
- Other tenets are particularly complex or relevant in terms of palliative care.
  - Patients receiving palliative care may have compromised DMC, thus making informed consent difficult to obtain. This situation is not unique to palliative care patients, however.
  - The value of palliative care research needs to take into account not only duration of life but also quality.
  - Patients at the end of life may be vulnerable, but this should not preclude them from taking part in research.
  - Any research protocol involves risks and potential benefits. Patients receiving palliative care may have greater need to achieve a potential benefit because of the seriousness of their illness while at the same time having diminished opportunity by virtue of their life expectancy.
- Evidence-based medicine is justifiably highly valued, but it may not sufficiently take into account individual patient variation. Some of the measures used in EBM may not optimally recognize the specific needs of the palliative care population.
- There exists lingering uncertainty as to the impact of Phase I trial participation on hospice enrollment, but these should be able to occur simultaneously if they are both consonant with a patient's goals and the patient's life expectancy meets hospice requirements.
- Compassionate use of non-FDA approved drugs can offer hope to seriously ill patients, but these patients need to recall that such drugs have yet to be proven superior to the standard of care. An equitable system for allocation of such scarce resources needs to be established.

References

Abigail Alliance v. von Eschenbach, F.3d (D.C. Cir. 2007).

Agrawal, M., & Emanuel, E. J. (2003). Ethics of phase 1 oncology studies: Reexamining the arguments and data. *JAMA, 290*(8), 1075–1082. doi:10.1001/jama.290.8.1075

Altman, D. G., & Bland, J. M. (1995). Absence of evidence is not evidence of absence. *BMJ, 311*(7003), 485.

Amberson, J. B., McMahon, B. T., & Pinner, M. (1931). A clinical trial of sanocrysin in pulmonary tuberculosis. *Amer Rev Tuberc, 24*(4), 401–435.

Angell, M. (2000). Investigators' responsibilities for human subjects in developing countries. *N Engl J Med, 342*(13), 967–969. doi:10.1056/NEJM200003303421309

Annas, G. J., & Grodin, M. A. (1992). *The Nazi doctors and the Nuremberg Code: Human rights in human experimentation*. New York: Oxford University Press.

Appelbaum, P. S., Grisso, T., Frank, E., O'Donnell, S., & Kupfer, D. J. (1999). Competence of depressed patients for consent to research. *Am J Psychiatry, 156*(9), 1380–1384. doi:10.1176/ajp.156.9.1380

Appelbaum, P. S., Roth, L. H., Lidz, C. W., Benson, P., & Winslade, W. (1987). False hopes and best data: Consent to research and the therapeutic misconception. *Hastings Cent Rep, 17*(2), 20–24.

Beauchamp, T. L., & Childress, J. F. (2009). *Principles of biomedical ethics* (6th ed.). New York: Oxford University Press.

Beecher, H. K. (1966). Ethics and clinical research. *N Engl J Med, 274*(24), 1354–1360. doi:10.1056/NEJM196606162742405

Behl, D., & Jatoi, A. (2010). What do oncologists say about chemotherapy at the very end of life? Results from a semiqualitative survey. *J Palliat Med, 13*(7), 831–835. doi:10.1089/jpm.2009.0414

Bernacki, R. E., & Block, S. D. (2014). Communication about serious illness care goals: A review and synthesis of best practices. *JAMA Intern Med, 174*(12), 1994–2003 doi:10.1001/jamainternmed.2014.5271

Bradley, F., & Field, J. (1995). Evidence-based medicine. *Lancet, 346*(8978), 838–839.

Breitbart, W., Bruera, E., Chochinov, H., & Lynch, M. (1995). Neuropsychiatric syndromes and psychological symptoms in patients with advanced cancer. *J Pain Symptom Manage, 10*(2), 131–141.

Breitbart, W., Marotta, R., Platt, M. M., Weisman, H., Derevenco, M., Grau, C., . . . Jacobson, P. (1996). A double-blind trial of haloperidol, chlorpromazine, and lorazepam in the treatment of delirium in hospitalized AIDS patients. *Am J Psychiatry, 153*(2), 231–237. doi:10.1176/ajp.153.2.231

Broomhead, A., Kerr, R., Tester, W., O'Meara, P., Maccarrone, C., Bowles, R., & Hodsman, P. (1997). Comparison of a once-a-day sustained-release morphine formulation with standard oral morphine treatment for cancer pain. *J Pain Symptom Manage, 14*(2), 63–73.

Bruera, E., Franco, J. J., Maltoni, M., Watanabe, S., & Suarez-Almazor, M. (1995). Changing pattern of agitated impaired mental status in patients with advanced cancer: Association with cognitive monitoring, hydration, and opioid rotation. *J Pain Symptom Manage, 10*(4), 287–291. doi:10.1016/0885-3924(95)00005-J

Bruera, E., Hui, D., Dalal, S., Torres-Vigil, I., Trumble, J., Roosth, J., . . . Tarleton, K. (2013). Parenteral hydration in patients with advanced cancer: A multicenter, double-blind, placebo-controlled randomized trial. *J Clin Oncol, 31*(1), 111–118. doi:10.1200/JCO.2012.44.6518

Bruera, E., Sala, R., Rico, M. A., Moyano, J., Centeno, C., Willey, J., & Palmer, J. L. (2005). Effects of parenteral hydration in terminally ill cancer patients: A preliminary study. *J Clin Oncol, 23*(10), 2366–2371. doi:10.1200/JCO.2005.04.069

Bruera, E., Schoeller, T., & MacEachern, T. (1992). Symptomatic benefit of supplemental oxygen in hypoxemic patients with terminal cancer: The use of the N of 1 randomized controlled trial. *J Pain Symptom Manage, 7*(6), 365–368.

Byock, I., & Miles, S. H. (2003). Hospice benefits and phase I cancer trials. *Ann Intern Med, 138*(4), 335–337.

Caplan, A., & Moch, K. (2014, August 27). Rescue me: The challenge of compassionate use in the social media era. *Health Affairs.*

Caplan, A. L. (2015). Does "right to try" new drugs really mean "right to beg?" Retrieved from http://www.medscape.com/viewarticle/853876

Casarett, D. (2005). Ethical considerations in end-of-life care and research. *J Palliat Med, 8*(Suppl. 1), S148–S160. doi:10.1089/jpm.2005.8.s-148

Casarett, D., Karlawish, J., Sankar, P., Hirschman, K. B., & Asch, D. A. (2001). Open label extension studies and the ethical design of clinical trials. *IRB, 23*(4), 1–5.

Casarett, D. J., & Karlawish, J. H. (2000). Are special ethical guidelines needed for palliative care research? *J Pain Symptom Manage, 20*(2), 130–139.

Casarett, D. J., Karlawish, J. H., Henry, M. I., & Hirschman, K. B. (2002). Must patients with advanced cancer choose between a phase I trial and hospice? *Cancer, 95*(7), 1601–1604. doi:10.1002/cncr.10820

Casarett, D. J., Karlawish, J. H., & Moreno, J. D. (2002). A taxonomy of value in clinical research. *IRB, 24*(6), 1–6.

Chaput de Saintonge, D. M., & Herxheimer, A. (1994). Harnessing placebo effects in health care. *Lancet, 344*(8928), 995–998.

Concato, J., Shah, N., & Horwitz, R. I. (2000). Randomized, controlled trials, observational studies, and the hierarchy of research designs. *N Engl J Med, 342*(25), 1887–1892. doi:10.1056/NEJM200006223422507

Cook, A. S., & Bosley, G. (1995). The experience of participating in bereavement research: Stressful or therapeutic? *Death Stud, 19*(2), 157–170. doi:10.1080/07481189508252722

Council for International Organizations of Medical Sciences. (2002). *International ethical guidelines for biomedical research involving human subjects.* Retrieved from https://cioms.ch/wp-content/uploads/2016/08/International_Ethical_Guidelines_for_Biomedical_Research_Involving_Human_Subjects.pdf

Dalal, S. (2014). Assessment and management of opioid side effects. In E. Bruera, I. Higginson, C. F. Von Gunten, & T. Morita (Eds.), *Textbook of palliative medicine and supportive care* (2nd ed., pp. 409–422). Boca Raton, FL: Taylor & Francis.

Dartmouth Institute for Health Policy and Clinical Practice. (2016). The Dartmouth atlas of health care. Retrieved from http://www.dartmouthatlas.org/

Department of Health and Human Services. (1981). Code of Federal Regulations, Title 45 Public Welfare CFR 46.

de Raeve, L. (1994). Ethical issues in palliative care research. *Palliat Med, 8*(4), 298–305.

de Stoutz, N. D., Bruera, E., & Suarez-Almazor, M. (1995). Opioid rotation for toxicity reduction in terminal cancer patients. *J Pain Symptom Manage, 10*(5), 378–384.

Derogatis, L. R., Morrow, G. R., Fetting, J., Penman, D., Piasetsky, S., Schmale, A. M., . . . Carnicke, C. L. Jr. (1983). The prevalence of psychiatric disorders among cancer patients. *JAMA, 249*(6), 751–757.

Diehl, H. S., Baker, A. B., & Cowan, D. W. (1938). Cold vaccines: An evaluation based on a controlled study. *JAMA, 111*, 1168–1173.

Duke, S., & Bennett, H. (2010). Review: A narrative review of the published ethical debates in palliative care research and an assessment of their adequacy to inform research governance. *Palliat Med, 24*(2), 111–126. doi:10.1177/0269216309352714

Dy, S. M., Kiley, K. B., Ast, K., Lupu, D., Norton, S. A., McMillan, S. C., . . . Casarett, D. J. (2015). Measuring what matters: Top-ranked quality indicators for hospice and palliative care from the American Academy of Hospice and Palliative Medicine and Hospice and Palliative Nurses Association. *J Pain Symptom Manage, 49*(4), 773–781. doi:10.1016/j.jpainsymman.2015.01.012

Dyregrov, K. (2004). Bereaved parents' experience of research participation. *Soc Sci Med, 58*(2), 391–400.

Eisenach, J. C., DuPen, S., Dubois, M., Miguel, R., & Allin, D. (1995). Epidural clonidine analgesia for intractable cancer pain. The Epidural Clonidine Study Group. *Pain, 61*(3), 391–399.

Emanuel, E. J., Wendler, D., & Grady, C. (2000). What makes clinical research ethical? *JAMA, 283*(20), 2701–2711.

Enzinger, A. C., Zhang, B., Weeks, J. C., & Prigerson, H. G. (2014). Clinical trial participation as part of end-of-life cancer care: Associations with medical care and quality of life near death. *J Pain Symptom Manage, 47*(6), 1078–1090. doi:10.1016/j.jpainsymman.2013.07.004

Ernst, E., & Resch, K. L. (1995). Concept of true and perceived placebo effects. *BMJ, 311*(7004), 551–553.

Faithfull, S. (1996). How many subjects are needed in a research sample in palliative care? *Palliat Med, 10*(3), 259–261.

Farrar, J. T., Cleary, J., Rauck, R., Busch, M., & Nordbrock, E. (1998). Oral transmucosal fentanyl citrate: Randomized, double-blinded, placebo-controlled trial for treatment of breakthrough pain in cancer patients. *J Natl Cancer Inst, 90*(8), 611–616.

Fibiger, J. (1898). Om Serumbehandling af Difteri. *Hospitalstidende, 6*, 309–325, 337–350.

Fine, P. G. (2003). Maximizing benefits and minimizing risks in palliative care research that involves patients near the end of life. *J Pain Symptom Manage, 25*(4), S53–S62.

Fine, P. G. (2004). The ethics of end-of-life research. *J Pain Palliat Care Pharmacother, 18*(1), 71–78.

Freedman, B. (1987a). Equipoise and the ethics of clinical research. *N Engl J Med, 317*(3), 141–145. doi:10.1056/NEJM198707163170304

Freedman, B. (1987b). Scientific value and validity as ethical requirements for research: A proposed explication. *IRB, 9*(6), 7–10.

Fu, S., McQuinn, L., Naing, A., Wheler, J. J., Janku, F., Falchook, G. S., . . . Kurzrock, R. (2013). Barriers to study enrollment in patients with advanced cancer referred to a phase I clinical trials unit. *Oncologist, 18*(12), 1315–1320. doi:10.1634/theoncologist.2013-0202

Gagnon, P., Allard, P., Masse, B., & DeSerres, M. (2000). Delirium in terminal cancer: A prospective study using daily screening, early diagnosis, and continuous monitoring. *J Pain Symptom Manage, 19*(6), 412–426.

Gallup. (2015). Americans' views of pharmaceutical industry take a tumble. Retrieved from http://www.gallup.com/poll/185432/americans-views-pharmaceutical-industry-tumble.aspx

Gawande, A. (2014). *Being mortal: Medicine and what matters in the end* (1st ed.). Toronto: Doubleday.

Gelfman, L. P., & Morrison, R. S. (2008). Research funding for palliative medicine. *J Palliat Med, 11*(1), 36–43. doi:10.1089/jpm.2006.0231

Greenhalgh, T., Howick, J., Maskrey, N., & Evidence Based Medicine Renaissance Group. (2014). Evidence based medicine: A movement in crisis? *BMJ, 348*, g3725. doi:10.1136/bmj.g3725

Gysels, M., Shipman, C., & Higginson, I. J. (2008). "I will do it if it will help others:" Motivations among patients taking part in qualitative studies in palliative care. *J Pain Symptom Manage*, *35*(4), 347–355. doi:10.1016/j.jpainsymman.2007.05.012

Hallenbeck, J. (2008). Evidence-based medicine and palliative care. *J Palliat Med*, *11*(1), 2–4. doi:10.1089/jpm.2008.9998

Hannan, E. L. (2008). Randomized clinical trials and observational studies: Guidelines for assessing respective strengths and limitations. *JACC Cardiovasc Interv*, *1*(3), 211–217. doi:10.1016/j.jcin.2008.01.008

Hardy, J. R. (1997). Placebo-controlled trials in palliative care: The argument for. *Palliat Med*, *11*(5), 415–418.

Harmon, A. (2010a, September 18). New drugs stir debate on rules of clinical trials. *New York Times*.

Harmon, A. (2010b, September 19). New drugs stir debate on rules of clinical trials. *New York Times*.

High, D. M., Whitehouse, P. J., Post, S. G., & Berg, L. (1994). Guidelines for addressing ethical and legal issues in Alzheimer disease research: A position paper. National Institute on Aging. *Alzheimer Dis Assoc Disord*, *8*(Suppl. 4), 66–74.

Hill, A. B. (1965). The environment and disease: Association or causation? *Proc R Soc Med*, *58*, 295–300.

Hopayian, K. (2000). Snakes and statistics: Association does not prove causation. *Br J Gen Pract*, *50*(456), 578.

Horstmann, E., McCabe, M. S., Grochow, L., Yamamoto, S., Rubinstein, L., Budd, T., . . . Grady, C. (2005). Risks and benefits of phase 1 oncology trials, 1991 through 2002. *N Engl J Med*, *352*(9), 895–904. doi:10.1056/NEJMsa042220

Jordan, E. O. (1897). Sanarelli's work upon yellow fever. *Science*, *31*(6), 981–985.

Karlawish, J. H., & Hall, J. B. (1996). The controversy over emergency research: A review of the issues and suggestions for a resolution. *Am J Respir Crit Care Med*, *153*(2), 499–506. doi:10.1164/ajrccm.153.2.8564087

Kathol, R. G., Mutgi, A., Williams, J., Clamon, G., & Noyes, R. Jr. (1990). Diagnosis of major depression in cancer patients according to four sets of criteria. *Am J Psychiatry*, *147*(8), 1021–1024. doi:10.1176/ajp.147.8.1021

Kaufman, S. R. (2005). —*And a time to die: How American hospitals shape the end of life*. New York: Scribner.

Keim-Malpass, J., Hart, T. G., & Miller, J. R. (2013). Coverage of palliative and hospice care for pediatric patients with a life-limiting illness: A policy brief. *J Pediatr Health Care*, *27*(6), 511–516. doi:10.1016/j.pedhc.2013.07.011

Kirkham, S. R., & Abel, J. (1997). Placebo-controlled trials in palliative care: The argument against. *Palliat Med*, *11*(6), 489–492.

Kreicbergs, U., Valdimarsdottir, U., Onelov, E., Henter, J. I., & Steineck, G. (2004). Talking about death with children who have severe malignant disease. *N Engl J Med*, *351*(12), 1175–1186. doi:10.1056/NEJMoa040366

Lind, J. (1757). *A treatise on the scurvy* (2nd ed.). London: A. Millar.

Lynn, J., Baily, M. A., Bottrell, M., Jennings, B., Levine, R. J., Davidoff, F., . . . James, B. (2007). The ethics of using quality improvement methods in health care. *Ann Intern Med*, *146*(9), 666–673.

Mack, J. W., Wolfe, J., Cook, E. F., Grier, H. E., Cleary, P. D., & Weeks, J. C. (2007). Hope and prognostic disclosure. *J Clin Oncol*, *25*(35), 5636–5642. doi:10.1200/JCO.2007.12.6110

McQuay, H., Carroll, D., & Moore, A. (1996). Variation in the placebo effect in randomised controlled trials of analgesics: All is as blind as it seems. *Pain*, *64*(2), 331–335.

Medical Research Council. (1934). The serum treatment of lobar pneumonia. *BMJ Qual Saf*, *1*, 241–245.

Melnick, V. L., Dubler, N. N., Weisbard, A., & Butler, R. N. (1984). Clinical research in senile dementia of the Alzheimer type: Suggested guidelines addressing the ethical and legal issues. *J Am Geriatr Soc*, *32*(7), 531–536.

Meropol, N. J., Weinfurt, K. P., Burnett, C. B., Balshem, A., Benson, A. B. 3rd, Castel, L., . . . Schulman, K. A. (2003). Perceptions of patients and physicians regarding phase I cancer clinical trials: Implications for physician-patient communication. *J Clin Oncol*, *21*(13), 2589–2596. doi:10.1200/JCO.2003.10.072

Miller, C. K., O'Donnell, D. C., Searight, H. R., & Barbarash, R. A. (1996). The Deaconess Informed Consent Comprehension Test: An assessment tool for clinical research subjects. *Pharmacotherapy*, *16*(5), 872–878.

Morrison, R. S., Dietrich, J., Ladwig, S., Quill, T., Sacco, J., Tangeman, J., & Meier, D. E. (2011). Palliative care consultation teams cut hospital costs for Medicaid beneficiaries. *Health Aff (Millwood), 30*(3), 454–463. doi:10.1377/hlthaff.2010.0929

Mount, B. M., Cohen, R., MacDonald, N., Bruera, E., & Dudgeon, D. J. (1995). Ethical issues in palliative care research revisited. *Palliat Med, 9*(2), 165–166.

National Commission for the Protection of Human Subjects of Biomedical and Behavioral Research. (1978). *The Belmont report: Ethical principles and guidelines for the protection of human subjects of research*. Bethesda, MD: U.S. Government Printing Office.

National Comprehensive Cancer Network. (2014). Clinical practice guidelines in oncology. Retrieved from https://www.nccn.org/about/nhl.pdf

NYU Medical Center. (2015). NYU Langone Medical Center Working Group on Compassionate Use and Pre-Approval Access. Retrieved from http://www.med.nyu.edu/pophealth/divisions/medical-ethics/compassionate-use

Parmelee, P. A., Smith, B., & Katz, I. R. (1993). Pain complaints and cognitive status among elderly institution residents. *J Am Geriatr Soc, 41*(5), 517–522.

Participants in the Conference on Ethical Aspects of Research in Developing Countries. (2002). Fair benefits for research in developing countries. *Science, 298*(5601), 2133–2134. doi:10.1126/science.1076899

Peppercorn, J. M., Weeks, J. C., Cook, E. F., & Joffe, S. (2004). Comparison of outcomes in cancer patients treated within and outside clinical trials: Conceptual framework and structured review. *Lancet, 363*(9405), 263–270. doi:10.1016/S0140-6736(03)15383-4

PhRMA. (2015). Principles on conduct of clinical trials: Communication of clinical trials results. Retrieved from http://phrma.org/sites/default/files/pdf/042009_clinical_trial_principles_final_0.pdf

Prasad, V., Gall, V., & Cifu, A. (2011). The frequency of medical reversal. *Arch Intern Med, 171*(18), 1675–1676. doi:10.1001/archinternmed.2011.295

Quill, T. E., & Abernethy, A. P. (2013). Generalist plus specialist palliative care—creating a more sustainable model. *N Engl J Med, 368*(13), 1173–1175. doi:10.1056/NEJMp1215620

Rahimzadeh, V., Bartlett, G., Longo, C., Crimi, L., Macdonald, M. E., Jabado, N., & Ells, C. (2015). Promoting an ethic of engagement in pediatric palliative care research. *BMC Palliat Care, 14*, 50. doi:10.1186/s12904-015-0048-5

Randall, F., & Downie, R. S. (1999). *Palliative care ethics: A companion for all specialties* (2nd ed.). New York: Oxford University Press.

Ranieri, V. M., Thompson, B. T., Barie, P. S., Dhainaut, J. F., Douglas, I. S., Finfer, S., . . . Wiliams, M. D. (2012). Drotrecogin alfa (activated) in adults with septic shock. *N Engl J Med, 366*(22), 2055–2064. doi:10.1056/NEJMoa1202290

Reed, W., & Carroll, J. (1901). The prevention of yellow fever. *Public Health Pap Rep, 27*, 113–129.

Robertson, R. (1807). *Observations on fevers which arise from marsh miasmata, and from other causes, in Europe, Africa, the West Indies, and Newfoundland*. London: Printed for T. Cadell and W. Davies.

Ross, D. S. (2006). The two-faced angel: Do phase I clinical trials have a place in modern hospice? *Penn Bioeth J, 2*(2), 46–49.

Sackett, D., Strauss, S., & Richardson, W. (2000). *Evidence-based medicine: How to practice and teach EBM* (2nd ed.). Edinburgh, UK: Churchill Livingstone.

Sackett, D. L., Rosenberg, W. M., Gray, J. A., Haynes, R. B., & Richardson, W. S. (1996). Evidence based medicine: What it is and what it isn't. *BMJ, 312*(7023), 71–72.

Saunders, C. (1960). Drug treatment of patients in the terminal stages of cancer. *Curr Med Drugs, 1*, 16–28.

Shapiro, A. K., & Shapiro, E. (1984). Patient-provider relationships and the placebo effect. In J. D. Matarazzo, S. M. Weiss, A. J. Herd, N. E. Miller, & S. M. Weiss (Eds.), *Behavioural health: A handbook of health enhancement and disease prevention* (pp. 371–383). New York: Wiley-Interscience.

Smith, T. J., Temin, S., Alesi, E. R., Abernethy, A. P., Balboni, T. A., Basch, E. M., . . . Von Roenn, J. H. (2012). American Society of Clinical Oncology provisional clinical opinion: The integration of palliative care into standard oncology care. *J Clin Oncol, 30*(8), 880–887. doi:10.1200/JCO.2011.38.5161

Song, F., Parekh, S., Hooper, L., Loke, Y. K., Ryder, J., Sutton, A. J., . . . Harvey, I. (2010). Dissemination and publication of research findings: An updated review of related biases. *Health Technol Assess, 14*(8), iii, ix–xi, 1–193. doi:10.3310/hta14080

Steinhauser, K. E., Christakis, N. A., Clipp, E. C., McNeilly, M., McIntyre, L., & Tulsky, J. A. (2000). Factors considered important at the end of life by patients, family, physicians, and other care providers. *JAMA*, *284*(19), 2476–2482.

Sternberg, G. (1898). The bacillus icteroides (Sanarelli) and bacillus X (Sternberg). *Trans Assoc Amer Physicians, 13,* 71.

SUPPORT Principal Investigators. (1995). A controlled trial to improve care for seriously ill hospitalized patients: The study to understand prognoses and preferences for outcomes and risks of treatments (SUPPORT). *JAMA, 274*(20), 1591–1598.

Takesaka, J., Crowley, R., & Casarett, D. (2004). What is the risk of distress in palliative care survey research? *J Pain Symptom Manage, 28*(6), 593–598. doi:10.1016/j.jpainsymman.2004.03.006

Temel, J. S., Greer, J. A., Muzikansky, A., Gallagher, E. R., Admane, S., Jackson, V. A., . . . Lynch, T. J. (2010). Early palliative care for patients with metastatic non-small-cell lung cancer. *N Engl J Med, 363*(8), 733–742. doi:10.1056/NEJMoa1000678

Turner, J. A., Deyo, R. A., Loeser, J. D., Von Korff, M., & Fordyce, W. E. (1994). The importance of placebo effects in pain treatment and research. *JAMA, 271*(20), 1609–1614.

Twain, M. (1906). *Chapters from my autobiography*. London; New York: Harper.

Vanderpool, H. Y. (1996). *The ethics of research involving human subjects: Facing the 21st century*. Frederick, MD: University Publishing Group.

Velleman, P. (2008). Truth, damn truth, and statistics. *J Stat Educ, 16*(2).

Wee, B., Hadley, G., & Derry, S. (2008). How useful are systematic reviews for informing palliative care practice? Survey of 25 Cochrane systematic reviews. *BMC Palliat Care, 7,* 13. doi:10.1186/1472-684X-7-13

Weinfurt, K. P., Sulmasy, D. P., Schulman, K. A., & Meropol, N. J. (2003). Patient expectations of benefit from phase I clinical trials: Linguistic considerations in diagnosing a therapeutic misconception. *Theor Med Bioeth, 24*(4), 329–344.

White, R. M. (2002). The Tuskegee syphilis study. *Hastings Cent Rep, 32*(6), 4–5; author reply 5.

Whoriskey, P., & Keating, D. (2014, December 26). Dying and profits: The evolution of hospice. *Washington Post*.

Wilkinson, D., Karim, S. S., & Coovadia, H. M. (1999). Short course antiretroviral regimens to reduce maternal transmission of HIV. *BMJ, 318*(7182), 479–480.

World Medical Association. (2013). Declaration of Helsinki. Retrieved from http://www.wma.net/en/30publications/10policies/b3/

18

Clinical Practice
of Palliative Care

This textbook has addressed a variety of specific topics (such as physician-assisted dying and palliative sedation) and particular contexts (such as the prenatal period and various developmental stages of childhood). There are, however, core concepts that pervade and influence every aspect of the practice of palliative care. Precisely because they influence the choices patients and families make, they should not be overlooked or taken for granted. Quite the contrary, they demand thoughtful analysis in order to best equip patients—as well as the families who love them and the clinicians who care for them—to make the best decisions.

The first core concept is communication, which is inherently a relational process and thus is complex and full of potential pitfalls. The words the physician uses, the concepts she chooses to disclose and emphasize, and the way she responds to patient inquiries all significantly impact the treatment plan. At the same time, what the patient understands is more relevant than what the physician says (or intends to say). Unless the patient has an accurate understanding of the medical situation and the relevant options, he cannot make a decision based on his goals and values.

Why a patient is making a particular decision is just as important as the decision he has made. When it comes to one's own health, choices generally are not made based on a detached analysis of medical facts. Background, beliefs, and feelings play a crucial role, which is the reason physicians ought to inquire about a patient's goals and fears (Bernacki & Block, 2014). These often extend beyond the patient to the patient's family and broader community, who might hold profound beliefs about how much information is shared and what should be done with it. These beliefs might reflect cultural mores or values, as well as spiritual convictions and religious obligations.

One might question whether communication, culture, and spirituality are "ethical" issues. Yet that question would never arise with regard to patient autonomy, the obligation of informed consent, or the right to refuse treatment. The foundation of all of these are the patient's goals, which are often profoundly influenced by his view of the world and his place in it (i.e., his spirituality), as well as the culture that formed him. Physicians thus have an ethical obligation to understand and respect the patient's values, which may differ from the physician's own. Navigating this complex terrain of communication, culture, and spirituality requires significant nuance.

Role of Communication in Palliative Care
Case Study

A seventy-five-year-old man has been experiencing abdominal pain for several months. He was reluctant to see his physician—both out of a general disregard for "fancy modern medicine" and also perhaps out of fear of what the doctor might find—but his two daughters prevail upon him to be evaluated. His physician refer him to the local hospital for radiological evaluation, and a CT scan reveals advanced pancreatic cancer.

The physician is about to convey this information to the patient when his oldest daughter—who is his presumed surrogate, in the absence of a durable power of attorney for health care—inquires about the findings. Both daughters have been part of all medical discussions up to that point, and the physician recognizes how much the patient (whose wife died several years earlier) relies on them. She therefore discloses the diagnosis, hoping that the daughters will be an emotional support to their father.

The daughters understand the gravity of the diagnosis and express a wish to take the patient home on hospice care. So as not to "take away his hope," however, they demand that no one tell the patient his diagnosis. The physician is troubled by this request and is unsure how to respond.

Historicolegal Evolution

The term "palliative" comes from the Latin word *pallium*—which means "cloak"—and for many years palliative care was more about cloaking the *nature* of the patient's condition rather than the symptoms associated with it (Randall & Downie, 2006). Patients were generally not informed of their diagnosis or prognosis, especially if it was serious (Field & Copp, 1999). As Glaser and Strauss wrote in 1965, "[A]merican physicians ordinarily do not tell patients outright that death is probable or inevitable. . . . [F]amilies also tend to guard the secret."

A combination of court decisions, rights movements, fragmentation within the medical profession, and well-publicized lapses in research ethics all led to a shift from parentalism to autonomy (p. 5). Instead of withholding the truth from patients, physicians began to inform patients of their condition, and rather than independently determining the plan of care, physicians would seek the patient's consent for recommended treatments.

As the years went on, though, the pendulum may have swung too far: rather than feeling no obligation to disclose a patient's diagnosis, physicians often viewed any failure to disclose all relevant details (even at the request of the patient or family) as unethical. Out of fear of infringing on the patient's autonomy, physicians would often provide extensive descriptions of various treatment options that frequently entailed multiple combinations and permutations. Written "consent forms" came to take the place of thoughtful conversations, even though these forms are often written at a college level (Hopper, TenHave, Tully, & Hall, 1998), beyond the capabilities of most patients.

Lost among the details was confirmation that the patient truly understood the situation he was facing (Braddock, Edwards, Hasenberg, Laidley, & Levinson, 1999). This is particularly true for patients with diminished health literacy—which the Institute of Medicine defines as "the capacity to obtain, process, and understand basic health information and services needed to make appropriate health decisions" (Nielsen-Bohlman & Institute of Medicine Committee on Health Literacy, 2004)—for whom even familiar terms such as "cardiopulmonary resuscitation" may be misunderstood. Such diminished health literacy is a strong predictor for poor health outcomes (Baker, Parker, Williams, Clark, & Nurss, 1997), as patients manifest less understanding of their disease and ability to care for themselves (Gazmararian, Williams, Peel, & Baker, 2003).

This is particularly a problem for patients with limited English proficiency, an increasingly common occurrence in a multicultural society. Language barriers create ethical issues all their own, as it is often more convenient to ask a family member—or an available staff person who happens to speak the patient's language—to interpret. This can be detrimental, however. Staff who are not trained as interpreters may lack the skills to function as an intermediary between the medical team and the patient, as medical interpretation involves far more than simply shifting words from one language to another without regard for nuance or cultural impact. Relying on a family member to interpret puts that person in an impossible position, balancing the need of the patient to understand with the family member's own emotions upon hearing information and then having to relay it. (There have been reports of young children being asked to interpret for a physician communicating a serious diagnosis to that child's parent.) For all these reasons, patients and their families should be offered language services by trained interpreters (Wilson-Stronks & Galvez, 2017).

But even where health literacy and English proficiency are not barriers, communication in palliative care remains a challenge by virtue of its complexity and nuance. The subject matter is literally life and death, involving clinically complex and emotionally wrenching decisions. Physicians often struggle with these topics, especially those who have not received specific training in communication (Ha & Longnecker, 2010). Palliative care teams are therefore frequently consulted to assist in optimizing communication, overcoming relational obstacles, and creating a forum for open dialogue. Some have gone so far as to proclaim the family meeting as the "procedure of palliative care," as so much of palliative care stems from accurate understanding and appropriate goal-setting (Cahill, Lobb, Sanderson, & Phillips, 2016).

Disclosure

Even once disclosure of relevant information became a standard expectation, there remained exceptions. The one that is universally accepted is *patient waiver*, whereby "a medical doctor need not make disclosures of risks when the patient requests that he not be so informed" (*Cobbs v. Grant*, 1972). The physician should, of course, verify that the patient is indeed waiving his right to full information and also sensitively inquire as to the reason for doing so (which might reveal previously unrecognized areas of anxiety or concern). The physician should document in the chart precisely what the patient waived his right to, while continuing to revisit the matter, since the patient always has the right to rescind the waiver and learn whatever he wants to know.

For many years, another exception to the obligation of disclosure was *therapeutic privilege*. This refers to a situation where the physician believes that "disclosure poses such a serious psychological threat of detriment to the patient as to be medically contraindicated" (Judicial Council of the American Medical Association, 1984). Some state laws interpreted this narrowly as referring to information that would render the patient incompetent, which itself would preclude the possibility of offering informed consent or refusal. Other states took a broader view which encompassed anything considered "counter-therapeutic," seeming to permit nondisclosure in practically any situation.

While once frequently practiced and initially endorsed by the American Medical Association, as patient autonomy became the cornerstone of American bioethics, the notion of therapeutic privilege fell into disfavor. Justice Byron White famously observed: "Informed consent provisions . . . may produce some anxiety in the patient and influence her in her choice. This is in fact their reason for existence, and . . . it is an entirely salutary reason" (*Thornburgh v. American College of Obstetricians*, 1986). Recent revisions of the American Medical Association (2010–2011) Code of Ethics have therefore deemed the practice "ethically unacceptable."

Less technical than "invoking therapeutic privilege," a more human response to disclosure is to withhold information out of concern that candor about a patient's diagnosis or prognosis will "take away hope." Families often—as in this section's case study—want to protect their loved one from something that might sap his fighting spirit or taint his final days.

This approach is also flawed, for studies have shown that frank prognostic disclosure not only provides a patient with a more realistic sense of his life expectancy but does not cause increased sadness or anxiety (Enzinger, Zhang, Schrag, & Prigerson, 2015). This has also been shown in the pediatric population (Mack et al., 2007), reinforcing the concept that patients and their families appreciate compassionate candor (and also often know more than physicians give them credit for). These studies underscore the multifaceted nature of hope which encompasses more than cure and long-term survival (Feudtner, 2009). Indeed, one of the primary tasks of palliative care is "reframing" hope in terms that are achievable, such as mending relationships or experiencing a peaceful death. As Robert Frost once said, "Hope does not lie in a way out, but in a way through."

Given medicine's history of withholding information from patients, an obvious remedy would be to strive for full and immediate disclosure in every case, to avoid even the appearance of parentalism. This, however, is frequently short-sighted, because some information—especially regarding treatment options—may clearly be inconsistent with the patient's stated goals. For instance, if a patient—upon being informed that he has cancer—expresses a desire to do everything possible to "beat it" because life is that precious to him, it may not be necessary at that time to explore what a purely comfort-directed plan of care might look like. By the same token, a seriously ill patient whose quality of life (by his own estimation) is extremely poor and expresses a desire to simply be kept comfortable and live out his remaining days in peace does not require an in-depth discussion of the risks and benefits of CPR. This would be at best a waste of his limited time and at worst counterproductive in terms of the patient's emotional well-being as well as the physician-patient relationship. Some have described this approach as being "economical with the truth" (Randall & Downie, 2006).

Even when information is relevant to a patient's condition or treatment options, disclosure need not occur all at once. To present all possible information may ignore the emotional impact of that information. It is often said that when a patient hears the word "cancer" for the first time, he is unable to hear—or, at least, remember—anything else that is said in that particular conversation. For this reason, it may be advisable to use a "staged" model of informed consent, whereby information is parceled out at appropriate times and contexts (Wear, 1998).

So rather than "protecting" the patient from the truth on the one hand and engaging in an "information dump" (Aulisio, 2016) on the other, a more nuanced response to a family's request for nondisclosure is called for. The patient in this section's case study clearly is not requesting a waiver, and it would not be practical to inquire whether he would seek one in relation to his terminal diagnosis. (A question along the lines of "If you had cancer, would you like to know?" would itself be revelatory.) The patient has also not communicated clear goals of care which might render certain treatment options irrelevant.

But neither is the physician seeking to withhold information based on a parentalistic sense of therapeutic privilege. It is the patient's daughters—who know the patient well and clearly care for him—who are seeking to safeguard his sense of hope, introducing a further layer of complexity into the relationship of hope and prognostic disclosure.

So rather than responding with an indignant defense of the primacy of patient autonomy, it is advisable to seek greater understanding of the family's reason for requesting nondisclosure (Hallenbeck & Arnold, 2007). The medical team should empathize with the family's desire to protect the patient at a time of extreme vulnerability and express their own views as simply that: opinions and the beginning of a deeper dialogue. This would allow the team to sensitively inquire whether the family's request stems from a desire to shield the patient from demoralizing information—an understandable if perhaps misguided motive—or from previous requests the patient may have made to not be informed about his health (or family norms to that effect) (Hallenbeck, 2003).

The latter represents the best rationale for nondisclosure. Far from being a violation of patient autonomy, not informing the patient of his diagnosis could rightly be considered an expression of respect for that autonomy (i.e., the patient's right *not* to know). To be sure, the clinician needs sufficient evidence to reach that conclusion, and nondisclosure should never stem from the clinician's human reluctance to share bad news. But previous statements could represent something of an "implicit waiver" of full disclosure, albeit one that still requires thoughtful exploration in order to confirm.

The most reliable source of this information is the patient himself, through sensitive open-ended inquiry. The medical team could thoughtfully inquire as to his understanding of his medical condition, which might reveal a deeper grasp than previously suspected. (This would itself largely resolve the perceived ethical dilemma.) If the patient was unaware of his condition, the team might inquire as to his preferred manner of communication between the medical team and either him or his family. Without divulging information the patient may not welcome, this allows the physician to confirm just how much information the patient wishes to know.

Several possibilities may follow from this approach. The patient may request full disclosure, which the physician may then in good conscience provide. Alternatively, the patient may already understand on some level what is happening to him but prefer not to bring it out into the open. Glaser and Strauss (1965) refer to this as "closed awareness." And if the patient reiterates the family's request to provide information to them directly—which they can choose to relay to the patient, or not—then that is the patient's wish, and honoring it also honors his autonomy.

This, then, represents a third legitimate reason for nondisclosure, in addition to explicit waiver and clear incompatibility with the patient's expressed treatment goals: inconsistency with the patient's *values*. Full disclosure to the patient may be a bedrock principle of American bioethics, but not every patient wants to know everything about his medical condition or treatment options. To be sure, a thoughtful exploration of the situation is required before reaching this conclusion, in order to ensure that failure to disclose is not a reflection of the physician's own reluctance or external pressures from a family whose values the patient does not share. But for a patient who truly would not wish to know about his prognosis, *not* directly informing him—after the thoughtful exploration described earlier—better respects his autonomy than foisting unwanted information upon him.

Return to the Case

Following Hallenbeck and Arnold's (2007) methodology, the team avoids overreacting to a supposed violation of patient autonomy by inquiring as to the family's explanatory model of the patient's illness and validating the care and concern that drove them to make this request. The physician then describes the normative decision-making model in the United States—which is something of a global outlier in demanding full disclosure to the patient—and then asks the family if it would be acceptable to them if she inquired of the patient (in a very open-ended way) the degree to which he would like to be involved in learning about and determining his own health care.

The family agrees, and when asked the patient expresses a preference that the team provide medical information to the family, rather than directly to him. The physician has the sense that the patient has good understanding of his diagnosis ("closed awareness") but is choosing not to openly discuss it. The patient clearly trusts his family and seems content relying on them for treatment decisions. Before concluding the conversation, the physician reassures the patient that he can re-engage in the conversations at any time.

Role of Culture in Palliative Care
Case Study

A sixty-five-year-old woman who recently emigrated from Vietnam is admitted to the hospital for abdominal pain, subsequently determined to be Stage 4 colon cancer. Through a translator, the oncologist informs the patient of her diagnosis and seeks to engage her in exploring treatment options, which include disease-modifying therapy or hospice.

Throughout the conversation, however, the patient remains mostly silent and communicates no preferences. Soon thereafter her eighty-year-old uncle arrives and informs the oncologist that as the eldest male family member, he will be making all medical decisions for the patient. The oncologist is conflicted, wanting to respect the patient's autonomy but also whatever cultural beliefs might impact her approach to care.

Culture—which has been defined as "that set of learned values, beliefs, customs, and behaviors that is shared by a group of interacting individuals" (Ruhnke et al., 2000)—shapes and defines one's beliefs about and perceptions of the world. Illness and approaching death are two areas where cultural beliefs and customs play an extremely important role.

For this reason, "care at the end of life should recognize, assess, and address the psychological, social, spiritual/religious issues, and cultural taboos realizing that different cultures may require significantly different approaches" (American Academy of Family Physicians, 2003). Culture is such an important consideration in palliative care that the National Consensus Project established a distinct domain for it (Colby, Dahlin, Lantos, Carney, & Christopher, 2010).

Any discussion of culture needs to find a balance between two extremes. One extreme is stereotyping, where it is assumed that one's cultural or ethnic background determines one's beliefs. For instance, it would be insensitive and inaccurate to assert that every Latino believes a certain way or every Japanese patient has the same values. To do so would reduce culture to "a series of isolated acontextual beliefs or practices characterized by ethnic origin" (Kagawa-Singer & Blackhall, 2001). Just because it is more likely, for instance, that a patient of Chinese descent might feel a certain way, does not meant that *every* patient of Chinese descent feels that way. Further, not every patient of Chinese descent is equivalent; the sociocultural forces present in Hong Kong, Taiwan, and mainland China are distinct. Studies have shown, for instance, that patients in Hong Kong value autonomy as highly as those in the United States (Fielding & Hung, 1996), while those from mainland China generally do not. The impact of culture must, therefore, be taken in context.

The other extreme—which is equally misguided—is to completely ignore the role of culture in the name of political correctness. One might be so concerned about stereotyping that culture is overlooked entirely, leading to a disregard for "culture's fundamental function of giving meaning to life and of providing guidelines for living" (Kagawa-Singer & Blackhall, 2001). To ignore the fact that a patient is a recent immigrant from another part of the world limits one's ability to optimally respect and care for that patient.

For the purposes of this discussion, assertions about beliefs held by certain cultural groups should be viewed not as blanket stereotypes but rather as empirically based observations about beliefs which have been shown to be common in those groups. Of course, each patient and family should be queried as to the degree to which they adhere to that belief. In that respect, culture represents not a conclusion but rather a jumping-off point for discussion, after which targeted inquiries can be made. As Kagawa-Singer and Blackhall (2001) quote a patient saying:

> If you don't know a person, you got to find out his identity, go where he lives, where he goes, where he was born, who's in his family. And he's got to open up, and tell you these things. Because the more you know about this person, his family, then that'll make you know more about you.

Cultural differences lead to diversity of opinion in many aspects of health care, including the balance of individualism versus collectivism, the definition of "family," assignment of gender roles, communication patterns, and views of physicians, suffering, and the afterlife

(Searight & Gafford, 2005). Three primary areas where culture significantly affects palliative care—with potential resulting ethical dilemmas—involve communication of prognosis, the locus of decision-making, and attitudes toward advance care planning (ACP) and end-of-life (EOL) care.

Communication of Prognosis

The ethical imperative—with some exceptions, as previously noted—to disclose to the patient her diagnosis is a very American notion. In many other countries, it is assumed that the family will definitely be informed of the diagnosis, with some debate about whether the patient should be informed too (Fallowfield, Jenkins, & Beveridge, 2002).

If the patient is informed, the manner of disclosure demands sensitivity, as culture-specific connotations of specific diagnoses can also lead to misunderstandings. Certain terms (like "cancer") may be taken as death sentences, even if the physician is quick to note that treatments are available. For a patient who holds such cultural beliefs, being informed that she has cancer could therefore be misleading because of the personal and cultural overlays of that term. In such cultures—which tend to prioritize beneficence over individual autonomy—preferred terminology might include "growth," "mass," or "blood disease." Examples of these cultures include African, Japanese, and Native American (Loue & Sajatovic, 2012).

This example highlights the fact that the significance of one's diagnosis is what it means for that patient going forward in terms of life expectancy, quality of life, and treatment options. The American emphasis on autonomy logically carries over from disclosure of diagnosis to that of prognosis, which necessarily impacts the treatment plan. Indeed, this is the basis of ACP, because in the absence of prognostic awareness a patient and her family cannot plan for the future and make informed treatment decisions.

With regard to prognosis, some cultures emphasize non-maleficence over autonomy. This applies not only to refraining from inflicting physical harm in the context of medical procedures but also psychic or spiritual harm. The mere mention of "death" may be viewed as inherently harmful, perhaps because such discussions burden a patient or are thought to increase the likelihood that negative events will come to pass (Holland, Geary, Marchini, & Tross, 1987). Some patients of Chinese descent, for example, believe that the elderly are vulnerable to being upset by bad news (Carrese & Rhodes, 1995; Yeo & Hikuyeda, 2000). Such patients, it is thought, should not be burdened unnecessarily by discussion of unwanted outcomes, which helps explain why people who hold this view are reluctant to complete advance directives (ADs, p. 99). In these situations, nonverbal communication assumes great importance, both to relate ideas that words are felt inappropriate and also to allow the patient to "save face" by not being confronted with information she would prefer not to discuss, or even be aware of. Other cultures where disclosure might be deemed harmful include Latino, Pakistani, Bosnian, Italian, and Filipino (Searight & Gafford, 2005).

In order to address prognosis in a culturally sensitive way, it is imperative that the team recognize the patient and family's cultural underpinnings of illness and disease. The most direct way of accomplishing this is to inquire of the patient and family about specific beliefs they may hold which would impact how they process medical information and decisions. So rather than feeling an ethical obligation to clearly state the technical diagnosis (such as "cancer"), the team's emphasis should be on expressing a concept that accurately reflects—in the patient's own language and understanding—what the patient's likely future is. A delicate balance may have to be struck between accommodating the patient and family's cultural needs on the one hand and the professional's obligation to provide information that is necessary to make important medical decisions on the other.

Locus of Decision-Making

As stated earlier (p. 4), for most of the history of Western medicine the locus of decision-making was the physician. Over the course of the twentieth century in the United States, that locus shifted to the patient, although recently there has been a renewed quest for balance in the form of "shared decision-making." In some cultures—such as much of eastern Europe—this shift has not occurred, leaving the physician as the primary decision-maker. Patients and families may look to the physician to make treatment decisions based on beneficence, not expecting to be integrally involved in the process. Indeed, for the physician to expect a patient or family to make a specific treatment decision—especially in the absence of a recommendation—would be viewed as unusual at best and unprofessional at worst.

In other cultures a different locus of decision-making exists: the family. To be sure, family is important to patients in every culture because the web of interrelationships impacts one's sense of self, as well as the decisions one makes. Mount (1985) describes the family as a "mobile": removal of any one element (even a small one) impacts everything else. But in some cultures—such as Korean and Mexican-American—the family is not merely involved in decision-making for a patient; they are responsible for it. This might be accomplished as a group or by one family member whom the rest defer to, which is often the patriarch (Blackhall, Murphy, Frank, Michel, & Azen, 1995). In that context, it would be viewed as disrespectful to direct information and queries to anyone other than the culturally appropriate decision-maker. And attempts to speak with the patient alone—often done out of good intentions to safeguard the patient's "autonomy" from family influence—may be unwelcome.

In still other cultures—such as many in Asia—there is a balance between physician and family. The decision is made jointly, in a more robust version of "shared decision-making" than is often practiced in the United States, despite the frequent use of that term (Moazam, 2000).

Given the diversity in the locus of decision-making, it is important for clinicians to determine how the patient wants decisions to be made. Just as in the case of diagnosis where the appropriate question to the patient might be, "How much do you want to know about your health condition?," in this case the follow-up question might be, "How would you like decisions about your health care to be made?"

Recognizing the importance of the decisions to be made, the patient may request that someone from her family be present, which could raise concerns for potential coercion. If so, the team might reassure the patient that the conversation is not so much about what medical decisions need to be made but rather *how* to make those decisions. The patient may then be willing to meet in private, but if this is not possible, the team will need to thoughtfully evaluate the degree—if any—to which the patient may be making decisions for the benefit of others rather than based on her own value system.

Ultimately, the patient may request that she make her own decisions or defer to another person (with varying degrees of continued involvement). The latter would represent a form a waiver of informed consent for future treatment and is already a component of many AD forms which allow a patient to defer decisional authority to her agent immediately upon signing, without requiring a loss of decision-making capacity (DMC, Vermont Ethics Network, 2017).

Potentially more problematic would be a patient's request that the physician make subsequent medical decisions, as this runs contrary to the predominant American model of patient autonomy. Even waiver of informed consent—which may also be unsettling—still establishes a "check-and-balance" between the physician's primary focus on the patient's best interests and the surrogate's sense of the patient's goals (stemming as they might from cultural values). But when the patient completely defers the decision itself to the physician, the physician may feel that he holds undue power, especially as the classic check-and-balance of beneficence and autonomy is no longer in place.

Faced with such a request, the physician should specifically confirm with the patient that she wants the physician to make decisions for her and that this is not merely polite deference or a feeling of her voice not being heard. (This should be clearly documented in the chart as well.) Alternatives—such as naming a surrogate decision-maker or deferring to one's family—should be explored.

But if the patient is resolute in her wish that the physician decide, this is not necessarily wrong. Just because the societal pendulum in the United States has swung all the way to the side of "radical autonomy" does not mean that this is every patient's preference. Rather than doing simply what he feels is best, however, the physician could take time to explore the patient's overall goals (unrelated to the medical procedure). Just as one would with a patient who *does* want to make her own decisions, identifying the patient's hopes and fears—as well as what she's willing to go through to achieve her goals and the level of family involvement she wants (Bernacki & Block, 2014)—can lead to a thoughtful recommendation. Although in this case the recommendation will automatically become the treatment plan, the fact remains that it is patient-centered and reflective of the patient's values.

It would actually be inconsistent with patient- and family-centered care to require the patient (or family) to explicitly consent to the proposed plan if she does not wish to. One might sensitively note that the patient is free to disagree with the rec-ommendation, essentially seeking informed assent (p. 382) although in a much less clear-cut situation than this approach is typically used. The patient, though, may be unwilling to do even that. At that point the physician should feel confident that he has involved the patient in the decision-making progress to the fullest extent that the pa-tient wishes, and then proceed with the treatment plan, while also assuring the patient that she can always become more involved in decision-making at a later time, should she wish to.

Attitudes toward End-of-Life Care and Advance Care Planning

There is significant variation across cultures regarding ADs and EOL care. One of the best-documented pertains to African-Americans, who in multiple studies have been shown to be significantly less likely to have an AD—and significantly more likely to opt for CPR—than white Americans (Bullock, 2011; Degenholtz, Thomas, & Miller, 2003; Johnstone & Kanitsaki, 2009; Kwak & Haley, 2005). African-Americans are also less likely to enroll in hospice, representing 13% of the American population but only 8% of hospice patients.

Several reasons have been posited for this difference. The first is the history of prejudice and oppression, ranging from the era of slavery well into the twentieth cen-tury, as exemplified by the Tuskegee syphilis experiments (p. 7). Second, African-Americans are more likely than white Americans to espouse religious views, which often lead patients and families to see life as a gift from God that is inherently valuable. Death should be on God's terms, it is argued, not as a result of limitation of treatment, leading conservative Christians to request more aggressive treatment at the end of life (Phelps et al., 2009). Third, depictions of medical care in the media—such as the un-realistically high percentage of positive outcomes resulting from CPR (Diem, Lantos, & Tulsky, 1996)—may contribute to opting for maximal treatment. Finally, there con-tinue to exist significant discrepancies and access to care, thus engendering a sense of mistrust among populations that have historically been denied adequate medical care, especially when the treating clinicians are predominantly of a different race (Cabral & Smith, 2011).

Other cultures also have beliefs that impact EOL care. Specifically, the understanding of what constitutes a "good death" often determines treatment decisions. Many people in Spain for instance, recognize the concept of *agonía*, "the gradual slipping away of the senses when life is extinguishing gradually and somnolence is acceptable, even preferable" (Nunez-Olarte & Gracia, 2001). By contrast, in northern Europe there is greater emphasis on awareness and the need to resolve psychological "business" (Wilkinson, 1999). And while in some cultures medically administered nutrition and hydration (p. 481) is viewed as obligatory because of the sacred nature of feeding, in others it is not so. "Many cultures see stopping eating as a sign of dying and not its cause. They never even consider the use of a feeding tube" (Dunn, 2009).

While some cultural beliefs inform ACP, others may impede it. The very concept of an AD composed and signed by a patient is, obviously, a very individualistic notion. While this comports well with the American emphasis on autonomy, cultures where the locus of decision-making is shared or deferred may not appreciate the importance (or even applicability) of an AD. Put simply, if the patient was never the primary decision-maker, her losing DMC does not create any added complexity in ongoing decision-making activities.

Examples of cultures where ACP may not be as great an emphasis include some Latino cultures which have a strong notion of collective responsibility that may preclude the completion of an AD by an individual patient (Blackhall et al., 1995). Similarly, many Asian cultures emphasize filial piety (*hsiao*) to the degree that broaching EOL decisions with an elder could be seen as disrespectful (Yeo & Hikuyeda, 2000).

This variation concerning ACP is illustrated on an international scale by the wide variation in the use of ADs. In many countries, ADs either have no legal basis, require court approval, or are simply seldomly used based on the inherent values of the culture. This variation can be explained not only by the opinions of patients but also by those of physicians. Even within Europe, the range of physicians who are willing to write a Do Not Resuscitate order ranges from less than 10% in Italy to over 90% in the Netherlands (Blank, 2011).

It is crucial that the palliative care physician recognize the impact of culture on EOL care and ACP. One size does not fit all, though. The reasons that one cultural group may be reluctant to engage in ACP may be much different than those of another group. In the case of African-Americans—who are disproportionately deprived of the benefits of hospice care—this might lead to focused initiatives to address specific reservations. Concerns about discrimination require reassurance of the universal application of ACP, which can be framed in terms of the right of self-determination. Establishing a trusting relationship with patients, clarifying potential misconceptions about the benefits and burdens of certain procedures, and thoughtfully engaging the spiritual beliefs that underlie treatment decisions may also be helpful.

But for patients from other backgrounds, respect for their culture may require a modification of the standard approach. Rather than encouraging them to engage in traditional ACP, available tools could be utilized to help them achieve their individual goals. If the locus of decision-making is not the patient, this could be documented in a proxy directive. If the patient wishes the physician to be the decision-maker, this should be clearly documented in the chart, as well as the conversation about the patient's goals and the reasons for the physician's decision regarding treatment. Respect for the patient's cultural beliefs may, therefore, require the physician to modify his own culturally determined expectations, in order to empower the patient to receive the appropriate care on whatever terms are most acceptable to her.

Return to the Case

After hearing the family's request to make all medical decisions for the patient, the physician asks the patient to meet in private to confirm this is what the patient wants too. There is initially some reluctance, but the physician reassures the patient that the discussion will only be about how decisions will be made, not what those particular decisions will be. Agreeing to meet privately, the patient confirms that she would prefer her family to make all decisions and to be fully informed of subsequent developments. She does not want to be present for the discussions, trusting her family to inform her of whatever she needs to know.

The physician respects the patient's wishes, while taking the opportunity to re-assure the patient that she can change her mind at any point. He recommends that the patient describe her preferred method of decision-making in an AD, to ensure that it is respected across all venues of care. The patient appreciates the respect the physician has shown her and is willing to complete a proxy directive. Future medical decisions are made by the family.

Role of Spirituality in Palliative Care
Case Study

A seventy-year-old man with multiple medical problems (including emphysema and congestive heart failure) has suffered a serious stroke, and the medical team believes he is likely never to regain consciousness. Even if he does, he will require around-the-clock care, which the family is not able to provide at home. He has previously said that he would never want to be placed in a nursing home. Given that it is not medically possible to achieve the patient's stated goals, the team recommends shifting the focus to comfort.

The family refuses, however, citing their belief that God will perform a miraculous healing. The team is unsure how to respond to the family's position.

For most of the history of Western medicine, spirituality and health were closely linked. The Hippocratic Oath, after all, is explicitly directed to the gods: "I swear by Apollo the physician, by Aesculapius, Hygeia, and Panacea, and I take to witness all the gods, all the goddesses, to keep according to my ability and my judgment the following oath." It was widely believed that many physical symptoms had a spiritual cause and thus were treated with religious rituals. Until the relatively recent past, religious orders provided the bulk of medical care. The first hospices were explicitly religious ventures, and the roles of physician and priest were often combined (Koenig, 2000).

This connection had profound implications for EOL care. Conceptions of death frequently involved religious symbols and rituals, with specific prayers to be said and even particular postures to be assumed in the last moments of life (p. 12). A sudden, unexpected death (*mors improvisa*) was the worst kind, as it did not permit adequate contrition for sins committed in this life or preparation for the next (Rawcliffe, 1995).

In the post-Enlightenment era, things changed. Descartes' famous dictum—"I think, therefore I am"—ushered in a dualistic philosophy where the body was viewed as distinct from the mind or the spirit. Greater understanding of the pathophysiology of disease explained phenomena that previously were attributed to supernatural causes. Decreasing religiosity in Western societies reduced the importance of sacred observance. At the same time, death became "medicalized," more frequently occurring in hospitals or other health care facilities, rather than at home (Ariès, 1974).

With increased diversity and secularization, death rituals—which used to involve prayer and contrition—are now comprised of CPR (Timmermans, 2017) and a physician's proclamation of the "time of death," as seen on television. And rather than dreading *mors improvisa*, many people in the modern world—and a disproportionate number of physicians—prefer a sudden, unexpected death, at least in comparison to a protracted battle with terminal illness (Gallo et al., 2003).

With fewer people espousing explicitly religious faith (Pew Research Center, 2015), spirituality has taken a more prominent role in people's lives and also in their health care decisions. Defined as "the personal quest for understanding answers to ultimate questions about life, about meaning, and about relationship to the sacred or transcendent, which may (or may not) lead to or arise from the development of religious rituals and the formation of community" (King & Koenig, 2009), spirituality is more difficult to quantify and also less standardized compared to codified religious faiths with specific expectations of adherents. While it would be unwise to make extensive assumptions about a patient's values simply because he self-describes, for instance, as Buddhist or Roman Catholic, it is *impossible* to do so when a person simply describes himself as "spiritual."

Even though it is difficult to define, spirituality inevitably comes into play when a patient is facing serious illness, which Sulmasy (1999) has rightly termed "a spiritual event." He goes on to observe that "illness grasps persons by the soul and by the body and disturbs them both. Illness ineluctably raises troubling questions of a transcendent nature—questions about meaning, value, and relationship. These are spiritual questions." A great many patients view their illness through the lens of spirituality—*Why did this happen to me?*—as they also view their future: *How does my spiritual well-being affect my physical health? What will happen to me when I die?* Understandably, patients and families want health care professionals to inquire about their spiritual questions and concerns (Ehman, Ott, Short, Ciampa, & Hansen-Flaschen, 1999; McCord et al., 2004). Despite this, the majority of patients report that their spiritual needs are at best minimally met by the medical system (Balboni et al., 2010).

This is precisely the reason that spiritual, religious, and existential aspects of care is one of the domains of palliative care, according to the National Consensus Project (Colby et al., 2010). Consistent with the notion of "transdisciplinary care," all members of the palliative care team should have at least a basic understanding of spiritual distress and frequently reported spiritual issues. Physicians are expected to be able to perform a spiritual assessment in order to understand core components of a patient's or family's religious or spiritual outlook, with multiple tools available (Anandarajah & Hight, 2001; Borneman, Ferrell, & Puchalski, 2010). More complex issues are the domain of the chaplain on the palliative care team, who should be familiar with the patient's particular tradition and able to speak to it (or, at least, engage the patient in it).

Given the pervasiveness of spiritual beliefs and the impact they have on medical decision-making (especially at the end of life), it is important for clinicians to understand the impact of faith on a patient's goals, and the appropriate response when the patient's spiritual beliefs seem to conflict with the medical model of illness. This is particularly true in relationship to a belief in miracles, religious "mandates" for life-sustaining medical treatment, and specific concepts of suffering.

Miracles

One of the most challenging areas related to religion (arguably more than spirituality) in palliative care has to do with an expectation of a miracle. While it may be difficult for physicians to accurately estimate a patient's prognosis (p. 84), there are definitely situations when it appears clear either that a patient will not survive, or that he will not achieve his clearly stated goals. In situations like this, standard procedure is to communicate this to the appropriate surrogate decision-maker and explore a shift in goals to comfort.

For understandable emotional reasons, patients and families often have a difficult time assimilating this information. Especially when the disease represents an acute change in the patient's condition, it can be very difficult to accept the news that he does not have long to live. And even when to external observers it may appear that the patient has experienced a steady decline over a significant period of time, it is not unusual for the patient or family to express surprise (or even dismay) at the limited prognosis.

These well-known emotional phenomena are appropriately addressed through empathy, reflective listening, and ongoing emotional support. Patients and families are usually able to achieve more accurate prognostic awareness, although this can take some time. Meanwhile, maintaining hope for cure (even in the face of evidence to the contrary) is a recognized coping mechanism. As the old adage in spiritual care goes, even if denial is a crutch, it should not be taken away from the patient until he finds something else to prop himself up with, or else he will fall down.

Sometimes when faced with a dire prognosis families will say they are "hoping for a miracle." In this context, the word "miracle"—which comes from the Latin *miraculum* meaning a wonder, marvel, or wonderful thing—can refer to many different things. It may be the family's way of expressing their incomplete acceptance of the patient's stated prognosis. It may also reflect a hope that their loved one could be among the rare known survivors with the aid of medical treatment (Back, Arnold, & Quill, 2003). Reference to miracles may also reflect anger or frustration over some aspect of the patient's medical care, as the family seeks a proportional response to the dire prognostication of the medical team (Delisser, 2009).

Actual "faith in miracles" is fundamentally different. This reflects an explicit recognition of the medical prognosis, without undue reliance on exceptional cases at the optimistic end of the bell-shaped curve (if any even exist). True faith in miracles involves a trust that *divine* intervention will lead to cure (Widera, Rosenfeld, Fromme, Sulmasy, & Arnold, 2011). While some argue that this involves a "violation of the law of nature" (Hume, 1985), from a faith perspective a miracle is more properly viewed as contrary to the *order* of nature (Thomas, 1975). In other words, if God is truly omnipotent, then "nature" is really just a human observation of the normal workings of the world around us, which God can choose to intervene in in exceptional ways, should God so choose (Sulmasy, 2007).

To be sure, many religious traditions have a history of miraculous cures. Conservative Christians and some Orthodox Jews, for instance, acknowledge—and hope for—their existence (Pawlikowski, 2007; Rushton & Russell, 1996; Sulmasy, 2007). Non-orthodox Jews, Muslims, and mainline Christians tend not to (Khan, 2007; Mackler, 2007; Pinches, 2007). Within—or even outside—these religious groups, patients or families who have had previous experiences with purported miracles or view this as a test of faith may be more likely to hope that a miracle will occur (Orr, 2007).

Such hope is remarkably common, even in an increasingly secular society. While younger people espouse fewer explicitly religious beliefs than older people, nearly eight out of ten Americans—irrespective of age—believe that miracles still occur (Pew Research Center, 2010). With specific reference to medical care, the majority of lay people believe that miracles can occur in specific clinical situations—such as for patients in a persistent vegetative state—whereas only 20% of medical professionals do. This discrepancy highlights the potential communication and relational difficulties involved in establishing an appropriate treatment plan (Jacobs, Burns, & Bennett Jacobs, 2008).

Because of the focus on divine rather than medical intervention, a belief in miracles may impact patient and family requests for treatment. Since a miracle is, by definition, a violation of the natural order, worsening physiologic (i.e., measurable) indicators are not likely to dissuade patients and families from believing that a miracle may still occur. Such a deterioration may instead be viewed as either irrelevant—because an omnipotent God can heal anyone, no matter how ill—or as a test of faith, further solidifying the family's expectation of an impending miracle. This is especially true in situations where the patient or family believes not only that God could perform a miracle but actually has promised to perform one in that particular case. If such a patient were to die, then the family would not only grieve his loss but possibly also the loss of their own faith, as well.

Studies have confirmed that faith in miracles impacts clinical decision-making, including an increased likelihood of requesting "full code" status (True et al., 2005). Such faith may also lead to less confidence in clinicians' predictions of futility, based (as they are) on medical rather than spiritual criteria (Zier et al., 2009). In one out of five cases, a patient or family's faith plays a greater role in their understanding of prognosis than their personal observations or even medical predictions (Boyd et al., 2010).

This can create deep angst within the medical team, especially if the decision is made by a surrogate rather than the patient himself. This indicates that the patient lacks DMC and may also suggest that he is suffering as a result of his underlying disease (or even the ineffective treatment he is receiving). Attempts to forge consensus may be unsuccessful because two conversations are occurring in parallel. One is the medical/scientific dialogue which recognizes his worsening clinical condition and poor prognosis. The other is a more spiritual conversation focusing on faith and the possibility of miracle. When a patient/family fails to respond as expected to news of clinical deterioration—such as by refusing to redirect care toward comfort—it may feel to the clinical team that the patient/family is in denial or is simply incapable of assimilating the necessary information. Quite the contrary, the patient or family is generally able to grasp the medical facts, but these are not the ultimate factors in reaching their decision.

In addressing the situation, a structured approach may help. One example is the "AMEN Protocol," which outlines a step-by-step approach (Cooper, Ferguson, Bodurtha, & Smith, 2014). The first step is for the medical team to Affirm the patient and family's belief in miracles, because what physician would not also hope for a miraculous recovery? This shows respect for the patient or family's spiritual beliefs, while also acknowledging in a very humble way that miracles are God's domain and it is entirely up to God to decide whether to perform one. Rather than establishing an antagonistic position, this may help align both "sides" behind a common hope, even if they have radically different senses of the likelihood (or even possibility) of it coming to pass.

The second step is to Meet the patient and family where they are, seeking greater understanding of what their beliefs are and precisely why they believe a miracle will occur in this case. The team should then also ask the patient and family to meet them where *they* are, by Educating the patient and family about the team's professional role. Even if the family believes a miracle may occur, this does not negate the team's obligation to offer only medically indicated interventions and to relieve suffering (Truog et al., 2008).

The last step is to reaffirm that No matter what happens, the team is committed to supporting the family. This promise—even in the midst of profound disagreement—is crucial, as abandonment is one of the things that families in these situations fear the most (Steinhauser, Clipp, et al., 2000).

It may be necessary to afford the family additional time to assimilate information and place it into a faith context. In the meantime, it is important to explore what "miracle" means to a family, given its many potential references (Rushton & Russell, 1996). Depending on their perspective, it may be helpful—rather than denying the possibility of a miracle—to reframe what a miracle might look like. For instance, a miracle might have already occurred, in the form of family reconciliation related to the patient's illness. Alternatively, a miracle could occur in a different way, such as in the relief of suffering rather than healing of the physical body (Brett & Jersild, 2003; Connors & Smith, 1996).

One might also consider exploring the precise relationship between medical treatment and divine intervention. This may take the form of accepting the inherently supernatural basis of miracles, and observing that if God were to perform a miracle, God would not require human interventions such as mechanical ventilators to do it. Viewed in this light, withdrawing the ventilator—as the team may recommend—is not a sign of unbelief. Quite the contrary, it could actually reflect ongoing faith that a miracle might still occur, without the assistance of a human invention (Delisser, 2009).

Another alternative is to invert the standard interpretation of what is God's will, based on the presumption—held by many religious people who are anticipating a miracle for their loved one—that life does not end with bodily death but rather continues for eternity in a state of perpetual bliss (i.e., heaven). Given that context, it is interesting that conservative Christians—who recognize the finitude of earthly life and live in anticipation of something better—are *more* likely to request aggressive treatment (Phelps et al., 2009). Likely this is due to a profound belief in life as a gift from God, such that a person should value its sacredness and not relinquish it lightly.

Given this context, it may be possible to reorient the discussion from one viewing continued treatment as respect for the sacredness of life to viewing it instead as clinging to something ephemeral, and possibly a sign of a lack of trust in the afterlife. In this vein, a chaplain colleague sometimes refers to CPR as "swatting God's hand away" as God tries to "bring the patient home."

Whichever approach is chosen, a conversation about miracles is explicitly a *spiritual* conversation. As such, it demands the expertise of a spiritual care professional and should not question the patient or family's understanding. They likely comprehend the medical facts and recognize the clinical team's views, but in *their* worldview, a spiritual reality takes precedence.

In some situations, consensus will not be reached. The team is then faced with the decision of whether to unilaterally withhold treatment or continue interventions which could lead to significant moral distress (p. 514) on the part of the staff. The extent of the patient's suffering is particularly relevant, as the team may be willing to continue treatment if they feel the patient is not suffering (either by virtue of the extent of his disease or their ability to treat any symptoms). If the institution has a relevant policy, this may be utilized to help distinguish between truly futile treatment and that which is "potentially nonbeneficial" (chapter 14). Throughout the process, in addition to attending to the complex emotional needs of both family and staff (Widera et al., 2011), consultation with the hospital ethics committee can be extremely helpful.

Religious "Mandates" for Continuing Life Sustaining Medical Treatment

From a purely *religious* point of view, there are specific situations where a patient or family may feel that continued potentially curative treatment is "mandated" by their faith. A general example pertains to conservative Christians who may feel obligated to pursue maximal treatment out of respect for the "sanctity of life" (Phelps et al., 2009). Even if the patient or family does not specifically espouse a belief that a miracle will occur, they may view medical technology as itself a gift from God which should be utilized to its fullest extent.

This is more of a spiritual dilemma than an ethical one, because patients make decisions for all sorts of reasons: emotional, psychological, social, as well as spiritual. As long as a patient has sufficient DMC, his requests must be taken seriously and his refusals respected. From a purely spiritual point of view, however, many of the same approaches that can be helpful in addressing a trust in miracles are also relevant here. Acknowledging the impact of one's faith on medical decisions brings faith into the discussion, rather than minimizing its importance. Engaging the patient on a spiritual level—especially out of his own particular faith tradition—can be very helpful, such as by sensitively pointing out that placing ultimate value on the ability of medical technology to extend life as long as possible might constitute idolatry, rather than faith (Drane, 2006).

A specific example of possibly mandated medical intervention is the use of medically administered nutrition and hydration (MANH) for patients of the Roman Catholic tradition. Traditionally, the Church has distinguished between ordinary treatments (which are obligatory) and extraordinary ones (which are optional), with an emphasis on avoiding excessive burdens on the patient. As Pope Pius XII (1958) stated, "Life, health and all temporal activities are subordinate to spiritual ends."

According to the Ethical and Religious Directives (ERDs) of the Catholic Church, there is a moral obligation to accept proportionate (the newer term for "ordinary") treatments, which refers to interventions "that in the judgment of the patient offer a reasonable hope of benefit and do not entail an excessive burden or impose excessive expense on the family or the community." By contrast, there is no obligation to accept treatments that are disproportionate, which do not offer a reasonable hope or represent excessive burden (United States Conference of Catholic Bishops, 2009).

The next directive (number 58) directly addresses MANH. In earlier editions of the ERDs, this directive declared that there was a "presumption in favor of providing nutrition and hydration to all patients." However, in 2004 Pope John Paul II asserted in an allocution that MANH was "normal care" and thus obligatory without reference to the balance of benefits and burdens. He even went so far as to say that withholding MANH constituted "euthanasia by omission."

As a result, ERD 58 was modified to read: "In principle, there is an *obligation* to provide patients with food and water, including medically assisted nutrition and hydration for those who cannot take food orally" (emphasis added). The directive specifically applies to patients "in chronically and presumably irreversible conditions (e.g., the 'persistent vegetative state')" but could reasonably be applied to patients in analogous circumstances. Exceptions to this requirement include situations where MANH would not prolong life and where it would be excessively burdensome (United States Conference of Catholic Bishops, 2009). As a result of this perceived shift in Church doctrine, some Roman Catholic patients—under the guidance of their local clergy or broader declarations—might feel morally obligated to receive MANH, even when they would otherwise wish not to.

There are several ways of responding to this sense of moral obligation. The first is to address the applicability of Pope John Paul's statement and the resulting revision of the ERDs. It is important to note that not every word spoken by a pope is viewed as infallible. Encyclicals and infallible pronouncements carry the greatest weight, with "allocutions" among the least authoritative papal statements. In fact, a pope claimed infallibility only once in twentieth century (Bradley, 2009).

Statements that carry greater weight than an allocution—such as the Congregation for the Doctrine of the Faith's *Declaration on Euthanasia*—continue to affirm the historic proportionate/disproportionate distinction. Commentators have reasonably questioned whether Pope John Paul II was really trying to overturn five hundred years of tradition. For if he was, an allocution would seem an unusual—and ineffective—way of doing so (Hamel, 2007).

Another approach is to take the pope's statement at face value, noting that ERD 58 begins with the words "in principle." This could reasonably be understood not as proclaiming a rule that must be applied in every case but rather a general guideline that needs to be interpreted in light of other factors such as the degree of burden that would ensue (Repenshek & Slosar, 2004).

It is also relevant to note that Pope John Paul II refused a permanent feeding tube even as his own health declined as a result of advanced Parkinson's disease. A nasogastric tube was finally inserted three days before his death, long past the point where supplemental nutrition and hydration would have had a substantial impact on life expectancy. His condition certainly met the criteria of "chronic" and "irreversible" that ERD 58 addresses, and thus the pope's choice to forgo MANH over nearly the entire course of his illness suggests a level of contextuality to his earlier comments. A reasonable inference would be that he did not intend to modify Catholic moral teaching on this topic, or else he would have applied the same standards to his own care.

The medical team could, therefore, explore with a Roman Catholic patient whether the Church is really requiring him to accept a treatment that he would not otherwise want. This obviously requires significant theological nuance, highlighting the need for a chaplain or local clergyperson who is able to thoughtfully explore the complexities of the tradition. This could be pivotal for a patient who is truly inquisitive about the specifics of church teaching, which he feels obligated to follow. Some patients, however, may be so concerned about violating a requirement that they opt to "err on the side of safety"—or, in this case, burden—by accepting additional treatments to avoid any risk of falling short of ecclesiastical expectations. In both cases, a thoughtful exploration may empower the patient to wrestle with his own tradition in a way that helps him make peace with it—and his own goals—from within that tradition.

Concepts of Suffering

A basic tenet of palliative care is the amelioration of suffering. While many of the seminal discoveries in the field involved ways to treat physical pain (Saunders, 1960, 1963), palliative care has always focused on other forms of suffering as well, such as social, psychological, and spiritual. These forms are not entirely distinct, as each type can impact the other(s). For instance, a patient in great physical pain is not able to participate in as many pleasurable activities, may feel more isolated as a result, and may wonder why he is suffering so intensely. By the same token, studies have shown that feelings of isolation, abandonment, and depression may increase perception of physical pain (Bar et al., 2005).

Recognizing this complex interrelationship, the concept of "total pain" was formulated, later followed by that of "total suffering" which recognizes that pain thresholds differ and the various types of pain interact in such a way that a specific patient could be said to "suffer" with less physical pain than someone with greater (Strang, Strang, Hultborn, & Arner, 2004). This recognition underscores palliative medicine's focus on ameliorating suffering in all its varied forms.

Treating one source of suffering may, however, worsen another. Sedation, for example, is a common side effect of opioids and is further exacerbated if benzodiazepines are simultaneously used to treat anxiety. Studies have shown that when confronted with a choice of analgesia or lucidity, physicians tend to value the former, especially with recent increased attention on pain as "the fifth vital sign" (Davis & Walsh, 2004). Many patients, however, prioritize lucidity even at the price of physical discomfort. Other areas of divergence between patients and physicians include the former more highly valuing being at peace with God, being able to help others, and not being a burden to their family (Steinhauser, Christakis, et al., 2000).

Certain groups stress the importance of lucidity, particularly at the end of life. In Buddhism, for example, suffering is a core element of life, the recognition of which is the first step on the path to enlightenment. For many Buddhists, pharmacologic amelioration of physical suffering is not as important as the struggle to understand and cope with that suffering. Given the Buddhist notion of reincarnation and karma, there is significant need to be awake and aware at the end of life in order to permit appropriate rituals preceding and following death (Bauer-Wu, Barrett, & Yeager, 2007).

Other religious groups hold what might termed a "redemptive" view of suffering. One example is the Flagellants, who in the thirteenth and fourteenth centuries whipped themselves in repentance for sins which they felt caused the Black Death.[1] This concept was revived in the period between the two world wars and was termed "dolorism"—from the Latin word for pain, *dolor*—by journalist Julian Teppe. Pain was viewed as a defense mechanism that would prompt defensive action, as well as a means of self-discovery and a way to understand basic truth in relation to oneself. As Teppe writes, "Pain . . . does not allow for cheating, or compromise . . . I consider extreme anguish, particularly that of somatic origin, as the perfect incitement for developing pure idealism, created anew in each individual" (Rey, 1995).

Christian theology often forms the basis of these beliefs, focusing on the suffering of Jesus on the Cross which his followers are called to emulate. In the gospel of Matthew, Jesus calls his disciples to "take up [their] cross and follow [him]" (Matthew 16:24), which some have interpreted as an endorsement—or even a command—of suffering. As the first letter to Peter states: "Christ also suffered for [us], leaving [us] an example so that [we] should follow in his steps" (1 Peter 2:21). The author of the Epistle to the Colossians says much the same thing: "Now I rejoice in what was suffered for you, and I fill up in my flesh what is still lacking in regard to Christ's afflictions, for the sake of his body, which is the church" (Colossians 1:24).

Patients espousing such beliefs may refuse symptomatic relief not so much out of a desire to remain lucid but rather out of a sense that they deserve the pain they are experiencing by virtue of sins they have committed. They may also view suffering as necessary to achieve some greater goal or meaning, either for themselves or others.

There are also many nonspiritual reasons a patient might refuse symptomatic treatment (p. 214). After excluding (or addressing) any medical or psychological reasons for refusal, the next step is to identify the specific spiritual tradition out of which this view arises, so as to appropriately address it from within that tradition. In the case of Christianity, for example, there are many Scriptural and theological references that call into question the redemptive nature of suffering. For every time that Jesus speaks of carrying one's cross in the gospels, he also speaks of his yoke being easy and his burden light (Matthew 11:30). Granted, Jesus refused a sedative while on the Cross, but this does not necessarily mean that patients need to refuse analgesia. According to Christian belief, Jesus was the savior of the world bearing the sins of all of humankind; hopefully patients do not carry that much weight upon their shoulders. And much of his ministry was dedicated to healing and comforting, not extolling the intrinsic value of suffering.

Often a desire to engage in redemptive suffering is a sign of a lack of self-forgiveness, which can be addressed from both psychological and spiritual angles. This might involve confessing one's sins to—and being proclaimed absolved by—a member of the clergy or reaching out and expressing contrition to whomever the patient believes he may have wronged. It could also involve discussion of a compromise, whereby the patient would accept some manner of symptomatic relief but still be aware of the suffering.

---

1. Of note, the Flagellants were later condemned by the Catholic Church as heretics.

In the end, if medical professionals truly take the notion of "total suffering" seriously, they may have to respect the patient's need to endure physical pain in order to experience spiritual meaning. It may be easier to accept in cases where the goal is lucidity in order to fully experience the final transition in life (as in Buddhism), rather than to appease the demands of a seemingly retributive deity (as in certain interpretations of Christianity). When confronted with a patient's refusal of symptomatic treatment, all steps should be taken to address this issue from medical, psychological, and spiritual perspectives. But if the patient experiences greater meaning and fulfillment through a balance of pain and relief that most other patients would not tolerate, that is his choice. The dilemma here is spiritual, not pharmacological.

Return to the Case

Before addressing explicitly spiritual concerns, the team explores the family's understanding of "miracle," to make sure they are not referring to an unlikely physical recovery or expressing frustration with some aspect of care. Once an explicitly spiritual meaning of the term is verified, rather than conversing in parallel—with the medical team speaking clinically and the family speaking spiritually—the team decides to engage the family directly on a spiritual level. Using the AMEN protocol, the team **A**ffirms the family's hope for a miracle. They also **M**eet the family where they are, seeking deeper understanding of what a miracle might look like while also trying to reframe that understanding. At the same time, they **E**ducate the family about the team's professional role and stress that **N**o matter what happens, they will always stand by the patient and family.

Despite this thoughtful approach, tensions remain high as the patient continues to decline and the family persists in their request for maximal treatment. The team consults the ethics committee to impartially to review the family's requests in light of professional obligations. The team ultimately decides that CPR would not be appropriate. While the family disagrees, when offered a meeting with an interdisciplinary committee as delineated in the institution's nonbeneficial treatment policy, the family does not actively contest the decision. The team also puts into place a Do Not Escalate Treatment order (p. 119) because they feel that additional interventions will not influence the overall outcome.

There is further discussion of withdrawing typically burdensome interventions, but the team feels that the patient's condition is so poor—and the level of analgesia adequate—that he is not suffering. They conclude that such an adversarial position would heighten the family's suffering without significantly minimizing the patient's, so current treatment is continued.

The patient eventually dies peacefully, and while the family is left to grapple with the miracle that never arrived, they deeply appreciate the caring concern of the medical team.

Summary Points

- In addition to specific ethical dilemmas that clinicians face, the core concepts of communication, culture, and spirituality pervade and influence every aspect of the practice of palliative care.
- Historically, physicians often concealed serious diagnoses and prognoses from patients in order to minimize harm ("therapeutic privilege") and avoid damaging hope. The former concern is parentalistic and the latter is misplaced, and neither are ethically acceptable.
- Communication
    - Disclosure of relevant information is an ethical obligation, but this need not occur all at once or include treatment options that are clearly incompatible with the patient's stated goals.
- Culture
    - In certain cultures, specific disease names may carry unreliable connotations, and speaking about death is thought to make it more likely to occur. The clinician's obligation is not to use particular terms but rather to communicate the significance of a patient's condition in a culturally appropriate way.
    - In certain cultures, rather than the patient making medical decisions, this responsibility could be shared with—or deferred to—either the family or the physician.
    - Patients clearly have the right to delegate authority to someone else, although physicians may be reluctant to assume this burden. Prior to doing so, the physician should identify the patient's goals and values in order to apply them to a particular situation, reminding the patient that she always has the right to resume participation in treatment decisions.
    - Certain groups are less likely to avail themselves of hospice and palliative care. It is therefore crucial to identify existing barriers and present the option of palliative care in a culturally sensitive manner.
- Spirituality
    - When a patient or family demands continued treatment in the hopes of a "miracle," this may reflect incomplete clinical understanding, hope for a highly unlikely outcome, or true belief in supernatural intervention. If the latter, the AMEN protocol—affirm the family's hope, meet the family where they are, explain professional responsibilities, and no matter what happens stand by the family—can be helpful.
    - Perceived religious "mandates" for specific treatments are often not quite as clear as they may seem and should be addressed thoughtfully from within that religious tradition.
    - Ameliorating "total suffering" includes addressing spiritual sources. Some patients may have spiritual reasons for refusing symptomatic treatment, which should

be addressed from within that spiritual tradition and may ultimately need to be respected, in order to prevent greater overall suffering.

References

American Academy of Family Physicians. (2003). Positions and policies: Cultural proficiency guidelines. Retrieved from http://www.aafp.org/x6701.xm

American Medical Association. (2010–2011). *Code of medical ethics, annotated current opinions* (1076-3996). Chicago: American Medical Association.

Anandarajah, G., & Hight, E. (2001). Spirituality and medical practice: Using the HOPE questions as a practical tool for spiritual assessment. *Am Fam Physician, 63*(1), 81–89.

Ariès, P. (1974). *Western attitudes toward death: From the Middle Ages to the present.* Baltimore: Johns Hopkins University Press.

Aulisio, M. P. (2016). "So what you want us to do?" Patient's rights, unintended consequences, and the surrogate's role. In S. J. Youngner & R. M. Arnold (Eds.), *The Oxford handbook of ethics at the end of life* (pp. 27–41). New York: Oxford University Press.

Back, A. L., Arnold, R. M., & Quill, T. E. (2003). Hope for the best, and prepare for the worst. *Ann Intern Med, 138*(5), 439–443.

Baker, D. W., Parker, R. M., Williams, M. V., Clark, W. S., & Nurss, J. (1997). The relationship of patient reading ability to self-reported health and use of health services. *Am J Public Health, 87*(6), 1027–1030.

Balboni, T. A., Paulk, M. E., Balboni, M. J., Phelps, A. C., Loggers, E. T., Wright, A. A., . . . Prigerson, H. G. (2010). Provision of spiritual care to patients with advanced cancer: Associations with medical care and quality of life near death. *J Clin Oncol, 28*(3), 445–452. doi:10.1200/JCO.2009.24.8005

Bar, K. J., Brehm, S., Boettger, M. K., Boettger, S., Wagner, G., & Sauer, H. (2005). Pain perception in major depression depends on pain modality. *Pain, 117*(1–2), 97–103. doi:10.1016/j.pain.2005.05.016

Bauer-Wu, S., Barrett, R., & Yeager, K. (2007). Spiritual perspectives and practices at the end-of-life: A review of the major world religions and application to palliative care. *Indian J Palliat Care, 13*(2).

Bernacki, R. E., & Block, S. D. (2014). Communication about serious illness care goals: A review and synthesis of best practices. *JAMA Intern Med, 174*(12), 1994–2003 doi:10.1001/jamainternmed.2014.5271

Blackhall, L. J., Murphy, S. T., Frank, G., Michel, V., & Azen, S. (1995). Ethnicity and attitudes toward patient autonomy. *JAMA, 274*(10), 820–825.

Blank, R. H. (2011). End-of-life decision making across cultures. *J Law Med Ethics, 39*(2), 201–214. doi:10.1111/j.1748-720X.2011.00589.x

Borneman, T., Ferrell, B., & Puchalski, C. M. (2010). Evaluation of the FICA tool for spiritual assessment. *J Pain Symptom Manage, 40*(2), 163–173. doi:10.1016/j.jpainsymman.2009.12.019

Boyd, E. A., Lo, B., Evans, L. R., Malvar, G., Apatira, L., Luce, J. M., & White, D. B. (2010). "It's not just what the doctor tells me:" Factors that influence surrogate decision-makers' perceptions of prognosis. *Crit Care Med, 38*(5), 1270–1275. doi:10.1097/CCM.0b013e3181d8a217

Braddock, C. H., Edwards, K. A., Hasenberg, N. M., Laidley, T. L., & Levinson, W. (1999). Informed decision making in outpatient practice: Time to get back to basics. *JAMA, 282*(24), 2313–2320.

Bradley, C. T. (2009). Roman Catholic doctrine guiding end-of-life care: A summary of the recent discourse. *J Palliat Med, 12*(4), 373–377. doi:10.1089/jpm.2008.0162

Brett, A. S., & Jersild, P. (2003). "Inappropriate" treatment near the end of life: Conflict between religious convictions and clinical judgment. *Arch Intern Med, 163*(14), 1645–1649. doi:10.1001/archinte.163.14.1645

Bullock, K. (2011). The influence of culture on end-of-life decision making. *J Soc Work End Life Palliat Care, 7*(1), 83–98. doi:10.1080/15524256.2011.548048

Cabral, R. R., & Smith, T. B. (2011). Racial/ethnic matching of clients and therapists in mental health services: A meta-analytic review of preferences, perceptions, and outcomes. *J Couns Psychol, 58*(4), 537–554. doi:10.1037/a0025266

Cahill, P. J., Lobb, E. A., Sanderson, C., & Phillips, J. L. (2016). What is the evidence for conducting palliative care family meetings? A systematic review. *Palliat Med, 31*(3), 197–211. doi:10.1177/0269216316658833

Carrese, J. A., & Rhodes, L. A. (1995). Western bioethics on the Navajo reservation. Benefit or harm? *JAMA, 274*(10), 826–829.

Cobbs v. Grant. (1972). 8 Cal. 3d 229, 502 P.2d 1, 104 Cal. Rptr. 505.

Colby, W. H., Dahlin, C., Lantos, J., Carney, J., & Christopher, M. (2010). The National Consensus Project for Quality Palliative Care clinical practice guidelines Domain 8: Ethical and legal aspects of care. *HEC Forum, 22*(2), 117–131. doi:10.1007/s10730-010-9128-3

Connors, R. B. Jr., & Smith, M. L. (1996). Religious insistence on medical treatment: Christian theology and re-imagination. *Hastings Cent Rep, 26*(4), 23–30.

Cooper, R. S., Ferguson, A., Bodurtha, J. N., & Smith, T. J. (2014). AMEN in challenging conversations: Bridging the gaps between faith, hope, and medicine. *J Oncol Pract, 10*(4), e191–195. doi:10.1200/JOP.2014.001375

Davis, M. P., & Walsh, D. (2004). Cancer pain: How to measure the fifth vital sign. *Cleve Clin J Med, 71*(8), 625–632.

Degenholtz, H. B., Thomas, S. B., & Miller, M. J. (2003). Race and the intensive care unit: Disparities and preferences for end-of-life care. *Crit Care Med, 31*(5 Suppl.), S373–S378. doi:10.1097/01.CCM.0000065121.62144.0D

Delisser, H. M. (2009). A practical approach to the family that expects a miracle. *Chest, 135*(6), 1643–1647. doi:10.1378/chest.08-2805

Diem, S. J., Lantos, J. D., & Tulsky, J. A. (1996). Cardiopulmonary resuscitation on television: Miracles and misinformation. *N Engl J Med, 334*(24), 1578–1582. doi:10.1056/NEJM199606133342406

Drane, J. F. (2006). Stopping nutrition and hydration technologies: A conflict between traditional Catholic ethics and church authority. *Christ Bioeth, 12*(1), 11–28. doi:10.1080/13803600600629876

Dunn, H. (2009). *Hard choices for loving people: CPR, artificial feeding, comfort measures only, and the elderly patient* (5th ed.). Lansdowne, VA: A & A Publishing.

Ehman, J. W., Ott, B. B., Short, T. H., Ciampa, R. C., & Hansen-Flaschen, J. (1999). Do patients want physicians to inquire about their spiritual or religious beliefs if they become gravely ill? *Arch Intern Med, 159*(15), 1803–1806.

Enzinger, A. C., Zhang, B., Schrag, D., & Prigerson, H. G. (2015). Outcomes of prognostic disclosure: Associations with prognostic understanding, distress, and relationship with physician among patients with advanced cancer. *J Clin Oncol, 33*(32), 3809–3816. doi:10.1200/JCO.2015.61.9239

Fallowfield, L. J., Jenkins, V. A., & Beveridge, H. A. (2002). Truth may hurt but deceit hurts more: Communication in palliative care. *Palliat Med, 16*(4), 297–303.

Feudtner, C. (2009). The breadth of hopes. *N Engl J Med, 361*(24), 2306–2307. doi:10.1056/NEJMp0906516

Field, D., & Copp, G. (1999). Communication and awareness about dying in the 1990s. *Palliat Med, 13*(6), 459–468.

Fielding, R., & Hung, J. (1996). Preferences for information and involvement in decisions during cancer care among a Hong Kong Chinese population. *Psychooncology, 5*(4), 321–329.

Gallo, J. J., Straton, J. B., Klag, M. J., Meoni, L. A., Sulmasy, D. P., Wang, N. Y., & Ford, D. E. (2003). Life-sustaining treatments: What do physicians want and do they express their wishes to others? *J Am Geriatr Soc, 51*(7), 961–969.

Gazmararian, J. A., Williams, M. V., Peel, J., & Baker, D. W. (2003). Health literacy and knowledge of chronic disease. *Patient Educ Couns, 51*(3), 267–275.

Glaser, B. G., & Strauss, A. L. (1965). *Awareness of dying.* Chicago: Aldine.

Ha, J. F., & Longnecker, N. (2010). Doctor-patient communication: A review. *Ochsner J, 10*(1), 38–43.

Hallenbeck, J. (2003). The explanatory model #26. *J Palliat Med, 6*(6), 931. doi:10.1089/109662103322654820

Hallenbeck, J., & Arnold, R. (2007). A request for nondisclosure: Don't tell mother. *J Clin Oncol, 25*(31), 5030–5034. doi:10.1200/JCO.2007.11.8802

Hamel, R. (2007). The Catholic Health Association's response to the Papal Allocution on Artificial Nutrition and Hydration. AMA Virtual Mentor. Retrieved from http://journalofethics.ama-assn.org/2007/05/oped1-0705.html

Holland, J. C., Geary, N., Marchini, A., & Tross, S. (1987). An international survey of physician attitudes and practice in regard to revealing the diagnosis of cancer. *Cancer Invest*, *5*(2), 151–154.

Hopper, K. D., TenHave, T. R., Tully, D. A., & Hall, T. E. (1998). The readability of currently used surgical/procedure consent forms in the United States. *Surgery*, *123*(5), 496–503. doi:10.1067/msy.1998.87236

Hume, D. (1985). *Of miracles*. La Salle, IL: Open Court.

Jacobs, L. M., Burns, K., & Bennett Jacobs, B. (2008). Trauma death: Views of the public and trauma professionals on death and dying from injuries. *Arch Surg*, *143*(8), 730–735. doi:10.1001/archsurg.143.8.730

Johnstone, M. J., & Kanitsaki, O. (2009). Ethics and advance care planning in a culturally diverse society. *J Transcult Nurs*, *20*(4), 405–416. doi:10.1177/1043659609340803

Judicial Council of the American Medical Association. (1984). Current opinions of Judicial Council of the American Medical Association. 2 vols. Chicago: American Medical Association.

Kagawa-Singer, M., & Blackhall, L. J. (2001). Negotiating cross-cultural issues at the end of life: "You got to go where he lives." *JAMA*, *286*(23), 2993–3001.

Khan, F. (2007). Miraculous medical recoveries and the Islamic tradition. *South Med J*, *100*(12), 1246–1251. doi:10.1097/SMJ.0b013e31815a9521

King, M. B., & Koenig, H. G. (2009). Conceptualising spirituality for medical research and health service provision. *BMC Health Serv Res*, *9*, 116. doi:10.1186/1472-6963-9-116

Koenig, H. G. (2000). Religion and medicine I: Historical background and reasons for separation. *Int J Psychiatry Med*, *30*(4), 385–398.

Kwak, J., & Haley, W. E. (2005). Current research findings on end-of-life decision making among racially or ethnically diverse groups. *Gerontologist*, *45*(5), 634–641.

Loue, S., & Sajatovic, M. (2012). *Encyclopedia of immigrant health*. New York: Springer.

Mack, J. W., Wolfe, J., Cook, E. F., Grier, H. E., Cleary, P. D., & Weeks, J. C. (2007). Hope and prognostic disclosure. *J Clin Oncol*, *25*(35), 5636–5642. doi:10.1200/JCO.2007.12.6110

Mackler, A. L. (2007). Eye on religion: A Jewish view on miracles of healing. *South Med J*, *100*(12), 1252–1254. doi:10.1097/SMJ.0b013e3181581b12

McCord, G., Gilchrist, V. J., Grossman, S. D., King, B. D., McCormick, K. E., Oprandi, A. M., . . . Srivastava, M. (2004). Discussing spirituality with patients: A rational and ethical approach. *Ann Fam Med*, *2*(4), 356–361.

Moazam, F. (2000). Families, patients, and physicians in medical decisionmaking: A Pakistani perspective. *Hastings Cent Rep*, *30*(6), 28–37.

Mount, B. (1985). Challenges in palliative care: Four clinical areas that confront and challenge hospice practitioners. *Am J Hosp Palliat Med*, *2*.

Nielsen-Bohlman, L., & Institute of Medicine Committee on Health Literacy. (2004). *Health literacy: A prescription to end confusion*. Washington, DC: National Academies Press.

Nunez-Olarte, J. M., & Gracia, D. (2001). Cultural issues and ethical dilemmas in palliative and end-of-life care in Spain. *Cancer Control*, *8*(1), 46–54.

Orr, R. D. (2007). Responding to patient beliefs in miracles. *South Med J*, *100*(12), 1263–1267. doi:10.1097/SMJ.0b013e31815a95cb

Pawlikowski, J. (2007). The history of thinking about miracles in the West. *South Med J*, *100*(12), 1229–1235. doi:10.1097/SMJ.0b013e3181581c79

Pew Research Center. (2010). Religion among the millennials: Less religiously active than older Americans, but fairly traditional in other ways. Retrieved from http://pewforum.org/uploadedFiles/Topics/Demographics/Age/millennials-report.pdf

Pew Research Center. (2015). U.S. public becoming less religious. Retrieved from http://www.pewforum.org/2015/11/03/u-s-public-becoming-less-religious/

Phelps, A. C., Maciejewski, P. K., Nilsson, M., Balboni, T. A., Wright, A. A., Paulk, M. E., . . . Prigerson, H. G. (2009). Religious coping and use of intensive life-prolonging care near death in patients with advanced cancer. *JAMA*, *301*(11), 1140–1147. doi:10.1001/jama.2009.341

Pinches, C. (2007). Miracles: A Christian theological overview. *South Med J*, *100*(12), 1236–1242. doi:10.1097/SMJ.0b013e31815843cd

Pius XII. (1958). The prolongation of life: Allocution to the International Congress of Anesthesiologists. *Pope Speaks*, *4*, 393–397.

Pope John Paul II. (2004). Address of Pope John Paul II to the participants in the International Congress on "Life-Sustaining Treatments and Vegetative State: Scientific Advances and Ethical Dilemmas." *NeuroRehabilitation, 19*(4), 273–275.

Randall, F., & Downie, R. S. (2006). *The philosophy of palliative care: Critique and reconstruction.* Oxford; New York: Oxford University Press.

Rawcliffe, C. (1995). *Medicine & society in later medieval England.* Stroud, UK: Alan Sutton.

Repenshek, M., & Slosar, J. P. (2004). Medically assisted nutrition and hydration: A contribution to the dialogue. *Hastings Cent Rep, 34*(6), 13–16.

Rey, R. (1995). *The history of pain.* Cambridge, MA: Harvard University Press.

Ruhnke, G. W., Wilson, S. R., Akamatsu, T., Kinoue, T., Takashima, Y., Goldstein, M. K., . . . Raffin, T. A. (2000). Ethical decision making and patient autonomy: A comparison of physicians and patients in Japan and the United States. *Chest, 118*(4), 1172–1182.

Rushton, C. H., & Russell, K. (1996). The language of miracles: Ethical challenges. *Pediatr Nurs, 22*(1), 64–67.

Saunders, C. (1960). Drug treatment of patients in the terminal stages of cancer. *Curr Med Drugs, 1*, 16–28.

Saunders, C. (1963). The treatment of intractable pain in terminal cancer. *Proc R Soc Med, 56*, 195–197.

Searight, H. R., & Gafford, J. (2005). Cultural diversity at the end of life: Issues and guidelines for family physicians. *Am Fam Physician, 71*(3), 515–522.

Steinhauser, K. E., Christakis, N. A., Clipp, E. C., McNeilly, M., McIntyre, L., & Tulsky, J. A. (2000). Factors considered important at the end of life by patients, family, physicians, and other care providers. *JAMA, 284*(19), 2476–2482.

Steinhauser, K. E., Clipp, E. C., McNeilly, M., Christakis, N. A., McIntyre, L. M., & Tulsky, J. A. (2000). In search of a good death: Observations of patients, families, and providers. *Ann Intern Med, 132*(10), 825–832.

Strang, P., Strang, S., Hultborn, R., & Arner, S. (2004). Existential pain—an entity, a provocation, or a challenge? *J Pain Symptom Manage, 27*(3), 241–250. doi:10.1016/j.jpainsymman.2003.07.003

Sulmasy, D. P. (1999). Is medicine a spiritual practice? *Acad Med, 74*(9), 1002–1005.

Sulmasy, D. P. (2007). What is a miracle? *South Med J, 100*(12), 1223–1228. doi:10.1097/SMJ.0b013e31815a9784

Thomas, Aquinas. (1975). *Summa contra gentiles.* Notre Dame, IN: University of Notre Dame Press.

Thornburgh v. American College of Obstetricians (106 S.Ct. 2169 1986).

Timmermans, S. (2017). Resuscitating to save life or save death? *Am J Bioeth, 17*(2), 55–57. doi:10.1080/15265161.2016.1265164

True, G., Phipps, E. J., Braitman, L. E., Harralson, T., Harris, D., & Tester, W. (2005). Treatment preferences and advance care planning at end of life: The role of ethnicity and spiritual coping in cancer patients. *Ann Behav Med, 30*(2), 174–179. doi:10.1207/s15324796abm3002_10

Truog, R. D., Campbell, M. L., Curtis, J. R., Haas, C. E., Luce, J. M., Rubenfeld, G. D., . . . Kaufman, D. C. (2008). Recommendations for end-of-life care in the intensive care unit: a consensus statement by the American College [corrected] of Critical Care Medicine. *Crit Care Med, 36*(3), 953–963. doi:10.1097/CCM.0B013E3181659096

United States Conference of Catholic Bishops. (2009). *Ethical and religious directives for Catholic health care services* (5th ed.). Washington, DC: USCCB Publishing.

Vermont Ethics Network. (2017). Advance directive short form. Retrieved from http://vtethicsnetwork.org/forms/advance_directive_short_form.pdf

Wear, S. (1998). *Informed consent: Patient autonomy and clinician beneficence within health care* (2nd ed.). Washington, DC: Georgetown University Press.

Widera, E. W., Rosenfeld, K. E., Fromme, E. K., Sulmasy, D. P., & Arnold, R. M. (2011). Approaching patients and family members who hope for a miracle. *J Pain Symptom Manage, 42*(1), 119–125. doi:10.1016/j.jpainsymman.2011.03.008

Wilkinson, S. (1999). Palliative care in Europe: Ethics and communication. *Int J Pall Nurs, 5*(4), 160.

Wilson-Stronks, A., & Galvez, E. (2017). *Hospitals, language, and culture: A snapshot of the nation.* Retrieved from http://www.jointcommission.org/assets/1/6/hlc_paper.pdf

Yeo, G., & Hikuyeda, N. (2000). Cultural issues in end-of-life decision making among Asians and Pacific Islanders in the United States. In K. Braun, J. H. Pietsch, & P. L. Blanchette (Eds.), *Cultural issues in end-of-life decision making* (pp. 101–126). Thousand Oaks, CA: SAGE.

Zier, L. S., Burack, J. H., Micco, G., Chipman, A. K., Frank, J. A., & White, D. B. (2009). Surrogate decision makers' responses to physicians' predictions of medical futility. *Chest, 136*(1), 110–117. doi:10.1378/chest.08-2753

19

Final Thoughts

This textbook has examined the trajectories of both clinical ethics and palliative care, as well as the points at which they intersect. It has described a comprehensive approach to ethical dilemmas in palliative care, explored the nuances of prognostication and advance care planning, and explored death and dying in great detail. Far from an afterthought, pediatric-specific issues have been analyzed with respect to various stages of development, ranging from prenatal to adolescent. Other crucial topics—such as nonbeneficial treatment, neuropalliative care, organ donation, and clinical research—have been explored, as well as fundamental aspects of patient care that influence all medical decisions, including communication, culture, and spirituality. The overall approach set forth here will (hopefully) empower clinicians to reach the best—or, in some cases, "least bad" (Powderly, 2003)—resolution to ethical dilemmas.

A basic dictum of ethics is that "ought implies can," meaning that one cannot say a person *ought* to do something that he is unable to do (Buckwalter & Turri, 2015). This is highly significant because to apply the lessons of this textbook, three things are required:

1. palliative care team that is
   a. well-trained and well-equipped, and
   b. highly functioning
2. the power or authority to act on the thoughtful conclusions the team reaches

Absent any of these, it may be impossible formulate a response to a complex ethical dilemma or implement the response even if it can be formulated.

These three prerequisites are often not met, especially in the developing world. But rather than merely acknowledging that sad fact, it is imperative to take active steps to remedy the situation. The fact that one is unable to do what one otherwise ought to do is itself an ethical dilemma, especially when the end result is that patients suffering from life-limiting illness do not receive the care they desperately need and deserve.

Access to Palliative Care

As noted in more detail elsewhere (p. 36), American society emphasizes negative rights (i.e., the right to be left alone). Among the very few positive rights are police, fire, and military protection and education through grade twelve. Health care is notably absent from this list, which is quite unique—not to mention tragic—compared with other developed nations (Fisher, 2012).

By its very nature, ethics goes beyond commenting on what is the case to advocating for what *should* be the case in an ethically ideal situation. The complexities of health care delivery systems and financing are legion and therefore far beyond the scope of this textbook. But it is reasonable to consider—after going into such detail about the momentous and often confounding decisions facing patients in need of palliative care—whether these patients are truly receiving the care that they deserve (and, by extension, the opportunity to make an informed choice from among an appropriate slate of options). In other words, should palliative care be considered a basic human right, which governments therefore have a moral obligation not only to refrain from interfering with but also to actively provide?

To be sure, there are other worthy candidates for the mantle of "guaranteed health care," childhood immunizations and basic primary care among them. But perhaps the one certainty of life is that it will end, making dying a universal experience. Beyond that—as should be clear from the preceding pages—the potential for suffering at the end of life is profound, as is the possibility of meaning. Is it, therefore, really such a revolutionary claim to assert that "all people have a right to receive high quality care during serious illness and to a dignified death free of overwhelming pain and in line with their spiritual and religious needs" (World Health Organization, 2004)?

The matter of access is not merely a practical or political issue; it is also an *ethical* issue, because for all the debate about the "right to die"—which at one point meant refusal of life-sustaining medical treatment and now has come to mean active hastening of death, such as through physician-assisted dying (chapter 8)—the most fundamental right related to dying is to do so with comfort, companionship, and dignity. It follows that every patient has the right to basic elements of palliative care in the midst of serious illness and approaching death: respect for personal values, symptom management, psychosocial support, coordination of care, and (of course) ethical decision-making (Brennan, 2007).

This is not to say that every patient requires a highly trained, deeply experienced transdisciplinary care team. While this is the ideal, such an expectation would rapidly outpace resources in most of the world. From a clinical perspective, this is often unnecessary, with generalist palliative care sufficing in most situations (Quill & Abernethy, 2013), especially when specialist-level treatment modalities are not available. It is also impractical to expect universal specialist palliative care, given the workforce challenges noted later in this chapter. For this reason Randall and Downie (1999) rightly assert only a weak moral obligation to provide specialist palliative care to those whose basic needs otherwise could be served by generalists.

By contrast, they assert a strong moral obligation to provide specialist palliative care to meet the needs of the sickest patients. Here it is important to identify precisely what is meant by "need." The World Health Organization statement noted earlier takes a rather broad view of this term, essentially equating it with "capacity for benefit." On this understanding, one might consider the majority of elderly patients to be "in need" of palliative care, which presumably would be more nuanced and comprehensive coming from a specialist in the field. This is too broad, however, for in terms of allocation of limited resources, "the perfect is the enemy of the good" (Voltaire, 1923).

A more modest definition is offered by Beauchamp and Childress (2009): "something without which someone will be fundamentally harmed." This lowers the bar substantially in terms of when generalist palliative care is appropriate and sufficient, while also recognizing the potential for harm when specialist level care is required but not available.

Specialist level care is often required because of the multiplicity of complex options available to patients in the developed world. By contrast, in the developing world even the most basic palliative care interventions may not be available (and could make a huge difference if they were). Patients' rights should not change depending on where one lives, but the approach to meeting those needs—recognizing that clinical ethics must be practical (p. 42)—is distinct.

In the Developed World

In the developed world,[1] people are living longer: between 1900 and 2000 life expectancy in the United States rose from forty-seven to seventy-seven, equivalent to the gain from the Stone Age to that point, a period of 10,000 years (Meier, 2010). Technological discoveries have not only prolonged life but also raised novel and thorny questions, making at least the context and timing—if not the ultimately inevitability—of death in many cases a matter of choice. It is estimated that ninety million Americans are currently living with serious illness, of whom six million could benefit from palliative care (Center to Advance Palliative Care, 2014).

There was not, however, an equivalent growth in palliative care, at least in the first half of the twentieth century. Indeed, the term itself had not yet been coined (p. 3), and the modern hospice movement was still on the horizon. Over the past few decades, however, the field has literally exploded. For a clinical specialty that was only formally recognized in the twenty-first century, the growth of palliative care programs in the developed world (and especially in the United States) has been impressive. Palliative care has gone from an

---

1. This section uses the United States as the primary example of palliative care in the developed world, given the emphasis on American law and culture throughout the text. Some areas where the American context does not extend to other developed nations are noted.

esoteric term that few understood, to being equated with "giving up,"[2] to becoming a reasonable expectation with almost 90% of US hospitals of three hundred or more beds now having an identified palliative care program (Center to Advance Palliative Care, 2015). Admittedly, this bar is rather low, as having an "identified" palliative care program is no guarantee of availability, experience, or quality.

Beyond palliative care simply being "the right thing to do," there are many reasons for its growth. It fits perfectly with the "triple aim" of modern health care: improved patient experience, better population health, and reduced costs (Institute for Healthcare Improvement, 2017). Palliative care has been shown to improve family experience with serious illness (Casarett et al., 2010). Studies have documented increased survival with palliative care in certain conditions (p. 15). And in an era of exploding health care costs, palliative care consultation has been shown to save money: $4,000 in direct hospital costs for patients discharged alive and over $7,500 for those who die in the hospital (Morrison et al., 2011).

The need for improved palliative care is highlighted by the deficiencies of previous initiatives. The seminal SUPPORT study, for instance, found that advance directives were often not honored—or even identified—and patients frequently suffered at the end of life, even when focused education and institutional initiatives were implemented (SUPPORT Principal Investigators, 1995). Regulatory structures have attempted to recognize and promote the practice of palliative care, as evidenced by the introduction in 2011 of palliative care certification by the Joint Commission (2012).

From a legal standpoint, there have been several seminal developments in palliative care. Supreme Court decisions in *Vacco v. Quill* and *Washington v. Glucksberg* in 1997 not only examined physician-assisted dying (PAD); they also touched on the Rule of Double Effect, palliative sedation, and palliative care in general. Some have gone so far as to argue that these decisions essentially established a constitutional right to aggressive palliative care, by declaring that any state law deeming intensive symptom management as homicide is unconstitutional (Burt, 1997). At the same time, lower courts have found physicians liable for inadequate pain management, which has been interpreted as negligent care (*Bergman v. Chin*, 2001).

Lest one view the situation through rose-colored lenses, there is still a long way to go. The ratio of patients with serious illness to palliative care physicians (1,200:1) dwarfs that of newly diagnosed cancer patients to oncologists (141:1) or patients with cardiac disease to cardiologists (71:1) (Block, 2014). The United States has less than 15% of the hospice/palliative medicine specialists necessary to meet the needs of patients (Lupu & American Academy of Hospice & Palliative Medicine Workforce Task Force, 2010), and that deficit is likely to worsen now that completion of a fellowship is a requirement for board certification. Fewer than 250 physicians graduate from fellowship each year, vastly

---

2. A misperception that, sadly, persists in some quarters.

insufficient to make up for the estimated shortage of 18,000 palliative care physicians in the United States (Kamal et al., 2016).

Training is also a challenge in the provision of generalist palliative care. For while palliative care is receiving increasing attention in medical school, it is still not a required component in the curriculum, as are standard specialties such as obstetrics and gynecology (despite the fact that only half the population is female, yet 100% of the population will die one day). Several states have established requirements for continuing education in palliative care or pain management as a precondition for medical licensure (Federation of State Medical Boards, 2017), but the degree to which this impacts care has not been proven. And despite the significant cost savings associated with palliative care (at least on an inpatient basis), hospitals are often reluctant to invest in palliative care programs because they tend not to be "revenue generators" (Cassel, Kerr, Kalman, & Smith, 2015).

Regulatory issues also stand in the way of patients receiving optimal hospice or palliative care. The Medicare Hospice benefit is essentially unchanged since its introduction in 1982, requiring a prognosis of six months or less if the disease runs its normal course (Centers for Medicare and Medicaid Services, 2015). Despite data showing that expanding access to hospice actually *lowers* costs by as much as 22% (Krakauer, Spettell, Reisman, & Wade, 2009), governmental restrictions remain in place. This is one of the reasons why the median hospice admission is only eighteen days, and one-third of patients are referred to hospice in the last week of life (National Hospice and Palliative Care Organization, 2015).[3]

Political grandstanding also stands in the way of meaningful reform. A well-known example involved the 2009 debate about the bill that would eventually become the Affordable Care Act, or "Obamacare." The Advance Care Planning Consultation section of the bill authorized Medicare reimbursement for physicians who provided voluntary counseling regarding advance directives and treatment wishes. Given the time required to do this well, not reimbursing physicians for this service created a significant disincentive to providing it.

Given that advance care planning shows respect for patient autonomy, this section would not seem controversial. But its proximity in the written bill to a section that noted potential cost savings prompted sharp criticism. Betsy McCaughey, former Lt. Governor of New York, falsely asserted that this section would "absolutely require that every five years people in Medicare have a required counseling session that will tell them how to end their life sooner" (Politifact, 2009). Most (in)famously, former Alaska governor and vice presidential candidate Sarah Palin asserted that

---

3. The situation is fundamentally different for children, as the Affordable Care Act explicitly permits children with a prognosis of less than six months to receive disease-directed treatment (Lindley, 2011). Several states have also applied for Medicaid waivers to permit use of hospice funds for pediatric patients who may not be in the last six months of life (Dabbs, Butterworth, & Hall, 2007).

the America I know and love is not one in which my parents or my baby
with Down Syndrome will have to stand in front of Obama's "death panel" so
his bureaucrats can decide, based on a subjective judgment of their "level of
productivity in society," whether they are worthy of health care. Such a system is
downright evil. (Corn, 2009)

Despite being named the "Lie of the Year" by Politifact, the resulting media storm led
Congress to remove the Advance Care Planning Consultation section of the bill, de-
laying Medicare reimbursement for this crucial service until it was finally passed in 2016
(Dresser, 2016).

Cultural mores are another barrier. Some have described American culture as "death-
denying," in that it treats death "as a kind of accident, a contingent event that greater prevention, proven technology, and further research could do away with" (Callahan, 1995).
Slogans for major hospitals—such as one proclaiming that it is "making cancer history"
(MD Anderson Cancer Center, 2016)—feed into this perception. In evolutionary terms,
it is not really that long ago that some hospital administrators expressed reluctance to
participate in Elizabeth Kübler-Ross's (1969) groundbreaking research because supposedly no patients were dying in their facilities. Perhaps not as much has changed since then
as one would have hoped.

A variety of remedies have been proposed. One is so-called "open access" to hospice, thereby allowing patients whose life expectancy is greater than six months to qualify
for the Medicare hospice benefit. While some have shied away from such a proposal for
fear of uncontrolled expenditures—which, it should be noted, was the reason the original
hospice benefit began as a "demonstration project" and was proven unfounded (Davis,
1988)—preliminary studies should allay these concerns. For instance, when Aetna
allowed patients with up to one year to live to receive hospice care as well as some types of
antineoplastic treatment, hospice use increased, but acute (i.e., emergency department)
and critical care use *decreased* (Spettell et al., 2009). The end result was both cost savings
and higher quality care.

Training barriers also have to be addressed. The number of government-funded
training slots has remained level since the Balanced Budget Act of 1997, even in the face
of increasing numbers of medical school graduates. This has forced fellowship programs
to rely on philanthropy for funding, which may or may not be forthcoming. Because of
the dearth of board-certified palliative care clinicians, the bulk of palliative care is provided by nonspecialists. Working within the current system, innovative programs have
been developed to nurture basic palliative care skills (Hauser, Preodor, Roman, Jarvis, &
Emanuel, 2015), but systems-level change is still required.

Several steps could be taken to improve the situation. One is lifting the cap on
Graduate Medical Education funding and positions, prioritizing in-demand specialties
such as hospice and palliative medicine. Innovative fellowship models could be developed, which might include mid-career and part-time tracks (American Academy of

Hospice and Palliative Medicine, 2015). Political and social activism are clearly necessary in order to correct present—and prevent future—misconceptions about hospice and palliative medicine.

Many of these initiatives are components of the Palliative Care and Hospice Education and Training Act (2015), which was first introduced in Congress in 2012 and has broad bipartisan support. This bill would provide educational grants and career development awards, expand fellowship options, boost retention of current clinicians, and provide career incentive awards for non-physicians who agree to teach or practice palliative medicine in their respective specialties. It would also expand public awareness of hospice and palliative care, and increase research funding in this area (p. 453).

This cultural shift is critically important and already in evidence. Greater attention by the media (Moyers, 2000) and the lay press (Gawande, 2014) has heightened awareness of the need for—and benefit of—palliative care. Grassroots efforts—such as "death cafés" (Nelson, 2017) and the "Before I Die" art project (Chang, 2013)—are making it easier for people to discuss their health and mortality. Perhaps, then, the pendulum is beginning to swing back from "death denied" to death as a legitimate topic of conversation.

In the Developing World

In the technological world of the United States, it is easy to lose perspective. Caught up in ethical debates about PAD—which affects a tiny fraction of the population—one can easily forget that the majority of the world's population has limited access to morphine for pain and dyspnea at the end of life. North America and Europe consume 90% of the world's opioids, with lower- and middle-income countries using only 6%. Morphine is not even available in over 150 countries, and 80% of the world's population does not have access to basic pain treatment (Lamas & Rosenbaum, 2012).

This is in large part due to onerous prescribing regulations which are often based on the 1961 United Nations Single Convention on Narcotic Drugs (United Nations, 1972) which disproportionately focused on use of illicit drugs like heroin. The unintended consequence is that opioids are not a therapeutic option in many countries (Rajagopal & Joranson, 2007). For instance, a recent documentary noted that in India, regulatory restrictions are so draconian that physicians in all but one of the country's twenty-eight states simply avoid prescribing opioids altogether (Rajagopal, 2014).

Even if opioids were available, delivering them to patients in need can be challenging, especially in large countries with large rural (and underserved) areas. Many such countries are quite poor, limiting the ability of those in greatest need to advocate in the halls of power. Cultural acceptability is also an issue: in many countries, opioids are associated with drugs of abuse, and appropriate use of opioids at the end of life is not well-known (Manjiani, Paul, Kunnumpurath, Kaye, & Vadivelu, 2014).

Beyond the availability of medications, there also exists a deficit in clinician education. Forty-two percent of countries have little or no access to hospice and palliative care services, and only twenty countries have palliative care well integrated into the health system (Worldwide Palliative Care Alliance, 2014). Understandably, clinicians tending to seriously ill patients may be more focused on keeping them from dying from preventable diseases such as malaria or gastrointestinal illness. The end result, however, is that patients who cannot be saved are allowed to die painful deaths.

Recognizing the systems-level barriers to providing even basic palliative care, the European Association for Palliative Care issued the "Lisbon Challenge" in 2011. This challenge appeals to governments to modify health policies to meet the needs of patients with life-limiting illness, ensure access to essential medications, provide training in palliative care, and integrate palliative care into the health care delivery system (Radbruch, Payne, de Lima, & Lohmann, 2013). Various professional organizations have assisted in implementing these noble objectives (American Academy of Hospice and Palliative Medicine, 2017), and targeted philanthropy has also been of assistance (Cairdeas International Palliative Care Trust, 2017).

The purpose of this discussion is not to attempt to provide the "answer" to palliative care needs in the developing world. That is a vastly complex question which must take into account global politics, economic disparities, deficiencies in training, and deeply ingrained cultural beliefs. Rather, the purpose is to highlight the ethical imperative to provide at least primary palliative care to all patients in need, regardless of what country or context they may live in. For all the (hopefully) insightful and nuanced discussion in the preceding pages about fascinating ethical issues such as PAD and palliative sedation, these impact relatively few patients, while millions suffer needlessly for want of basic palliative care interventions (such as morphine). Just as ethics consultation is merely the tip of the iceberg of clinical ethics—highly visible yet proportionally small compared to the entire enterprise—so also "first-world problems" may attract a great deal of attention, but this should not distract from global issues that present a greater threat (in terms of suffering) to humanity in general.

Maintaining Highly Functioning Teams

Even if a palliative care team is accessible at some point—which, as noted, is a big *if*—this is no guarantee that the palliative care team will remain highly functioning over a prolonged period of time. Precisely because palliative care addresses very complex and emotionally charged issues, burnout and compassion fatigue are important concerns. Once again, the task here is not so much to attempt to solve those problems—which have proven very challenging—but to identify them and highlight their *ethical* importance. For if there exists an ethical obligation to provide high-quality palliative care to patients in need, then there must also exist a parallel ethical obligation to safeguard the well-being of those tasked with providing that care, so as to maintain provision of that care over time.

Personal challenges begin early in medicine. Between 21% and 43% of residents (Mata et al., 2015)—and one out of four medical students (Rotenstein et al., 2016)—show signs of depression. Once in practice, the pressure only increases. While varying to degrees, every medical specialty is seeing increasing rates of burnout (Shanafelt et al., 2015), which refers to "a form of mental distress manifested in normal individuals who experience decreased work performance resulting from negative attitudes and behaviors" (Kearney, Weininger, Vachon, Harrison, & Mount, 2009). Physicians are significantly more likely to commit suicide (Council on Scientific Affairs, 1987) and experience divorce (Sotile & Sotile, 1996) than other professions.

Burnout is quite common among physicians caring for patients at the end of life, with up to 60% of oncologists showing signs of it. Its characteristic symptoms—such as numbness, detachment, and avoidance of emotionally charged situations—have a direct impact on the care provided (Kearney et al., 2009). It is also a stronger predictor of poor job satisfaction than is depression and can lead to a variety of health complications, including increased risk of heart attack, stroke, and sleep disturbance (Melamed, Shirom, Toker, Berliner, & Shapira, 2006). This has led some to expand the "triple aim" of health care to a quadruple aim, adding improving the work lives of clinicians and those who provide care (Bodenheimer & Sinsky, 2014).

A related concept is compassion fatigue, which has been defined as "a formal caregiver's reduced capacity or interest in being empathetic or bearing witness to the suffering of patients and is the emotional state that results from knowing about the traumatizing events that another human being experienced" (Figley, 1983). Whereas burnout arises out of the work environment, compassion fatigue is the result of the physician-patient relationship. Described by some as the "cost of caring" for people in distress, it can be quite pronounced in palliative care (O'Mahony et al., 2017). Frequently it is the result of secondary or vicarious traumatization, as the clinician—out of a noble attempt to actively engage with the patient's own suffering—suffers himself, as well. This can lead to symptoms of posttraumatic stress disorder including hyperarousal, avoidance, and re-experiencing.

A variety of solutions to burnout and compassion fatigue have been proposed, often focusing on self-care outside of the work place. By itself, though, this is not enough, as it overlooks the institutional and structural factors which led to these conditions in the first place. As Kearney et al. (2009) write, "Physicians with burnout who use self-care without self-awareness may feel as though they are drowning and barely able to come up for air, whereas self-care with self-awareness is like learning to breathe underwater."

Institutional factors also need to be taken into account. Studies have shown that it is not so much the amount of work that contributes to burnout and compassion fatigue but rather the proportion of time spent on meaningful activities. In an increasingly automated and technological medical environment (Hill, Sears, & Melanson, 2013), physicians are spending more and more time on administrative and regulatory tasks, rather than on the human elements of patient care that brought them to the profession in the first place. Institutions would do well, therefore, to establish an acceptable balance between these competing obligations.

On a personal level, the way to treat—and, ideally, prevent—burnout and compassion fatigue involves both self-care and self-awareness. Clinicians must recognize the stressors that are inherent in the practice of palliative care and seek to engage with the patient's suffering, while also recognizing that it is something other than one's own. Steps shown to build self-awareness include Balint groups (Rabinowitz, Kushnir, & Ribak, 1996), reflective writing (Frisina, Borod, & Lepore, 2004), and mindfulness meditation (Shanafelt et al., 2005).

Such self-awareness allows the clinician to simultaneously take into consideration the patient, the work environment, and himself. Rather than withdrawing from emotionally charged patient encounters, the clinician leans *into* the encounter, daring to engage in what the trauma literature calls "exquisite empathy" through full engagement with the patient. This enables the development of "compassionate satisfaction"—rather than fatigue—through a measure of "bi-directionality." Instead of weighing the clinician down with vicarious suffering, exquisite empathy enlivens the clinician through witnessing the meaning the patient and family may ultimately derive from the care they receive. This, then, leaves clinicians "invigorated rather than depleted by their intimate professional connections with traumatized clients" (Harrison & Westwood, 2009).

It is not enough to merely acknowledge the need for palliative care in a certain population and then initially train a team to address that need. That team requires ongoing support to do the noble and challenging work of palliative care, which includes permission to engage in self-care. Beyond that, though, the team needs to be equipped with the tools of self-awareness in order to avoid burnout and compassion fatigue. To attend to one's own needs as a palliative care clinician is not selfish; rather, as a necessary component of continuing to care for people in need over a prolonged period of time, it is an ethical obligation.

Moral Distress

This textbook has attempted to describe a thoughtful approach to various ethical dilemmas, ideally leading to the optimal resolution. But the mere fact of arriving at an insightful conclusion is no guarantee of being able to implement it. The inability to do so may lead to "moral distress," which has been defined as "one or more negative self-directed emotions or attitudes that arise in response to one's perceived involvement in a situation that [one] perceives to be morally undesirable" (Campbell, Ulrich, & Grady, 2016).[4]

The most common reasons for experiencing moral distress are acceding to a family's request for treatment that is felt to be contrary to the patient's best interest and continuing treatment that seems to merely be prolonging death (Austin, Saylor, & Finley, 2017).

---

4.   It is important to note that while "moral distress" is often used to refer to moral uncertainty (i.e., lack of clarity as to what is the best course of action), this is not what the term actually means.

These are specifically cited by nurses as the cause of their moral distress (Ferrell, 2006; Solomon et al., 2005), and also affect resident trainees (Dzeng et al., 2016).

The concept of moral distress was first formulated by Jameton (1984) in the nursing literature of the 1980s. Both the timing and context are understandable. Medical technologies were rapidly expanding, as was the patients' rights movement. In the not so distant past, there was relatively little one could do to sustain critically ill patients. Now, though, not only is there a wide range of therapeutic options, but patients are also given the choice of whether to accept them or not. The complexity of decision-making has markedly increased, as has the likelihood that a clinician might be called upon to execute a treatment plan that he fundamentally disagrees with.

That the concept of moral distress grew out of the nursing literature is also not surprising. Physicians are logically less susceptible to suffering moral distress because they generally formulate the treatment plans that the team is then tasked with carrying out. For all the talk of interdisciplinary team care, physician instructions are still called "orders." To be sure, external forces may compromise a physician's ability to do what he feels he should, but other members of the team may feel even more powerless.

In addition, while physicians—in the intensive care unit (ICU), for instance—check on their patients regularly, they are often caring for a great many patients, and thus individual encounters tend to be relatively brief and extremely focused. An ICU nurse, on the other hand, is generally assigned only one or two patients to care for throughout an entire eight-to twelve-hour shift. This offers a much more intimate vantage point on the patient experience, thus heightening distress if the patient seems to be suffering unduly or unnecessarily. It also creates additional opportunities for deeper and less directed conversation, over the course of which patient hopes and doubts might arise that were not identified in the more focused "rounding" of physicians. This may help explain the limited concordance between physicians' and nurses' perception of "futility" in specific clinical cases, leading to different conclusions as to what should be done for a particular patient (Neville et al., 2015).

Given that a major task of palliative care is identifying the patient's goals and formulating a treatment plan that is consonant with them, staff moral distress may reflect inadequate palliative care participation in patient care. Admittedly, the palliative care team may have been involved but was unable to forge consensus, or the family did not heed their recommendations (Cavinder, 2014). But in many cases palliative care is not consulted until death is imminent (Von Roenn, Voltz, & Serrie, 2013), which may reflect clinicians' misunderstanding of what palliative care really is. It also depends on the clinician's sense of when death is actually approaching, which has been shown to often be unreliable (p. 84).

Moral distress not only prevents the patient or family from getting what they need; it also threatens the personal integrity of the professional (Carse, 2013) by undermining integrity and authenticity (McCue, 2010). To know—or at least *believe* one knows—what the right thing to do is and not be able to do it is disempowering and demoralizing.

Not surprisingly, moral distress plays a major role in job dissatisfaction (Cavaliere, Daly, Dowling, & Montgomery, 2010), burnout (Sundin-Huard & Fahy, 1999), and attrition (Corley, 2002). Its effects are long-lasting, creating what some have called "moral residue" (Epstein & Hamric, 2009).

A comprehensive review of steps that can be taken to prevent or alleviate moral distress is outside the scope of this textbook and can be found elsewhere (Rushton, Kaszniak, & Halifax, 2013). From a purely ethical standpoint, though, several points are in order. An important potential cause of moral distress is a lack of complete information about the rationale behind a specific clinical decision and the thoughtfulness of the steps taken in reaching it. Especially in the case of burdensome treatment without likelihood of benefit, staff who did not participate in—or may not even be aware of—the discussions between the clinical team and the family may assume that the burdens were not explained or the minimal likelihood of benefit was not appreciated. Updating staff on the conversations that took place and the rationale for the decision—as well as welcoming dissenting views and eliciting suggestions for moving forward—can help staff feel empowered and thus minimize moral distress. Steps should also be taken to involve staff in those conversations on an ongoing basis, in order to prevent moral distress from developing in the first place.

Another proactive step is the involvement of a palliative care team. This is by no means a panacea, but it does reflect the primary team's intention of using every tool at their disposal to establish an appropriate treatment plan and to mediate conflict. It can also serve as reassurance to other staff, who may interpret a lack of palliative care involvement as a failure to acknowledge the patient's true condition or likely prognosis.

Despite such thoughtful steps, moral distress is inevitable in the world of modern medicine, replete as it is with strong opinions and profound needs. Constructive approaches to dealing with moral distress are therefore necessary, which acknowledge its importance, inevitability, and preventive interventions. This includes self-regulation which empowers a clinician to maintain his boundaries and distinguish problems that he is responsible for from those that he is not. Ethical competence is also crucial, which empowers the clinician to thoughtfully analyze dilemmas and constructively work through them (Rushton, 2017). Nurturing such skills fosters the development of "moral resilience," which refers to "the capacity of an individual to sustain or restore their integrity in response to moral complexity, confusion, distress, or setbacks" (Rushton, 2016).

The last important quality in relationship to moral distress is self-awareness. As noted, one of the primary reasons cited for moral distress is a perception that a certain treatment plan conflicts with the patient's best interests. But this is clearly a value judgment, which should prompt the person experiencing moral distress to reflect on what values have led him to the conclusion that the patient's best interests are not being served.

On some very deep level, the problem may not be so much with the team making the "wrong choice" as much as the fact that no good choice exists. This is precisely the dilemma that constitutes much of modern medical ethics: the search for the "least bad option." There may not, therefore, be *any* acceptable treatment plan. This is difficult to acknowledge, as it confronts the clinician experiencing moral distress with the inevitability—and some would say universality—of suffering. Framed in the context of palliative care, the specialty tasked with ameliorating suffering in certain cases seems powerless to do so. What the patient endures directly, the staff—particularly the empathic and passionate advocates that people would most want caring for them at critical moments of their lives—experiences vicariously.

Ultimately, clinicians may need to become more comfortable with "sitting with suffering" (Rattner & Berzoff, 2016) and acknowledging their relative powerlessness to ameliorate—let alone eradicate—it. This does not mean one should take suffering lightly or stand idly by when there are available means of minimizing it. But sometimes patients and families make choices that are very difficult for others to accept, yet nevertheless represent very heartfelt values (Macauley, 2011). An example might be refusal of optimal analgesia, in order to achieve some greater goal (p. 214).

In such situations, a clinician would do well to reflect on precisely *whose* suffering is causing his moral distress: the patient's, the family's, or perhaps his own. If the last of these, it is not the patient's understanding or the team's process that requires attention but rather the clinician's own internal state (and preconceptions). By fostering self-awareness as well as self-regulation, clinicians can minimize and navigate moral distress, ideally preventing the burnout and compassion fatigue that often accompanies it.

This represents a fitting conclusion to a textbook that has examined complex situations from a wide variety of viewpoints, striving to offer a coherent and consistent—though certainly not universally shared—perspective throughout. In the ethics of palliative care, precious few clinical dilemmas yield "obvious" answers. In all the others, the clinician is tasked with bringing all of his knowledge, experience, and insight to bear on a fearfully complex situation, ideally engaging with—and risking being changed by—team members in the transdisciplinary model that palliative care strives for. Ultimately, in some situations what may be asked of that clinician is not certainty and success, but rather humility and relinquishment of control, acknowledging that the patient does not wish to do what the clinician believes is "right" for him.

But that in no way minimizes the clinician's obligation to care for that patient. Quite the contrary, it asks *more* of the clinician: to bear witness to the patient's suffering, to enter into it with empathy and self-awareness, and to find healthy ways to cope with his own pain so as to ensure that the patient and family are never abandoned.

References

American Academy of Hospice and Palliative Medicine. (2015). Aligning graduate medical education with the changing health care landscape. Retrieved from http://aahpm.org/uploads/advocacy/AAHPM_GME_Policy_Statement_and_Recommendations_06_2015.pdf

American Academy of Hospice and Palliative Medicine. (2017). International physician scholarship. Retrieved from http://aahpm.org/scholarships/developing-countries

Austin, C. L., Saylor, R., & Finley, P. J. (2017). Moral distress in physicians and nurses: Impact on professional quality of life and turnover. *Psychol Trauma, 9*(4), 399–406.

Beauchamp, T. L., & Childress, J. F. (2009). *Principles of biomedical ethics* (6th ed.). Ncare and eew York: Oxford University Press.

Bergman v. Chin, No. H205732-1 (Alameda County Ct 2001).

Block, S. D. (2014). Palliative care. In T. Quill & F. G. Miller (Eds.), *Palliative care and ethics* (pp. 34–46). New York: Oxford.

Bodenheimer, T., & Sinsky, C. (2014). From triple to quadruple aim: Care of the patient requires care of the provider. *Ann Fam Med, 12*(6), 573–576. doi:10.1370/afm.1713

Brennan, F. (2007). Palliative care as an international human right. *J Pain Symptom Manage, 33*(5), 494–499. doi:10.1016/j.jpainsymman.2007.02.022

Buckwalter, W., & Turri, J. (2015). Inability and obligation in moral judgment. *PLoS One, 10*(8), e0136589. doi:10.1371/journal.pone.0136589

Burt, R. A. (1997). The Supreme Court speaks—not assisted suicide but a constitutional right to palliative care. *N Engl J Med, 337*(17), 1234–1236. doi:10.1056/NEJM199710233371712

Cairdeas International Palliative Care Trust. (2017). Global palliative care. Retrieved from https://cairdeas.org.uk/global-palliative-care

Callahan, D. (1995). Frustrated mastery: The cultural context of death in America. *West J Med, 163*(3), 226–230.

Campbell, S. M., Ulrich, C. M., & Grady, C. (2016). A broader understanding of moral distress. *Am J Bioeth, 16*(12), 2–9. doi:10.1080/15265161.2016.1239782

Carse, A. (2013). Moral distress and moral disempowerment. *Narrat Inq Bioeth, 3*(2), 147–151. doi:10.1353/nib.2013.0028

Casarett, D., Shreve, S., Luhrs, C., Lorenz, K., Smith, D., De Sousa, M., & Richardson, D. (2010). Measuring families' perceptions of care across a health care system: Preliminary experience with the Family Assessment of Treatment at End of Life Short form (FATE-S). *J Pain Symptom Manage, 40*(6), 801–809. doi:10.1016/j.jpainsymman.2010.03.019

Cassel, J. B., Kerr, K. M., Kalman, N. S., & Smith, T. J. (2015). The business case for palliative care: Translating research into program development in the U.S. *J Pain Symptom Manage, 50*(6), 741–749. doi:10.1016/j.jpainsymman.2015.06.013

Cavaliere, T. A., Daly, B., Dowling, D., & Montgomery, K. (2010). Moral distress in neonatal intensive care unit RNs. *Adv Neonatal Care, 10*(3), 145–156. doi:10.1097/ANC.0b013e3181dd6c48

Cavinder, C. (2014). The relationship between providing neonatal palliative care and nurses' moral distress: An integrative review. *Adv Neonatal Care, 14*(5), 322–328. doi:10.1097/ANC.0000000000000100

Center to Advance Palliative Care. (2014). Palliative care facts and stats. Retrieved from https://media.capc.org/filer_public/68/bc/68bc93c7-14ad-4741-9830-8691729618d0/capc_press-kit.pdf

Center to Advance Palliative Care. (2015). America's care of serious illness. Retrieved from https://reportcard.capc.org/wp-content/uploads/2015/08/CAPC-Report-Card-2015.pdf

Centers for Medicare and Medicaid Services. (2015). Medicare benefit policy manual. Retrieved from https://www.cms.gov/Regulations-and-Guidance/Guidance/Manuals/downloads/bp102c09.pdf

Chang, C. (2013). *Before I die.* New York: St. Martin's Griffin.

Corley, M. C. (2002). Nurse moral distress: A proposed theory and research agenda. *Nurs Ethics, 9*(6), 636–650. doi:10.1191/0969733002ne557oa

Corn, B. W. (2009). Ending end-of-life phobia—a prescription for enlightened health care reform. *N Engl J Med, 361*(27), e63. doi:10.1056/NEJMp0909740

Council on Scientific Affairs. (1987). Results and implications of the AMA-APA Physician Mortality Project: Stage II. *JAMA, 257*(21), 2949–2953.

Davis, F. A. (1988). Medicare hospice benefit: Early program experiences. *Health Care Financ Rev, 9*(4), 99–111.

Dresser, R. (2016). Medicare and advance planning: The importance of context. *Hastings Cent Rep, 46*(3), 5–6. doi:10.1002/hast.583

Dzeng, E., Colaianni, A., Roland, M., Levine, D., Kelly, M. P., Barclay, S., & Smith, T. J. (2016). Moral distress amongst american physician trainees regarding futile treatments at the end of life: A qualitative study. *J Gen Intern Med, 31*(1), 93–99. doi:10.1007/s11606-015-3505-1

Epstein, E. G., & Hamric, A. B. (2009). Moral distress, moral residue, and the crescendo effect. *J Clin Ethics*, *20*(4), 330–342.

Federation of State Medical Boards. (2017). Continuing medical education. Retrieved from https://www.fsmb.org/Media/Default/PDF/FSMB/Advocacy/GRPOL_CME_Overview_by_State.pdf

Ferrell, B. R. (2006). Understanding the moral distress of nurses witnessing medically futile care. *Oncol Nurs Forum*, *33*(5), 922–930. doi:10.1188/06.ONF.922-930

Figley, C. (1983). Catastrophes: An overview of family reaction. In C. Figley & A. McCubbin (Eds.), *Stress and the family* (vol. 11, pp. 3–20). New York: Brunner/Mazel.

Fisher, M. (2012, June 28). Here's a map of the countries that provide universal health care (America's still not on it). *The Atlantic*.

Frisina, P. G., Borod, J. C., & Lepore, S. J. (2004). A meta-analysis of the effects of written emotional disclosure on the health outcomes of clinical populations. *J Nerv Ment Dis*, *192*(9), 629–634.

Gawande, A. (2014). *Being mortal: Medicine and what matters in the end* (1st ed.). Toronto: Doubleday.

Harrison, R. L., & Westwood, M. J. (2009). Preventing vicarious traumatization of mental health therapists: Identifying protective practices. *Psychotherapy (Chic)*, *46*(2), 203–219. doi:10.1037/a0016081

Hauser, J. M., Preodor, M., Roman, E., Jarvis, D. M., & Emanuel, L. (2015). The evolution and dissemination of the education in palliative and end-of-life care program. *J Palliat Med*, *18*(9), 765–770. doi:10.1089/jpm.2014.0396

Hill, R. G. Jr., Sears, L. M., & Melanson, S. W. (2013). 4000 clicks: A productivity analysis of electronic medical records in a community hospital ED. *Am J Emerg Med*, *31*(11), 1591–1594. doi:10.1016/j.ajem.2013.06.028

Institute for Healthcare Improvement. (2017). Triple aim for health care. Retrieved from http://www.ihi.org/Topics/TripleAim/Pages/default.aspx

Jameton, A. (1984). *Nursing practice: The ethical issues*. Englewood Cliffs, NJ: Prentice Hall.

Joint Commission. (2012). Clarification: Eligibility for advanced certification for palliative care. *Jt Comm Perspect*, *32*(2), 4.

Kamal, A. H., Bull, J., Wolf, S., Samsa, G. P., Swetz, K. M., Myers, E. R., . . . Abernethy, A. P. (2016). Characterizing the hospice and palliative care workforce in the U.S.: Clinician demographics and professional responsibilities. *J Pain Symptom Manage*, *51*(3), 597–603. doi:10.1016/j.jpainsymman.2015.10.016

Kearney, M. K., Weininger, R. B., Vachon, M. L., Harrison, R. L., & Mount, B. M. (2009). Self-care of physicians caring for patients at the end of life: "Being connected . . . a key to my survival." *JAMA*, *301*(11), 1155–1164. doi:10.1001/jama.2009.352

Krakauer, R., Spettell, C. M., Reisman, L., & Wade, M. J. (2009). Opportunities to improve the quality of care for advanced illness. *Health Aff (Millwood)*, *28*(5), 1357–1359. doi:10.1377/hlthaff.28.5.1357

Kübler-Ross, E. (1969). *On death and dying*. New York: Macmillan.

Lamas, D., & Rosenbaum, L. (2012). Painful inequities—palliative care in developing countries. *N Engl J Med*, *366*(3), 199–201. doi:10.1056/NEJMp1113622

Lupu, D., & American Academy of Hospice & Palliative Medicine Workforce Task Force. (2010). Estimate of current hospice and palliative medicine physician workforce shortage. *J Pain Symptom Manage*, *40*(6), 899–911. doi:10.1016/j.jpainsymman.2010.07.004

MD Anderson Cancer Center. (2016). Making cancer history. Retrieved from http://makingcancerhistory.com/home.html

Macauley, R. (2011). Patients who make "wrong" choices. *J Palliat Med*, *14*(1), 13–16. doi:10.1089/jpm.2010.0318

Manjiani, D., Paul, D. B., Kunnumpurath, S., Kaye, A. D., & Vadivelu, N. (2014). Availability and utilization of opioids for pain management: Global issues. *Ochsner J*, *14*(2), 208–215.

Mata, D. A., Ramos, M. A., Bansal, N., Khan, R., Guille, C., Di Angelantonio, E., & Sen, S. (2015). Prevalence of depression and depressive symptoms among resident physicians: A systematic review and meta-analysis. *JAMA*, *314*(22), 2373–2383. doi:10.1001/jama.2015.15845

McCue, C. (2010). Using the AACN framework to alleviate moral distress. *Online J Issues Nurs*, *16*(1), 9. doi:10.3912/OJIN.Vol16No01PPT02

Meier, D. E. (2010). The development, status, and future palliative care. In D. E. Meier, S. L. Isaacs, & R. G. Hughes (Eds.), *Palliative care: Transforming the care of serious illness* (1st ed., pp. 3–75). San Francisco: Jossey-Bass.

Melamed, S., Shirom, A., Toker, S., Berliner, S., & Shapira, I. (2006). Burnout and risk of cardiovascular disease: Evidence, possible causal paths, and promising research directions. *Psychol Bull, 132*(3), 327–353. doi:10.1037/0033-2909.132.3.327

Morrison, R. S., Dietrich, J., Ladwig, S., Quill, T., Sacco, J., Tangeman, J., & Meier, D. E. (2011). Palliative care consultation teams cut hospital costs for Medicaid beneficiaries. *Health Aff (Millwood), 30*(3), 454–463. doi:10.1377/hlthaff.2010.0929

Moyers, B. (2000). *On our own terms: Moyers on dying* [DVD]. Athena.

National Hospice and Palliative Care Organization. (2015). NHPCO's facts and figures. Retrieved from https://www.nhpco.org/sites/default/files/public/Statistics_Research/2014_Facts_Figures.pdf

Nelson, R. (2017). Discussing death over coffee and cake: The emergence of the death cafe. *Am J Nurs, 117*(2), 18–19. doi:10.1097/01.NAJ.0000512293.80522.67

Neville, T. H., Wiley, J. F., Yamamoto, M. C., Flitcraft, M., Anderson, B., Curtis, J. R., & Wenger, N. S. (2015). Concordance of nurses and physicians on whether critical care patients are receiving futile treatment. *Am J Crit Care, 24*(5), 403–410. doi:10.4037/ajcc2015476

O'Mahony, S., Ziadni, M., Hoerger, M., Levine, S., Baron, A., & Gerhart, J. (2017). Compassion fatigue among palliative care clinicians. *Am J Hosp Palliat Care*, 1049909117701695. doi:10.1177/1049909117701695

Palliative Care and Hospice Education and Training Act. (2015). Retrieved from https://www.congress.gov/bill/114th-congress/house-bill/3119

Politifact. (2009). Retrieved from http://www.politifact.com/truth-o-meter/statements/2009/jul/23/betsy-mccaughey/mccaughey-claims-end-life-counseling-will-be-requi/

Powderly, K. E. (2003). Ethical issues for risk managers. In F. Kavaler & A. D. Spiegel (Eds.), *Risk management in health care institutions* (2nd ed.). Sudbury, MA: Jones and Bartlett.

Quill, T. E., & Abernethy, A. P. (2013). Generalist plus specialist palliative care—creating a more sustainable model. *N Engl J Med, 368*(13), 1173–1175. doi:10.1056/NEJMp1215620

Rabinowitz, S., Kushnir, T., & Ribak, J. (1996). Preventing burnout: Increasing professional self efficacy in primary care nurses in a Balint Group. *AAOHN J, 44*(1), 28–32.

Radbruch, L., Payne, S., de Lima, L., & Lohmann, D. (2013). The Lisbon challenge: Acknowledging palliative care as a human right. *J Palliat Med, 16*(3), 301–304. doi:10.1089/jpm.2012.0394

Rajagopal, M. R. (2014). *The pain project.*

Rajagopal, M. R., & Joranson, D. E. (2007). India: opioid availability: An update. *J Pain Symptom Manage, 33*(5), 615–622. doi:10.1016/j.jpainsymman.2007.02.028

Randall, F., & Downie, R. S. (1999). *Palliative care ethics: A companion for all specialties* (2nd ed.). New York: Oxford University Press.

Rattner, M., & Berzoff, J. (2016). Rethinking suffering: Allowing for suffering that is intrinsic at end of life. *J Soc Work End Life Palliat Care, 12*(3), 240–258. doi:10.1080/15524256.2016.1200520

Rotenstein, L. S., Ramos, M. A., Torre, M., Segal, J. B., Peluso, M. J., Guille, C., . . . Mata, D. A. (2016). Prevalence of depression, depressive symptoms, and suicidal ideation among medical students: A systematic review and meta-analysis. *JAMA, 316*(21), 2214–2236. doi:10.1001/jama.2016.17324

Rushton, C. H. (2016). Moral resilience: A capacity for navigating moral distress in critical care. *AACN Adv Crit Care, 27*(1), 111–119. doi:10.4037/aacnacc2016275

Rushton, C. H. (2017). Cultivating moral resilience. *Am J Nurs, 117*(2 Suppl. 1), S11–S15. doi:10.1097/01.NAJ.0000512205.93596.00

Rushton, C. H., Kaszniak, A. W., & Halifax, J. S. (2013). Addressing moral distress: Application of a framework to palliative care practice. *J Palliat Med, 16*(9), 1080–1088. doi:10.1089/jpm.2013.0105

Shanafelt, T. D., Hasan, O., Dyrbye, L. N., Sinsky, C., Satele, D., Sloan, J., & West, C. P. (2015). Changes in burnout and satisfaction with work-life balance in physicians and the general US working population between 2011 and 2014. *Mayo Clin Proc, 90*(12), 1600–1613. doi:10.1016/j.mayocp.2015.08.023

Shanafelt, T. D., West, C., Zhao, X., Novotny, P., Kolars, J., Habermann, T., & Sloan, J. (2005). Relationship between increased personal well-being and enhanced empathy among internal medicine residents. *J Gen Intern Med, 20*(7), 559–564. doi:10.1111/j.1525-1497.2005.0108.x

Solomon, M. Z., Sellers, D. E., Heller, K. S., Dokken, D. L., Levetown, M., Rushton, C., . . . Fleischman, A. R. (2005). New and lingering controversies in pediatric end-of-life care. *Pediatrics*, *116*(4), 872–883. doi:10.1542/peds.2004-0905

Sotile, W. M., & Sotile, M. O. (1996). *The medical marriage: A couple's survival guide*. Secaucus, NJ: Carol Publishing Group.

Spettell, C. M., Rawlins, W. S., Krakauer, R., Fernandes, J., Breton, M. E., Gowdy, W., . . . Brennan, T. A. (2009). A comprehensive case management program to improve palliative care. *J Palliat Med*, *12*(9), 827–832. doi:10.1089/jpm.2009.0089

Sundin-Huard, D., & Fahy, K. (1999). Moral distress, advocacy and burnout: Theorizing the relationships. *Int J Nurs Pract*, *5*(1), 8–13.

SUPPORT Principal Investigators. (1995). A controlled trial to improve care for seriously ill hospitalized patients: The study to understand prognoses and preferences for outcomes and risks of treatments (SUPPORT). *JAMA*, *274*(20), 1591–1598.

United Nations. (1972). Single convention on narcotic drugs. Retrieved from https://www.unodc.org/pdf/convention_1961_en.pdf

Voltaire. (1923). *L'œuvre de Voltaire*. Paris: Bibliothèque des curieux.

Von Roenn, J. H., Voltz, R., & Serrie, A. (2013). Barriers and approaches to the successful integration of palliative care and oncology practice. *J Natl Compr Canc Netw*, *11*(Suppl. 1), S11–S16.

World Health Organization. (2004). *Palliative care: The solid facts*. Retrieved from http://www.euro.who.int/__data/assets/pdf_file/0003/98418/E82931.pdf

Worldwide Palliative Care Alliance. (2014). Global atlas of palliative care at the end of life. Retrieved from http://www.who.int/nmh/Global_Atlas_of_Palliative_Care.pdf

Frequently Used Abbreviations

AAHPM	American Academy of Hospice and Palliative Medicine
AAN	American Academy of Neurology
AAP	American Academy of Pediatrics
ABMS	American Board of Medical Specialties
ACP	Advance care planning
AD	Advance directive
ALS	Amyotrophic lateral sclerosis, or Lou Gehrig's disease
AMA	American Medical Association
AND	Allow natural death
BiPAP	Bilevel positive airway pressure
COPD	Chronic obstructive pulmonary disease
CSU	Continuous sedation to unconsciousness
DMC	Decision-making capacity
DNAR	Do not attempt resuscitation
DNET	Do not escalate treatment
DNI	Do not intubate
DNR	Do not resuscitate
ECMO	Extracorporeal membrane oxygenation
HD	Huntington's disease
IND	Investigational new drug
LSMT	Life-sustaining medical treatment
MANH	Medically administered nutrition and hydration
PAD	Physician-assisted dying

PD	Parkinson's disease
PPS	Palliative Performance Scale
PSDA	Patient Self Determination Act
PVS	Persistent vegetative state
RCT	Randomized controlled trial
SCI	Spinal cord injury
TLT	Time-limited trial
UWS	Unresponsive wakefulness syndrome

Glossary

Advance directive A document completed by a patient which may describe treatments the patient does (or does not) want if that patient were to lose decision-making capacity ("treatment directive") and/or identify a person to make medical decisions for that patient in the event of incapacity ("proxy directive").

Agent A surrogate decision-maker named by a patient in an advance directive.

Amniocentesis A procedure usually performed between sixteen and eighteen weeks of pregnancy, involving inserting a needle into the uterus to take a sample of amniotic fluid in order to check for chromosomal (and other) abnormalities.

Aneuploidy An abnormal number of chromosomes, such as Trisomy 21 (Down syndrome).

Antenatal steroids Steroids administered to a pregnant woman prior to premature delivery, which have been shown to accelerate lung maturity. Administration forty-eight or more hours before delivery is considered "full" pre-treatment.

Antisialogogue A medication which reduces secretions, commonly used in end of life care to lessen respiratory distress.

Asystole Absence of cardiac contraction causing pulselesness.

Benzodiazepine A class of medications used primarily for anxiety, ranging from very short-acting (Alprazolam [Xanax]) to medium-acting (Midazolam [Versed]) to longer acting (Lorazepam [Ativan] or Diazepam [Valium]). Benzodiazepines are essential medicines in a palliative care "took kit" and are also the most common medication used for palliative sedation (chapter 9).

Bilevel positive airway pressure Noninvasive positive pressure ventilation accomplished through a tight-fitting mask over the nose or nose and mouth. This can be quite uncomfortable and lead to skin breakdown. It is not, therefore, generally a long-term solution but rather a "bridge" to either improved respiratory function or invasive ventilation.

Chronotrope A medication to increase heart rate (e.g., epinephrine), often used during resuscitation but also frequently in the operating room to stabilize a patient.

Clinical equipoise Referring to the situation where available evidence does not show that one intervention in a research study is superior to the other(s).

Clinical trial A methodical inquiry into whether a certain intervention is safe and effective. A Phase I trial focuses on the safety of a given drug (at a specific dose). In Phase II, the efficacy of the intervention to treat the condition is measured. In Phase III, the intervention is compared against either a placebo or an established treatment (or both) to measure its relative effectiveness.

COPD Chronic obstructive pulmonary disease, referring to either chronic bronchitis or emphysema, both of which compromise lung function and are often associated with smoking. In advanced stages, COPD constitutes a terminal diagnosis.

Craniectomy Removal of one or more skull plates to allow neurosurgical access or to decompress brain swelling.

Delirium An acute disturbance of consciousness that compromises clarity of awareness and ability to focus, leading to increased distractibility and change in cognition.

Dementia A progressive decline in memory and at least one other cognitive area, such as attention, orientation, judgment, abstract thinking, or personality.

DNR order A clinician's order directing that a patient not receive resuscitative interventions in the event of cardiopulmonary arrest. Also called a DNAR order (Do Not Attempt Resuscitation) and, by some, an AND order (Allow Natural Death).

Dystonic reaction Intermittent spasmodic or sustained involuntary muscle contractions, which can be a side effect of certain medications.

Extracorporeal membrane oxygenation A treatment that uses a pump to circulate blood through an artificial lung back into the bloodstream, for prolonged support of patients whose lungs are not able to effectively oxygenate the blood.

Gastrostomy A tube placed through the abdominal wall into the stomach, to permit direct infusion of hydration and nutrition.

Gavage feeds Nutrition infused directly into the gastrointestinal tract of a neonate or infant who is unable to swallow.

Hydrocephalus Literally "water-brain," this condition is often caused by an obstruction to the flow of cerebrospinal fluid causing brain swelling. If the skull plates are not fused (as in a fetus or neonate), the head expands. If the skull plates are fused, this leads to severe headache. Hydrocephalus is often a part of a larger syndrome, such as Trisomy 13.

Hypovolemia Decreased blood volume within the body, which will result from voluntarily stopping eating and drinking or refusal of medically administered nutrition and hydration.

Ischemic Referring to lack of blood flow—and thus oxygen delivery—to a part of the body.

Myoclonus Spasmodic jerky contraction of groups of muscles.

Nasogastric tube A temporary tube placed through the nose into the stomach to provide medically administered nutrition and hydration.

Opioid A class of medications that act on the mu-receptor, thereby diminishing pain and often causing euphoria. Negative side effects include respiratory depression, itching, constipation, and sedation.

Opioid-induced hyperalgesia A condition whereby increasing doses of opioids lead to *increased* rather than reduced pain. It can be very difficult in practice to tell whether escalating pain in the face of increasing opioids is an indication of advancing disease (which would require further increased doses) or a side effect of the opioids (which would require *decreased* doses, with possible switch to another opioid).

PaCO$_2$ Partial pressure of carbon dioxide, an elevation of which should stimulate the patient to breathe if the brain stem is functioning properly.

Pacemaker-dependent Some patients benefit intermittently from pacemakers, which maintain heart rhythm during intervals when the patient's intrinsic electrophysiology is insufficient. Other patients are truly pacemaker-dependent, meaning that the only impetus for their heart to beat comes from their pacemaker. For such a patient, deactivation of the pacemaker will cause asystole and death.

Palliative sedation "The use of sedative medications to relieve intolerable suffering from refractory symptoms by a reduction in patient consciousness" (de Graeff & Dean, 2007).

Parentalism A less patriarchal term for "paternalism," referring to the practice of a physician deciding what is best for the patient and not asking for the patient's consent before pursuing a given treatment.

Parenteral Route of medication administration that does not involve the gastrointestinal (i.e., enteral) route. This includes intravenous, intranasal, and subcutaneous routes.

Placebo An intervention that is physiologically ineffective or not specifically effective for the symptom or condition it is being used for.

Pressor A medication to increase blood pressure, such as dopamine, dobutamine, or epinephrine.

prn Abbreviation for Latin *pro re nata*, meaning "as needed".

Pulse oximetry Noninvasive measurement of the percentage of blood cells carrying oxygen, accomplished by clipping or taping a small probe, usually to a patient's finger.

Sedation vacation The practice of regularly lightening sedation for a patient undergoing burdensome treatment (such as mechanical ventilation), in order to reduce complications and maximize communication.

Sick sinus syndrome A condition where the sinoatrial node of the heart is insufficient to create a regular heart rhythm, potentially necessitating a pacemaker.

Substituted judgment The standard by which a surrogate decision-maker optimally makes decisions for a patient, based on what the patient would have wanted in that situation rather than the personal beliefs or values of the surrogate.

Tracheostomy A short tube placed through an incision in the neck into the lungs, to permit long-term mechanical ventilation.

Trisomy Normally people have twenty-three pairs of chromosomes (forty-six in total). "Trisomy" refers to a condition where one of the twenty-three "pairs" actually has three chromosomes, for a total of forty-seven. The number (e.g., Trisomy 13) refers to which chromosome has an extra copy.

Tocolytic A medication used to moderate or delay labor, such as magnesium and terbutaline.

Uremia The build-up of toxins in the body when the kidneys do not have enough fluid with which to filter them out, leading to depressed consciousness. The end result of voluntary stopping eating and drinking or refusal of medically administered nutrition and hydration.

Vegetative state A state of unaware wakefulness that may give the false impression that the patient is responding to external stimuli. A more precise term that also avoids any pejorative connotations is "unresponsive wakefulness syndrome."

Vital organ An organ without which a person cannot live, such as heart or liver.

Legal Cases

Index

Page references for figures are indicated by *f*, for tables by *t*, for boxes by *b*, and for notes by *n*.